Evaluations of Drug Interactions

The extent of human suffering and death caused by drug interactions is not precisely known, but there is adequate evidence that the magnitude demands the serious attention of all medical practitioners involved in the prescribing, dispensing, and administration of drugs, as well as the awareness of members of the public who engage in autotherapy.

One of the major projects of the American Pharmaceutical Association during the 1970's is to contribute to the understanding of the general mechanisms involved in drug interactions and their clinical significance, and to make evaluated information about known drug interactions available to all practitioners in a convenient form.

The Association undertook this project because it believes that if during their professional careers, each of the more than 100,000 practicing pharmacists personally contributes to the saving of only one life, the return on the APhA investment will benefit society beyond monetary comparison.

In the words of Thomas Henry Huxley, "If a little knowledge is dangerous, where is the man who has so much as to be out of danger." Certainly, when it comes to drug interactions, every medical professional involved in treating patients has more to learn. The objective of the pharmacist is not only to become better informed about drug interactions, but to share this vital information with colleagues in the other health professions in their efforts to avoid needless suffering and even death itself.

William S. Apple, Ph.D.
Executive Director
American Pharmaceutical Association

June 1976

Evaluations of Drug Interactions

SECOND EDITION

Prepared by the American Pharmaceutical Association
with the cooperation and assistance of

The American Dental Association
The American Podiatry Association
The American Society of Hospital Pharmacists
The Food and Drug Administration
The National Library of Medicine

1976

Publisher:

American
Pharmaceutical
Association

The National
Professional Society
of Pharmacists

2215 Constitution Avenue, N.W., Washington, DC 20037

Notice

This publication does not purport to include all reported drug interactions. All expressions of opinion and statements presented in this publication concerning the incidence and severity of possible drug interactions—as well as recognition, side effects, and treatment of such interactions—represent the consensus of the panel involved with the preparation of specific material and do not reflect any endorsement on the part of the American Pharmaceutical Association or the cooperating organizations, including pharmaceutical manufacturers.

The inclusion in this publication of the drug in respect to which patent or trademark rights may exist shall not be deemed, and is not intended as, a grant of, or authority to exercise, any right or privilege protected by such patent or trademark. All such rights and privileges are vested in the patent or trademark owner, and no other person may exercise the same without express permission, authority, or license secured from such patent or trademark owner.

ISBN   0-917330-10-2

Library of Congress Number 76-14501

© Copyright 1976; all rights reserved
American Pharmaceutical Association
2215 Constitution Avenue, N.W.
Washington, DC 20037

Table
of
Contents

Steering Committee

Frank J. Ascione, Pharm.D.,
  ex officio
  American Pharmaceutical Association
  Washington, D.C.

O'Neill Barrett, Jr., M.D.
  University of South Florida
  College of Medicine
  Tampa, Fla.

Donald O. Fedder, B.S.
  University of Maryland
  Baltimore, Md.

Lorne K. Garrettson, M.D.
  Medical College of Virginia
  Richmond, Va.

Daniel A. Hussar, Ph.D.
  Philadelphia College of Pharmacy
    and Science
  Philadelphia, Pa.

John F. Kerege, Pharm.D.
  (August 1974–September 1975)
  Student American Pharmaceutical
    Association
  Washington, D.C.

William F. McGhan, Pharm.D.
  Academy of Pharmaceutical Sciences
  Washington, D.C.

Mary Jo Reilly, M.S.
  American Society of Hospital
    Pharmacists
  Bethesda, Md.

Fred J. Salter, Pharm.D.
  Medical College of Virginia
  Richmond, Va.

Ronald L. Williams, B.S.
  Academy of Pharmacy Practice
  Washington, D.C.

Staff

Program Director: Frank J. Ascione, Pharm.D.

Project Editor: L. Luan Corrigan, B.S.

Production Editor: Margaret F. Rose, B.A.

Traffic Coordinator: Marcia T. Jay, B.A.

Research Assistants: Heidi Alperovich, B.S., R.Ph.
                    James P. Caro, B.S., R.Ph.

Director of Publications: Leland J. Arney, M.A.

Program Advisor: Edward G. Feldmann, Ph.D.

How to use EDI

Introduction

The unique format of EDI enables the reader to obtain the depth and type of drug interaction information desired or needed and to extract this information quickly.

By following a stepwise progression, the reader may choose to stop reading when the desired information is reached or may continue on through additional steps which increasingly provide broader and more detailed information.

The arrangement of material has been designed for consistency and convenience. However, this arrangement may not immediately reveal the wealth of information presented in EDI. In particular, the Monograph titles may not convey that chemically and pharmacologically related drugs are discussed *(e.g.,* the Monograph entitled *Warfarin — Chlordiazepoxide* also discusses various drugs related to warfarin and chlordiazepoxide).

TO LOCATE INFORMATION IN EDI
The following pages provide an easy four-step guide about how to use EDI effectively.

One...REFER TO THE INDEX   Information on a suspected

drug interaction can be located most quickly using the *nonproprietary drug name*. The reader will find all suspected drug interactions discussed in EDI listed in the Index by their nonproprietary name as follows:

Amitriptyline
—Alcohol, 1
—Bethanidine, 83

This listing is reversed to allow access to desired drug interaction information by using the nonproprietary name of either interacting drug:

Alcohol
—Amitriptyline, 1

If the reader uses a major *drug trade name* to find the suspected drug interaction in EDI, the Index entry for this term will refer to the nonproprietary drug name:

Elavil Hydrochloride—see
Amitriptyline

If the reader uses a *"class like"* term *(e.g.,* Tricyclic antidepressants) to find the suspected interaction in EDI, the Index entry for this term will refer to the nonproprietary name of the drugs in that class:

Tricyclic Antidepressants—*see*
Amitriptyline, Desipramine,
Doxepin, Imipramine,
Nortriptyline, Protriptyline

Note: Index entries followed by (R) direct the reader to the **Recommendations** section of the Monograph first. Entries followed by (SI) direct the reader to the Supplemental Information. For example:

Alcohol
—Ethchlorvynol, 47 (R)
—Phenytoin, 444 (SI)

TWO ... TURN TO THE MONOGRAPH   The location of the

Monograph is indicated by the page number listed by the Index entry for the suspected drug interaction. The Monograph discusses more than the drugs listed in the title.

Chemically and pharmacologically related drugs expected to interact in a similar manner also are included.

Related drugs are identified by boldface entries under the **Related Drugs** section of the Monograph.

Drugs that interact similarly but that are not chemically and pharmacologically related are often mentioned in the **Recommendations** section.

Note: At this point, the reader may wish to verify that the suspected drug interaction sought is, in fact, discussed in the Monograph. If the reader initially used a major drug trade name to find the interaction in EDI, the **Nonproprietary and Trade Names** section should be checked. If the reader had used a "class like" term or a nonproprietary name that is not listed in the Monograph title, then the **Related Drugs** section should be checked.   ▶

Three ...READ OR STUDY THE MONOGRAPH

The reader now has a choice between studying the Monograph to obtain in-depth information or quickly extracting the specific information desired.

FOR IN-DEPTH INFORMATION: The reader may study the Monograph by reading the information in the order in which it is presented, which leads the reader through a step-by-step logical presentation. However, the Monograph format is designed to allow the reader to study the information in any order that is chosen.

FOR QUICK INFORMATION: The best approach for the reader to obtain limited information quickly is to read each section of the Monograph in the following order which is based on a level of decreasing clinical importance. The reader may proceed as far as the need for information is required:

1. To obtain the essential elements about the suspected drug interaction, gaining a concise overview of the entire Monograph, the reader should first examine the **Summary.**

2. To obtain guidance on how to avoid or manage the suspected interaction, next read the **Recommendations.**

3. To review the clinical basis used by the pertinent expert panel to assess the interaction, then read the **Evaluation of Clinical Data,** which concludes with a judgment of the validity of these data—as identified with the symbol ■.

4. To gain an understanding of the pharmacology involved and, particularly, for an explanation of the mechanism causing the interaction, the reader should then review the discussion under the heading **Pharmacological Effect and Mechanism.**

5. To determine the basis and source of statements made in the Monograph and/or to locate the original literature or report, a list of **References** is provided near the end of the Monograph. (Statements made throughout the Monograph are supported by scientific documentation as indicated by the accompanying parenthetical arabic numerals which are keyed to the **References** listed.)

6. To correlate trade or brand names with the "generic" or official names of drugs discussed in the Monograph, refer to the listing of **Nonproprietary and Trade Names of Drugs,** found at the end of each Monograph. (For brevity and consistency, only nonproprietary names are used throughout the Monograph.)

Tetracycline—Ferrous Sulfate

Summary—The oral administration of ferrous sulfate (200–600 mg) interferes with the absorption of tetracycline from the gastrointestinal (GI) tract and vice versa, leading to decreased serum levels of the antibiotic and the iron salt, respectively. If simultaneous administration is necessary, patients should receive tetracycline 3 hr after or 2 hr before iron administration.

Related Drugs—Of the tetracycline analogs, **doxycycline** (1, 2), **methacycline** (1), and **oxytetracycline** (1) have demonstrated a similar interaction with iron. Although there is no documentation, other **tetracycline analogs** theoretically can be expected to behave similarly.

Other salts of iron such as **ferrous fumarate** (3) and **ferrous gluconate** (3) have been shown to interact with tetracycline. Since the interaction between tetracycline and iron appears to be due to the ferrous or ferric ion, preparations such as **ferrocholinate** and **ferrous lactate** can also be expected to inhibit the absorption of tetra-

Pharmacological Effect and Mechanism—The oral administration of ferrous ion, like other polyvalent cations, decreases the GI absorption of tetracycline (1, 4) and tetracycline derivatives (1). The precise mechanism by which iron impairs tetracycline absorption is unclear. Since tetracycline binds with several divalent cations (5–7), two possible mechanisms have been proposed: tetracyclines may form chelates with ferrous ions, causing inhibition of absorption; or in the presence of ferrous ion,

Evaluation of Clinical Data—In a controlled study (1), five healthy subjects received either doxycycline (200 mg po), methacycline (300 mg po), oxytetracycline (500 mg po), or tetracycline (500 mg po). A similar group received the same dose of antibiotic plus ferrous sulfate (200 mg po). Concurrent iron administration decreased the maximum serum concentrations of tetracycline and oxytetracycline by approximately

■ Based on these reports, the concurrent administration of tetracycline or its analogs and ferrous sulfate results in a statistically significant reduction in the serum levels of the antibiotic and in the amount of iron absorbed. The amount of the reduction is dependent on many factors: formulation differences among ferrous sulfate dosage forms (10), type of iron salt used (3), the type of tetracycline compound used (1, 2), and the time interval between administration of these drugs (4). The drug interaction may be therapeutically significant in certain severe infections where high serum

Recommendations—Ferrous sulfate should not be given simultaneously with tetracycline or tetracycline analogs. In those situations in which it is necessary for patients to receive both iron and tetracycline therapy orally, this interaction may be avoided by administering the ferrous sulfate not less than 3 hr before or 2 hr after tetracycline.

References

(1) P. J. Neuvonen *et al.*, "Interference of Iron with the Absorption of Tetracyclines in Man," *Brit. Med., J., 4*, 532 (1970).

cycline to Macromolecules," *Nature*, *191*, 1156 (1961).
(6) A. Albert and C. W. Rees, "Avidity of the Tetracyclines for the Cations

[For additional information, see *Anti-Infective Therapy*, p. 388.]

Nonproprietary and Trade Names of Drugs

Chlortetracycline hydrochloride—
  Aureomycin
Demeclocycline—*Declomycin*
Doxycycline monohydrate—*Doxy-II Monohydrate, Doxychel, Vibramycin Monohydrate*

Oxytetracycline—*Dalimycin, Terramycin*
Oxytetracycline hydrochloride—
  Oxy-Kesso-Tetra, Oxy-Tetrachel,
  Terramycin Hydrochloride
Rolitetracycline—*Syntetrin*
Tetracycline—*Achromycin, Panmycin,*

▶

Four ... TURN TO SUPPLEMENTAL INFORMATION

To obtain additional information about the **therapeutic class** of the drugs discussed in the Monograph, the reader should refer to the Supplemental Information as directed by the bracketed statement pertaining to "Additional Information."

[For additional information, see *Anti-Infective Therapy*, p. 388.]

To derive a broad overview of the mechanisms of drug interactions, including a discussion of the pharmacokinetics and terminology related to drug interactions, refer to the **General Mechanisms** discussion in the beginning of the Supplemental Information, page 307.

To assess the significance of abnormal values of body physiology which may be encountered in drug interactions, the reader should compare those values with the normal range by consulting **Laboratory Tests and Clinical Values.** The tables which appear as part of the Supplemental Information, on page 461, provide standard or normal laboratory values.

EDI attempts to discuss all drug interactions about which there is a reasonable body of information in the drug literature, but the book is not all inclusive. For additional information concerning the scope of the book, please consult the Preface.

Evaluations of Drug Interactions:
Preface, Participants

Preface

The problems of how to detect and prevent the harmful effects caused by drug interactions have received increasing attention from the health-care professions and the public. The increased attention has generated intensive research and discussion among scientists and health-care practitioners to define the magnitude of the problem and to provide information about how to reduce the potential for harm.

The demand for useful drug interaction information resulted in the publication of numerous books, review articles, charts, and lists. Despite the availability of these publications, health-care practitioners continued to express concern about the quality and suitability of available information. This concern prompted the American Pharmaceutical Association to undertake a study to identify the best method to disseminate drug interaction information.

Three major subjective areas were defined.

First, an assessment must be made about the quality of the scientific literature about the drug interaction.

Second, a judgment may be necessary concerning the likelihood of the drug interaction occurring and its expected clinical effects.

Third, a practical and specific recommendation should be made relative to avoiding the harmful effects of the interaction.

Recognizing that useful drug interaction information can only be provided by utilizing these subjective aspects, APhA undertook to develop a process built on these requirements. The process would utilize an extensive review of the relevant literature by experts who would provide specific recommendations about how to avoid these interactions and their harmful effects. The process also would use a group of health-care practitioners to review the recommendations to ensure that they were practical and relevant.

To form these groups and to develop this process, APhA organized the Drug Interactions Evaluation Program (initially known as the Drug Interactions Project). The DIEP consists of individuals from dentistry, medicine, and pharmacy who are charged with the responsibility of providing a multidisciplinary consensus review of the pertinent scientific literature and recommending practical methods to avoid the potential adverse effects of drug interactions.

The conclusions emanating from the DIEP are communicated and disseminated primarily through *Evaluations of Drug Interactions* (EDI). In determining what EDI should contain, the DIEP was faced with two basic questions: how much information should be provided, and in what form should it be provided to enable health-care practitioners to make an authoritative judgment concerning the drug interaction. A monograph format was selected to present the more pertinent information about drug interactions and supplemental information was also added to include an overview of drug interaction mechanisms, general therapeutic information, and tables of normal values.

It is fully recognized that the approach to providing drug interaction information used in EDI will not be acceptable to all health-care professionals. Some may believe that more extensive information is necessary to understand an interaction. Conversely, others may suggest that EDI contains much more information than is really needed. However, most health-care professionals have found that the format used in EDI is flexible enough to provide information quickly and comprehensively.

Nevertheless, additional revisions of the EDI format will be made should these changes appear necessary and technically feasible. Users of EDI are invited to provide the DIEP with their suggestions for further improving the communication of drug interaction information.

History of EDI

The new edition represents the fourth publication produced by APhA and its Drug Interactions Evaluation Program. The first publication was the prototype booklet in 1971; more than 10,000 copies were distributed. The first complete edition was published in April 1973 and contained 104 monographs and 25 chapters. More than 80,000 copies were distributed worldwide and the book was translated into two foreign languages. In July 1974, a Supplement was published and contained 28 additional monographs; more than 60,000 copies were distributed.

The 132 monographs published in the first edition and its Supplement were combined into 115 monographs in this new edition for easier use. These monographs were all significantly updated and revised and 29 new monographs were added. Additionally, all supplemental information was updated and revised.

The second edition represents more than a 2-year effort by APhA and its DIEP to publish the first completely revised and updated version of EDI. (The material was updated through April 2, 1976.) This lengthy time was necessary because of the extensive amount of effort required to revise and update previously published material.

Significant changes in the format and content of EDI also were incorporated based on comments from users of previous editions. For example, comments from DIEP participants and others have focused on the need to provide easier access to specific drug interactions. Therefore, a more comprehensive index has been developed.

This edition of EDI is a culmination of more than 6 years of experience in providing useful drug interaction information for the health-care professions. Many individuals were involved in this effort and the content of EDI reflects the diversity of their input.

Organization of the DIEP

Organizationally, the Drug Interactions Evaluation Program includes a Steering Committee, a Scientific Review Panel, a Practitioner Panel, Participating Pharmaceutical Manufacturers, Cooperating Health-Related Organizations, and Ancillary Reviewers.

Organizational Structure Of DIEP

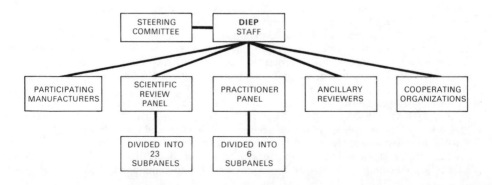

The Steering Committee, consisting of individuals from medicine and pharmacy, has the responsibility of providing overall direction and general guidance to the DIEP in the areas of program policy and future DIEP activities. The Steering Committee also has the responsibility for approving the drug interactions selected for evaluation, approving DIEP panel members recommended for appointment, and approving the final content of each edition of EDI.

It was recognized early in the development of EDI that two factors were equally important: the scientific accuracy of the material and the suitability of this material for everyday use. Therefore, the Scientific Review Panel and the Practitioner Panel were developed to ensure that these factors were considered carefully. These panels are subdivided to reduce the workload of participants.

The Scientific Review Panel consists of 23 subpanels divided by pharmacological classes of drugs and has approximately 150 members. This panel is responsible for ensuring the technical accuracy of EDI material.

The Practitioner Panel has approximately 50 members divided into six groups. This panel is responsible for assessing and reviewing the suitability of EDI content for everyday use by the health-care practitioner. The Practitioner Panel members also review the nonproprietary and trade names section of the EDI monographs to ensure that this section provides the most current and commonly used trade names of drugs discussed in the monographs.

Although the Scientific Review Panel and the Practitioner Panel are responsible for most of the content review of EDI, assistance is also provided by the participating manufacturers, cooperating health-related organizations, and the ancillary reviewers. The participating manufacturers—15 were involved in the publication of EDI—review selected EDI monographs and provide the DIEP with information about their products.

Cooperating health-related organizations are the American Dental Association, the American Podiatry Association, the American Society of Hospital Pharmacists, the Food and Drug Administration, and the National Library of Medicine. These organizations provide assistance to the DIEP based on their professional functions.

To round out the personnel involved with the generation of EDI material, ancillary reviewers were incorporated into the review process. These individuals review selected monographs related to their area of expertise.

DIEP Review Process

The DIEP review process is designed to emphasize the group approach to the evaluation of drug interaction information. The review process begins when a preliminary list of reported drug interactions is submitted to the DIEP Steering Committee for its approval. The list is usually prepared by the Program Director. It is based upon recommendations from the DIEP staff, individual Steering Committee members, program participants, and other interested professionals.

For a drug interaction to be selected one of the following criteria must be met:

(1) The drug interaction is thought to be potentially clinically significant.

(2) The drug interaction is not likely to be clinically significant and has enough scientific documentation to support this conclusion.

(3) There is insufficient evidence to evaluate a particular drug interaction but it has gained "notoriety" by being discussed frequently in other reference sources on drug interactions.

After the preliminary list of drug interactions has been approved, the Program Director assigns the monograph to a member of the appropriate Scientific Review Subpanel. This person is responsible for researching and evaluating the scientific literature about the assigned drug interaction and preparing a monograph draft based on this investigation. To assist these efforts, a starter bibliography on the drug interaction is given to the author. After the rough draft is prepared, it is submitted to the Program Director.

When the author's monograph is received by the DIEP staff, it is reviewed both for accuracy, content, and consistency in writing style. Care is taken to avoid altering significantly the author's concepts about the drug interaction, but the draft is usually revised to make it consistent with DIEP writing guidelines and to make the presented material clear. After the monograph has been revised, it is sent to the pertinent sub-panel, participating manufacturers, cooperating organizations, and appropriate ancillary reviewers for the initial review and evaluation.

The DIEP staff compiles all comments and suggestions received from the program participants about the monograph. The staff, rather than the monograph author, then revises the monograph draft based on these comments and suggestions. In prior EDI publications, the monograph author was responsible for revising the monograph draft, but the DIEP staff found that this approach was time consuming and resulted in revised monographs inconsistent with DIEP writing guidelines. The revised monograph draft is then sent for a second time to all appropriate program participants for the final review and evaluation.

At this point, it is appropriate to discuss the key role that the subpanel chairperson plays in the review process. The chairperson may be called upon to act as a final arbitrator in any serious difference of opinion occurring among reviewers and also may recommend, with appropriate documentation, the withholding of any monograph draft from publication.

When the final comments of the reviewers are received, they are evaluated and the monograph is revised accordingly. During this final revision, the DIEP staff reviews the monograph to ensure that all important statements are documented and that the monograph is as concise as possible and easy to read. An attempt is made to ensure that the subpanel's recommendations are definitive and practical. Any unresolved questions are referred to the appropriate subpanel chairperson for a decision. At this stage, most major revisions of the content of the monograph are usually completed.

A final list of monographs is then submitted to the Steering Committee for approval. The Steering Committee is also asked at that time to approve the final content of the book. The last step of the DIEP review process is done in-house and primarily involves the physical aspects of production.

This extensive review process, in which each monograph is reviewed twice by at least 20 persons, often produces a monograph that has been so significantly revised that there is little, if any, resemblance to the initial monograph draft. Because of this comprehensive review, the subpanel as a whole, not just one person, assumes overall responsibility—as well as credit—for preparing the monograph when it is eventually published.

Scope and Content of EDI

EDI is designed to provide the health-care practitioner with enough information that he or she may detect and prevent the harmful effects of drug interactions. This information is presented primarily in the drug interaction monographs but also is summarized in the Supplemental Information section.

Although a definition of a drug interaction is not included in EDI, certain types of "drug interactions" are discussed. These include (a) drug interactions that are well documented to cause harmful effects to the patient (e.g., digitalis–chlorothiazide), (b) drug interactions that are not well documented but are still potentially harmful (e.g., warfarin–quinidine), (c) drug interactions that have a beneficial effect (e.g., guanethidine–hydrochlorothiazide), (d) drug interactions that have sufficient documentation to show that a clinically significant drug interaction does not occur (e.g., probenecid–chlorothiazide), and (e) drug interactions that are generally regarded as hazardous but, upon critical evaluation of the literature, are found to be without accepted clinical evidence (*e.g.,* allopurinol–iron).

The DIEP has received requests from health-care practitioners to include a ranking or rating of the severity of each drug interaction. After careful consideration, it was decided that such a system would be impractical and misleading.

First, a system based on severity or incidence would be confusing. For example, how does one comparatively rate a drug interaction that occurs very rarely but with fatal results with a drug interaction that occurs frequently but with only minor adverse effects?

Second, the severity of a drug interaction is often determined by the environment in which it occurs. Would not a drug interaction that causes potentially harmful effects be considered less harmful in a closely supervised hospital setting than in socially isolated situations?

Third, different practitioners often use different criteria to rate a drug interaction. Would a drug interaction be more severe if it was difficult to detect, was difficult to treat, or required additional laboratory tests?

Therefore, it was decided to include the full spectrum of reported drug interactions and not to confuse the practitioner with any definitions or ranking of the drug interactions—an approach that encourages the health-care practitioner to exercise professional judgment.

Terminology Used in EDI

In the course of the review and evaluation of drug interaction information, it became apparent that many scientific terms might be used inconsistently or might have multiple meanings; indiscriminate use of such terms could be misleading in EDI. In some cases, the use of these ambiguous terms was eliminated, or they were replaced by more specific terms. In other cases, the terms were used in a consistent manner throughout EDI in order not to add any additional ambiguity to their meaning.

For example, the adjective used to describe the levels of drug in the blood has been either "serum," "plasma," or "blood." A review of a number of scientific journals indicated that these terms were often used interchangeably. The DIEP decided that it would be less confusing to the reader if only one term was used. The adjective "serum" was selected and is used in most cases to describe drug levels unless a specific different meaning is intended, requiring that another adjective be used.

The terms "concurrently" and "simultaneously" are often used interchangeably. However, the DIEP believed that these terms have different meanings and should be used differently. The term "simultaneously" is used in EDI to describe events occurring at the same point in time or within about 30 minutes of each other. The term "concurrently" would not mean at the same point in time but within a 24-hour period.

The terms "additive," "antagonistic," and "potentiation" originally had very specific meanings. However, these terms are currently used less precisely and may be very confusing. The DIEP has decided to avoid using these terms whenever possible and to use less specific, but also less confusing, terms such as "enhance," "intensify," "prevent," or "block."

The DIEP is not attempting to standardize scientific language. Indeed, such an effort would require a separate publication. Nevertheless, it is believed that brief mention of the rationale behind the use of some important terms in EDI may avoid confusing the user.

Organization of EDI

The monograph section is the most important part of this book. The monographs are followed by supplemental information and the index. Additional suggestions and guidance on how to use this book can be found on pages ix–xiv.

Monographs

The number of drug interactions discussed in the monographs is much greater than the 144 monograph titles would indicate. Although specific drugs of a certain pharmacological class are selected as title drugs, other drugs of that class are discussed in the monograph body, particularly in the **Related Drugs** section. The monographs are unique in that they discuss drug interactions by specific drugs rather than by general pharmacological or chemical class. This approach is used in order not to incriminate unfairly those drugs of the same class for which there is no documentation of an interaction.

The monograph format is designed to allow various health-care practitioners to extract a wide range of information depending on their interest. The monograph is divided into distinct sections as follows.

Monograph Title—The drugs selected for the monograph title are the drugs most frequently discussed in the drug interaction literature. For example, the title of a monograph on the interaction between tricyclic antidepressants and monoamine oxidase inhibitors would be imipramine–tranylcypromine because they are the most common drugs discussed in the literature. The order of the drugs in the title may also be important. If sufficient information is available about the mechanism, the first drug given in the title is usually the drug whose pharmacological action is being modified, while the second drug in the title is the drug usually responsible for that modification (*e.g.*, the monograph entitled Warfarin–Aspirin means that aspirin is modifying the hypoprothrombinemic effect of warfarin). In many drug interactions, this mechanism is not known; in others, the interaction occurs without such a direct cause and effect relationship.

Summary—The summary provides concise information about the main points of the drug interaction including its clinical significance. It usually includes brief instructions for reducing or preventing the harmful effects associated with the drug interaction.

Related Drugs—This section broadens the scope of the monograph by including those drugs that are pharmacologically and chemically related and are expected to interact in a similar manner. The section further differentiates those related drugs that have been shown to interact from those where the interaction is only theoretically possible.

Pharmacological Effect and Mechanism—The pharmacological background necessary to understand the mechanism of the drug interaction and its expected clinical effects is discussed.

Evaluation of Clinical Data—This section contains abbreviated discussions of the pertinent published reports about the drug interaction and those of any related drugs. Only data obtained from observations in humans are discussed. Particular attention is given to study design, methods employed, the statistical significance of the results, and the numerical values of the results. The last paragraph(s) of this section is set off by the symbol ■; it provides a summary of the clinical data about the drug interaction. This summary also reflects the DIEP participants' judgment about the validity of the clinical data and also attempts to determine, based on these data, if a clinically significant drug interaction occurs.

Recommendations—Specific courses of action for avoiding the potential hazardous effects of the drug interaction are given. These recommendations may include utilization of certain laboratory tests to monitor the patient, suggestions for alternative drugs, or methods to treat any toxic effects occurring as a result of the drug interaction.

References—Literature documentation for the information and recommendations presented are also included. This section enables the reader to consult the most pertinent original information sources for further details. The references are not intended to be exhaustive, particularly for the more extensively studied interactions. An attempt is made to use only the most current references with particular emphasis on the use of primary reference sources.

Nonproprietary and Trade Names of Drugs—The listing of drugs at the end of the monograph provides a general guide to the drugs and drug products involved in or related to the interaction. In general, only major trade names of single entity products are listed. The United States Adopted Names (USAN) have been used throughout the publication.

Supplemental Information

The Supplemental Information section contains an overview of the mechanisms of drug interactions (pages 307–326). Additionally, general discussions regarding the pharmacology and therapeutics of each class of drugs and an overview of the drug interactions that occur in that class are provided (pages 327–458). The discussions are intended to supply sufficient related information to enable health-care practitioners with varied backgrounds and training to understand the pharmacological and therapeutic implications of the drug interaction, as well as to assist health-care practitioners in developing alternative therapy.

Tables of Normal Values are also included to provide a standard reference of laboratory values that can be used to compare the values cited in the EDI monographs (pages 461–476).

Future Editions

Since the amount of drug interaction information is constantly growing, a completely revised edition of EDI is expected to be published every few years with supplements during the intervening period. Future supplements are planned to contain evaluations of over-the-counter (nonprescription) drug interactions, drug–laboratory test interactions, drug–pesticide interactions, and drug–food interactions. Pharmaceutical incompatibilities, such as those that might be encountered in preparing intravenous admixtures, do not constitute drug interactions within the scope of this publication.

Planning for the next edition of EDI is now under way. Readers who are interested and so inclined should contact the DIEP office if they would like to be considered for participation.

Significance of EDI

It is appropriate to question whether EDI, particularly this new edition, is really unique among the numerous publications about drug interactions. The answer is an emphatic "yes"!

First, unlike other publications on drug interactions, EDI represents a group evaluation rather than the opinion of one or two individuals.

Second, because this collective evaluation is a continual process, EDI represents a dynamic, rather than a static, source of information about drug interactions.

Third, EDI provides more information about drug interactions than any other publication, but it is designed to be flexible enough to provide selected information quickly and concisely. For instance, EDI not only includes information about the drug interaction but also includes recommendations for controlling or avoiding the harmful effects associated with the interaction. Additionally, EDI provides full literature references on which the evaluation is based.

And fourth, EDI content reflects diverse input of all segments of the health-care professions and therefore is designed to be useful to all such groups.

Another question is whether a unique publication like EDI is really necessary. Again, we respond affirmatively. Although numerous publications about drug interactions have been published in the last few years, and EDI has existed as a full edition

since 1973, the amount of misleading or inaccurate information about drug interactions is still substantial. It was hoped that the publication of a definitive book like
EDI would serve to reduce this misinformation significantly. However, this has not
been the case. When one "mythical" drug interaction is discredited, another arises
to take its place. Therefore, the DIEP now recognizes that the problem of eliminating misleading information about drug interactions may be its greatest challenge and
may be where EDI will make its greatest contribution.

The DIEP and EDI are best equipped to deal with this challenge because the
group evaluation process provides a forum to discuss the controversial aspects of a
reported drug interaction and allows significant input from individuals with various
backgrounds and experience. Additionally, the format used in EDI allows the health-
care practitioner to examine the basis for any evaluations or recommendations contained in the book and provides him or her with the opportunity to arrive at an
independent decision if desired.

A major objective of the DIEP review is to promote in-depth discussion about
the clinical significance of a drug interaction and to encourage the expression of
differences of opinion. It is hoped that EDI will serve to focus on these differences
and to stimulate new research and discussion about drug interactions.

Hence, while the immediate and most obvious contribution of EDI will be as
a tool for the health-care practitioner to detect and prevent the harmful effects due
to drug interactions, the ultimate impact of the book is expected to extend much
further. By combining a group evaluation process with a multidisciplinary approach
to the problem, EDI should come to be the standard reference source for authoritative drug interaction information for academia, the health-care professions, the pharmaceutical industry, and the government.

Acknowledgments

The publication of a book with the quality and scope of EDI requires substantial input from many individuals. These contributions represent a diversity of backgrounds with a common goal: to provide authoritative drug interaction information
to the health-care professions. The numerous participants in this effort gave freely
of their time, most often on a volunteer basis, with little hope for significant personal recognition. However, they can derive immense personal satisfaction with the
knowledge that they have contributed in a very meaningful way to the public health
and welfare through the dissemination of accurate drug interaction information.

Unfortunately, space does not permit us to acknowledge each participant individually. Nevertheless, we want to extend our sincere thanks to all DIEP participants
listed on pp. xxvii–xliii. Without their dedication and efforts, this publication would
not exist.

The 23 Scientific Review Panel Chairpersons deserve special recognition. They
were asked to act as final arbitrators on all differences of opinion that arose among
the subpanel members and to review the monographs and supplemental therapeutic
information assigned to their subpanel to ensure that the information contained therein
was consistent. They performed this difficult task exceptionally well and deserve our
special commendation.

Many outside groups contributed their expertise to the effort to publish EDI.
However, certain groups were outstanding in this function. Special thanks is given
to the American Dental Association, the American Society of Hospital Pharmacists,
the Bureau of Drugs of the Food and Drug Administration, and the participating
pharmaceutical manufacturers.

Special appreciation is also given the members of the DIEP Steering Committee.
These individuals readily assumed the responsibility of providing direction and insight into the activities of the DIEP and the publication of EDI. Not only did they
approve of the makeup of the panels and the content of EDI, but they also gave

constructive criticism and helpful recommendations throughout the course of the publication of EDI.

Ultimately, however, the success of any publication is dependent upon the abilities and the assistance rendered by the staff responsible for that publication. The DIEP has been fortunate to have staff members whose selfless dedication and superior achievement exceeded what could be reasonably expected from any employee. Ms. L. Luan Corrigan must be singled out for particular praise. As project editor of EDI since its development, she has been able to provide a valuable perspective about the activities of the DIEP and the publication of EDI. It is through her conscientious efforts and her organizational talents that publication deadlines were met and that the high standards for EDI content were maintained.

As secretary to the DIEP, Ms. Marcia T. Jay assisted most competently. She had the very important, but thankless task, of keeping track of the large amount of paper generated by the DIEP review process. She performed this task most admirably.

The DIEP research assistants, Ms. Heidi Alperovich and later Mr. James P. Caro, performed most valuably throughout the publication of EDI. They had the responsibility of maintaining the DIEP information base, evaluating and verifying the comments of the DIEP participants, and revising the EDI content accordingly. The fact that they performed this function exceptionally well is reflected by the outstanding quality of the EDI content. Sincere appreciation is also extended to Ms. Margaret F. Rose and Ms. Janet D. Shoff who provided considerable assistance in the final stages of EDI production. The Program Director wishes to express his deepest gratitude to these individuals for their outstanding efforts.

The Program Director would be remiss if special thanks were not given to other members of the APhA staff who gave freely of their advice and considerable expertise. Dr. Edward G. Feldmann, APhA Associate Executive Director for Scientific Affairs, was administratively responsible for the development of the DIEP and served as a valuable counsel throughout the publication of EDI. Mr. Leland J. Arney, APhA Director of Publications, provided much insight into the publication and production aspects. Dr. Pierre S. Del Prato, APhA Director of Clinical Practice, as the previous Program Director, gave an important perspective of the evolution of some activities of the DIEP and of the development of the content for the first edition.

Finally, the Program Director wishes to give special recognition to his wife Patty, who has patiently accepted the sharing of her husband with the preparation of this book and who I thank for having provided me with love and understanding while I completed this challenging task.

Frank J. Ascione
May 2, 1976

Flow Diagram for EDI Monographs

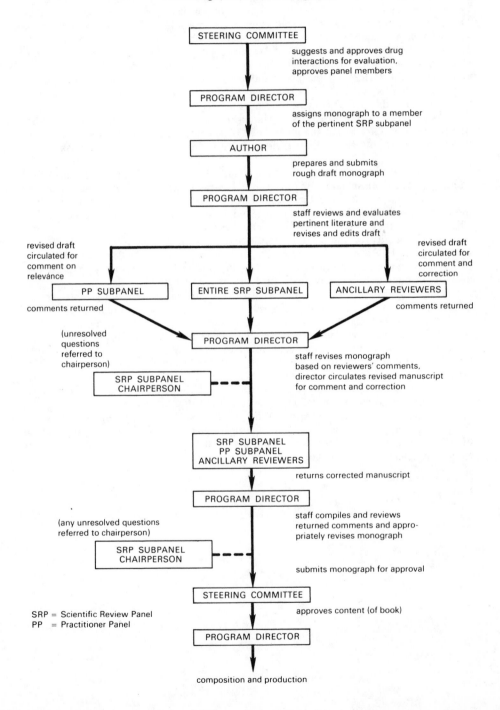

STEERING COMMITTEE

suggests and approves drug
interactions for evaluation,
approves panel members

PROGRAM DIRECTOR

assigns monograph to a member
of the pertinent SRP subpanel

AUTHOR

prepares and submits
rough draft monograph

PROGRAM DIRECTOR

staff reviews and evaluates
pertinent literature and
revises and edits draft

revised draft
circulated for
comment on
relevance

revised draft
circulated for
comment and
correction

PP SUBPANEL   ENTIRE SRP SUBPANEL   ANCILLARY REVIEWERS

comments returned   comments returned

(unresolved
questions
referred to
chairperson)

PROGRAM DIRECTOR

staff revises monograph
based on reviewers' comments,
director circulates revised manuscript
for comment and correction

SRP SUBPANEL
CHAIRPERSON

SRP SUBPANEL
PP SUBPANEL
ANCILLARY REVIEWERS

returns corrected manuscript

PROGRAM DIRECTOR

staff compiles and reviews
returned comments and appropriately revises monograph

(any unresolved questions
referred to chairperson)

SRP SUBPANEL
CHAIRPERSON

submits monograph for approval

STEERING COMMITTEE

approves content (of book)

SRP = Scientific Review Panel
PP = Practitioner Panel

PROGRAM DIRECTOR

composition and production

Scientific
Review
Panel

Acid–Base Balance Agents

Morris D. Faiman, Ph.D., *Chairperson*
  University of Kansas
  Lawrence, Kan.

J. Edward Bell, Pharm.D.
  University of Michigan
  Ann Arbor, Mich.

Monte S. Cohon, Pharm.D.
  University of Wisconsin
  Madison, Wis.

Peter P. Lamy, Ph.D.
  University of Maryland
  Baltimore, Md.

Daniel A. Nona, Ph.D.
  American Council on
    Pharmaceutical Education
  Chicago, Ill.

Noel I. Robin, M.D.
  Stamford Hospital
  Stamford, Conn.

David M. Stuart, Ph.D.
  Ohio Northern University
  Ada, Ohio

Robert S. Thompson, Ph.D.
  Temple University
  Philadelphia, Pa.

Analgesics

Carl C. Hug, Jr., M.D., Ph.D., *Chairperson*
  Emory University School of Medicine
  Atlanta, Ga.

John Adriani, M.D.
  Charity Hospital of Louisiana
  New Orleans, La.

William H. Barr, Pharm.D., Ph.D.
  Medical College of Virginia
  Richmond, Va.

William L. Dewey, Ph.D.
  Medical College of Virginia
  Richmond, Va.

John C. Drach, Ph.D.
  University of Michigan
  Ann Arbor, Mich.

Max Fink, M.D.
  State University of New York
  Stony Brook, N.Y.

William H. Forrest, Jr., M.D.
  Stanford University
  Stanford, Calif.

·Ira W. Hillyard, Ph.D.
  ICN Pharmaceutical Co.
  Irvine, Calif.

Stephen G. Hoag, Ph.D.
  North Dakota State University
  Fargo, N.D.

Paul A. Jablon, Ph.D.
  Albany College of Pharmacy
  Albany, N.Y.

Ronald L. Katz, M.D.
  University of California
  Los Angeles, Calif.

Arthur H. Kibbe, Ph.D.
  University of Mississippi
  University, Miss.

Joseph V. Levy, Ph.D.
  Pacific Medical Center
  San Francisco, Calif.

Ralph W. Morris, Ph.D.
  University of Illinois Medical Center
  Chicago, Ill.

Ronald E. Nagata, Jr., Pharm.D.
  Veterans Administration Hospital
  Palo Alto, Calif.

Thomas E. Needham, Jr., Ph.D.
  University of Georgia
  Athens, Ga.

Nathan R. Strahl, Ph.D.
  University of Mexico
  Albuquerque, N.M.

David M. Stuart, Ph.D.
  Ohio Northern University
  Ada, Ohio

Morton A. Winner, D.D.S.
  Roosevelt Hospital
  New York, N.Y.

Richard L. Wynn, Ph.D.
University of Kentucky
Lexington, Ky.

Anesthetics
Ronald D. Miller, M.D., *Chairperson*
University of California
San Francisco, Calif.

John Adriani, M.D.
Charity Hospital of Louisiana
New Orleans, La.

Ervin E. Bagwell, Ph.D.
Medical University of South Carolina
Charleston, S.C.

Burnell R. Brown, Jr., M.D., Ph.D.
University of Arizona
Tucson, Ariz.

Sebastian G. Ciancio, D.D.S.
State University of New York
Buffalo, N.Y.

Carlton K. Erickson, Ph.D.
University of Kansas
Lawrence, Kan.

John T. Frank, Pharm.D.
Cedars-Sinai Medical Center
Los Angeles, Calif.

Adolph H. Giesecke, Jr., M.D.
University of Texas
Dallas, Tex.

Michael B. Gormley, D.D.S.
Dorchester General Hospital
Cambridge, Md.

Ronald L. Katz, M.D.
University of California
Los Angeles, Calif.

Frank M. McCarthy, M.D., D.D.S.
University of Southern California
Los Angeles, Calif.

Robert N. Miller, M.D.
Washington University
St. Louis, Mo.

Robert E. Pearson, M.S.
David Wastchak & Associates
Phoenix, Ariz.

Morton A. Winner, D.D.S.
Roosevelt Hospital
New York, N.Y.

Richard L. Wynn, Ph.D.
University of Kentucky
Lexington, Ky.

Antiarrhythmic Agents
John J. Curry, M.D., *Chairperson*
Georgetown University
Washington, D.C.

Ervin E. Bagwell, Ph.D.
Medical University of South Carolina
Charleston, S.C.

James E. Berger, Ph.D.
Butler University
Indianapolis, Ind.

Young W. Cho, M.D.
University of North Carolina
Chapel Hill, N.C.

Arthur H. Hayes, Jr., M.D.
Milton S. Hershey Medical Center
Hershey, Pa.

Osamu James Inashima, Ph.D.
Northeastern University
Boston, Mass.

Joseph V. Levy, Ph.D.
Pacific Medical Center
San Francisco, Calif.

Helmut M. Redetzki, M.D.
Louisiana State University
Shreveport, La.

Harold I. Silverman, D.Sc.
Massachusetts College of Pharmacy
Boston, Mass.

Theodore G. Tong, Pharm.D.
University of California
San Francisco, Calif.

Anticoagulants
Murdo G. MacDonald, M.D., *Chairperson*
University of Vermont
Burlington, Vt.

O'Neill Barrett, Jr., M.D.
University of South Florida
College of Medicine
Tampa, Fla.

Madison J. Cawein, M.D.
Merrell-National Laboratories
Cincinnati, Ohio

William G. Crouthamel, Ph.D.
University of Maryland
Baltimore, Md.

Tommy W. Gage, Ph.D., D.D.S.
Baylor University
Dallas, Tex.

Philip P. Gerbino, Pharm.D.
Philadelphia College of Pharmacy
and Science
Philadelphia, Pa.

Daniel A. Hussar, Ph.D.
Philadelphia College of Pharmacy
and Science
Philadelphia, Pa.

Martin J. Jinks, Pharm.D.
Health Applications Systems, Inc.
Burlingame, Calif.

Edward F. LaSala, Ph.D.
Massachusetts College of Pharmacy
Boston, Mass.

Leonard L. Naeger, Ph.D.
St. Louis College of Pharmacy
St. Louis, Mo.

E. Don Nelson, Pharm.D.
University of Cincinnati
Cincinnati, Ohio

Larry E. Patterson, Pharm.D.
South Dakota State University
Brookings, S.D.

Fred J. Salter, Pharm.D.
Medical College of Virginia
Richmond, Va.

Walter F. Stanaszek, Ph.D.
University of Oklahoma
Norman, Okla.

Ronald B. Stewart, M.S.
University of Florida
Gainesville, Fla.

Gordon L. Strommen, M.S.
North Dakota State University
Fargo, N.D.

Robert S. Thompson, Ph.D.
Temple University
Philadelphia, Pa.

Lee A. Wanke, M.S.
State University of Oregon
Corvallis, Ore.

Anticonvulsants
Richard K. Richards, M.D., *Chairperson*
Stanford University
Stanford, Calif.

Ann B. Amerson, Pharm.D.
University of Kentucky
Lexington, Ky.

Alex A. Cardoni, M.S.
University of Connecticut
Hartford, Conn.

Gregory M. Chudzik, Pharm.D.
Bristol Laboratories
Syracuse, N.Y.

Ernest A. Daigneault, Ph.D.
Louisiana State University
New Orleans, La.

Morris D. Faiman, Ph.D.
University of Kansas
Lawrence, Kan.

Lorne K. Garrettson, M.D.
Medical College of Virginia
Richmond, Va.

Douglas Goldman, M.D.
University of Cincinnati
Cincinnati, Ohio

F. James Grogan, Pharm.D.
Chicago, Ill.

Lawrence Isaac, Ph.D.
University of Illinois Medical Center
Chicago, Ill.

Louis C. Littlefield, Pharm.D.
University of Texas
San Antonio, Tex.

Fred J. Salter, Pharm.D.
Medical College of Virginia
Richmond, Va.

Byron F. Schweigert, Pharm.D.
Memorial Hospital Medical Center
Long Beach, Calif.

Antihistamines
I. Leonard Bernstein, M.D., *Chairperson*
Cincinnati General Hospital
Cincinnati, Ohio

Donald E. Cadwallader, Ph.D.
University of Georgia
Athens, Ga.

Elliot F. Ellis, M.D.
National Jewish Hospital and
Research Center
Denver, Colo.

Lawrence Isaac, Ph.D.
University of Illinois Medical Center
Chicago, Ill.

A. Vincent Lopez, Ph.D.
Mercer University
Atlanta, Ga.

Joseph F. Palumbo, M.S.
Northeastern University
Boston, Mass.

Richard K. Richards, M.D.
Stanford University
Stanford, Calif.

Brandt Rowles, Ph.D.
Ferris State College
Big Rapids, Mich.

Nathan R. Strahl, Ph.D.
University of New Mexico
Albuquerque, N.M.

Antihypertensive Agents
Joseph P. Buckley, Ph.D., *Chairperson*
University of Houston
Houston, Tex.

Ervin E. Bagwell, Ph.D.
  Medical University of South Carolina
  Charleston, S.C.

Young W. Cho, M.D.
  University of North Carolina
  Chapel Hill, N.C.

Monte S. Cohon, Pharm.D.
  University of Wisconsin
  Madison, Wis.

Michael A. Commarato, Ph.D.
  Warner-Lambert Research Institute
  Morris Plains, N.J.

John J. Curry, M.D.
  Georgetown University
  Washington, D.C.

Earl W. Dunham, Ph.D.
  University of Minnesota
  Minneapolis, Minn.

Arthur H. Hayes, Jr., M.D.
  Milton S. Hershey Medical Center
  Hershey, Pa.

Lawrence Isaac, Ph.D.
  University of Illinois
    Medical Center
  Chicago, Ill.

Joseph V. Levy, Ph.D.
  Pacific Medical Center
  San Francisco, Calif.

Louis C. Littlefield, Pharm.D.
  University of Texas
  San Antonio, Tex.

Thomas E. Needham, Jr., Ph.D.
  University of Georgia
  Athens, Ga.

Helmut M. Redetzki, M.D.
  Louisiana State University
  Shreveport, La.

Michael A. Riddiough, Pharm.D.
  University of California
  San Francisco, Calif.

Diana F. Rodriguez-Calvert, Pharm.D.
  University of New Mexico
  Albuquerque, N.M.

Harold I. Silverman, D.Sc.
  Massachusetts College of Pharmacy
  Boston, Mass.

Donald W. Stansloski, Ph.D.
  Ohio Northern University
  Ada, Ohio

Gordon L. Strommen, M.S.
  North Dakota State University
  Fargo, N.D.

Victor A. Yanchick, Ph.D.
  University of Texas
  Austin, Tex.

Anti-Infectives
Lawrence H. Block, Ph.D., *Chairperson*
  Duquesne University
  Pittsburgh, Pa.

Ann B. Amerson, Pharm.D.
  University of Kentucky
  Lexington, Ky.

Bill B. Butcher, M.S.
  Good Samaritan Hospital
  Phoenix, Ariz.

Donald E. Cadwallader, Ph.D.
  University of Georgia
  Athens, Ga.

Madison J. Cawein, M.D.
  Merrell-National Laboratories
  Cincinnati, Ohio

Gregory A. Chudzik, Pharm.D.
  Bristol Laboratories
  Syracuse, N.Y.

Sebastian G. Ciancio, D.D.S.
  State University of New York
  Buffalo, N.Y.

Isidore Cohn, Jr., M.D.
  Louisiana State University
  New Orleans, La.

Monte S. Cohon, Pharm.D.
  University of Wisconsin
  Madison, Wis.

William G. Crouthamel, Ph.D.
  University of Maryland
  Baltimore, Md.

Raymond E. Dann, Ph.D.
  Norwich Pharmacal Co.
  Norwich, N.Y.

Nancy N. Huang, M.D.
  Temple University
  Philadelphia, Pa.

Gary L. Manley, Pharm.D.
  Medical College of Virginia
  Richmond, Va.

Edward A. Mock, Pharm.D.
  Veterans Administration Hospital
  San Francisco, Calif.

Charles N. Nightingale, Ph.D.
  University of Connecticut
  Storrs, Conn.

Richard Quintiliani, M.D.
  Hartford Hospital
  Hartford, Conn.

Diana F. Rodriguez-Calvert, Pharm.D.
  University of New Mexico
  Albuquerque, N.M.

Byron F. Schweigert, Pharm.D.
  Memorial Hospital Medical Center
  Long Beach, Calif.

David S. Tatro, Pharm.D.
  Stanford University
  Stanford, Calif.

Robert S. Thompson, Ph.D.
  Temple University
  Philadelphia, Pa.

Flynn W. Warren, Jr., M.S.
  Medical College of Georgia
  Augusta, Ga.

Lawrence R. Weiss, Ph.D.
  Food and Drug Administration
  Washington, D.C.

Antineoplastic Agents
James A. Visconti, Ph.D., *Chairperson*
  (January 1976–   )
  Ohio State University Hospitals
  Columbus, Ohio

J. Worth Estes, M.D., *Chairperson*
  (March 1974–December 1975)
  Boston University
  Boston, Mass.

O'Neill Barrett, Jr., M.D.
  University of South Florida
  Tampa, Fla.

Isidore Cohn, Jr., M.D.
  Louisiana State University
  New Orleans, La.

Raymond E. Dann, Ph.D.
  Norwich Pharmacal Co.
  Norwich, N.Y.

John C. Drach, Ph.D.
  University of Michigan
  Ann Arbor, Mich.

Clarence L. Fortner, M.S.
  National Cancer Institute
  Baltimore, Md.

Ronald B. Kluza, Ph.D.
  Massachusetts College of Pharmacy
  Boston, Mass.

Edward F. LaSala, Ph.D.
  Massachusetts College of Pharmacy
  Boston, Mass.

Larry E. Patterson, Pharm.D.
  South Dakota State University
  Brookings, S.D.

Robert E. Pearson, M.S.
  David Wastchak & Associates
  Phoenix, Ariz.

M. Peter Pevonka, M.S.
  University of Florida
  Gainesville, Fla.

Larry J. Powers, Ph.D.
  T. R. Evans Research Center
  Painesville, Ohio

Antitussive Agents
Lawrence R. Weiss, Ph.D., *Chairperson*
  Food and Drug Administration
  Washington, D.C.

A. Vincent Lopez, Ph.D.
  Mercer University
  Atlanta, Ga.

Joseph F. Palumbo, M.S.
  Northeastern University
  Boston, Mass.

Autonomic Agents
John P. Long, Ph.D., *Chairperson*
  University of Iowa
  Iowa City, Iowa

James E. Berger, Ph.D.
  Butler University
  Indianapolis, Ind.

Floyd E. Bloom, M.D.
  The Salk Institute
  San Diego, Calif.

Bill B. Butcher, M.S.
  Good Samaritan Hospital
  Phoenix, Ariz.

Bernard J. Carroll, M.D., Ph.D.
  University of Michigan
  Ann Arbor, Mich.

Michael A. Commarato, Ph.D.
  Warner-Lambert Research Institute
  Morris Plains, N.J.

Erminio Costa, M.D.
  National Institute of Mental Health
  Washington, D.C.

Ernest A. Daigneault, Ph.D.
  Louisiana State University
  New Orleans, La.

Balwant N. Dixit, Ph.D.
  University of Pittsburgh
  Pittsburgh, Pa.

Arnold J. Friedhoff, M.D.
  New York University Medical Center
  New York, N.Y.

Tommy W. Gage, Ph.D., D.D.S.
  Baylor University
  Dallas, Tex.

Ira W. Hillyard, Ph.D.
  ICN Pharmaceutical Co.
  Irvine, Calif.

O. L. Lorenzetti, Ph.D.
Alcon Laboratories, Inc.
Fort Worth, Tex.

John H. McNeill, Ph.D.
University of British Columbia
Vancouver, Canada

Ralph W. Morris, Ph.D.
University of Illinois
Medical Center
Chicago, Ill.

Daniel A. Nona, Ph.D.
American Council on Pharmaceutical
Education
Chicago Ill.

Noel I. Robin, M.D.
Stamford Hospital
Stamford, Conn.

Gerald P. Sherman, Ph.D.
University of Kentucky
Lexington, Ky.

Harold I. Silverman, D.Sc.
Massachusetts College of Pharmacy
Boston, Mass.

Fridolin Sulser, M.D.
Vanderbilt University
Nashville, Tenn.

Cardiac Glycosides
Gary L. Lage, Ph.D., *Chairperson*
University of Wisconsin
Madison, Wis.

William H. Barr, Ph.D.
Medical College of Virginia
Richmond, Va.

Joseph P. Buckley, Ph.D.
University of Houston
Houston, Tex.

John J. Curry, M.D.
Georgetown University
Washington, D.C.

Arthur H. Hayes, Jr., M.D.
Milton S. Hershey Medical Center
Hershey, Pa.

Osamu James Inashima, Ph.D.
Northeastern University
Boston, Mass.

Ronald E. Nagata, Jr., Pharm.D.
Veterans Administration Hospital
Palo Alto, Calif.

Gerald P. Sherman, Ph.D.
University of Kentucky
Lexington, Ky.

Ronald B. Stewart, M.S.
University of Florida
Gainesville, Fla.

James A. Visconti, Ph.D.
Ohio State University Hospitals
Columbus, Ohio

Flynn W. Warren, Jr., M.S.
Medical College of Georgia
Augusta, Ga.

Victor A. Yanchick, Ph.D.
University of Texas
Austin, Tex.

Diuretics
Leonard L. Naeger, Ph.D., *Chairperson*
St. Louis College of Pharmacy
St. Louis, Mo.

Ann B. Amerson, Pharm.D.
University of Kentucky
Lexington, Ky.

J. Edward Bell, Pharm.D.
University of Michigan
Ann Arbor, Mich.

Donald E. Cadwallader, Ph.D.
University of Georgia
Athens, Ga.

Osamu James Inashima, Ph.D.
Northeastern University
Boston, Mass.

Gary L. Lage, Ph.D.
University of Wisconsin
Madison, Wis.

Gary L. Manley, Pharm.D.
Medical College of Virginia
Richmond, Va.

Edward A. Mock, Pharm.D.
Veterans Administration Hospital
San Francisco, Calif.

M. Peter Pevonka, M.S.
University of Florida
Gainesville, Fla.

Gordon L. Strommen, M.S.
North Dakota State University
Fargo, N.D.

Environmental Agents
Robert E. Pearson, M.S., *Chairperson*
David Wastchak & Associates
Phoenix, Ariz.

Ernest A. Daigneault, Ph.D.
Louisiana State University
New Orleans, La.

Raymond E. Dann, Ph.D.
Norwich Pharmacal Co.
Norwich, N.Y.

Mostafa S. Fahim, Ph.D.
University of Missouri
Columbia, Mo.

Morris D. Faiman, Ph.D.
  University of Kansas
  Lawrence, Kan.

Lorne K. Garrettson, M.D.
  Medical College of Virginia
  Richmond, Va.

Diana F. Rodriguez-Calvert, Pharm.D.
  University of New Mexico
  Albuquerque, N.M.

Hypoglycemic Agents
John A. Owen, Jr., M.D., *Chairperson*
  University of Virginia
  Charlottesville, Va.

J. Edward Bell, Pharm.D.
  University of Michigan
  Ann Arbor, Mich.

Balwant N. Dixit, Ph.D.
  University of Pittsburgh
  Pittsburgh, Pa.

Daniel A. Hussar, Ph.D.
  Philadelphia College of Pharmacy
    and Science
  Philadelphia, Pa.

Peter P. Lamy, Ph.D.
  University of Maryland
  Baltimore, Md.

A. Vincent Lopez, Ph.D.
  Mercer University
  Atlanta, Ga.

Edward D. Mock, Pharm.D.
  Veterans Administration Hospital
  San Francisco, Calif.

Daniel Nona, Ph.D.
  American Council on Pharmaceutical
    Education
  Chicago, Ill.

Arthur C. Solomon, M.S.
  Nuclear Pharmacy, Inc.
  Atlanta, Ga.

Walter F. Stanaszek, Ph.D.
  University of Oklahoma
  Norman, Okla.

David S. Tatro, Pharm.D.
  Stanford University Medical Center
  Stanford, Calif.

Victor A. Yanchick, Ph.D.
  University of Texas
  Austin, Tex.

Hypolipidemic Agents
Young W. Cho, M.D., *Chairperson*
  University of North Carolina
  Chapel Hill, N.C.

Stephen G. Hoag, Ph.D.
  North Dakota State University
  Fargo, N.D.

John A. Owen, Jr., M.D.
  University of Virginia
  Charlottesville, Va.

Noel I. Robin, M.D.
  Stamford Hospital
  Stamford, Conn.

Brandt Rowles, Ph.D.
  Ferris State College
  Big Rapids, Mich.

Donald W. Stansloski, Ph.D.
  Ohio Northern University
  Ada, Ohio

Muscle Relaxants
Adolph H. Giesecke, Jr., M.D., *Chairperson*
  University of Texas
  Dallas, Tex.

John Adriani, M.D.
  Charity Hospital of Louisiana
  New Orleans, La.

Sidney Goldstein, D.Sc.
  Merrell-National Laboratories
  Cincinnati, Ohio

Ronald L. Katz, M.D.
  University of California
  Los Angeles, Calif.

Ronald D. Miller, M.D.
  University of California
  San Francisco, Calif.

Joseph F. Palumbo, M.S.
  Northeastern University
  Boston, Mass.

Lawrence R. Weiss, Ph.D.
  Food and Drug Administration
  Washington, D.C.

Morton A. Winner, D.D.S.
  Roosevelt Hospital
  New York, N.Y.

Psychotropic Agents
Baron Shopsin, M.D., *Chairperson*
    (May 1975–   )
  New York University Medical Center
  New York, N.Y.

Nathan S. Kline, M.D., *Chairperson*
    (March 1973–April 1975)
  Rockland Research Center
  Orangeburg, N.Y.

Frank J. Ayd, Jr., M.D.
  Taylor Manor Hospital
  Ellicott City, Md.

Thomas A. Ban, M.D.
McGill University
Montreal, Canada

John P. Bederka, Ph.D.
University of Illinois Medical Center
Chicago, Ill.

Kenneth J. Bender, Pharm.D., M.A.
University of Illinois Medical Center
Chicago, Ill.

Alex A. Cardoni, M.S.
University of Connecticut
Hartford, Conn.

K. D. Charalampous, M.D.
Baylor College of Medicine
Houston, Tex.

Mervin L. Clark, M.D.
University of Oklahoma
Norman, Okla.

John M. Davis, M.D.
Illinois State Psychiatric Institute
Chicago, Ill.

Herman C. B. Denber, M.D., Ph.D.
University of Louisville
Louisville, Ky.

William L. Dewey, Ph.D.
Medical College of Virginia
Richmond, Va.

Carl W. Driever, Ph.D.
University of Houston
Houston, Tex.

Jack Durell, M.D.
The Psychiatric Institute of
Washington, D.C.
Washington, D.C.

Donald M. Gallant, M.D.
Tulane University
New Orleans, La.

Samuel Gershon, M.D.
New York University Medical Center
New York, N.Y.

Albert A. Kurland, M.D.
Maryland Psychiatric Research Center
Baltimore, Md.

Morris A. Lipton, M.D., Ph.D.
University of North Carolina
Chapel Hill, N.C.

Jack M. Rosenberg, Pharm.D.
Brooklyn College of Pharmacy
Brooklyn, N.Y.

George M. Simpson, M.D.
Rockland Research Center
Orangeburg, N.Y.

Robert B. Sloane, M.D.
Los Angeles County/U.S.C. Medical
Center
Los Angeles, Calif.

Arthur C. Solomon, M.S.
Nuclear Pharmacy, Inc.
Atlanta, Ga.

A. Arthur Sugerman, M.D.
Carrier Clinic Foundation
Belle Meade, N.J.

Fridolin Sulser, M.D.
Vanderbilt University
Nashville, Tenn.

Joseph M. Tobin, M.D.
Northwest Psychiatric Clinic
Eau Claire, Wis.

Lee A. Wanke, M.S.
State University of Oregon
Corvallis, Ore.

Richard J. Wyatt, M.D.
National Institute of Mental Health
Washington, D.C.

Sedative–Hypnotics

Helmut M. Redetzki, M.D., *Chairperson*
Louisiana State University
Shreveport, La.

Kenneth J. Bender, Pharm.D., M.A.
University of Illinois Medical Center
Chicago, Ill.

Frank M. Berger, M.D.
University of Louisville Medical School
Louisville, Ky.

Henry Brill, M.D.
Pilgrim Psychiatric Center
West Brentwood, N.Y.

Enoch Callaway, M.D.
Langley Porter Neuropsychiatric
Institute
San Francisco, Calif.

Bernard J. Carroll, M.D., Ph.D.
University of Michigan
Ann Arbor, Mich.

Sebastian G. Ciancio, D.D.S.
State University of New York
Buffalo, N.Y.

Carl W. Driever, Ph.D.
University of Houston
Houston, Tex.

Carlton K. Erickson, Ph.D.
University of Kansas
Lawrence, Kan.

Mostafa S. Fahim, Ph.D.
University of Missouri
Columbia, Mo.

Max Fink, M.D.
  State University of New York
  Stony Brook, N.Y.

William H. Forrest, Jr., M.D.
  Stanford University
  Stanford, Calif.

Eric Goldstein, Pharm.D.
  University of Florida
  Gainesville, Fla.

Frank M. McCarthy, M.D., D.D.S.
  University of Southern California
  Los Angeles, Calif.

Sidney Merlis, M.D.
  Central Islip State Hospital
  Central Islip, N.Y.

Charles H. Nightingale, Ph.D.
  University of Connecticut
  Storrs, Conn.

Richard K. Richards, M.D.
  Stanford University
  Stanford, Calif.

Jack M. Rosenberg, Pharm.D.
  Brooklyn College of Pharmacy
  Brooklyn, N.Y.

Charles Shagass, M.D.
  Eastern Pennsylvania Psychiatric
    Institute
  Philadelphia, Pa.

Steroids
Paul A. Jablon, Ph.D., *Chairperson*
  Albany College of Pharmacy
  Albany, N.Y.

William H. Barr, Ph.D.
  Medical College of Virginia
  Richmond, Va.

I. Leonard Bernstein, M.D.
  Cincinnati General Hospital
  Cincinnati, Ohio

Bill B. Butcher, M.S.
  Good Samaritan Hospital
  Phoenix, Ariz.

Elliot F. Ellis, M.D.
  National Jewish Hospital and
    Research Center
  Denver, Colo.

Mostafa S. Fahim, Ph.D.
  University of Missouri
  Columbia, Mo.

John T. Frank, Pharm.D.
  Cedars-Sinai Medical Center
  Los Angeles, Calif.

Gary L. Lage, Ph.D.
  University of Wisconsin
  Madison, Wis.

John A. Owen, Jr., M.D.
  University of Virginia
  Charlottesville, Va.

Tai-Chan Peng, M.D.
  University of North Carolina
  Chapel Hill, N.C.

Theodore G. Tong, Pharm.D.
  University of California
  San Francisco, Calif.

Uricosuric Agents
David M. Stuart, Ph.D., *Chairperson*
  Ohio Northern University
  Ada, Ohio

Paul A. Jablon, Ph.D.
  Albany College of Pharmacy
  Albany, N.Y.

Martin J. Jinks, Pharm.D.
  Health Application Systems, Inc.
  Burlingame, Calif.

Louis C. Littlefield, Pharm.D.
  University of Texas
  San Antonio, Tex.

Leonard L. Naeger, Ph.D.
  St. Louis College of Pharmacy
  St. Louis, Mo.

Ronald E. Nagata, Jr., Pharm.D.
  Veterans Administration Hospital
  Palo Alto, Calif.

Nelson Rivers, Pharm.D.
  University of Tennessee
  Memphis, Tenn.

Vitamins
Charles H. Nightingale, Ph.D., *Chairperson*
  University of Connecticut
  Storrs, Conn.

Enoch Callaway, M.D.
  Langley Porter Neuropsychiatric Institute
  San Francisco, Calif.

Philip P. Gerbino, Pharm.D.
  Philadelphia College of Pharmacy
    and Science
  Philadelphia, Pa.

Nancy N. Huang, M.D.
  Temple University
  Philadelphia, Pa.

Martin J. Jinks, Pharm.D.
  Health Applications Systems, Inc.
  Burlingame, Calif.

Peter P. Lamy, Ph.D.
  University of Maryland
  Baltimore, Md.

Tai-Chan Peng, M.D.
University of North Carolina
Chapel Hill, N.C.

Paul G. Pierpaoli, M.S.
McCook Hospital
Hartford, Conn.

Byron F. Schweigert, Pharm.D.
Memorial Hospital Medical Center
Long Beach, Calif.

Theodore G. Tong, Pharm.D.
University of California
San Francisco, Calif.

Practitioner Panel

Subpanel I

David E. Bailey, M.S.
Massachusetts General Hospital
Boston, Mass.

Vincent E. Bouchard, M.S.
University of Michigan
Ann Arbor, Mich.

James R. Hayward, D.D.S.
University of Michigan
Ann Arbor, Mich.

Michael L. Kleinberg, M.S.
Ohio State University Hospitals
Columbus, Ohio

William E. Lotterhos, M.D.
Medical College of Georgia
Augusta, Ga.

William A. Miller, Pharm.D.
University of Tennessee
Memphis, Tenn.

Darrell R. Newcomer, M.S.
Henry Ford Hospital
Detroit, Mich.

William H. Randall, Jr., B.S.
Practicing Pharmacist
Lillington, N.C.

Sara Jane White, M.S.
University of Kansas Medical Center
Kansas City, Kan.

Subpanel II

Thomas G. Baumgartner, M.Ed.
Stockton, Calif.

Robert L. Church, Pharm.D.
Family Health Center, Inc.
Kalamazoo, Mich.

David V. DeGruy, B.S.
Mobile Mental Health Center
Mobile, Ala.

Mario Forcione, M.S.
Beth Israel Hospital
Boston, Mass.

Stanley H. Freeman, Pharm.D.
Lee Memorial Hospital
Fort Myers, Fla.

James M. Moss, M.D.
Georgetown University
Washington, D.C.

Joseph A. Romano, Pharm.D.
Columbia University
New York, N.Y.

Julius M. Tesi, M.D.
Ohio State University
Columbus, Ohio

Kay Yamagata, Pharm.D.
Alta Bates Hospital
Berkeley, Calif.

Subpanel III

Kenneth J. Bykowski, B.S.
Silver Cross Hospital
Joliet, Ill.

Eugene Elkin, M.S.
Kustner's Pharmacy
Riverside, Calif.

William R. Grove, B.S.
Baltimore Cancer Research Center
Baltimore, Md.

Arthur J. Hadler, M.D.
Veterans Administration Outpatient Clinic
Boston, Mass.

William J. Hossley, M.D.
Family Practice Physician
Deming, N.M.

Gary M. McCart, Pharm.D.
University of California
San Francisco, Calif.

Lee M. Quon, Pharm.D.
Cedars of Lebanon Hospital
Los Angeles, Calif.

Earnest E. Roehrs†, B.S.
Sandusky Memorial Hospital
Sandusky, Ohio

Arthur F. Shinn, Pharm.D.
William Beaumont Hospital
Royal Oak, Mich.

Subpanel IV

Robert C. Barger, M.S.
Providence Hospital
Southfield, Mich.

---

† Deceased.

Robert P. Fudge, B.S.
Ohio State University Hospitals
Columbus, Ohio

Harold N. Godwin, M.S.
University of Kansas Medical Center
Kansas City, Kan.

Gerald D. Griffin, Pharm.D.
Universidad Autonoma de Ciudad Juarez
El Paso, Tex.

Richard A. Henry, M.D.
University of Florida
Gainesville, Fla.

Ernest H. Luther, B.S.
Hospital Pharmacist
Arlington, Va.

C. Ronald Stephen, M.D.
Washington University
St. Louis, Mo.

Garf Thomas, M.S.
University of Missouri
Columbia, Mo.

Alan M. Weissman, Pharm.D.
Appalachian Regional Hospital
South Williamson, Ky.

Subpanel V
Steven L. Barriere, Pharm.D.
University of California
San Francisco, Calif.

Harry E. Dascomb, M.D.
Louisiana State University
New Orleans, La.

Bill B. Ferguson, M.D.
Practicing Physician
Hillsboro, Ore.

Thomas J. Garrison, B.S.
Center for Health Science Hospital
Kansas City, Mo.

William D. Mastin, B.S.
High Street Pharmacy
Blue Island, Ill.

Russell R. Miller, Pharm.D., Ph.D.
New England Medical Center Hospital
Boston, Mass.

Martin Rein, B.S.
Fisk and Pfennig Pharmacy
Williamsville, N.Y.

Andrew W. Roberts, M.S.
University of Minnesota Hospital
Minneapolis, Minn.

Anthony J. Silvagni, Pharm.D.
Massachusetts College of Pharmacy
Boston, Mass.

Subpanel VI
Joel Covinsky, Pharm.D.
Kansas City General Hospital
and Medical Center
Kansas City, Mo.

Dennis F. Dziczkowski, B.S.
Menizer Pharmacy
Hales Corner, Wis.

Ronald D. Kaufmann, B.S.
Kaufmann's Pharmacy
Philadelphia, Pa.

Marc F. Laventurier, B.S.
Paid Prescriptions
Burlingame, Calif.

Edward L. Platcow, Ph.D.
Lilly Research Laboratories
Indianapolis, Ind.

Charles N. Shalhoob, B.S.
Veterans Hospital
St. Louis, Mo.

N. Ty Smith, M.D.
University Hospital of
San Diego County
San Diego, Calif.

Lloyd Y. Young, Pharm.D.
Washington State University
Spokane, Wash.

Ancillary Reviewers

E. F. Domino, M.D.
  University of Michigan
  Ann Arbor, Mich.

Nathan S. Kline, M.D.
  Rockland Research Center
  Orangeburg, N.Y.

Paolo Morselli, M.D.
  Synthelabo
  Paris, France

Rodolfo Paoletti, M.D.
  Università di Milano
  Milan, Italy

Jerome Ryan, M.D.
  Tulane University
  New Orleans, La.

Edward M. Sellers, M.D., Ph.D.
  Addiction Research Foundation
  Toronto, Canada

Gianni Tognoni, M.D.
  Istituto de Ricerche
    di Farmacologiche
  "Mario Negri"
  Milan, Italy

Cooperating Organizations and Agencies and their Designated Representatives

American Dental Association
  Edgar W. Mitchell, Ph.D.
  Chicago, Ill.

American Podiatry Association
  Chester L. Rossi, D.P.M.
  Washington, D.C.

American Society of Hospital Pharmacists
  Mary Jo Reilly, M.S.
  Bethesda, Md.

Food and Drug Administration
  Vincent J. Gagliardi, M.D.
  Rockville, Md.

National Library of Medicine
  Joan M. Burnside, B.S.
  Bethesda, Md.

Participating Pharmaceutical Manufacturers and their Designated Representatives

Abbott Laboratories
Fredric B. Bauer, M.D.
North Chicago, Ill.

Bristol Laboratories
Louis A. Farchione, M.D.
Syracuse, N.Y.

Burroughs Wellcome & Co.
Richard M. Welch, Ph.D.
Research Triangle Park, N.C.

Hoechst Pharmaceutical Co.
Harold R. Dettelbach, Ph.D.
Somerville, N.J.

Lederle Laboratories
Alexander Thomson, M.D.
Pearl River, N.Y.

Eli Lilly & Co.
S. O. Waife, M.D.
Indianapolis, Ind.

Merck Sharp & Dohme
James P. Hoffman, M.D.
West Point, Pa.

Norwich Pharmacal Co.
William F. Hewitt, Ph.D.
Norwich, N.Y.

Roche Laboratories
Jack I. Boyland, B.S.
Nutley, N.J.

William H. Rorer, Inc.
Robert R. Smith, M.D.
Fort Washington, Pa.

Sandoz Pharmaceuticals
William F. Westlin, M.D.
Hanover, N.J.

G. D. Searle
Robert L. Alberti, M.D.
Chicago, Ill.

Smith Kline and French Laboratories
Robert C. Hoppe, M.D.
Philadelphia, Pa.

The Upjohn Company
Marvin Guthaus, M.S.
Kalamazoo, Mich.

Winthrop Laboratories
G. Warren McCarl, M.D.
New York, N.Y.

Participants

John Adriani, *New Orleans, La.*
Robert L. Alberti, *Chicago, Ill.*
Heidi Alperovich, *Ramat Gan, Israel*
Ann B. Amerson, *Lexington, Ky.*
William S. Apple, *Washington, D.C.*
Leland J. Arney, *Washington, D.C.*
Frank J. Ascione, *Washington, D.C.*
Frank J. Ayd, Jr., *Ellicott City, Md.*
Ervin E. Bagwell, *Charleston, S.C.*
David E. Bailey, *Boston, Mass.*
Thomas A. Ban, *Montreal, Canada*
Robert C. Barger, *Southfield, Mich.*
William H. Barr, *Richmond, Va.*
O'Neill Barrett, Jr., *Tampa, Fla.*
Steven L. Barriere, *San Francisco, Calif.*
Fredric B. Bauer, *North Chicago, Ill.*
Thomas G. Baumgartner, *Stockton, Calif.*
John P. Bederka, *Chicago, Ill.*
J. Edward Bell, *Ann Arbor, Mich.*
Kenneth J. Bender, *Chicago, Ill.*
Frank M. Berger, *Louisville, Ky.*
James E. Berger, *Indianapolis, Ind.*
I. Leonard Bernstein, *Cincinnati, Ohio*
Lawrence H. Block, *Pittsburgh, Pa.*
Floyd E. Bloom, *San Diego, Calif.*
David R. Bohardt, *Washington, D.C.*
Vincent E. Bouchard, *Ann Arbor, Mich.*
Jack I. Boyland, *Nutley, N.J.*
Henry Brill, *West Brentwood, N.Y.*
Burnell R. Brown, Jr., *Tucson, Ariz.*
Paul Bryan, *Rockville, Md.*
Joseph P. Buckley, *Houston, Tex.*
Erika H. Burch, *Washington, D.C.*
Joan M. Burnside, *Bethesda, Md.*
Bill B. Butcher, *Phoenix, Ariz.*
Kenneth J. Bykowski, *Joliet, Ill.*
Donald E. Cadwallader, *Athens, Ga.*
Enoch Callaway, *San Francisco, Calif.*
Alex A. Cardoni, *Hartford, Conn.*
James P. Caro, *Washington, D.C.*
Allan D. Carpenter, *Washington, D.C.*
Bernard J. Carroll, *Ann Arbor, Mich.*
Madison J. Cawein, *Cincinnati, Ohio*
K. D. Charalampous, *Houston, Tex.*
Young W. Cho, *Chapel Hill, N.C.*
Gregory Chudzik, *Syracuse, N.Y.*
Robert L. Church, *Kalamazoo, Mich.*
Sebastian G. Ciancio, *Buffalo, N.Y.*
Mervin L. Clark, *Norman, Okla.*
Isidore Cohn, Jr., *New Orleans, La.*
Monte S. Cohon, *Madison, Wis.*

Michael A. Commarato, *Morris Plains, N.J.*
L. Luan Corrigan, *Washington, D.C.*
Erminio Costa, *Washington, D.C.*
Joel O. Covinsky, *Kansas City, Mo.*
William G. Crouthamel, *Baltimore, Md.*
John J. Curry, *Washington, D.C.*
Ernest A. Daigneault, *New Orleans, La.*
Raymond E. Dann, *Norwich, N.Y.*
Harry E. Dascomb, *New Orleans, La.*
John M. Davis, *Chicago, Ill.*
David V. DeGruy, *Mobile, Ala.*
Pierre S. Del Prato, *Washington, D.C.*
Herman C. B. Denber, *Louisville, Ky.*
Harold R. Dettelbach, *Somerville, N.J.*
William L. Dewey, *Richmond, Va.*
Balwant N. Dixit, *Pittsburgh, Pa.*
E. F. Domino, *Ann Arbor, Mich.*
John C. Drach, *Ann Arbor, Mich.*
Carl W. Driever, *Houston, Tex.*
Earl W. Dunham, *Minneapolis, Minn.*
Jack Durell, *Washington, D.C.*
Dennis F. Dziczkowski, *Hales Corner, Wis.*
Eugene Elkin, *Riverside, Calif.*
Elliot F. Ellis, *Denver, Colo.*
Carlton K. Erickson, *Lawrence, Kan.*
J. Worth Estes, *Boston, Mass.*
Mostafa S. Fahim, *Columbia, Mo.*
Morris D. Faiman, *Lawrence, Kan.*
Louis A. Farchione, *Syracuse, N.Y.*
Donald O. Fedder, *Baltimore, Md.*
Edward G. Feldmann, *Washington, D.C.*
Bill B. Ferguson, *Hillsboro, Ore.*
Max Fink, *Stony Brook, N.Y.*
Mario Forcione, *Boston, Mass.*
William H. Forrest, Jr., *Stanford, Calif.*
Clarence L. Fortner, *Baltimore, Md.*
John T. Frank, *Los Angeles, Calif.*
Stanley H. Freeman, *Fort Myers, Fla.*
Arnold J. Friedhoff, *New York, N.Y.*
Robert P. Fudge, *Columbus, Ohio*
Tommy W. Gage, *Dallas, Tex.*
Vincent Gagliardi, *Rockville, Md.*
Donald M. Gallant, *New Orleans, La.*
Lorne K. Garrettson, *Richmond, Va.*
Thomas J. Garrison, *Kansas City, Mo.*
Philip P. Gerbino, *Philadelphia, Pa.*
Samuel Gershon, *New York, N.Y.*
Adolph H. Giesecke, *Dallas, Tex.*
Harold N. Godwin, *Kansas City, Kan.*
Douglas Goldman, *Cincinnati, Ohio*
Eric Goldstein, *Gainesville, Fla.*

George S. Goldstein, *New York, N.Y.*
Sidney Goldstein, *Cincinnati, Ohio*
Michael B. Gormley, *Cambridge, Md.*
Herb Graber, *Washington, D.C.*
Gerald D. Griffin, *El Paso, Tex.*
F. James Grogan, *Chicago, Ill.*
William R. Grove, *Baltimore, Md.*
Marvin Guthaus, *Kalamazoo, Mich.*
Arthur J. Hadler, *Boston, Mass.*
Phillip A. Harris, *Los Angeles, Calif.*
Arthur H. Hayes, Jr., *Hershey, Pa.*
James R. Hayward, *Ann Arbor, Mich.*
Richard Henry, *Gainesville, Fla.*
Vicki Hershiser, *Washington, D.C.*
William F. Hewitt, *Norwich, N.Y.*
Ira W. Hillyard, *Irvine, Calif.*
Stephen G. Hoag, *Fargo, N.D.*
James P. Hoffman, *West Point, Pa.*
Robert C. Hoppe, *Philadelphia, Pa.*
William J. Hossley, *Deming, N.M.*
Nancy N. Huang, *Philadelphia, Pa.*
Carl C. Hug, *Clarkston, Ga.*
Daniel A. Hussar, *Philadelphia, Pa.*
Osamu James Inashima, *Boston, Mass.*
Lawrence Isaac, *Chicago, Ill.*
Paul A. Jablon, *Albany, N.Y.*
Marcia T. Jay, *Washington, D.C.*
Martin J. Jinks, *Burlingame, Calif.*
Susan Kallem, *Washington, D.C.*
Samuel H. Kalman, *Washington, D.C.*
Ronald L. Katz, *Los Angeles, Calif.*
Ronald D. Kaufmann, *Philadelphia, Pa.*
John F. Kerege, *Baton Rouge, La.*
Arthur H. Kibbe, *University, Miss.*
Michael L. Kleinberg, *Columbus, Ohio*
Nathan S. Kline, *Orangeburg, N.Y.*
Ronald B. Kluza, *Boston, Mass.*
Edward Kravitz, *Rockville, Md.*
Albert A. Kurland, *Baltimore, Md.*
Gary L. Lage, *Madison, Wis.*
Peter P. Lamy, *Baltimore, Md.*
Edward F. LaSala, *Boston, Mass.*
Marc F. Laventurier, *Burlingame, Calif.*
Diana T. Leggett, *Washington, D.C.*
Joseph V. Levy, *San Francisco, Calif.*
Morris A. Lipton, *Chapel Hill, N.C.*
Louis C. Littlefield, *San Antonio, Tex.*
John P. Long, *Iowa City, Iowa*
A. Vincent Lopez, *Atlanta, Ga.*
O. J. Lorenzetti, *Fort Worth, Tex.*
William E. Lotterhos, *Augusta, Ga.*
Ernest H. Luther, *Arlington, Va.*
Murdo G. MacDonald, *Burlington, Vt.*
Gary L. Manley, *Richmond, Va.*
William D. Mastin, *Blue Island, Ill.*
G. Warren McCarl, *New York, N.Y.*
Gary M. McCart, *San Francisco, Calif.*
Frank M. McCarthy, *Los Angeles, Calif.*
William F. McGhan, *Washington, D.C.*
John H. McNeill, *Vancouver, Canada*

Sidney Merlis, *Central Islip, N.Y.*
Robert N. Miller, *St. Louis, Mo.*
Ronald D. Miller, *San Francisco, Calif.*
Russell R. Miller, *Boston, Mass.*
William A. Miller, *Memphis, Tenn.*
Edgar W. Mitchell, *Chicago, Ill.*
Edward D. Mock, *San Francisco, Calif.*
Ralph W. Morris, *Chicago, Ill.*
Paolo Morselli, *Paris, France*
James M. Moss, *Washington, D.C.*
Leonard L. Naeger, *St. Louis, Mo.*
Ronald E. Nagata, Jr., *Palo Alto, Calif.*
Thomas E. Needham, Jr., *Athens, Ga.*
E. Don Nelson, *Cincinnati, Ohio*
Darrell R. Newcomer, *Detroit, Mich.*
Paul J. Niebergall, *Kansas City, Mo.*
Charles H. Nightingale, *Storrs, Conn.*
Daniel A. Nona, *Chicago, Ill.*
John A. Owen, Jr., *Charlottesville, Va.*
R. E. Owens, *Oklahoma City, Okla.*
Joseph F. Palumbo, *Boston, Mass.*
Rodolfo Paoletti, *Milan, Italy*
Larry E. Patterson, *Brookings, S.D.*
Robert E. Pearson, *Phoenix, Ariz.*
Tai-Chan Peng, *Chapel Hill, N.C.*
Richard P. Penna, *Washington, D.C.*
Joanne Peters, *Washington, D.C.*
M. Peter Pevonka, *Gainesville, Fla.*
Paul G. Pierpaoli, *Hartford, Conn.*
Edward L. Platcow, *Indianapolis, Ind.*
Deborah Pomerance, *Washington, D.C.*
Larry J. Powers, *Painesville, Ohio*
Joyce Pristavec, *Washington, D.C.*
Richard Quintiliani, *Hartford, Conn.*
Lee M. Quon, *Los Angeles, Calif.*
William H. Randall, *Lillington, N.C.*
Helmut M. Redetzki, *Shreveport, La.*
Mary Jo Reilly, *Bethesda, Md.*
Martin Rein, *Williamsville, N.Y.*
Richard K. Richards, *Stanford, Calif.*
Michael A. Riddiough, *San Francisco, Calif.*
Nelson P. Rivers, *Little Rock, Ark.*
Andrew W. Roberts, *Minneapolis, Minn.*
Carl Roberts, *Washington, D.C.*
Noel I. Robin, *Stamford, Conn.*
Diana Rodriguez-Calvert, *Albuquerque, N.M.*
Earnest E. Roehrs †, *Sandusky, Ohio*
Joseph A. Romano, *New York, N.Y.*
Margaret F. Rose, *Washington, D.C.*
Jack M. Rosenberg, *Brooklyn, N.Y.*
Chester L. Rossi, *Washington, D.C.*
Brandt Rowles, *Big Rapids, Mich.*
Jerome R. Ryan, *New Orleans, La.*
Fred J. Salter, *Richmond, Va.*
Foster Sansbury, *Washington, D.C.*
Elora A. Sayre, *Washington, D.C.*
Byron F. Schweigert, *Long Beach, Calif.*
Edward M. Sellers, *Toronto, Canada*

---

† Deceased.

Charles Shagass, *Philadelphia, Pa.*
Charles N. Shalhoob, *St. Louis, Mo.*
Gerald P. Sherman, *Lexington, Ky.*
Arthur F. Shinn, *Royal Oak, Mich.*
Janet D. Shoff, *Washington, D.C.*
Baron Shopsin, *New York, N.Y.*
Anthony J. Silvagni, *Boston, Mass.*
Harold I. Silverman, *Boston, Mass.*
George M. Simpson, *Orangeburg, N.Y.*
Robert B. Sloane, *Los Angeles, Calif.*
N. Ty Smith, *San Diego, Calif.*
Robert R. Smith, *Fort Washington, Pa.*
Arthur C. Solomon, *Atlanta, Ga.*
Thomas C. Springer, *Washington, D.C.*
Walter F. Stanaszek, *Norman, Okla.*
Donald W. Stansloski, *Ada, Ohio*
C. Ronald Stephen, *St. Louis, Mo.*
Ronald B. Stewart, *Gainesville, Fla.*
Nathan R. Strahl, *Albuquerque, N.M.*
Gordon L. Strommen, *Fargo, N.D.*
David M. Stuart, *Ada, Ohio*
A. Arthur Sugerman, *Belle Meade, N.J.*
Fridolin Sulser, *Nashville, Tenn.*
David S. Tatro, *Stanford, Calif.*

Julius M. Tesi, *Columbus, Ohio*
Garf P. Thomas, *Columbia, Mo.*
Robert S. Thompson, *Philadelphia, Pa.*
Alexander Thomson, *Pearl River, N.Y.*
Joseph M. Tobin, *Eau Claire, Wis.*
Gianni Tognoni, *Milan, Italy*
Theodore G. Tong, *San Francisco, Calif.*
James A. Visconti, *Columbus, Ohio*
S. O. Waife, *Indianapolis, Ind.*
Lee A. Wanke, *Corvallis, Ore.*
Flynn W. Warren, Jr., *Augusta, Ga.*
Lawrence R. Weiss, *Washington, D.C.*
Alan M. Weissman, *South Williamson, Ky.*
Richard M. Welch,
  Research Triangle Park, N.C.
William F. Westlin, *East Hanover, N.J.*
Sara Jane White, *Kansas City, Kan.*
Ronald L. Williams, *Washington, D.C.*
Morton A. Winner, *New York, N.Y.*
Richard J. Wyatt, *Washington, D.C.*
Richard L. Wynn, *Lexington, Ky.*
Kay Yamagata, *Berkeley, Calif.*
Victor A. Yanchick, *Austin, Tex.*
Lloyd Y. Young, *Spokane, Wash.*

Evaluations
of
Drug
Interactions:
Monographs

The following monographs are comprehensive assessments of reported drug interactions prepared, evaluated, and reviewed by participants from dentistry, medicine, and pharmacy. Each monograph includes a summary of the interaction, the interaction potential of related drugs, the pharmacological effects and mechanisms of the drugs pertinent to the interaction, a critical evaluation of published reports, a summary of the clinical data (designated with the symbol ■), recommendations for avoiding and managing the interaction, references, and nonproprietary and trade names.

Alcohol—Amitriptyline

Summary—The effects of amitriptyline and related tricyclic antidepressants on alcohol are unpredictable. Various studies have reported that tricyclic antidepressants enhance, prevent, or do not affect the central nervous system (CNS) depressant effects of alcohol. The most hazardous effect is enhanced CNS depression induced by alcohol. Patients receiving amitriptyline should avoid concurrent use of alcohol and should be warned about driving an automobile or operating hazardous machinery after concurrent ingestion of these drugs.

Related Drugs—**Doxepin** (1, 2) and **nortriptyline** (2, 3) may interact with alcohol. Although not supported by clinical evidence, the other tricyclic antidepressants expected to interact with alcohol in a manner similar to amitriptyline are **desipramine, imipramine,** and **protriptyline.** Nonspecific sedative effects vary among the tricyclic antidepressants; amitriptyline is the most potent and protriptyline is the weakest (4).

Pharmacological Effect and Mechanism—Amitriptyline is an antidepressant drug which also has sedative effects (5, 6). In a double-blind clinical study (6) in which doses of 25, 50, and 75 mg of amitriptyline were compared with each other, with 100- or 200-mg doses of secobarbital, and with a placebo, 25 mg of amitriptyline produced an overall quality of sleep between the 100- and 200-mg doses of secobarbital (based on patient responses to a questionnaire). Because alcohol is a CNS depressant, the enhanced sedation produced by the short-term ingestion of alcohol and amitriptyline probably results from the combined effects of the two agents (1).

In contrast, the results of another study (2) suggest that tricyclic antidepressants antagonize the sedative effects of alcohol. This effect was noted while evaluating the subjects' performances using a driving simulator.

Evaluation of Clinical Data—The effects of concurrent alcohol and amitriptyline ingestion on skills related to driving behavior were studied by appropriate tests in a double-blind manner (7). Twenty-one healthy subjects were randomized into one of three treatment groups. One group received amitriptyline (0.8 mg/kg po) on both the night before and the morning of the tests. Another group received a placebo the night before the tests and amitriptyline (0.8 mg/kg po) on the morning of the tests. The remaining group received a placebo on both occasions. All three groups were given a calculated amount of alcohol sufficient to produce a blood alcohol level of approximately 80 mg/100 ml. Both groups pretreated with amitriptyline showed an impairment in the motor skills related to driving when compared with the group pretreated with the placebo.

An additional double-blind study (8) was undertaken to determine the effect of 5 days of pretreatment with amitriptyline (50 mg po every 12 hr) or placebo in normal subjects and to examine how driving skills are affected with and without similar blood alcohol levels as in the previous study (7). There were no significant differences in test performances in a simulated driving test between the amitriptyline-treated and placebo groups. Furthermore, no significant decrease in motor function performance was observed after the concurrent ingestion of alcohol and amitriptyline (8).

Sixteen subjects were given nortriptyline (20–50 mg/day po) alone 1 day before the test and during ingestion of enough alcohol to achieve a blood alcohol level of 50 mg/100 ml (approximately 90 ml of whiskey ingested in 30 min) (3). Nortriptyline did not significantly increase or decrease the effects of alcohol on the subjects' performances in a delayed audiofeedback test. However, after nortriptyline administration, the subjects' performance scores tended to revert toward their scores prior to alcohol ingestion. The results suggest a slight antagonism of the depressant effects of alcohol.

Twenty-two healthy subjects received doxepin (2) (12–25 mg/m^2) concurrently with enough alcohol to achieve intoxication (mean blood alcohol level, 73.6 mg/100 ml). Their performance scores in a simulated driving test were much better than the scores of a control group of 12 subjects who received a similar quantity of alcohol alone.

Forty subjects were randomly given amitriptyline, clomipramine, doxepin, and nortriptyline in a double-blind crossover trial (1). The doses of amitriptyline, doxepin, and nortriptyline were 30 mg/day po for the first 7 days and then 60 mg/day po for the next 7 days. The dose of clomipramine was 30 mg/day po for the first 7 days and then 75 mg/day po for the next 7 days. On Days 7 and 14, alcohol was ingested in sufficient quantities to reach a peak blood alcohol level of 47 mg/100 ml (0.5 g/kg). Amitriptyline and doxepin significantly increased the impairment of psychomotor skills caused by alcohol on the seventh day of treatment but showed minor effects on the 14th day, indicating that this drug interaction may become less harmful with continued administration. The results after clomipramine or nortriptyline was given concurrently with alcohol were only slightly modified.

■ The clinical evidence is too contradictory to predict the effects of concurrent ingestion of tricyclic antidepressants and alcohol. Various studies reported that tricyclic antidepressants enhance, prevent, or do not affect the CNS depressant effects of alcohol. The most hazardous effect would be enhanced CNS depression induced by alcohol. Concurrent ingestion of unstated quantities of alcohol and therapeutic doses of amitriptyline has been associated with two deaths (9) and is also thought to impair gastrointestinal activity (10). However, there are insufficient clinical data to support these speculations.

Recommendations—Although the clinical effects of this drug interaction are unpredictable, it would be prudent to advise a patient receiving amitriptyline or other tricyclic antidepressants to avoid alcoholic beverages. The patient also should be cautioned about driving an automobile or operating hazardous machinery after concurrent ingestion of these agents.

References

(1) T. Seppala *et al.*, "Effect of Tricyclic Antidepressants and Alcohol on Psychomotor Skills Related to Driving," *Clin. Pharmacol. Ther.*, *17*, 515 (1975).

(2) G. Milner and A. Landauer, "The Effects of Doxepin, Alone and Together with Alcohol, in Relation to Driving Safety," *Med. J. Aust.*, *1*, 837 (1973).

(3) F. W. Hughes and R. B. Forney, "Delayed Audiofeedback (DAF) for Induction of Anxiety. Effect of Nortriptyline, Ethanol, or Nortriptyline-Ethanol Combinations on Performance with DAF," *J. Amer. Med. Ass.*, *185*, 556 (1963).

(4) D. J. Greenblatt, "Rational Use of Psychotropic Drugs," *Amer. J. Hosp. Pharm.*, *32*, 59 (1975).

(5) E. Hartmann, "The Effect of Four Drugs on Sleep Patterns in Man," *Psychopharmacologia*, *12*, 346 (1968).

(6) K. F. Urbach, "Hypnotic Properties of Amitriptyline: Comparison with Secobarbital," *Anesth. Analg.*, *46*, 835 (1967).

(7) A. A. Landauer *et al.*, "Alcohol and Amitriptyline Effects on Skills Related to Driving Behavior," *Science*, *163*, 1467 (1969).

(8) J. Patman *et al.*, "The Combined Effect of Alcohol and Amitriptyline on Skills Similar to Motor-Car Driving," *Med. J. Aust.*, *2*, 946 (1969).

(9) M. F. Lockett and G. Milner, "Combining the Antidepressant Drugs," *Brit. Med. J.*, *1*, 921 (1965).

(10) G. Milner, "Gastro-Intestinal Side Effects and Psychotropic Drugs," *Med. J. Aust.*, *2*, 153 (1969).

[For additional information, see *Antidepressant Therapy*, p. 373.]

Nonproprietary and Trade Names of Drugs

Alcohol—*Various products and beverages*
Amitriptyline hydrochloride—*Elavil Hydrochloride and various combination products*
Desipramine hydrochloride—*Norpramin, Pertofrane*
Doxepin hydrochloride—*Adapin, Sinequan*

Imipramine hydrochloride—*Presamine, Tofranil, Tofranil PM*
Nortriptyline hydrochloride—*Aventyl Hydrochloride*
Protriptyline hydrochloride—*Vivactil Hydrochloride*

Prepared and evaluated by the Scientific Review Subpanel on Psychotropic Agents and reviewed by Practitioner Panel I.

Allopurinol—Aminophylline

Summary—Although the chemical relationship of allopurinol (a hypoxanthine derivative) and aminophylline (a methylxanthine) suggests a possible interaction, it has not been documented in the literature. Concurrent therapy with these agents appears to present no problems.

Related Drugs—Aminophylline is a soluble salt containing about 85% theophylline and 15% ethylenediamine. Related preparations include **dyphylline, oxtriphylline, theophylline, theophylline olamine, theophylline sodium acetate,** and **theophylline sodium glycinate. Theobromine** and its salts are used for similar purposes.

Pharmacological Effect and Mechanism—Based on animal and *in vitro* work, allopurinol has been shown to be a competitive inhibitor of xanthine oxidase in low concentrations and a noncompetitive inhibitor of xanthine oxidase in high concentrations. Allopurinol itself is a substrate for xanthine oxidase and is converted to oxypurinol (alloxanthine). Oxypurinol is a xanthine oxidase inhibitor that exerts a slightly weaker but longer inhibitory effect than allopurinol on xanthine oxidase (1). Another factor contributing to the therapeutic action of allopurinol is the increase in reutilization of hypoxanthine and xanthine, which are not oxidized in the presence of allopurinol (2). This action, through a negative feedback mechanism, decreases purine biosynthesis (3, 4).

As a diuretic, aminophylline inhibits sodium reabsorption in a pattern similar to the thiazide diuretics (5). Thiazides are known inhibitors of uric acid excretion, but theophylline does not affect the levels of uric acid excretion (6). However, unless laboratory tests are specific for uric acid, theophylline and other methylxanthines can give false-positive values for uric acid (7). In addition, allopurinol interferes with the UV spectrophotometric determination of theophylline (8).

Urinary excretion of epinephrine is increased as much as threefold in many persons by aminophylline, possibly due to stimulation of catecholamine release by the adrenal medulla (9). Epinephrine stimulates the oxidation of hypoxanthine by xanthine oxidase (10). Furthermore, epinephrine decreases the clearance of urate, possibly due to a vasoconstrictive alteration of renal blood flow (11). Thus, it is theoretically possible that aminophylline could reduce the net effect of allopurinol inhibition of xanthine oxidase. Xanthine oxidase is not involved in the metabolism of methylxanthine (12, 13).

Evaluation of Clinical Data—No clinical report specifically relating to an allopurinol–aminophylline interaction is available.

■ The listing of xanthines under agents that antagonize the "uricosuric action" of allopurinol in several reviews on drug interactions is misleading. The term uricosuric pertains to agents promoting uricosuria. Allopurinol is not in this sense a uricosuric agent but is an inhibitor of an enzyme responsible for the formation of uric acid. Available information does not support the existence of any clinically significant interaction between allopurinol and aminophylline.

Recommendations—Since aminophylline does not affect uric acid excretion or appear to have any effect on allopurinol activity, concurrent therapy with these agents appears to pose no problem. Concurrent administration also does not affect aminophylline activity.

References

(1) R. W. Rundles et al., "Allopurinol in the Treatment of Gout," Ann. Intern. Med., 64, 229 (1966).

(2) R. Pomales et al., "Augmentation of the Incorporation of Hypoxanthine into Nucleic Acids by the Administration of an Inhibitor of Xanthine Oxidase," Biochim. Biophys. Acta, 72, 119 (1963).

(3) R. J. McCollister et al., "Pseudofeedback Inhibition of Purine Synthesis by 6-Mercaptopurine Ribonucleotide and Other Purine Analogues," J. Biol. Chem., 239, 1560 (1964).

(4) T.-F. Yu and A. B. Gutman, "Effect of Allopurinol (4-Hydroxypyrazolo-(3,4-d)pyrimidine) on Serum and Urinary Uric Acid in Primary and Secondary Gout," Amer. J. Med., 37, 885 (1964).

(5) B. R. Nechay, "Aminophylline and Its Relationship to Some Other Diuretic Agents in Dogs," J. Pharmacol. Exp. Ther., 132, 339 (1961).

(6) H. H. Cornish and A. A. Christman, "A Study of the Metabolism of Theobromine, Theophylline, and Caffeine in Man," J. Biol. Chem., 228, 315 (1957).

(7) H. E. Paulus et al., "Clinical Significance of Hyperuricemia in Routinely Screened Hospitalized Men," J. Amer. Med. Ass., 211, 277 (1970).

(8) J. W. Jenne et al., "Pharmacokinetics of Theophylline: Application to Adjustment of the Clinical Dose of Aminophylline," Clin. Pharmacol. Ther., 13, 349 (1972).

(9) N. Atuk et al., "Effect of Aminophylline on Urinary Excretion of Epinephrine and Norepinephrine in Man," Circulation, 35, 745 (1967).

(10) D. M. Valerino and J. J. McCormack, "Xanthine Oxidase-Mediated Oxidation of Epinephrine," Biochem. Pharmacol., 20, 47 (1971).

(11) F. E. Demartini, "Hyperuricemia Induced by Drugs," Arthritis Rheum., 8, 823 (1965).

(12) B. B. Brodie et al., "Metabolism of Theophylline (1,3-Dimethylxanthine) in Man," J. Biol. Chem., 194, 215 (1952).

(13) F. Bergmann and S. Dikstein, "Studies on Uric Acid and Related Compounds III. Observations on the Specificity of Mammalian Xanthine Oxidases," J. Biol. Chem., 223, 765 (1956).

[For additional information, see Uricosuric Therapy, p. 447.]

Nonproprietary and Trade Names of Drugs

Allopurinol—Zyloprim
Aminophylline—Various manufacturers
Dyphylline—Dilor, Lufyllin, Neothylline
Oxtriphylline—Choledyl
Theobromine—Various manufacturers
Theophylline—Elixophyllin, Liquophylline, Optiphyllin

Theophylline olamine—Fleet Theophylline, Monotheamin
Theophylline sodium acetate—Various manufacturers
Theophylline sodium glycinate—Glynazan, Synophylate, Theoglycinate

Prepared and evaluated by the Scientific Review Subpanel on Uricosuric Agents and reviewed by Practitioner Panel I.

Allopurinol—Iron

Summary—Studies in humans do not support earlier animal data indicating that allopurinol and iron interact adversely. Since it is unlikely that a clinically important drug interaction occurs, no additional precautions are necessary when these drugs are given concurrently.

Related Drugs—Various iron-containing products are available including **ferrous fumarate, ferrous gluconate, ferrous lactate,** and **ferrous sulfate.**

Pharmacological Effect and Mechanism—The enzyme xanthine oxidase was hypothesized to play an essential role in the release of iron from its storage form ferritin (hemosiderin) (1). Several animal studies (1–3) and the report of an individual with decreased hepatic xanthine oxidase activity and hemosiderosis (4) indicated that altered iron metabolism may occur concurrently with the inhibition of xanthine oxidase activity.

According to this hypothesis, iron is stored in the liver in the oxidized or ferric state and is tightly bound to protein as ferric ferritin. Xanthine oxidase appears to be involved in the conversion of ferric ferritin to ferrous ferritin. The reduced form of iron is less tightly bound to ferritin and thus is more easily released for utilization. Therefore, a possible inverse relationship between hepatic xanthine oxidase activity and hepatic iron storage exists. Theoretically, the xanthine oxidase inhibitor allopurinol should decrease the activity of xanthine oxidase and increase hepatic iron storage (3, 5).

Evaluation of Clinical Data—Although several reports (1--4) support an allopurinol–iron interaction, other animal studies (5–7) failed to document it. Most importantly, there is no evidence from other reports in humans (5, 8–11) that inhibition of xanthine oxidase by allopurinol in therapeutic doses has any demonstrable effect on iron metabolism. These observations were not influenced by the length of allopurinol administration or the dietary intake of the subjects (5).

■ Most reported data indicate that there is little likelihood that allopurinol, in thera-peutic doses, inhibits the metabolism of iron. The study (3) supporting this inter-action utilized a small number of animals and used doses much greater on a weight basis than the dose range of allopurinol normally administered in humans. Addi-tionally, the case report (4) substantiating this hypothesis is now thought to have been caused by other factors (7). Moreover, it has been proven that a very sub-stantial decrease (probably greater than 99%) in xanthine oxidase activity would be required to affect iron metabolism (5, 7). Since the degree of inhibition of xanthine oxidase by allopurinol is seldom more than 50% (12), it is highly unlikely that any noticeable effect occurs in humans.

Recommendations—Although the package literature of the manufacturer of allo-purinol warns that these two drugs should not be administered concurrently (13), clinical studies do not support the existence of an interaction. Therefore, no additional precautions are required when these drugs are given concurrently.

References

(1) S. Green and A. Mazur, "Relation of Uric Acid Metabolism to Release of Iron from Hepatic Ferritin," *J. Biol. Chem., 227,* 653 (1957).

(2) A. Mazur *et al.,* "Mechanism of Release of Ferritin Iron *In Vivo* by Xanthine Oxidase," *J. Clin. Invest., 37,* 1809 (1958).

(3) L. W. Powell, "Effects of Allopurinol on Iron Storage in the Rat," *Ann. Rheum. Dis.*, *25*, 697 (1966).

(4) J. H. Ayvazian, "Xanthinuria and Hemochromatosis," *N. Engl. J. Med.*, *270*, 18 (1964).

(5) R. Green *et al.*, "The Effect of Allopurinol on Iron Metabolism," *S. Afr. Med. J.*, *42*, 776 (1968).

(6) V. Udall and D. Deller, "Allopurinol Symposium, 1966," *Ann. Rheum. Dis.*, *25*, 704 (1966).

(7) C. Kozma *et al.*, "Chronic Allopurinol Administration and Iron Storage in Mice," *Life Sci.*, *7*, 341 (1968).

(8) R. W. Rundles *et al.*, "Allopurinol in the Treatment of Gout," *Ann. Intern. Med.*, *64*, 229 (1966).

(9) B. T. Emmerson, "Effects of Allopurinol on Iron Metabolism in Man," *Ann. Rheum. Dis.*, *25*, 700 (1966).

(10) P. S. Davis and D. J. Deller, "Effect of a Xanthine-Oxidase Inhibitor (Allopurinol) on Radioiron Absorption in Man," *Lancet*, *ii*, 470 (1966).

(11) N. W. Levin and O. L. Abrahams, "Allopurinol in Patients with Impaired Renal Function," *Ann. Rheum. Dis.*, *25*, 681 (1966).

(12) G. H. Hitchings, "Effects of Allopurinol in Relation to Purine Biosynthesis," *Ann. Rheum. Dis.*, *25*, 601 (1966).

(13) "Physicians' Desk Reference," 29th ed., Medical Economics, Inc., Oradell, NJ 07649, 1975, p. 677.

[For additional information, see *Uricosuric Therapy*, p. 447.]

Nonproprietary and Trade Names of Drugs

Allopurinol—*Zyloprim*
Ferrocholinate—*Chel-Iron, Ferrolip*

Ferrous fumarate, gluconate, lactate, and sulfate—*Various manufacturers, available alone or as a fixed combination*

Prepared and evaluated by the Scientific Review Subpanel on Uricosuric Agents and reviewed by Practitioner Panel II.

Allopurinol—Probenecid

Summary—Concurrent use of allopurinol and probenecid may decrease the effectiveness of allopurinol in the treatment of chronic hyperuricemia associated with primary and secondary gout. However, the clinical significance of this effect has not been established, and concurrent therapy is useful in therapeutic situations requiring both a maximum reduction in uric acid production and a maximum increase in uric acid excretion (*e.g.,* congenital overproduction of uric acid). A fluid intake of approximately 3 liters/day and alkalinization of the urine should be recommended to ensure that the total amount of urinary acids presented to the kidney does not exceed the ability of the kidney to excrete it.

Related Drugs—Allopurinol is unique in its ability to inhibit xanthine oxidase, and currently there are no drugs on the market with a similar mechanism of action, although many compounds have uricosuric activity.

Pharmacological Effect and Mechanism—Allopurinol inhibits xanthine oxidase, the enzyme that catalyzes the conversion of xanthine to uric acid (1). It is metabolized to oxypurinol (alloxanthine), a metabolite that exerts a slightly weaker but longer inhibitory effect than allopurinol on xanthine oxidase. Oxypurinol appears to contribute significantly to the overall therapeutic reduction of serum urate levels (2). As blood and urine levels of uric acid decrease, there is an increase (although not proportional) in the blood and urine levels of the uric acid precursors hypoxanthine and xanthine (1). These compounds are more soluble than uric acid and are less likely to precipitate in the kidney (3).

Various mechanisms have been proposed for the allopurinol–probenecid interaction. Allopurinol may inhibit the metabolism of probenecid, thereby prolonging the half-life of the uricosuric agent (4, 5). Similarly, probenecid may increase the renal excretion of oxypurinol, resulting in a decrease in the overall inhibition of uric acid production (2). This increase would cause increased blood levels of xanthine and hypoxanthine and possibly result in their precipitation in body tissues. Moreover, administering probenecid with allopurinol produces a greater increase in the excretion of uric acid than is produced with allopurinol alone. This effect could lead to uric acid crystallization in the kidney and would be especially detrimental to patients with impaired renal function (1).

Evaluation of Clinical Data—In one study (1), 19 patients received allopurinol (200–600 mg/day po) and either probenecid (0.5–1.0 g/day po) or sulfinpyrazone (200–600 mg/day po). The addition of the uricosuric agent resulted in an appreciably increased renal excretion of uric acid from a mean of 364 mg/24 hr (allopurinol alone) to a mean of 571 mg/24 hr. The combined action of the drugs was accompanied by a further decline in serum urate levels from a mean of 7.1 mg% to a mean of 6.1 mg%.

Probenecid (2–3 g/day po) and sulfinpyrazone (800 mg/day po) on different occasions were added to the allopurinol drug regimen of one patient with gout and one with xanthinuria (6). A decrease in the excretion of hypoxanthine and xanthine was noted in both patients.

In two other studies (2, 7), a substantial increase in the excretion of the metabolite of allopurinol, oxypurinol, occurred in four patients who had also received probenecid (1 g/day po).

■ The clinical significance of this interaction has not been demonstrated. Although the addition of probenecid to allopurinol therapy has been shown to increase the serum levels of hypoxanthine and xanthine significantly (2, 4, 7), no data have been presented to indicate that the levels reached were close to the saturation levels of these compounds in the plasma (6). Additionally, the extent of the effect of probenecid on oxypurinol excretion has never been firmly established (2). Even in the studies showing a significant increase in uric acid secretion caused by the allopurinol–probenecid interaction as compared to allopurinol alone, the investigators concluded that this effect would not be detrimental to the well-hydrated patient with normal renal function and that it may actually be the desired effect in certain clinical situations (1, 6).

Recommendations—Concurrent administration of allopurinol and probenecid should be approached with caution in patients with impaired renal function because of the danger of precipitation of urate or urate precursors in the kidney. Moreover, fluid intake should be maintained at a level of 3 liters/day in all patients taking these drugs. Alkalinization of the urine may also be desirable as a means of promoting and ensuring adequate xanthine clearance through the kidney (8). Sodium bicarbonate (4–8 g/day) is the alkalinizing agent of choice for this purpose (9, 10).

Other uricosuric agents, such as sulfinpyrazone (1), can be expected to have an effect similar to that of probenecid.

References

(1) T.-F. Yu and A. B. Gutman, "Effect of Allopurinol (4-Hydroxypyrazolo(3,4-d)pyrimidine) on Serum and Urinary Uric Acid in Primary and Secondary Gout," *Amer. J. Med.*, *37*, 885 (1964).

(2) G. B. Elion *et al.*, "Metabolic Studies of Allopurinol, an Inhibitor of Xanthine Oxidase," *Biochem. Pharmacol.*, *15*, 863 (1966).

(3) "The Pharmacological Basis of Thera-peutics," 5th ed., L. S. Goodman and A. Gilman, Eds., Macmillan, New York, NY 10022, 1975, p. 353.

(4) T.-F. Yu, in "Gout," A. B. Gutman, Ed., Medcom, Burroughs-Wellcome, Research Triangle Park, N. C., 1971, p. 79.

(5) T. B. Tjandramaga et al., "Observations on the Disposition of Probenecid in Patients Receiving Allopurinol," Pharmacology, 8, 259 (1972).

(6) S. Goldfinger et al., "The Renal Excretion of Oxypurines," J. Clin. Invest., 44, 623 (1965).

(7) G. B. Elion et al., "Renal Clearance of Oxipurinol, the Chief Metabolite of Allopurinol," Amer. J. Med., 45, 69 (1968).

(8) A. Rastegar and S. O. Thier, "The Treatment of Hyperuricemia in Gout," Ration. Drug Ther., 8 (3), 1 (1974).

(9) M. D. Kogut et al., "Disorder of Purine Metabolism Due to Partial Deficiency of Hypoxanthine-Guanine Phosphoribosyltransferase. A Study of a Family," Amer. J. Med., 48, 148 (1970).

(10) "Drugs of Choice 1974–1975," W. Modell, Ed., Mosby, St. Louis, Mo., 1974, p. 482.

[For additional information, see *Uricosuric Therapy*, p. 447.]

Nonproprietary and Trade Names of Drugs

Allopurinol—*Zyloprim*
Probenecid—*Benemid*

Sulfinpyrazone—*Anturane*

Prepared and evaluated by the Scientific Review Subpanel on Uricosuric Agents and reviewed by Practitioner Panel III.

Amitriptyline—Chlordiazepoxide

Summary—At least three cases of impaired motor function have been attributed to the concurrent administration of amitriptyline and chlordiazepoxide. However, the occurrence of a clinically significant interaction appears uncommon, patients receiving these drugs concurrently should be warned about possible enhanced central nervous system (CNS) depression.

Related Drugs—Other tricyclic antidepressants which are structurally and pharmacologically related to amitriptyline include **desipramine, doxepin, imipramine, nortriptyline,** and **protriptyline.** Benzodiazepines related to chlordiazepoxide include **clonazepam, clorazepate, diazepam, flurazepam, nitrazepam,** and **oxazepam.**

Pharmacological Effect and Mechanism—The antidepressant action of the tricyclic compounds is believed to be the result of a depression of inhibitory functions in the brain rather than due to a euphoric action as produced by the monoamine oxidase inhibitors (1). Nonspecific sedative effects vary among the tricyclics from amitriptyline (the strongest) to protriptyline (the weakest) (2). The depressant effects of amitriptyline and other tricyclic antidepressants may enhance the sedation produced by chlordiazepoxide and other tranquilizers or sedatives.

Amitriptyline also has some anticholinergic activity and may produce dry mouth and other atropine-like effects at high doses. There is little evidence that chlordiazepoxide is an active anticholinergic (3), but its depressant effects might enhance this activity of amitriptyline. There are no animal data to support the enhanced depressant action observed in humans (4–6).

Evaluation of Clinical Data—There have been at least three case reports of serious adverse effects attributed to the concurrent use of amitriptyline and chlordiazepoxide. One patient taking amitriptyline (150 mg/day po) and chlordiazepoxide (40 mg/day po) showed ataxia, tremors, and some impairment of motor coordination (4). Two other patients, each taking amitriptyline (75 mg/day po) and chlordiazepoxide (30 mg/day po) showed slurred speech, loss of memory, drowsiness, and motor impairment (5). When the same doses of amitriptyline and chlordiazepoxide were given for shorter periods in two double-blind studies (7, 8) attempting to determine if the concurrent use of the two drugs was better than amitriptyline by itself, the incidence or severity of the side effects was not statistically greater than with amitriptyline alone. One patient who had taken amitriptyline (75 mg/day po) and diazepam (6 mg/day po) for 6 months died of apparent acute hepatic necrosis. These drugs could not definitely be established as the causative agents of the necrosis but a number of pathologists felt the association was significant (6).

Two subsequent clinical studies (9, 10) measured the effect of a benzodiazepine (chlordiazepoxide, diazepam, or oxazepam) on the serum levels of a tricyclic antidepressant (amitriptyline or nortriptyline). No detectable change in the serum levels of the tricyclic antidepressant occurred. Additional studies showed that these drugs can be used safely in the treatment of depression accompanied by anxiety (11–13).

■ Concurrent administration of amitriptyline and chlordiazepoxide reportedly has caused impairment of motor function in three patients (4, 5). However, these observations have not been confirmed in controlled clinical trials (7–13). Concurrent use of amitriptyline and chlordiazepoxide has been suggested (14, 15) as safe therapy for the treatment of depression with concurrent anxiety, but the therapeutic efficacy of such therapy in treating depression has not been proven to be superior to tricyclic antidepressants alone (16).

Recommendations—Although the occurrence of a clinically significant interaction appears uncommon, a few patients may experience symptoms of CNS depression (*e.g.*, drowsiness, loss of memory, motor impairment, and slurred speech) when amitriptyline is given concurrently with chlordiazepoxide. Patients receiving these drugs concurrently should be advised of these effects.

References

(1) D. O. Lewis, "The Pharmacodynamics of Depression and Its Relation to Therapy," *Brit. J. Clin. Pract., 28*, 21 (1974).

(2) D. J. Greenblatt, "Rational Use of Psychotropic Drugs," *Amer. J. Hosp. Pharm., 32*, 59 (1975).

(3) L. F. Droppleman and D. M. McNair, "Screening for Anticholinergic Effects of Atropine and Chlordiazepoxide," *Psychopharmacologia, 12*, 164 (1968).

(4) F. J. Kane and T. W. Taylor, "A Toxic Reaction to Combined Elavil–Librium Therapy," *Amer. J. Psychiat., 119*, 1179 (1963).

(5) F. A. Abdou, "Elavil–Librium Combination," *Amer. J. Psychiat., 120*, 1204 (1964).

(6) M. L. Cunningham, "Acute Hepatic Necrosis following Treatment with Amitriptyline and Diazepam," *Brit. J. Psychiat., 111*, 1107 (1965).

(7) I. Haider, "A Comparative Trial of Ro 4-6270 and Amitriptyline in Depressive Illness," *Brit. J. Psychiat., 113*, 993 (1967).

(8) General Practitioner Research Group, "Chlordiazepoxide with Amitriptyline in Neurotic Depression," *Practitioner, 202*, 437 (1969).

(9) G. Silverman and R. A. Braithwaite, "Benzodiazepines and Tricyclic Antidepressant Plasma Levels," *Brit. Med. J., 3*, 18 (1973).

(10) L. F. Gram *et al.*, "Influence of Neuroleptics and Benzodiazepines on Metabolism of Tricyclic Antidepressants in Man," *Amer. J. Psychol., 131*, 863 (1974).

(11) C. R. Beber, "Treating Anxiety and Depression in the Elderly. A Double Blind Crossover Evaluation of Two Widely Used Tranquilizers," *J. Fla. Med. Ass., 58*, 35 (1971).

(12) W. L. Wingfield *et al.*, "A Double Blind, Phase I Clinical Study of Oxazepam and Protriptyline Combined," *Curr. Ther. Res.*, *15*, 97 (1973).

(13) J. Yamamoto *et al.*, "Double-Blind Drug Study in Depressed Outpatients," *Rocky Mountain Med. J.*, *69*, 71 (1971).

(14) N. S. Kline, "Psychochemotherapeutic Drug Combinations," *J. Amer. Med. Ass.*, *210*, 1928 (1969).

(15) H. P. Hare, "Comparison of Chlordiazepoxide-Amitriptyline Combination with Amitriptyline Alone in Anxiety-Depressive States," *J. Clin. Pharmacol. J. New Drugs*, *11*, 456 (1971).

(16) D. J. Greenblatt and R. I. Shader, "Benzodiazepines in Clinical Practice," Raven, New York, NY 10003, 1974, pp. 78–82.

[For additional information, see *Antidepressant Therapy*, p. 373.]

Nonproprietary and Trade Names of Drugs

Amitriptyline hydrochloride—*Elavil Hydrochloride and various combination products*
Chlordiazepoxide—*Libritabs*
Chlordiazepoxide hydrochloride — *Librium and various combination products*
Clonazepam—*Clonopin*
Clorazepate dipotassium—*Tranxene*
Desipramine hydrochloride — *Norpramin, Pertofrane*
Diazepam—*Valium*

Doxepin hydrochloride—*Adapin, Sinequan*
Flurazepam hydrochloride—*Dalmane*
Imipramine hydrochloride—*Presamine, Tofranil, Tofranil PM*
Nitrazepam—*Mogadon*
Nortriptyline hydrochloride — *Aventyl Hydrochloride*
Oxazepam—*Serax*
Protriptyline hydrochloride—*Vivactil Hydrochloride*

Prepared and evaluated by the Scientific Review Subpanel on Psychotropic Agents and reviewed by Practitioner Panel II.

Amphetamine—Furazolidone

Summary—The antibacterial action of furazolidone is accompanied by progressive and generalized inhibition of monoamine oxidase and the concurrent or subsequent administration of amphetamine could result in a hypertensive crisis. Although no clinical reports of a hypertensive crisis caused by concurrent administration of these drugs have appeared, they should not be used concurrently.

Related Drugs—**Tyramine** has also been reported to interact with furazolidone (1) and **tyramine-containing foods** (*e.g.*, broad bean pods, aged cheeses, beer, wine, pickled herring, unrefrigerated chicken livers, fermented products, and foods susceptible to artificial protein breakdown) should be avoided. Other similarly acting sympathomimetics include **cyclopentamine, dextroamphetamine, dopamine, ephedrine, metaraminol, methamphetamine, methylphenidate, phenylephrine,** and **pseudoephedrine.** The primarily direct-acting sympathomimetics such as **epinephrine, isoproterenol, levarterenol,** and **methoxamine** apparently are not affected by furazolidone (1).

Other nitrofuran drugs do not possess monoamine oxidase inhibitory activity (2).

Pharmacological Effect and Mechanism—Although it is used as an antibacterial agent, furazolidone is also an inhibitor of monoamine oxidase in animals (2) and humans (1). A cumulative effect would result in a hypertensive reaction if amphetamine is administered during prolonged (longer than 5 days) furazolidone therapy.

Amphetamine is an indirect-acting sympathomimetic amine; its hypertensive activity results from its ability to promote release of norepinephrine from adrenergic neurons. Inhibition of monoamine oxidase causes a supersensitivity to amphetamine apparently because of an increased amount of norepinephrine released at the adrenergic neuron terminals (3). Inhibition of the metabolic inactivation of amines plays only a minor role in this supersensitivity phenomenon (3).

Furazolidone does not inhibit monoamine oxidase *in vitro*, suggesting that this action is the result of a metabolite (possibly a hydrazine) (2, 4). Furthermore, the effect persists in rats where a 60–70% increase in brain norepinephrine and 5-hydroxytryptamine (serotonin) was observed from 10 days to 3 weeks after administration was discontinued.

Evaluation of Clinical Data—Furazolidone caused a dose-related inhibition of monoamine oxidase in humans (1). After this inhibition was achieved, a concomitant enhancement of the pressor response was observed following the intravenous administration of tyramine and amphetamine (dose not reported) but not following levarterenol (norepinephrine) administration. Direct confirmation of this monoamine oxidase inhibitory action of furazolidone was obtained by measurements of monoamine oxidase activity in jejunal mucosal biopsy material. The degree of monoamine oxidase inhibitory activity of furazolidone was comparable to that of the monoamine oxidase inhibitor pargyline. However, no psychic stimulation, sleep pattern disturbances, or blood pressure changes were noted in these patients receiving furazolidone (400 or 800 mg/day po).

■ Monoamine oxidase inhibition by furazolidone (administered systemically) exposes patients to the hazards of a potential hypertensive crisis if amphetamine or other amine-releasing agents are taken concurrently. Since the monoamine oxidase inhibitory action of furazolidone is cumulative, this hazard is increased by prolonged use, especially if the therapy extends beyond the recommended 5 days (1). Although no clinical reports of a hypertensive crisis caused by the concurrent administration of amphetamine and furazolidone have appeared, this reaction has been reported to occur in patients receiving amphetamine with other monoamine oxidase inhibitors (see *Phenylpropanolamine–Tranylcypromine,* p. 188).

Recommendations—Tyramine-containing foods, amphetamines, and other indirect-acting sympathomimetic agents and those sympathomimetics whose action is partly associated with the release of norepinephrine are contraindicated in patients receiving furazolidone. A drug history should be taken prior to instituting furazolidone therapy to ensure that these agents were not being taken. Patients receiving furazolidone should be warned of the potential interaction with sympathomimetic substances.

References

(1) W. A. Pettinger *et al.*, "Inhibition of Monoamine Oxidase in Man by Furazolidone," *Clin. Pharmacol. Ther., 9,* 442 (1968).

(2) D. Palm *et al.*, "Hemmung der Monoaminoxydase durch Bakteriostatisch Wirksame Nitrofuran-Derivate," *Naunyn-Schmiedebergs Arch. Pharmakol. Exp. Pathol., 256,* 281 (1967).

(3) W. A. Pettinger and J. A. Oates, "Supersensitivity to Tyramine during Monoamine Oxidase Inhibition in Man," *Clin. Pharmacol. Ther., 9,* 341 (1968).

(4) I. J. Stern *et al.*, "The Anti-Monoamine Oxidase Effects of Furazolidone," *J. Pharmacol. Exp. Ther., 156,* 492 (1967).

[For additional information, see *Adrenergic Therapy,* p. 332, and *Phenylpropanolamine– Tranylcypromine,* p. 188.]

Nonproprietary and Trade Names of Drugs

Amphetamine complex—*Biphetamine*
Amphetamine sulfate—*Benzedrine*
Cyclopentamine hydrochloride—*Clopane Hydrochloride*
Dextroamphetamine sulfate—*Dexedrine and various combination products*
Dopamine hydrochloride—*Intropin*
Ephedrine—*Various manufacturers*
Epinephrine hydrochloride—*Adrenalin Chloride*
Furazolidone—*Furoxone*
Isoproterenol hydrochloride—*Isuprel Hydrochloride*

Levarterenol bitartrate—*Levophed Bitartrate*
Metaraminol bitartrate—*Aramine*
Methamphetamine hydrochloride—*Desoxyn, Norodin Hydrochloride, Syndrox*
Methoxamine hydrochloride—*Vasoxyl*
Methylphenidate hydrochloride—*Ritalin Hydrochloride*
Phenylephrine hydrochloride—*Neo-Synephrine Hydrochloride and various combination products*
Pseudoephedrine hydrochloride—*Sudafed*
Tyramine—*Various foods and beverages*

Prepared and evaluated by the Scientific Review Subpanel on Autonomic Agents and reviewed by Practitioner Panel VI.

Ascorbic Acid—Aspirin

Summary—The administration of aspirin (>600 mg/day po) for more than 1 week results in decreased plasma and leukocyte levels of ascorbic acid. These decreased levels are just in excess of those associated with ascorbic acid deficiency. Since the clinical effects of this drug interaction have not been documented, supplemental ascorbic acid therapy is not recommended as routine therapy. Nevertheless, patients receiving large doses of aspirin who show symptoms of ascorbic acid deficiency (*e.g.,* bleeding gums, petechial tongue lesions, drowsiness, lethargy, and skin pigmentation) should be evaluated for this deficiency.

Related Drugs—The administration of **sodium salicylate** appears to result in a similar interaction with ascorbic acid (1). Therefore, the administration of other **salicylates,** either alone or in combination products, may produce a similar interaction with ascorbic acid.

Pharmacological Effect and Mechanism—Ascorbic acid is a water-soluble vitamin which must be supplied to humans at levels sufficient to prevent the development of scurvy. Maintenance of tissue saturation with ascorbic acid by supplementary administration of an adequate dose of the vitamin may be capable of producing improved tissue growth and nutrition through its anabolic effect (1), but this treatment was discarded because of insufficient evidence to justify the possible therapeutic benefit (2). It has, however, been shown that the dose of exogenous ascorbic acid adequate to maintain uniform plasma, leukocyte, and tissue levels varies under different physiological and pathological conditions (3–6). Decreased leukocyte levels of the vitamin have been demonstrated in many pathological states (3, 4). These include peptic ulceration, gastrointestinal (GI) disease, and surgery (3); cardiovascular disorders and diseases of the hemopoietic system (4); upper respiratory inflammation (7); bone and joint diseases (7–9); pressure sores and burns in the skin (4); malignant cancerous states (4, 10, 11); some mental diseases (12–18); and some iatrogenic conditions (19).

Ascorbic acid is stored in the leukocytes (20) and platelets (21). The concentration in the leukocytes provides a measure of its status in the body tissues. Changes in the plasma concentration give an indication of its transfer between the tissues and leukocytes for metabolic utilization and storage, respectively (5).

Aspirin blocks the uptake of ascorbic acid into leukocytes *in vitro* and *in vivo* (22). Simultaneously with the fall in leukocyte levels, the plasma concentration of ascorbic acid rises as the dose of aspirin is increased (23). Leukocyte absorption of ascorbic acid is almost completely inhibited by a 600-mg dose of aspirin. Concurrent administration of ascorbic acid (500–2000 mg po) does not prevent this inhibitory action of aspirin.

Leukocyte stores of ascorbic acid are depleted to levels just in excess of those associated with ascorbic acid deficiency after administration of aspirin (600 mg) for 4–7 days (22). Administration of high aspirin doses to healthy subjects significantly reduced platelet ascorbic acid levels (8). As a result, increased excretion of ascorbic acid has been observed after aspirin administration in children (24), in healthy young adults (22), and in animals (25). This increase is attributed to the increased availability of ascorbic acid in the plasma, resulting from its arrested uptake into tissue stores, and inhibition of reabsorption from the kidney tubule (22).

The mechanism responsible for the inhibition of ascorbic acid uptake into the leukocytes when aspirin is administered is not fully understood. However, it was shown that aspirin does not cause cell membrane damage (22), thus discounting the possibility of leakage of ascorbic acid out of the leukocytes.

Evaluation of Clinical Data—In one study (22), aspirin almost completely blocked the uptake of ascorbic acid into leukocytes in an unreported number of healthy subjects. The administration of aspirin (600 mg po) with ascorbic acid (500 mg po) resulted in a 200% increase of ascorbic acid in the plasma over control values after 1 hr ($p < 0.01$) whereas leukocyte levels remained virtually unchanged over the same period. When aspirin alone was continued for four doses, the 24-hr urinary excretion of ascorbic acid increased by 100% over the quantity excreted during the previous 24-hr period when no aspirin was given. When aspirin alone (2.4 g/day po) was continued for 7 days, plasma ascorbic acid levels decreased to 87% of the original level. The level of ascorbic acid in the leukocytes dropped from 48 to 10 μg/10^8 cells, slightly higher than that associated with symptoms of ascorbic acid deficiency (3). However, none of these subjects exhibited such symptoms.

Platelet ascorbic acid levels were significantly reduced in comparison to control values ($p < 0.001$) in 14 patients with rheumatoid arthritis receiving 12 or more aspirin tablets daily (dose not reported) (8). Seven of these patients were also receiving corticosteroids, which may have affected the results. Ten other patients taking less than 12 tablets/day or no aspirin at all showed significantly lower than normal plasma ascorbic acid levels but not significantly different platelet levels. There was no correlation between serum salicylate levels and platelet or plasma ascorbic acid levels.

A significantly lower mean leukocyte ascorbic acid level was found in 40 patients with GI hemorrhage who had taken either aspirin or alcohol, or both, the week prior to hospitalization (26). Leukocyte ascorbic acid levels in patients with GI hemorrhage who had taken aspirin were not significantly different than those who had taken alcohol. Administration of aspirin (300 mg/day po for 1 week) to four healthy subjects had no effect on the leukocyte ascorbic acid levels.

An increase in the urinary excretion of ascorbic acid was reported in three children, 4–6 years old, who were given two 150-mg doses of aspirin 3 days apart (24).

A study in six normal subjects showed that a low dose of aspirin (600 mg) inhibited the uptake of ascorbic acid completely in the leukocytes when ascorbic acid (500–1000 mg/day po) was given concurrently (23). Increasing the dose of ascorbic acid did not increase the leukocyte levels of ascorbic acid. None of these subjects manifested any symptoms of ascorbic acid deficiency.

■ Clinical evidence indicates that long-term (>1 week) administration of aspirin (>600 mg/day) results in decreased plasma and leukocyte levels of ascorbic acid and in increased urinary excretion of ascorbic acid. However, there is no conclusive clinical documentation that this drug interaction precipitated symptoms of ascorbic acid deficiency in any subject tested. The concurrent administration of ascorbic acid and aspirin helps raise plasma levels of ascorbic acid but may not result in significantly higher tissue body stores of the vitamin (22, 23).

Recommendations—Although supplemental administration of ascorbic acid to patients receiving aspirin (>600 mg/day po for 1 week) has been suggested (8, 22, 23), such therapy should not be given routinely. If ascorbic acid supplementation is desirable, it probably will not increase leukocyte vitamin stores but only the plasma levels (22, 23). High plasma levels of ascorbic acid without a similar increase in leukocyte stores is insufficient to relieve any symptoms due to ascorbic acid deficiency. Large doses of ascorbic acid (>2 g/day po) should be discouraged not only because most of the vitamin will be excreted in the urine (23), but also because large doses may also be harmful. Excretion of large amounts of ascorbic acid lowers the pH of the urine (27–30) and could cause a low enough urine pH to increase the tubular reabsorption of aspirin significantly and result in an increase in serum salicylate levels (31).

The most prudent course of action would be to evaluate carefully each patient who receives chronic high doses (>600 mg/day po for more than 1 week) of aspirin and exhibits ascorbic acid deficiency [e.g., bleeding gums, petechial tongue lesions, drowsiness, lethargy, and skin pigmentation (3)] or who has other conditions (e.g., bone and joint diseases) associated with decreased body tissue stores of ascorbic acid. Even if patients receive ascorbic acid supplementation, they should be monitored closely for similar symptoms, because such supplementation will not necessarily correct the aspirin-induced ascorbic acid depletion.

The effect of other anti-inflammatory agents on the tissue stores of ascorbic acid is not known. Indomethacin (dose not reported) may have decreased the leukocyte levels of ascorbic acid in two patients (8), but more clinical data are needed before an authoritative evaluation of its effects on leukocyte ascorbic acid levels can be made.

References

(1) R. S. Williams and R. E. Hughes, "Dietary Protein, Growth and Retention of Ascorbic Acid in Guinea-Pigs," *Brit. J. Nutr.*, *28*, 167 (1972).

(2) R. B. Alfin-Slater, "Fats, Essential Fatty Acids and Ascorbic Acid, Three Essential Nutrients," *J. Amer. Diet. Ass.*, *64*, 168 (1974).

(3) C. W. M. Wilson, "Vitamin C: Tissue Saturation, Metabolism and Desaturation," *Practitioner*, *212*, 481 (1974).

(4) C. W. M. Wilson, "Vitamin C: Tissue Metabolism, Over-Saturation, Desaturation and Compensation," in "Vitamin C, Recent Aspects of Its Physiological and Technological Importance," G. G. Birch and K. Parker, Eds., Applied Science Publishers, London, England, 1974, pp. 203–220.

(5) C. W. M. Wilson, "Clinical Pharmacological Aspects of Ascorbic Acid," *Ann. N.Y. Acad. Sci.* (2nd Symposium on Vitamin C), 1975, in press.

(6) C. W. M. Wilson, "Ascorbic Acid and the Common Cold," *Practitioner*, *215*, 343 (1975).

(7) C. W. M. Wilson, "Ascorbic Acid Metabolism and Functions during Colds," *Ann. N.Y. Acad. Sci.* (2nd Symposium on Vitamin C), 1975, in press.

(8) M. A. Sahud and R. J. Cohen, "Effect of Aspirin Ingestion on Ascorbic-Acid Levels in Rheumatoid Arthritis," *Lancet*, *i*, 937 (1971).

(9) A. Mullen and C. W. M. Wilson, "The Metabolism of Ascorbic Acid in Rheumatoid Arthritis," *Proc. Nutr. Soc.*, *35*, 9A (1975).

(10) S. C. Kakar et al., "Plasma and Leuco-
cyte Ascorbic Acid Concentrations in
Acute Lymphoblastic Leukemia," Irish
J. Med. Sci., 144, 227 (1975).

(11) T. K. Basu et al., "Leucocyte Ascorbic
Acid and Urinary Hydroxyproline
Levels in Patients Bearing Breast
Cancer with Skeletal Metastases,"
Eur. J. Cancer, 10, 507 (1974).

(12) G. Milner, "Ascorbic Acid in Chronic
Psychiatric Patients—A Controlled
Trial," Brit. J. Psychiat., 109, 294
(1963).

(13) H. Vanderkamp, "A Biochemical Abnormality in Schizophrenia Involving
Ascorbic Acid," Int. J. Neuropsychiat.,
2, 204 (1966).

(14) M. H. Briggs, "Possible Relations of
Ascorbic Acid, Ceruloplasmin and
Toxic Aromatic Metabolites in Schizo-
phrenia," N. Z. Med. J., 61, 229 (1962).

(15) N. Hayarbic, "Studies on Cerulo-
Plasmic Metabolism in Mental Diseases: Serum Ceruloplasmin Level in
Schizophrenics and the Relation of
Ascorbic Acid to Its Enzymatic Reactions," Vitamins (Kyoto), 16, 1
(1960).

(16) W. Salks and S. M. Simpson, "Ascorbic Acid in Levodopa Therapy,"
Lancet, i, 527 (1975).

(17) B. P. F. Adlard et al., "The Effect of
Age, Growth Retardation and As-
phyxia on Ascorbic Acid Concentrations in Developing Brain," J. Neurochem., 21, 877 (1973).

(18) E. Cameron and L. Pauling, "Ascorbic
Acid and the Glycosaminoglycans. An
Orthomolecular Approach to Cancer
and Other Diseases," Oncology, 27, 181
(1973).

(19) C. W. M. Wilson, "Vitamins and
Drug Metabolism with Particular
Reference to Vitamin C," Proc. Nutr.
Soc., 33, 231 (1974).

(20) H. S. Loh and C. W. M. Wilson,
"Relationship between Leukocyte and
Plasma Ascorbic Acid Concentra-
tions," Brit. Med. J., 3, 733 (1971).

(21) J. V. Lloyd et al., "Platelet Ascorbic
Acid Levels in Normal Subjects and
in Disease," J. Clin. Pathol., 25, 478
(1972).

(22) H. S. Loh et al., "The Effects of
Aspirin on the Metabolic Availability
of Ascorbic Acid in Human Beings," J.
Clin. Pharmacol., 13, 480 (1973).

(23) H. S. Loh and C. W. M. Wilson, "The
Interactions of Aspirin and Ascorbic
Acid in Normal Men," J. Clin. Phar-
macol., 15, 36 (1975).

(24) A. L. Daniels and G. J. Everson,
"Influence of Acetylsalicylic Acid
(Aspirin) on Urinary Excretion of
Ascorbic Acid," Proc. Soc. Exp. Biol.
Med., 35, 20 (1936).

(25) "Vitamin C Excretion," J. Pharmacol.
Exp. Ther., 68, 465 (1940).

(26) R. I. Russel et al., "Ascorbic-Acid
Levels in Leucocytes of Patients with
Gastrointestinal Haemorrhage," Lan-
cet, ii, 603 (1968).

(27) L. B. Travis et al., "Urinary Acidification with Ascorbic Acid," J. Pediat., 67,
1176 (1965).

(28) D. F. McDonald et al., "Bacteriostatic
and Acidifying Effects of Methionine,
Hydrolyzed Casein and Ascorbic Acid
on the Urine," N. Engl. J. Med., 261,
803 (1959).

(29) F. J. Murphy and S. Zelman, "Ascorbic Acid as a Urinary Acidifying
Agent. 1. Comparison with Ketogenic
Effect of Fasting," J. Urol., 94, 297
(1965).

(30) F. J. Murphy et al., "Ascorbic Acid as
a Urinary Acidifying Agent. 2. Its
Adjunctive Role in Chronic Urinary
Infection," J. Urol., 94, 300 (1965).

(31) G. Levy and J. R. Leonards, "Urine
pH and Salicylate Therapy," J. Amer.
Med. Ass., 217, 81 (1971).

[For additional information, see *Analgesic Therapy (Nonnarcotic)*, p. 341, and *Vitamin Therapy*, p. 449.]

Nonproprietary and Trade Names of Drugs

Aluminum aspirin—*Available in combination products*
Ascorbic acid — *Various manufacturers,
available alone or in combination products*
Aspirin—*Available alone or as a fixed combination in many trade name products,
especially over-the-counter preparations*
Calcium carbaspirin—*Calurin*
Carbethyl salicylate—*Sal-Ethyl Carbonate*

Choline salicylate—*Actasal, Arthropan*
Indomethacin—*Indocin*
Magnesium salicylate—*Various manufac-
turers*
Potassium salicylate—*Various manufac-
turers*
Salicylamide—*Various manufacturers*
Sodium salicylate—*Various manufacturers*

*Prepared and evaluated by the Scientific Review Sub-
panel on Vitamins and reviewed by Practitioner Panel VI.*

Aspirin—Alcohol

Summary—Concurrent ingestion of aspirin and alcohol may enhance occult blood loss and gastric damage induced by aspirin. Aspirin and alcohol, either alone or together, should be avoided by patients with a history of gastrointestinal (GI) bleeding. There is no evidence that concurrent use of aspirin and alcohol is more harmful than either drug alone in patients without GI problems, but the potential toxicity of either agent suggests that concurrent use be avoided whenever possible.

Related Drugs—Most forms of **salicylates** may interact with alcohol, although buffered preparations may be exceptions (1).

Pharmacological Effect and Mechanism—Aspirin depresses gastric acid secretion and mucus production by the gastric mucosa in humans and breaks the gastric mucosal barrier to hydrogen and other ions by acting locally on the human mucosa (2). Alcohol increases acid secretion in animals by direct effects on the mucosa and perhaps by systemic mechanisms. Alcohol (350 ml) in concentrations up to 6% (equivalent to 42 ml of 100-proof whiskey) did not stimulate acid secretion in humans (3). Aspirin (650–1300 mg) caused a 50% decrease in gastric potential difference (a test parameter used to measure damage to the gastric mucosa) in 3 min following ingestion (2). In a similar period, 25 and 50 ml of alcohol (80-proof bourbon) decreased the gastric potential by 30 and 50%, respectively (2).

It has been reported that 70% of healthy subjects lose from 0.2 to 13.5 ml of blood per day following the daily ingestion of 2–3 g of unbuffered aspirin (4). The site of blood loss is the stomach.

Solid dosage forms of aspirin with alkaline buffers exert a local effect around the dosage form to yield aspirin in its ionized form (pKa of aspirin is 3.5; at pH 3.5, 50% would be unionized and therefore absorbable). Aspirin in the ionized form is virtually unabsorbed by the stomach and does not damage the gastric mucosa (5). Alcohol reportedly causes acute superficial gastritis, but the gastric mucosa reverts to normal within 7–20 days. Whether or not changes of acute superficial gastritis lead to chronic gastritis is doubtful in nonalcoholics. Although the gastritis may subside if alcohol ingestion ceases, it is more often likely to progress to severe atrophic gastritis with continuing ingestion of large amounts of alcohol (6).

Evaluation of Clinical Data—Fecal blood loss was determined in 13 healthy adults after administration of unbuffered aspirin alone and with alcohol (7). In seven other adults, only alcohol was given. The total dose of aspirin was 2.1 g (administered in divided doses) and the quantity of alcohol was 180 ml (31.8% w/v). In each of the 13 subjects, the mean daily fecal blood loss was 3.2 ml after aspirin ingestion (normal daily blood loss, 0.4 ml). The addition of alcohol to this aspirin regimen increased the mean daily fecal blood loss to 5.3 ml. There was only a 0.2 ml/day increase in fecal blood loss in the seven patients receiving alcohol alone. The clinical significance of the increased blood loss was not determined.

Twenty-two healthy adults received a buffered aspirin product (containing aspirin sodium, 728 mg) with or without 142 ml of 40% alcohol (1). When compared to placebo administration, no significant change in fecal blood loss was found when buffered aspirin was given concurrently with alcohol.

An epidemiological study evaluated 817 patients who had been admitted to the hospital with an admission diagnosis of GI hemorrhage (8). Each patient was questioned soon after admission about the use of aspirin and alcohol with particular reference to the 72 hr before the diagnosis of bleeding. A control series of 300 patients was questioned similarly about aspirin intake and 113 of these patients were questioned about alcohol intake. A statistical comparison of the tested group with the control group showed a possible relationship between aspirin intake and bleeding. No such relationship was established with alcohol. The concurrent use of aspirin and alcohol showed a high correlation with bleeding.

Six healthy volunteers were given unbuffered aspirin alone in doses of 300 or 600 mg (9). Additionally, 100 ml of 15% alcohol was given separately with or without 600 mg of unbuffered aspirin. Buffered aspirin (containing aspirin sodium, 728 mg) also was administered, but on a different time schedule. The gastric potential difference was determined in each patient. Unbuffered aspirin caused a rapid and significant fall in the gastric potential difference that was greater with the 600-mg dose than with the 300-mg dose. Alcohol also caused a rapid and statistically significant fall in the gastric potential difference and when administered with aspirin (600 mg) the effects were additive. This decrease in the gastric potential difference indicates that the gastric mucosal barrier was broken and that gastric damage may occur. Buffered aspirin sodium did not reduce the gastric potential difference but actually increased it.

■ There is ample evidence that the ingestion of moderate amounts of alcohol can aggravate aspirin-induced fecal blood loss. Alcohol ingested alone (especially in amounts of 30–60 ml) does not seem to cause this effect. The toxic significance of this increased fecal blood loss has not been established definitely. One study noted an additive association between GI bleeding and concurrent ingestion of aspirin and alcohol (7), but this was a poorly controlled epidemiological study that did not adequately exclude other causative factors. This effect appears to be related to the dose of aspirin given and may only apply to unbuffered aspirin (7–9).

Recommendations—It seems prudent to avoid all aspirin products in patients with GI disorders (10) where there is a possibility of GI bleeding. If aspirin is to be given, low doses and the buffered form should be used if possible. Acetaminophen does not cause GI bleeding (11) and may be a useful alternative to aspirin for analgesia and antipyresis. Alcohol, particularly in large amounts, should be avoided.

Although there is no evidence that concurrent use of aspirin and alcohol in patients without GI problems is any more harmful than the use of either drug alone, the potential toxicity of either agent indicates that concurrent use should be avoided whenever possible. There appears to be some association between high doses of aspirin (2–3 g/day) and induction of severe GI bleeding, but the occurrence of this effect is rare (12).

References

(1) I. A. D. Bouchier and H. S. Williams, "Determination of Faecal Blood-Loss after Combined Alcohol and Sodium-Acetylsalicylate Intake," *Lancet, i*, 178 (1969).

(2) M. G. Geall *et al.*, "Profile of Gastric Potential Difference in Man. Effects of Aspirin, Alcohol, Bile and Endogenous Acid," *Gastroenterology, 58*, 437 (1970).

(3) A. R. Cooke and A. Birchall, "Absorption of Ethanol from the Stomach," *Gastroenterology, 57*, 269 (1969).

(4) K. K. Matsumoto and M. I. Grossman, "Quantitative Measurement of Gastrointestinal Blood Loss during Ingestion of Aspirin," *Proc. Soc. Exp. Biol. Med., 102*, 517 (1959).

(5) J. R. Leonards and G. Levy, "Biopharmaceutical Aspects of Aspirin-Induced Gastrointestinal Blood Loss in Man," *J. Pharm. Sci., 58*, 1277 (1969).

(6) A. R. Cooke, "Aspirin, Ethanol and the Stomach," *Australas. Ann. Med., 19*, 269 (1970).

(7) K. Goulston and A. R. Cooke, "Alcohol, Aspirin and Gastrointestinal Bleeding," *Brit. Med. J., 4*, 664 (1968).

(8) C. D. Needham *et al.*, "Aspirin and Alcohol in Gastrointestinal Hemorrhage," *Gut, 12*, 819 (1971).

(9) H. S. Murray *et al.*, "Effect of Several Drugs on Gastric Potential Difference in Man," *Brit. Med. J., 1*, 19 (1974).

(10) F. J. Inglefinger, "The Side Effects of Aspirin," *N. Engl. J. Med., 290*, 1196 (1974).

(11) "Side Effects of Drugs," L. Meyler and A. Herxheimer, Eds., Excerpta Medica Foundation, Amsterdam, The Netherlands, 1972, p. 158.

(12) M. Levy, "Aspirin Use in Patients with Major Upper Gastrointestinal Bleeding and Peptic-Ulcer Disease," *N. Engl. J. Med.*, *290*, 1158 (1974).

[For additional information, see *Analgesic Therapy (Nonnarcotic)*, p. 341.]

Nonproprietary and Trade Names of Drugs

Acetaminophen—*Datril, Nebs, SK-APAP, Tempra, Tenlap, Tylenol, Valadol, and various combination products*
Aluminum aspirin—*Available in combination products*
Alcohol—*Various products and beverages*
Aspirin—*Available alone or as a fixed combination in many trade name products, especially over-the-counter preparations*

Calcium carbaspirin—*Calurin*
Carbethyl salicylate—*Sal-Ethyl Carbonate*
Choline salicylate—*Actasal, Arthropan*
Magnesium salicylate—*Various manufacturers*
Potassium salicylate—*Various manufacturers*
Salicylamide—*Various manufacturers*
Sodium salicylate—*Various manufacturers*

Prepared and evaluated by the Scientific Review Subpanel on Analgesics and reviewed by Practitioner Panel I.

Aspirin—Hydrocortisone

Summary—Hydrocortisone may increase the renal excretion of aspirin and result in decreased salicylate levels during concurrent therapy, but the clinical significance of this interaction has not been established. A corresponding increase in serum salicylate levels may occur when hydrocortisone therapy is discontinued. Aspirin and hydrocortisone may theoretically exert combined deleterious effects on the gastric mucosa, but there are no reports of this combined effect occurring in clinical practice. Concurrent administration of aspirin and hydrocortisone need not be avoided, but patients receiving both drugs should be observed closely for adverse effects from either agent, especially when one drug is discontinued.

Related Drugs—Because of insufficient clinical data, the effects of the concurrent use of other **corticosteroids** and other **salicylates** in humans cannot be assessed. Until more data are available, these related drugs should be used together with caution.

Pharmacological Effect and Mechanism—Aspirin enhanced (1) or antagonized (2) the anti-inflammatory effects of hydrocortisone in rats. The different results may be due to the experimental designs used. This effect has not been reported in humans.

Aspirin, in doses 10 times greater than the therapeutic dose used in humans, displaced endogenous corticosteroids from plasma proteins of rats (3, 4), but it had minimal or no effect on the binding of hydrocortisone to plasma proteins in humans in normal and large doses (5, 6). Reduction in the hydrocortisone dose caused an increase in the serum salicylate levels in a small groups of humans (7); the increase was attributed to the reversal of the hydrocortisone-induced increased salicylate clearance.

The potential of aspirin to cause gastric ulceration has been attributed to an increased exfoliation of gastric surface cells without an accompanying increase in renewal rate (8). Aspirin may also disrupt the mucosal barrier, making the mucosa abnormally permeable to water-soluble compounds and ions (9). The disruption of the mucosal barrier has also been observed following parenteral aspirin (10).

Animal studies reporting the effects of adrenal corticoids on gastric mucosa suggest that steroids are capable of causing ulcers as well as aggravating preexisting ulcers (11). The effects of steroids on canine mucosa include decreased mucus formation (12), a decrease in renewal of surface epithelial cells (8), and an augmented secretory response to histamine (13).

Animal studies showed that adrenocorticotropic hormone (ACTH) (12), aspirin (9, 10), or corticosteroids (13) may damage the gastric mucosa. It has not been established if these agents alone or together cause gastric ulceration in humans.

Evaluation of Clinical Data—One study (5) showed that the concentrations of salicylate required to displace corticosteroids from plasma proteins in humans were much higher than the usual therapeutic concentrations of aspirin. Although the dosage of aspirin is sometimes quite high, elevated serum levels of unbound corticosteroids have not been associated with any clinical toxicity (14).

Four cases of increased serum salicylate levels were described after reduction of the corticosteroid dose (7). In one case, the serum salicylate level of a 5-year-old male rose to 88 mg% resulting in salicylate intoxication. The renal clearance of salicylate also was studied in three normal and two polyarthritic subjects during concurrent administration of hydrocortisone (240 mg/day po for 3 days) (7). Reversal of the hydrocortisone-induced increased salicylate clearance was suggested as the reason for the elevated serum salicylate levels.

The combined effects of aspirin and hydrocortisone on the gastric mucosa have not been studied in humans, but each agent has the potential to aggravate existing ulcers (11).

■ Interactions between aspirin and hydrocortisone involving displacement of hydrocortisone from protein binding sites or involving alteration of renal excretion rates of hydrocortisone have not been studied sufficiently. Hydrocortisone may increase the renal clearance of salicylate; and, when hydrocortisone is discontinued, serum salicylate levels may rise significantly. Since there is only a single report of salicylate toxicity, the clinical significance of this interaction remains in question.

Aspirin and hydrocortisone also may interact through combined effects on gastric mucosa, but the clinical significance of this drug interaction has yet to be evaluated.

Recommendations—Concurrent administration of aspirin and hydrocortisone does not appear to be contraindicated. However, these agents should be used concurrently with caution, and patients should be observed closely for adverse effects from either agent during therapy and especially when one agent is discontinued. It also may be necessary to reduce the salicylate dosage when steroid therapy is discontinued.

References

(1) K. F. Swingle *et al.*, "Interactions of Anti-Inflammatory Drugs in Carrageenan-Induced Foot Edema of the Rat," *J. Pharmacol. Exp. Ther., 172,* 423 (1970).

(2) C. G. Van Arman *et al.*, "Interactions of Aspirin, Indomethacin, and Other Drugs in Adjuvant-Induced Arthritis in the Rat," *J. Pharmacol. Exp. Ther., 187,* 400 (1973).

(3) R. P. Maickel *et al.*, "Interaction of Non-Steroidal Antiinflammatory Agents with Corticosterone Binding to Plasma Proteins in the Rat," *Arzneim.-Forsch., 19,* 1803 (1969).

(4) B. B. Brodie, "Displacement of One Drug by Another from Carrier or Receptor Sites," *Proc. Roy. Soc. Med., 58,* 946 (1965).

(5) J. B. Stenlake *et al.*, "The Effect of Acetylsalicylic Acid, Phenylbutazone and Indomethacin on the Binding of 11-Hydroxysteroids to Plasma Proteins in Patients with Rheumatoid Arthritis," *J. Pharm. Pharmacol., 20,* suppl., 248S (1968).

(6) J. B. Stenlake *et al.*, "The Effect of Anti-inflammatory Drugs on the Protein-Binding of 11-Hydroxysteroids in Human Plasma *In Vitro*," *J. Pharm. Pharmacol.*, *28*, 451 (1969).

(7) J. R. Klinenberg and F. Miller, "Effect of Corticosteroids on Blood Salicylate Concentration," *J. Amer. Med. Ass.*, *194*, 601 (1965).

(8) M. Max and R. Menguy, "Influence of Adrenocorticotropin, Cortisone, Aspirin, and Phenylbutazone on the Rate of Exfoliation and the Rate of Renewal of Gastric Mucosal Cells," *Gastroenterology*, *58*, 329 (1970).

(9) H. W. Davenport, "Salicylate Damage to the Gastric Mucosal Barrier," *N. Engl. J. Med.*, *276*, 1307 (1967).

(10) B. F. Overholt *et al.*, "Effect of the Vagus Nerve and Salicylate Administration on the Permeability Characteristics of the Rat Gastric Mucosal Barrier," *Gastroenterology*, *56*, 651 (1969).

(11) D. C. H. Sun, "Iatrogenic Gastrointestinal Diseases in the Aged," *Geriatrics*, *27* (3), 89 (1972).

(12) L. Desbaillets and R. Menguy, "Inhibition of Gastric Mucous Secretion by ACTH. An Experimental Study," *Amer. J. Dig. Dis.*, *12*, 582 (1967).

(13) E. D. Jacobson and W. E. Price, "Effect of Hydrocortisone on Gastric Mucosal Blood Flow and Secretion," *Gastroenterology*, *57*, 36 (1969).

(14) H. C. Elliott, "Reduced Adrenocortical Steroid Excretion Rates in Man following Aspirin Administration," *Metabolism*, *11*, 1015 (1962).

[For additional information, see *Analgesic Therapy (Nonnarcotic)*, p. 341.]

Nonproprietary and Trade Names of Drugs

Aluminum aspirin—*Various combination products*
Aspirin—*Available alone or as a fixed combination in many trade name products, especially over-the-counter preparations*
Betamethasone—*Celestone*
Calcium carbaspirin—*Calurin*
Carbethyl salicylate—*Sal-Ethyl Carbonate*
Choline salicylate—*Actasal, Arthropan*
Cortisone acetate—*Cortone Acetate*
Dexamethasone—*Decadron, Hexadrol*
Fludrocortisone acetate—*Florinef Acetate*
Fluprednisolone—*Alphadrol*
Hydrocortisone—*Various manufacturers*

Magnesium salicylate—*Various manufacturers*
Meprednisone—*Betapar*
Methylprednisolone—*Medrol*
Paramethasone acetate—*Haldrone*
Potassium salicylate—*Various manufacturers*
Prednisolone—*Delta-Cortef, Meticortelone, Sterane*
Prednisone—*Delta-dome, Deltasone, Deltra, Meticorten, Paracort*
Salicylamide—*Various manufacturers*
Sodium salicylate—*Various manufacturers*
Triamcinolone—*Aristocort, Kenacort*

Prepared and evaluated by the Scientific Review Subpanel on Analgesics and reviewed by Practitioner Panel III.

Chloral Hydrate—Alcohol

Summary—Concurrent ingestion of chloral hydrate and alcohol results in a greater central nervous system (CNS) depression than when either agent is taken alone, but there is no scientific evidence to support the idea that concurrent use has a particularly potent hypnotic action ("knock-out drops" or "Mickey Finn"). Occasionally, subjects receiving chloral hydrate may develop a vasodilation reaction after they ingest alcohol. All patients should be warned of possible enhanced CNS effects or of profound vasodilation occurring after concurrent ingestion of these agents.

Related Drugs—**Chloral betaine, triclofos,** and other products metabolized to yield trichloroethanol will interact with alcohol.

Pharmacological Effect and Mechanism—The concurrent ingestion of chloral hydrate and alcohol causes two clinically important interactions. One is an alleged marked enhancement of the CNS depressant effects of chloral hydrate and alcohol (1, 2); the other is a profound vasodilation (3).

The CNS depressant effects might be explained on the basis of altered production of centrally active metabolites. Chloral hydrate has a direct sedative effect but is converted rapidly by alcohol dehydrogenase to trichloroethanol which is responsible for the sustained hypnotic effect (4). Chloral hydrate is also converted to the hypnotically inactive trichloroacetic acid by aldehyde dehydrogenase. Alcohol is converted to acetaldehyde by liver alcohol dehydrogenase and subsequently to acetate by aldehyde dehydrogenase (5).

After concurrent ingestion, the metabolism of both chloral hydrate and alcohol is reduced (5). Blood alcohol levels are higher and more prolonged because the rate of alcohol oxidation is decreased by trichloroethanol's competitive inhibition of alcohol dehydrogenase (5). Since less alcohol is oxidized, blood acetaldehyde levels decrease. In contrast, serum trichloroethanol levels increase because alcohol induces the reduction of chloral hydrate to trichloroethanol. Clinically, these changes in blood levels of centrally active drugs or their active metabolites result in a greater CNS effect than after either agent alone (6).

The vasodilation interaction occurs infrequently in subjects who have received chloral hydrate (1 g) for more than 7 days and then ingest alcohol. They may experience a profound vasodilation reaction characterized by tachycardia, palpitations, facial flushing, and dysphoria (7). Although the symptoms are clinically indistinguishable from the alcohol–disulfiram reaction, they are not related to the increased acetaldehyde levels caused by concurrent ingestion of alcohol and disulfiram (3, 5, 8).

Evaluation of Clinical Data—In five human volunteers, the effects of concurrent ingestion of chloral hydrate (15 mg/kg or approximately 1 g) and alcohol (0.5 g/kg or approximately 70 ml of 100-proof whiskey) were studied. Small changes occurred in both chloral hydrate and alcohol metabolism after concurrent ingestion (3, 5). Concurrent ingestion produced a significantly greater impairment of the subjects' ability to perform complex motor tasks than ingestion of either drug alone.

One of these reports also detailed the consistent physiological changes that produced the vasodilation reaction associated with alcohol ingestion during chronic chloral hydrate usage (3). A few subjects became profoundly hypotensive with marked tachycardia.

■ There is no evidence for the mythical "knock-out drop" effect from the concurrent ingestion of chloral hydrate–alcohol when using typical dosages. Nevertheless, subjects ingesting both agents concurrently perform significantly worse on a complex motor task and an auditory vigilance test than after ingestion of either agent alone (3). Some patients also experience profound vasodilation after ingesting these drugs concurrently (3).

Recommendations—All patients taking chloral hydrate should be warned that the effects of both chloral hydrate and alcohol are increased by concurrent ingestion. In view of the changes in heart rate and blood pressure caused by the vasodilation that may occur with concurrent use of these agents, patients with cardiac disease should avoid alcohol if they receive chloral hydrate chronically.

References

(1) W. L. Adams, "The Comparative Toxicity of Chloral Alcoholate and Chloral Hydrate," *J. Pharmacol. Exp. Ther.*, *78*, 340 (1943).
(2) P. K. Gessner and B. E. Cabana,

"Chloral Alcoholate: Reevaluation of Its Role in the Interaction between Hypnotic Effects of Chloral Hydrate and Ethanol," *J. Pharmacol. Exp. Ther.*, *156*, 602 (1967).

(3) E. M. Sellers *et al.*, "Interaction of Chloral Hydrate and Ethanol in Man. II. Hemodynamics and Performance," *Clin. Pharmacol. Ther.*, *13*, 50 (1972).

(4) A. H. Owens *et al.*, "A Comparative Evaluation of the Hypnotic Potency of Chloral Hydrate and Trichloroethanol," *Bull. Johns Hopkins Hosp.*, *96*, 71 (1955).

(5) E. M. Sellers *et al.*, "Interaction of Chloral Hydrate and Ethanol in Man. I. Metabolism," *Clin. Pharmacol. Ther.*, *13*, 37 (1972).

(6) H. L. Kaplan *et al.*, "Chloral Hydrate and Alcohol Metabolism in Human Subjects," *J. Forensic Sci.*, *12*, 295 (1967).

(7) Z. Bardodej, "Intolerance Alkoholu po Chloralhydratu," *Cesk. Farm.*, *14*, 478 (1965).

(8) E. Asmussen *et al.*, "The Pharmacological Action of Acetaldehyde on the Human Organism," *Acta Pharmacol. Toxicol.*, *4*, 311 (1948).

[For additional information, see *Sedative–Hypnotic Therapy*, p. 442.]

Nonproprietary and Trade Names of Drugs

Alcohol—*Various products and beverages*
Chloral betaine—*Beta-Chlor*

Chloral hydrate—*Kessodrate, Noctec, Somnos*
Triclofos sodium—*Triclos*

Prepared and evaluated by the Scientific Review Subpanel on Sedative–Hypnotics and reviewed by Practitioner Panel IV.

———————————

Chloral Hydrate—Furazolidone

Summary—In addition to its antimicrobial action, furazolidone can inhibit monoamine oxidase and probably other enzymes. Therefore, it may theoretically inhibit the metabolism of chloral hydrate and enhance its central nervous system (CNS) depressant effects. However, since there are no reported clinical manifestations of this inhibition with concurrent use of chloral hydrate, there appears to be little need to exercise additional precautions whenever these drugs are given together.

Related Drugs—Other monoamine oxidase inhibitors are **isocarboxazid, pargyline, phenelzine,** and **tranylcypromine.**

Pharmacological Effect and Mechanism—Furazolidone is a synthetic antimicrobial nitrofuran with a broad antibacterial spectrum covering the majority of gastrointestinal tract pathogens (1). In addition to antibacterial activity, furazolidone also has monoamine oxidase-inhibiting activity when it is administered for more than 4–5 days (2). Because furazolidone itself does not inhibit monoamine oxidase *in vitro*, the monoamine oxidase inhibition observed after the oral administration of furazolidone to rats may result from a metabolite of furazolidone (3). The enzyme inhibition observed with furazolidone is also cumulative as a function of the total dose (4).

The monoamine oxidase inhibitors also inhibit many liver enzymes responsible for drug metabolism (5). Therefore, since chloral hydrate is normally metabolized by the liver enzyme systems, it could show exaggerated effects in the presence of monoamine oxidase inhibitors, primarily CNS depression (1).

Evaluation of Clinical Data—There are no specific reports of prolonged or enhanced CNS depression following administration of chloral hydrate in the presence of furazolidone.

■ Since the drug interaction between chloral hydrate and furazolidone is based on theoretical considerations and has not been documented in humans, the clinical significance of the drug interaction has not been established.

Recommendations—There appears to be little need to exercise additional precautions when chloral hydrate and furazolidone are given concurrently.

References

(1) "The Pharmacological Basis of Thera- peutics," 5th ed., L. S. Goodman and A. Gilman, Eds., Macmillan, New York, NY 10022, 1975, pp. 128, 1100.
(2) W. A. Pettinger *et al.*, "Monoamine-Oxidase Inhibition by Furazolidone in Man," *Clin. Res., 14,* 258 (1966).
(3) I. J. Stern *et al.*, "The Anti-Monoamine Oxidase Effects of Furazolidone," *J. Pharmacol. Exp. Ther., 156,* 492 (1967).

(4) W. A. Pettinger *et al.*, "Inhibition of Monoamine Oxidase in Man by Fura-zolidone," *Clin. Pharmacol. Ther., 9,* 442 (1968).
(5) M. M. Ghoneim, "Drug Interaction in Anaesthesia, A Review," *Can. Anaesth. Soc. J., 18,* 353 (1971).

[For additional information, see *Sedative–Hypnotic Therapy*, p. 442.]

Nonproprietary and Trade Names of Drugs

Chloral hydrate—*Kessodrate, Noctec, Som-nos*
Furazolidone—*Furoxone*
Isocarboxazid—*Marplan*

Pargyline hydrochloride—*Eutonyl and various combination products*
Phenelzine sulfate—*Nardil*
Tranylcypromine—*Parnate*

Prepared and evaluated by the Scientific Review Subpanel on Sedative–Hypnotics and reviewed by Practitioner Panel V.

Chlorcyclizine—Phenobarbital

Summary—Concurrent administration of chlorcyclizine and phenobarbital may enhance the central nervous system (CNS) depression caused by either drug. Although there is no clinical documentation that this enhanced effect occurs, patients should be cautioned that concurrent use of these drugs may cause drowsiness and could impair their ability to drive an automobile or endanger their safety in operating hazardous machinery.

Related Drugs—**Hexobarbital** (1), **pentobarbital** (2), and **thiopental** (3) are known to interact with antihistamines in the same manner as phenobarbital. Although undocu-mented, most **antihistamines** are thought to interact in a similar manner with **barbitu-rates. Phenindamine,** an antihistamine that reportedly does not cause CNS depression (4), could probably be excluded from this group.

Pharmacological Effect and Mechanism—Antihistamines act as pharmacological antagonists of histamine at most of the histamine receptor sites, although not by preventing the release of histamine (5). The hepatic microsomal enzyme-inducing properties of chlorcyclizine are well established in animals and have shortened the duration of action of some barbiturates as a result of enzyme induction (1, 6, 7).

Barbiturates act as general depressants of a wide range of biological functions. The CNS is particularly sensitive to their depressant activity, although it is not certain if their hypnotic effects are due to cellular or synaptic action (5). The barbiturates are one of the more potent classes of hepatic microsomal enzyme-inducing agents (3).

Although chlorcyclizine and diphenhydramine stimulate microsomal enzyme production in animals (2), the potential for enzyme induction causing increased metabolism of either drug is not believed to be of major clinical importance, particularly with regard to acute administration (8). Increased CNS depression is probably the predominant effect when these agents are administered concurrently.

Evaluation of Clinical Data—There are no clinical data on the interaction between chlorcyclizine and phenobarbital. The depressant effects of either agent are well documented (5, 8), and the increased depression produced by their concurrent use is the primary effect of their interaction.

■ Although clinical documentation is lacking, increased CNS depressant effects theoretically may occur when antihistamines and barbiturates are administered concurrently. An enzyme induction effect also has been demonstrated in animals, but this effect does not appear to be significant and has not been demonstrated in humans (8).

Recommendations—Patients receiving an antihistamine and a barbiturate concurrently should be cautioned about the possibility of drowsiness interfering with such activities as driving an automobile and operating hazardous machinery. The patient also should be reminded that antihistamines are present in certain nonprescription medications and that enhanced CNS depression may occur when these products are used concurrently with barbiturates.

Overdosage with antihistamines may cause convulsions in children, requiring treatment with a short-acting barbiturate or a benzodiazepine. In such cases, the smallest dose of barbiturate necessary to control the convulsions should be used, since the convulsions may superficially mask the additive depressant effects of the antihistamine and barbiturate (5).

References

(1) A. H. Conney et al., "Stimulatory Effect of Chlorcyclizine on Barbiturate Metabolism," *J. Pharmacol. Exp. Ther.*, *132*, 202 (1961).

(2) J. J. Burns et al., "Stimulatory Effects of Chronic Drug Administration on Drug-Metabolizing Enzymes in Liver Microsomes," *Ann. N.Y. Acad. Sci.*, *104*, 881 (1963).

(3) A. H. Conney, "Pharmacological Implications of Microsomal Enzyme Induction," *Pharmacol. Rev.*, *19*, 317 (1967).

(4) D. R. Mahan, "A Nasal Decongestant Unlikely to Cause Drowsiness," *Clin. Med.*, *79*, 28 (1972).

(5) "The Pharmacological Basis of Therapeutics," 5th ed., L. S. Goodman and A. Gilman, Eds., Macmillan, New York, NY 10022, 1975, pp. 102–123, 590–629.

(6) A. H. Conney and A. Klutch, "Increased Activity of Androgen Hydroxylases in Liver Microsomes of Rats Pretreated with Phenobarbital and Other Drugs," *J. Biol. Chem.*, *238*, 1611 (1963).

(7) A. H. Conney et al., "Drug Induced Changes in Steroid Metabolism," *Ann. N.Y. Acad. Sci.*, *123*, 98 (1965).

(8) "Histamines and Antihistamines," M. Schachter, Ed., International Encyclopedia of Pharmacology and Therapeutics, Pergamon Press, Oxford, England, 1973, p. 159.

[For additional information, see *Antihistamine Therapy*, p. 377.]

Nonproprietary and Trade Names of Drugs

Allobarbital—*Diadol*

Amobarbital—*Amytal and various combination products*

Aprobarbital—*Alurate*

Barbital—*Neurondia*

Brompheniramine maleate—*Dimetane and various combination products*

Butabarbital sodium—*Butisol Sodium*

Butalbital—*Available in various combination products*

Chlorcyclizine hydrochloride—*Available in various combination products*

Chlorpheniramine maleate—*Chlor-Trimeton Maleate, Teldrin, and various combination products*

Cyclizine hydrochloride—*Marezine Hydrochloride*

Dexbrompheniramine maleate—*Disomer and various combination products*

Dexchlorpheniramine maleate—*Polaramine*

Dimenhydrinate—*Dramamine*

Diphenhydramine hydrochloride—*Benadryl*

Hexobarbital—*Sombulex*

Mephobarbital—*Mebaral, Mebroin*

Methapyrilene hydrochloride—*Histadyl*

Metharbital—*Gemonil*

Methohexital sodium—*Brevital Sodium*

Pentobarbital—*Nembutal and various combination products*

Phenindamine tartrate—*Thephorin*

Phenobarbital—*Eskabarb, Luminal*

Promethazine hydrochloride—*Phenergan, Remsed*

Pyrilamine maleate—*Various manufacturers*

Secobarbital—*Seconal and various combination products*

Talbutal—*Lotusate*

Thiopental sodium—*Pentothal Sodium*

Tripelennamine hydrochloride—*Pyribenzamine Hydrochloride*

Prepared and evaluated by the Scientific Review Subpanel on Antihistamines and reviewed by Practitioner Panel VI.

Chlorpromazine—Aluminum and Magnesium Ions

Summary—Chlorpromazine absorption from the gastrointestinal (GI) tract may be altered by the simultaneous oral administration of gel-type antacids containing aluminum and magnesium ions, and this alteration results in decreased serum levels of the psychotropic drug. The drug interaction may have contributed to the decreased clinical effectiveness of chlorpromazine in one patient, but there are no other reports corroborating this effect. Simultaneous administration of these drugs should be avoided, and patients should receive the antacid at least 1 hr before or 2 hr after chlorpromazine administration.

Related Drugs—Although there is no literature documentation, all other **phenothiazines** theoretically can be expected to behave similarly. Since the interaction with chlorpromazine has been reported to occur with an aluminum hydroxide gel and **magnesium trisilicate** combination product and an aluminum hydroxide gel and **magnesium hydroxide** preparation, it can be expected that all similar gel-type antacids, such as those containing **aluminum phosphate** gel, may interact in a similar manner with chlorpromazine.

Chelation of promazine by magnesium ions has occurred *in vitro* (1). Therefore, all products containing magnesium ion (*e.g.*, **milk of magnesia**) could possibly interact with phenothiazine compounds in a similar manner.

Pharmacological Effect and Mechanism—The oral administration of gel-type antacids containing aluminum and magnesium ions decreases the GI absorption (2, 3) and lowers the serum levels (3) of chlorpromazine in humans. The urinary chlorpromazine excretion rate also was decreased by 10–45% when chlorpromazine was administered simultaneously with a gel-type antacid (3). Brain homogenates from rats given ^{14}C-labeled chlorpromazine orally with and without a gel-type antacid showed lower levels of the unchanged drug after receiving an antacid as compared to those that were not given a gel-type antacid (2).

Although the exact mechanism of this interaction is not known, it has been shown *in vitro* that chlorpromazine becomes highly bound to gel-type antacids at ratios of 50:1 and lower in 0.1 N HCl. This binding suggests that the gel-type antacid acts as a physical adsorbent of simultaneously administered chlorpromazine and decreases its absorption (4).

Aluminum- and magnesium-containing antacids increase urine pH in humans (5) and could theoretically affect the urinary excretion of chlorpromazine metabolites. However, there is no clinical evidence to support this theory.

Evaluation of Clinical Data—Six hospitalized psychiatric patients were given liquid chlorpromazine orally (dose not reported) alone and concurrently with 30 ml of an aluminum–magnesium gel-type antacid (2). Serum chlorpromazine levels after the antacid and chlorpromazine were 21% lower than after chlorpromazine alone ($p<0.01$). Another patient stabilized on chlorpromazine therapy had a relapse 3 days after being placed on a regular regimen of antacid therapy (dose not reported) (3). When the antacid was discontinued, chlorpromazine appeared to be clinically effective again.

Another study (4) showed the effect of simultaneous administration of 30 ml of an aluminum–magnesium hydroxide suspension on urinary chlorpromazine metabolite excretion in 10 patients receiving chronic chlorpromazine therapy (600–1200 mg/day po). Patients receiving chlorpromazine and antacids demonstrated a 10–45% decrease (mean 27%) in urinary excretion of chlorpromazine metabolites indicating a decreased absorption of chlorpromazine. Three of the patients also received the antacid at various intervals (time not reported) following chlorpromazine therapy; more chlorpromazine was absorbed when the antacids were not given concurrently.

■ Although the clinical data are limited, the concurrent administration of chlorpromazine and aluminum–magnesium gel-type antacids results in a reduction in the serum levels of the psychotropic drug. There has been only one case report of decreased effectiveness of chlorpromazine (3), but this interaction may become therapeutically significant in any psychiatric patient previously stabilized on chlorpromazine.

Recommendations—Gel-type antacids or other drug products containing aluminum or magnesium ions (*e.g.*, milk of magnesia) should not be given simultaneously with chlorpromazine or other phenothiazine derivatives but should be administered 1 hr before or 2 hr after chlorpromazine administration (4).

Although the ionic-type antacids (*e.g.*, calcium carbonate) have been suggested as alternatives to magnesium ion- or aluminum ion-containing antacids (4), there is no clinical documentation to support this recommendation. Moreover, *in vitro* studies indicated that chlorpromazine and calcium ions form metal chelates (1).

References

(1) K. S. Rajan *et al.*, "Studies on the Metal Chelation of Chlorpromazine and Its Hydroxylated Metabolites," in "The Phenothiazines and Structurally Related Drugs," I. S. Forrest *et al.*, Eds., Raven, New York, N. Y., 1974, p. 571.

(2) W. E. Fann *et al.*, "Chlorpromazine: Effects of Antacids on Its Gastrointestinal Absorption," *J. Clin. Pharmacol.*, *13*, 388 (1973).

(3) W. E. Fann *et al.*, "The Effects of Antacids on the Blood Levels of Chlorpromazine," abstract, *Clin. Pharmacol. Ther.*, *14*, 135 (1973).

(4) F. M. Forrest *et al.*, "Modification of Chlorpromazine Metabolism by Some Other Drugs Frequently Administered to Psychiatric Patients," *Biol. Psychiat.*, *2*, 53 (1970).

(5) M. Gibaldi *et al.*, "Effect of Antacids on pH of Urine," *Clin. Pharmacol. Ther.*, *16*, 520 (1974).

[For additional information, see *Antipsychotic Therapy*, p. 397.]

Nonproprietary and Trade Names of Drugs

Acetophenazine maleate—*Tindal*
Aluminum-, magnesium-, or calcium-
   containing products—*Aludrox, Alzinox,*
   Amphojel, A-M-T, Camalox, Creamalin,
   Dicarbosil, DiGel, Ducon, Gaviscon,
   Gelusil, Gelusil-M, Kolantyl Gel, Kudrox,
   Maalox, Malcogel, Mylanta, Oxaine-M,
   Phosphaljel, Robalate, Rolaids, Titralac,
   Trisogel, Tums, WinGel
Butaperazine maleate—*Repoise Maleate*
Carphenazine maleate—*Proketazine*
Chlorpromazine—*Chlor-PZ, Promapar,*
   Thorazine
Fluphenazine enanthate—*Prolixin*
   Enanthate

Fluphenazine hydrochloride—*Permitil,*
   Prolixin
Mesoridazine—*Serentil*
Perphenazine—*Trilafon and various com-*
   bination products
Piperacetazine—*Quide*
Prochlorperazine—*Compazine and various*
   combination products
Promazine hydrochloride—*Sparine*
Thiopropazate hydrochloride—*Dartal*
Thioridazine hydrochloride—*Mellaril*
Trifluoperazine hydrochloride—*Stelazine*
Triflupromazine hydrochloride—*Vesprin*

*Prepared and evaluated by the Scientific Review Subpanel on
Psychotropic Agents and reviewed by Practitioner Panel IV.*

Chlorpromazine—Amphetamine

Summary—Chlorpromazine and amphetamine are antagonistic relative to their effects on norepinephrine and dopamine receptors in the central nervous system (CNS). This antagonism can be exploited advantageously in the use of chlorpromazine as a treatment for amphetamine poisonings which involve excessive CNS stimulation. In any other situation, concurrent administration is not pharmacologically sound.

Related Drugs—The interactions between chlorpromazine and amphetamine, although not documented, may apply to other **phenothiazine** derivatives. However, since these agents vary in the degree of adrenergic blockade produced (chlorpromazine causes the strongest blockade) (1), the extent of the drug interaction would be different with each agent.

Other sympathomimetic stimulants that also are antagonized by chlorpromazine are **dextroamphetamine** (2), **methamphetamine** (2), and **phenmetrazine** (2). Other sympathomimetic stimulants (*e.g.*, **methylphenidate**) have not been studied but still may interact with chlorpromazine in a similar manner.

Pharmacological Effect and Mechanism—Chlorpromazine and other phenothiazines produce a postsynaptic block of both norepinephrine and dopamine receptors (3). Specific CNS pathways were shown to use one or another of these transmitters selectively. It is unclear whether the antipsychotic action of these drugs is mediated by inhibition of noradrenergic or dopaminergic synapses or by some unrelated mechanism. The other pharmacological action of antipsychotic drugs is to produce extrapyramidal reactions similar to parkinsonism. This action seems to be derived primarily from the blockade of dopamine receptors (3).

Amphetamine also operates through the catecholamine transmitters, norepinephrine and dopamine, probably by two separate mechanisms. Amphetamine increases the release of these transmitters (4, 5). Increased peripheral release of norepinephrine would account for the peripheral sympathomimetic effects of the drug; release of both norepinephrine and dopamine in the CNS could account for many central effects of the drug, including increased alertness, increased motor activity, dyskinetic or chewing movements (sometimes seen in amphetamine users), or the amphetamine psychosis (6).

In addition to the direct release of these catecholamines, amphetamine impairs their reuptake in the storage vesicles in specific nerve endings. This action resembles that of the tricyclic antidepressants (7). Thus, chlorpromazine and amphetamine have antagonistic effects on both noradrenergic and dopaminergic synapses.

Another interaction between these two types of drugs relates to the effect of chlorpromazine on the metabolism of amphetamine. Chlorpromazine and the tricyclic antidepressants inhibit the metabolism of amphetamine (8). With low doses of chlorpromazine, the accumulation of amphetamine in brains of rats exceeds the receptor-blocking effect, so that enhancement of amphetamine's effect occurs (8). Higher doses of chlorpromazine overcome the increased amphetamine levels, blocking the amphetamine effect (8).

Not all drugs that block the action of amphetamine at the receptors also decrease its metabolism. Haloperidol, in doses adequate to block completely amphetamine-induced stereotyped movements in rats, has no appreciable effect on the metabolism of amphetamine. Chlorpromazine, on the other hand, diminishes the metabolism of amphetamine at doses which fail to block this pharmacological effect (9). The potency of chlorpromazine and haloperidol in treating amphetamine intoxication in dogs was compared (10). Haloperidol was effective at a dose of 1 mg/kg iv while chlorpromazine required higher doses (10–18 mg/kg iv).

Evaluation of Clinical Data—Amphetamine abuse has led to an increasing number of reports of a paranoid psychosis strongly resembling paranoid schizophrenia (11). It is theoretically possible that amphetamine might counter the antipsychotic effects of chlorpromazine if the two are used concurrently. A controlled clinical trial in which dextroamphetamine (10–40 mg/day po) was added to the treatment regimen of 520 chronic schizophrenic patients treated with chlorpromazine (200–600 mg/day po) indicated some deterioration of the mental state, tending to confirm the supposition that the two drugs are antagonistic in this aspect (12).

In another study (13), pretreatment with chlorpromazine (150 mg/day po for 7 or 13 days) significantly decreased (about 40%) the euphoric state (measured by a self-rated scale) induced by amphetamine (200 mg iv) in eight former amphetamine abusers. A single dose of chlorpromazine (50 mg po) also decreased the euphoric effect (about 10%) in eight patients, but when 25 mg was used no antagonism occurred. In all cases, 4 hr elapsed between the time of the last dose of chlorpromazine and the administration of amphetamine.

The antagonism of these two drugs was used beneficially in cases of intoxication with amphetamine or similar drugs (dextroamphetamine, methamphetamine, and phenmetrazine). Chlorpromazine (usual initial dose, 1 mg/kg im; then 0.4–4.0 mg/kg im) given to 22 children with such poisonings dramatically ameliorated the signs of toxicity (2). Excess sedation was a problem only in those who were poisoned with a combination product containing a barbiturate and was managed by using a smaller dose of chlorpromazine (0.5 mg/kg im).

■ The concurrent use of phenothiazines and sympathomimetic stimulants of the amphetamine type should be discouraged. The use of chlorpromazine for treating poisonings with amphetamine-like drugs may be beneficial, and it is based on sound pharmacological evidence of an antagonistic effect at reasonable clinical doses.

Amphetamine should not be used in phenothiazine intoxication, because the dangers of adding the former drug do not seem justified by the benefits. Generally, such intoxications are best managed by supportive treatment rather than by an antagonist; under such management, the fatality rate is negligible.

Recommendations—Chlorpromazine may be used, along with general supportive measures, for treating overdoses of amphetamine in adults and children when excessive CNS stimulation is present. It has been recommended (2) that 1 mg/kg im of chlorpromazine be given, followed by 0.5 mg/kg im in 30 min if needed.

Animal studies indicate that haloperidol is effective in the treatment of amphetamine intoxication (9, 10). Haloperidol has antagonized the psychotic symptoms and the cardiovascular effects of amphetamine in humans (14), but it has not been used in treating amphetamine intoxication.

References

(1) "The Pharmacological Basis of Therapeutics," 5th ed., L. S. Goodman and A. Gilman, Eds., Macmillan, New York, NY 10022, 1975, pp. 157–164.

(2) D. E. Espelin and A. K. Done, "Amphetamine Poisoning. Effectiveness of Chlorpromazine," *N. Engl. J. Med.*, *278*, 1361 (1968).

(3) J. M. van Rossum *et al.*, in "The Neuroleptics, Modern Problems in Pharmacology 5," D. P. Bobon *et al.*, Eds., Karger, Basel, Switzerland, 1970, pp. 23–70.

(4) J. Axelrod, in "Amphetamines and Related Compounds," F. Costa and S. Garattini, Eds., Raven, New York, N. Y., 1970, p. 207.

(5) A. Carlsson, in "Amphetamines and Related Compounds," F. Costa and S. Garattini, Eds., Raven, New York, N. Y., 1970, pp. 289–300.

(6) J. M. van Rossum, "Mode of Action of Psychomotor Stimulant Drugs," *Int. Rev. Neurobiol.*, *12*, 307 (1970).

(7) K. M. Taylor and S. H. Snyder, "Amphetamine: Differentiation by d and l Isomers of Behavior Involving Brain Norepinephrine or Dopamine," *Science*, *168*, 1487 (1970).

(8) F. Sulser and J. V. Dingell, "Potentiation and Blockade of the Central Action of Amphetamine by Chlorpromazine," *Biochem. Pharmacol.*, *17*, 634 (1968).

(9) L. Lemberger *et al.*, "The Effects of Haloperidol and Chlorpromazine on Amphetamine Metabolism and Amphetamine Stereotype Behavior in the Rat," *J. Pharmacol. Exp. Ther.*, *174*, 428 (1970).

(10) J. D. Catravas *et al.*, "Haloperidol for Acute Amphetamine Poisoning: A Study in Dogs," letter to the editor, *J. Amer. Med. Ass.*, *231*, 1340 (1975).

(11) AMA Committee on Alcoholism and Addiction, "Dependence on Amphetamines and Other Stimulant Drugs," *J. Amer. Med. Ass.*, *197*, 1023 (1966).

(12) J. F. Casey *et al.*, "Combined Drug Therapy of Chronic Schizophrenics. Controlled Evaluation of Placebo, Dextro-amphetamine, Imipramine, Isocarboxazid, and Trifluoperazine Added to Maintenance Doses of Chlorpromazine," *Amer. J. Psychiat.*, *117*, 997 (1961).

(13) L. E. Jonsson, "Pharmacological Blockade of Amphetamine Effects in Amphetamine Dependent Subjects," *Eur. J. Clin. Pharmacol.*, *4*, 206 (1972).

(14) B. Angrist *et al.*, "The Antagonism of Amphetamine-Induced Symptomatology by a Neuroleptic," *Amer. J. Psychiat.*, *131*, 817 (1974).

[For additional information, see *Antipsychotic Therapy*, p. 397.]

Nonproprietary and Trade Names of Drugs

Acetophenazine maleate—*Tindal*
Amphetamine complex—*Biphetamine*
Amphetamine sulfate—*Benzedrine*
Butaperazine maleate—*Repoise Maleate*
Carphenazine maleate—*Proketazine*
Chlorpromazine—*Chlor-PZ, Promapar, Thorazine*
Dextroamphetamine sulfate—*Dexedrine and various combination products*
Fluphenazine enanthate—*Prolixin Enanthate*
Fluphenazine hydrochloride—*Permitil, Prolixin*
Mesoridazine—*Serentil*
Methamphetamine hydrochloride—*Desoxyn, Norodin Hydrochloride, Syndrox*

Methylphenidate hydrochloride—*Ritalin Hydrochloride*
Perphenazine—*Trilafon and various combination products*
Phenmetrazine hydrochloride—*Preludin*
Piperacetazine—*Quide*
Prochlorperazine—*Compazine and various combination products*
Promazine hydrochloride—*Sparine*
Thiopropazate hydrochloride—*Dartal*
Thioridazine hydrochloride—*Mellaril*
Trifluoperazine hydrochloride—*Stelazine*
Triflupromazine hydrochloride—*Vesprin*

Prepared and evaluated by the Scientific Review Subpanel on Psychotropic Agents and reviewed by Practitioner Panel IV.

Chlorpromazine—Benztropine

Summary—Chlorpromazine and benztropine interact by multiple mechanisms and cause various clinical effects. Benztropine is useless in treating the tardive dyskinesia caused by chlorpromazine and the possibility exists that it contributes to this adverse effect. Both chlorpromazine and benztropine produce anticholinergic effects, but the clinical outcome of these combined effects is unpredictable. Benztropine also may decrease chlorpromazine's therapeutic effectiveness possibly by decreasing the amount of chlorpromazine absorbed. Benztropine should not be given routinely for long-term prophylaxis against chlorpromazine-induced extrapyramidal reactions, but it may be useful for alleviation of phenothiazine-induced acute extrapyramidal effects.

Related Drugs—Other phenothiazines associated with tardive dyskinesia include **fluphenazine** (1), **perphenazine** (2), **prochlorperazine** (3), **thioridazine** (3), and **trifluoperazine** (4). Similarly acting **phenothiazines** would be expected to have the capability of producing dyskinesia.

In addition to benztropine, other centrally acting anticholinergic agents that may exacerbate tardive dyskinesia include **biperiden, cycrimine, procyclidine,** and **trihexyphenidyl.**

Pharmacological Effect and Mechanism—Concurrent use of benztropine and a phenothiazine drug such as chlorpromazine may aggravate phenothiazine-induced tardive dyskinesia (1, 5), but a causal relationship has not been established. Although tardive dyskinesia also may be related to other factors such as age and cerebral damage (6–8), phenothiazine-induced tardive dyskinesia is thought to be due to an excessive response to dopamine by neurons in the corpus striatum (9, 10).

Phenothiazines block the dopamine receptors in rats and, usually after long-term administration, cause a "denervation hypersensitivity" of these receptors (11). The atropine-like antiparkinsonian agents prevent the reuptake of dopamine into the rat corpus striatum (12) which would make more dopamine available to react with the "supersensitive" dopamine receptors and aggravate the symptoms of tardive dyskinesia (1). However, this theory has not been conclusively demonstrated in animals and has not been tested in humans.

Antiparkinsonian drugs and phenothiazines both exhibit anticholinergic effects, but the clinical outcome of these effects is difficult to measure because of variation in individual response (13–15), different degrees of anticholinergic activity among phenothiazines (16, 17), and difficulty in differentiating autonomic side effects of therapy from symptoms of ongoing illness (18). Although chlorpromazine enhances the anticholinergic central nervous system effects of scopolamine (19), the combined anticholinergic effects of phenothiazines and antiparkinsonian drugs are usually of minor clinical significance unless an underlying pathological process such as angle closure glaucoma exists (20), excessive doses are utilized (21), or a preexisting sensitivity to the autonomic effects of these drugs is present (22).

Lowered serum levels of chlorpromazine occurring when trihexyphenidyl was administered concurrently were suggested to be the result of the anticholinergic effect on gastric motility by the antiparkinsonian agent (23). It was suggested that the diminished gastric emptying would slow the transit of chlorpromazine and thus favor its metabolism in the intestine. Chlorpromazine is metabolized in the rat gut (24), but investigators have only speculated about this occurrence in humans (13, 14). An additional mechanism offered for lowered chlorpromazine levels is the possibility that long-term use of phenothiazines may induce hepatic microsomal enzymes and thus a large fraction of the dose may be metabolized and deactivated before it can reach the general circulation (25, 26).

Evaluation of Clinical Data—Benztropine or related drugs may precipitate toxic psychosis (27), increase mental confusion (28), and possibly exacerbate tardive dyskinesia (1, 5). Benztropine is ineffective in the treatment of phenothiazine-induced tardive dyskinesias and many patients suffer no ill effects when benztropine or similar drugs are withdrawn from the phenothiazine dosage regimen (29, 30). The lack of effectiveness of benztropine in the treatment of phenothiazine-induced tardive dyskinesia and the drug's potentially severe adverse effects discourage its long-term use with chlorpromazine or other phenothiazines.

Most descriptions of anticholinergic side effects occurring with concurrent phenothiazine–antiparkinsonian therapy arise from the observation of individual patients rather than from controlled population studies. Therefore, it is difficult to determine if the anticholinergic effects are due to the single agent or to both drugs. One report (31) described three patients who developed toxic confusional states from the respective regimens of benztropine mesylate (12 mg/day po), imipramine (150 mg/day po), and perphenazine (72 mg/day po); benztropine mesylate (6.0 mg/day po) and thioridazine (150 mg/day po); and benztropine mesylate (8.0 mg/day po) and chlorpromazine (800 mg/day po). In each patient, physostigmine salicylate was significantly superior to the placebo (total average, $p<0.0002$, t test) in alleviating the confusional state, thus indicating that confusion had resulted from anticholinergic toxicity.

Chlorpromazine's inhibitory effect on basal gastric secretion was enhanced by tricyclamol chloride (an anticholinergic) in five patients with chronic duodenal ulcer (32). In two control groups of five patients, the degree of inhibition of total acid output increased with increasing doses of each drug, chlorpromazine being significantly less potent than tricyclamol ($p<0.05$). The effect on inhibition was significantly greater with concurrent therapy than expected ($p<0.05$) and was interpreted as synergism. The inability (33) to duplicate previous results (32) using prochlorperazine was reported to be consistent with the differences in degree of autonomic and central effects of chlorpromazine and prochlorperazine.

Anticholinergic symptomatology and changes of perceptual ability were measured in 33 patients of mixed psychiatric diagnosis who received, singly and concurrently, chlorpromazine and atropine, chlorpromazine and piperidyl benzilate hydrochloride (an anticholinergic), promazine and piperidyl benzilate hydrochloride, and imipramine and piperidyl benzilate hydrochloride (34). When phenothiazines were administered with the anticholinergic agent, a significant ($p<0.05$) enhancement of sedation was observed based on neurological, consciousness, and perceptual areas. This enhancement did not occur when the anticholinergic drug was administered with imipramine, a drug that has a high degree of anticholinergic activity. The investigators concluded that an unknown mechanism of interaction between phenothiazines and anticholinergic agents—not involving combined anticholinergic properties—may have resulted in the enhancement of sedation.

A lowered serum phenothiazine level, resulting from the concurrent use of an atropine-like antiparkinsonian agent, was reported (23) in five patients taking trihexyphenidyl (6–8 mg/day po) concurrently with chlorpromazine (300–600 mg/day po). Two patients were given trihexyphenidyl for the first 2 weeks of chlorpromazine therapy, and an additional three patients received trihexyphenidyl as concurrent therapy from the third to the sixth week. This interval was chosen because of another report showing declining serum levels of chlorpromazine (300 mg/day po) in the third week of a 6-week regimen in 10 patients receiving no other medication (13). Chlorpromazine was administered as a liquid to minimize interferences with the absorption rate caused by a variable rate of drug release (14). Serum chlorpromazine levels were impaired when trihexyphenidyl was administered and improved when it was discontinued (no statistical test was given). To eliminate the possibility of intra-patient variation in serum levels and absorption reported to be significant by other investigators (13–15, 35), three of the five patients had serum chlorpromazine levels measured with and without trihexyphenidyl; results again indicated lowered serum levels with concurrent administration of trihexyphenidyl. Lack of clinical improvement (evaluated by The Brief Psychiatric Rating Scale) occurred in three of these patients and another patient's clinical state deteriorated after the serum chlorpromazine levels decreased. It was suggested that trihexyphenidyl delayed gastric emptying time and increased chlorpromazine metabolism in the gastrointestinal tract.

■ Four areas of concern arise from the data in regard to administering a phenothiazine such as chlorpromazine with an atropine-like antiparkinsonian agent such as benztropine. First, the antiparkinsonian agent is useless in treating tardive dyskinesia and the possibility exists that it has a contributing role in the precipitation of this adverse effect. Second, although both chlorpromazine and benztropine have anticholinergic activity, the clinical result from their concurrent use is unpredictable. Third, there is a possible interference of chlorpromazine absorption when an atropine-like antiparkinsonian agent is taken concurrently, leading to decreased serum chlorpromazine levels and less clinical efficacy. Finally, in many patients, antiparkinsonian agents do not have to be given chronically with phenothiazines to prevent extrapyramidal reactions.

Recommendations—Because of possible complications to antipsychotic phenothiazine therapy, atropine-like antiparkinsonian agents should not be given routinely as a long-term prophylactic measure for the extrapyramidal side effects of phenothiazine therapy. They may be used when required to alleviate phenothiazine-induced acute extrapyramidal effects but may be discontinued or adjusted in a significant number of patients without adverse effects.

A similar interaction occurs between butyrophenones such as haloperidol and atropine-like antiparkinsonian agents (36) and the same precautions should be followed when these drugs are used concurrently.

References

(1) L. G. Kiloh et al., "Antiparkinson Drugs as Causal Agents in Tardive Dyskinesia," *Med. J. Aust.*, 2, 591 (1973).

(2) L. Uhrband and A. Faurbye, "Reversible and Irreversible Dyskinesia after Treatment with Perphenazine, Chlorpromazine, Reserpine, and Electroconvulsive Therapy," *Psychopharmacologia*, 1, 408 (1960).

(3) G. E. Crane, "Tardive Dyskinesia in Patients Treated with Major Neuroleptics: A Review of the Literature," *Amer. J. Psychiat.*, 124, suppl., 40 (1968).

(4) J. H. Evans, "Persistent Oral Dyskinesia in Treatment with Phenothiazine Derivatives," *Lancet*, i, 458 (1965).

(5) R. Hunter et al., "An Apparently Irreversible Syndrome of Abnormal Movements following Phenothiazine Medication," *Proc. Roy. Soc. Med.*, 57, 758 (1964).

(6) W. R. Schmidt and L. W. Jarcho, "Persistent Dyskinesias following Phenothiazine Therapy," *Arch. Neurol.*, 14, 369 (1966).

(7) A. Faurbye et al., "Neurological Symptoms in Pharmacotherapy of Psychoses," *Acta Psychiat. Scand.*, 40, 10 (1964).

(8) N. S. Kline, "On the Rarity of 'Irreversible' Oral Dyskinesias following Phenothiazines," *Amer. J. Psychiat.*, 124, suppl., 48 (1968).

(9) J. M. van Rossum, "The Significance of Dopamine-Receptor Blockade for the Action of Neuroleptic Drugs," in "Neuro Psychopharmacology," W. Brill, Ed., Excerpta Medica Foundation, Amsterdam, The Netherlands, 1966, p. 321.

(10) R. Hunter et al., "Neuropathological Findings in Three Cases of Persistent Dyskinesia following Phenothiazine Medication," *J. Neurol. Sci.*, 7, 263 (1968).

(11) H. Nyback and G. Sedvall, "Regional Accumulation of Catecholamines Formed from Tyrosine-^{14}C in Rat Brain: Effect of Chlorpromazine," *Eur. J. Pharmacol.*, 5, 245 (1969).

(12) J. T. Coyle and S. H. Snyder, "Antiparkinsonian Drugs: Inhibition of Dopamine Uptake in the Corpus Striatum as a Possible Mechanism of Action," *Science*, 166, 899 (1969).

(13) G. Sakalis et al., "Physiologic and Clinical Effects of Chlorpromazine and Their Relationship to Plasma Level," *Clin. Pharmacol. Ther.*, 13, 931 (1972).

(14) S. H. Curry et al., "Factors Affecting Chlorpromazine Plasma Levels in Psychiatric Patients," Arch. Gen. Psychiat., 22, 209 (1970).

(15) S. H. Curry and J. H. L. Marshall, "Plasma Levels of Chlorpromazine and Some of Its Relatively Non-polar Metabolites in Psychiatric Patients," Life Sci., 7, 9 (1968).

(16) A. Dimasco et al., in "Recent Advances in Biological Psychiatry," vol. III, J. Wortis, Ed., Grune and Stratton, New York, N.Y., 1961, pp. 68–76.

(17) S. Jonas, "Miosis following Administration of Chlorpromazine and Related Agents," Amer. J. Psychiat., 115, 817 (1959).

(18) B. L. Busfield et al., "Depressive Symptom or Side Effect? A Comparative Study of Symptoms during Pre-Treatment and Treatment Periods of Patients on Three Antidepressant Medications," J. Nerv. Ment. Dis., 134, 339 (1962).

(19) J. S. Ketchum et al., "Atropine, Scopolamine, and Ditran: Comparative Pharmacology and Antagonists in Man," Psychopharmacologia, 28, 121 (1973).

(20) W. M. Grant, "Ocular Complications of Drugs. Glaucoma," J. Amer. Med. Ass., 207, 2089 (1969).

(21) M. R. Goldstein and R. Kasper, "Hyperpyrexia and Coma Due to Overdose of Benztropine," S. Med. J., 61, 984 (1968).

(22) E. C. Miller et al., "Gross Hematuria as a Complication in the Combination Use of Psychotropic Drugs," Amer. J. Psychiat., 124, 229 (1967).

(23) L. Rivera-Calimlim et al., "Effects of Mode of Management on Plasma Chlorpromazine in Psychiatric Patients," Clin. Pharmacol. Ther., 14, 978 (1973).

(24) S. H. Curry et al., "Destruction of Chlorpromazine during Absorption in the Rat In Vivo and In Vitro," Brit. J. Pharmacol., 42, 403 (1971).

(25) J. O. Cole, "Introduction," Dis. Nerv. Syst., 31, suppl., 5 (1970).

(26) R. L. Young et al., "Role of Liver in Metabolism of Chlorpromazine," Nature, 183, 1396 (1959).

(27) J. V. Ananth and R. C. Jain, "Benztropine Psychosis," Can. Psychiat. Ass. J., 18, 409 (1973).

(28) J. B. Dynes, "Oral Dyskinesias—Occurrence and Treatment," Dis. Nerv. Syst., 31, 854 (1970).

(29) C. J. Klett and E. Caffey, "Evaluating the Long-Term Need for Antiparkinson Drugs by Chronic Schizophrenics," Arch. Gen. Psychiat., 26, 374 (1972).

(30) P. Orlov et al., "Withdrawal of Antiparkinson Drugs," Arch. Gen. Psychiat., 25, 410 (1971).

(31) M. K. El-Yousef et al., "Reversal of Benztropine Toxicity by Physostigmine," letter to the editor, J. Amer. Med. Ass., 220, 125 (1972).

(32) D. C. H. Sun and H. Shay, "Synergistic Action of Chlorpromazine and Tricyclamol on Basal Gastric Secretion in Duodenal Ulcer Patients," Gastroenterology, 36, 245 (1959).

(33) A. J. Cummins, "Effect of Prochlorperazine and of Prochlorperazine-Isopropamide on Basal Gastric Secretion," Amer. J. Dig. Dis., 5, 523 (1960).

(34) S. Gershon et al., "Interaction between Some Anticholinergic Agents and Phenothiazines. Potentiation of Phenothiazine Sedation and Its Antagonism," Clin. Pharmacol. Ther., 6, 749 (1965).

(35) J. E. March et al., "Interpatient Variation and Significance of Plasma Levels of Chlorpromazine in Psychotic Patients," J. Med., 3, 146 (1972).

(36) M. M. Singh and J. M. Smith, "Reversal of Some Therapeutic Effects of an Antipsychotic Agent by an Antiparkinsonism Drug," J. Nerv. Ment. Dis., 157, 50 (1973).

[For additional information, see *Antipsychotic Therapy*, p. 397.]

Nonproprietary and Trade Names of Drugs

Acetophenazine maleate—*Tindal*

Benztropine mesylate—*Cogentin Mesylate*

Biperiden—*Akineton*

Butaperazine maleate—*Repoise Maleate*

Carphenazine maleate—*Proketazine*

Chlorpromazine—*Chlor-PZ, Promapar, Thorazine*

Cycrimine hydrochloride—*Pagitane Hydrochloride*

Fluphenazine enanthate—*Prolixin Enanthate*

Fluphenazine hydrochloride—*Permitil, Prolixin*

Haloperidol—*Haldol*

Mesoridazine—*Serentil*

Perphenazine—*Trilafon and various combination products*

Piperacetazine—*Quide*

Prochlorperazine—*Compazine and various combination products*

Procyclidine hydrochloride—*Kemadrin*

Promazine hydrochloride—*Sparine*

Thiopropazate hydrochloride—*Dartal*

Thioridazine hydrochloride—*Mellaril*

Trifluoperazine hydrochloride—*Stelazine*

Triflupromazine hydrochloride—*Vesprin*

Trihexyphenidyl hydrochloride—*Artane, Pipanol, Tremin*

Prepared and evaluated by the Scientific Review Subpanel on Psychotropic Agents and reviewed by Practitioner Panel V.

Chlorpromazine—Piperazine

Summary—Although there has been one clinical report of convulsions after administration of chlorpromazine following piperazine, corroborating evidence in humans or animals is lacking. Therefore, it is not possible to make any definite clinical evaluation. Concurrent use of these drugs need not be avoided, but close observation of the patient is required to avoid the occurrence of potentially harmful seizures.

Related Drugs—Numerous **phenothiazine** drugs are available and in clinical use.

Pharmacological Effect and Mechanism—A single clinical report suggested that piperazine exaggerated the extrapyramidal effects of chlorpromazine, precipitating convulsions (1). The convulsive effect also was observed in animals; a significant number of deaths occurred in dogs (four out of six) and goats (six out of nine) after concurrent administration of chlorpromazine (10 mg) and piperazine (220 mg/kg). A later animal study (2) carried out by the Food and Drug Administration and the same investigators failed to confirm these findings. The mechanism of the reported drug interaction is unknown at the present time, but chlorpromazine alone may also lower seizure threshold and precipitate convulsions (3).

Evaluation of Clinical Data—Insufficient information concerning the chlorpromazine–piperazine interaction was provided in the one reported case (1). This report stated that convulsions were observed in a child given chlorpromazine a few days after the administration of piperazine for a pinworm infection.

■ There is no explanation for the convulsive seizure reported in a child and the convulsive seizures and death observed in experimental animals (1). However, the possibility of an adverse effect due to a chlorpromazine–piperazine interaction should be considered when these drugs are administered concurrently. With only the two conflicting references pertaining to this specific interaction, it is not possible to make any definite clinical evaluation.

Recommendations—Because the clinical data are inconclusive, the concurrent use of chlorpromazine and piperazine need not be avoided. However, since some clinical and experimental evidence indicates that potentially dangerous seizures may occur, close observation of the patient is required.

References

(1) B. M. Boulos and L. E. Davis, "Hazard of Simultaneous Administration of Phenothiazine and Piperazine," *N. Engl. J. Med.*, *280*, 1245 (1969).
(2) B. H. Armbrecht, "Reaction between Piperazine and Chlorpromazine," *N. Engl. J. Med.*, *282*, 1490 (1970).
(3) "The Pharmacological Basis of Therapeutics," 5th ed., L. S. Goodman and A. Gilman, Eds., Macmillan, New York, NY 10022, 1975, p. 159.

[For additional information, see *Antipsychotic Therapy*, p. 397.]

Nonproprietary and Trade Names of Drugs

Acetophenazine maleate—*Tindal*
Butaperazine maleate—*Repoise Maleate*
Carphenazine maleate—*Proketazine*
Chlorpromazine—*Chlor-PZ, Promapar, Thorazine*
Fluphenazine enanthate—*Prolixin Enanthate*

Fluphenazine hydrochloride—*Permitil, Prolixin*
Mesoridazine—*Serentil*
Perphenazine—*Trilafon and various combination products*
Piperacetazine—*Quide*
Piperazine—*Antepar*

Piperazine calcium edetate—*Perin*
Piperazine citrate—*Multifuge Citrate*
Prochlorperazine—*Compazine and various combination products*
Promazine hydrochloride—*Sparine*

Thiopropazate hydrochloride—*Dartal*
Thioridazine hydrochloride—*Mellaril*
Trifluoperazine hydrochloride—*Stelazine*
Triflupromazine hydrochloride—*Vesprin*

Prepared and evaluated by the Scientific Review Subpanel on Psychotropic Agents and reviewed by Practitioner Panel V.

Chlorpropamide—Allopurinol

Summary—Some clinical data, although not conclusive, indicate that allopurinol may increase the serum half-life of chlorpropamide significantly. Until more clinical data are available, patients receiving these drugs concurrently should be observed closely for any unusual increases in the pharmacological effect or the serum half-life of chlorpropamide.

Related Drugs—The other sulfonylurea drugs such as **acetohexamide, tolazamide,** and **tolbutamide** have not been documented to interact with allopurinol but could theoretically be expected to interact similarly to chlorpropamide.

There are no drugs commercially available in the United States similar to allopurinol.

Pharmacological Effect and Mechanism—Chlorpropamide is the longest acting sulfonylurea compound and is metabolized and excreted slowly (1) either as parent compound or as metabolites (2, 3).

Allopurinol is a competitive inhibitor of and a substrate for xanthine oxidase and it inhibits the conversion of hypoxanthine to xanthine as well as xanthine to uric acid (4). Thus, the serum level of uric acid is lowered to normal or below, the renal excretion of uric acid is decreased, and the serum level and renal clearance of xanthine and hypoxanthine are increased. Xanthine stone formation in the kidneys during allopurinol therapy is a possibility, but this rarely occurs except in some children with the Lesch–Nyhan syndrome (5).

Although there have been no studies to support this conclusion, it has been hypothesized that allopurinol may competitively interfere with the renal transport of chlorpropamide, thereby increasing its half-life (6).

Evaluation of Clinical Data—The only clinical report of this drug interaction was a study of chlorpropamide in 20 patients with nephropathies and in 41 patients with normal renal function (6). In one patient with normal renal function treated with allopurinol for 10 days (dose not reported), the chlorpropamide half-life exceeded 200 hr. In two other patients receiving allopurinol, the chlorpropamide half-life reached 44 and 55 hr. In three additional patients who took allopurinol for a shorter period (1–2 days), the chlorpropamide half-life remained within normal limits.

■ Limited evidence supports the clinical significance of this drug interaction. The only clinical study was not well controlled, and allopurinol was not definitely implicated as the causative factor in the prolongation of the chlorpropamide half-life. If this drug interaction does occur, it appears to be influenced by the length of allopurinol administration.

Recommendations—The clinical outcome of this drug interaction cannot be predicted because of insufficient data. Nevertheless, any patient receiving these drugs concurrently should be observed closely for any symptoms of hypoglycemia caused by an increase in the serum chlorpropamide half-life. Patients with hepatic or renal disorders should be observed for any additional or unexpected increases in the chlorpropamide half-life.

If the half-life or the pharmacological effect of chlorpropamide increases, an appropriate reduction in the dose of the hypoglycemic agent should be made, or the patient should be switched to insulin therapy.

References

(1) P. M. Brotherton *et al.*, "A Study of the Metabolic Fate of Chlorpropamide in Man," *Clin. Pharmacol. Ther.*, **10**, 505 (1969).

(2) L. J. P. Duncan and B. F. Clarke, "Pharmacology and Mode of Action of the Hypoglycaemic Sulphonylureas and Diguanides," *Ann. Rev. Pharmacol.*, **5**, 151 (1965).

(3) J. A. Taylor, "Pharmacokinetics and Biotransformation of Chlorpropamide in Man," *Clin. Pharmacol. Ther.*, **13**, 710 (1972).

(4) "The Pharmacological Basis of Therapeutics," 5th ed., L. S. Goodman and A. Gilman, Eds., Macmillan, New York, NY 10022, 1975, pp. 352–353.

(5) S. Goldfinger *et al.*, "The Renal Excretion of Oxypurines," *J. Clin. Invest.*, **44**, 623 (1965).

(6) B. Petitpierre *et al.*, "Behavior of Chlorpropamide in Renal Insufficiency and under the Effect of Associated Drug Therapy," *Helv. Med. Acta, 36*, 245 (1972).

[For additional information, see *Hypoglycemic Therapy*, p. 422, and *Uricosuric Therapy*, p. 447.]

Nonproprietary and Trade Names of Drugs

Acetohexamide—*Dymelor*
Allopurinol—*Zyloprim*
Chlorpropamide—*Diabinese*

Tolazamide—*Tolinase*
Tolbutamide—*Orinase*

Prepared and evaluated by the Scientific Review Subpanels on Hypoglycemic Agents and Uricosuric Agents and reviewed by Practitioner Panel IV.

Chlorpropamide—Aspirin

Summary—The hypoglycemic activity of chlorpropamide may be enhanced by the concurrent administration of aspirin. Patients receiving both drugs should be monitored closely for symptoms of hypoglycemia and appropriate reductions in the chlorpropamide or the salicylate dose should be made.

Related Drugs—**Tolbutamide** has also been shown to interact with the salicylates (1). Although not documented, the other sulfonylureas **acetohexamide** and **tolazamide** are structurally similar to chlorpropamide and also should be expected to interact with the salicylates.

Since aspirin is metabolized to salicylic acid, which reportedly interacts with the sulfonylureas (1), other **salicylates** can be expected to interact in a similar manner.

Salicylamide, although not metabolized to salicylic acid, has many properties similar to the salicylates and could be expected to interact with the sulfonylureas (2).

Pharmacological Effect and Mechanism—As a result of concurrent administration of aspirin and chlorpropamide, the hypoglycemic effect of the latter drug may be increased, leading to a prolonged and protracted fall in serum glucose levels. It has been suggested (3) that this interaction results from a competitive interference in tubular secretion between chlorpropamide and salicylate. However, other *in vitro* data (4) indicate that the reaction is due to salicylate displacing chlorpropamide from its binding sites. This displacement would increase the amount of free (pharmacologically active) drug in circulation and greater hypoglycemia would result.

Large doses of aspirin may have intrinsic hypoglycemic activity when administered to diabetic patients (2, 5, 6). The exact mechanism of this effect is not completely understood. However, several mechanisms by which aspirin may decrease serum glucose levels have been postulated (5, 7) and include depletion of hepatic glycogen, increased glucose utilization, and uncoupling of oxidative phosphorylation with resulting peripheral tissue uptake of glucose. In the diabetic patient receiving well-controlled sulfonylurea therapy, this fall in the serum glucose level will decrease the oral dosage requirement.

Evaluation of Clinical Data—There are no well-controlled studies documenting the interaction between chlorpropamide and aspirin.

In one study (3), patients receiving chlorpropamide (500 mg po) simultaneously with aspirin (in quantities sufficient to produce serum salicylate levels of 10–26 mg/100 ml) had lower serum glucose levels than when chlorpropamide alone was ingested. The investigators suggested that chlorpropamide and aspirin compete for renal excretion, resulting in an increase in the amount of chlorpropamide in the body.

Another study (1) showed that salicylic acid (dose not reported) enhanced the symptoms of hypoglycemia caused by chlorpropamide (0.5–3 g po) or tolbutamide (0.5–3 g po) in 14 patients.

■ Since controlled clinical trials are few and isolated reports of an interaction between chlorpropamide and aspirin are infrequent, no quantitative statement can be made regarding the significance of this interaction. The available literature, however, indicates that the hypoglycemic activity of chlorpropamide may be enhanced by aspirin. In addition, this interaction may occur only when large doses (2–6 g/day) (5) of aspirin are administered. Additional studies are necessary to assess adequately the frequency, magnitude, and host-determining characteristics of this interaction.

Recommendations—The possible occurrence of this interaction is not a contraindication to concurrent administration of chlorpropamide and aspirin. Serum and urinary glucose levels can be measured rapidly and easily. When it is necessary to administer both drugs, the patient should be observed closely for signs and symptoms of hypoglycemia. Proper adjustments in the chlorpropamide dosage will prevent the occurrence of hypoglycemia. If reductions are made in the sulfonylurea dose when aspirin is added to the drug regimen, it should be realized that the dosage of the sulfonylurea may have to be increased when aspirin is discontinued.

If the serum glucose levels cannot be controlled adequately by the adjustment of the dose of the sulfonylureas, insulin therapy or strict dietary management should be used instead.

References

(1) E. Schulz, "Severe Hypoglycemic Reactions after Tolbutamide, Carbutamide, and Chlorpropamide," *Arch. Klin. Med.*, *214*, 135 (1968).
(2) "The Pharmacological Basis of Therapeutics," 5th ed., L. S. Goodman and A. Gilman, Eds., Macmillan, New York, NY 10022, 1975, pp. 332–333.
(3) J. M. Stowers *et al.*, "A Clinical and Pharmacological Comparison of Chlorpropamide and Other Sulfonylureas," *Ann. N.Y. Acad. Sci.*, 74, 689 (1959).
(4) H. Wishinsky *et al.*, "Protein Interactions of Sulfonylurea Compounds," *Diabetes, 2*, suppl., 18 (1962).

(5) Medical Staff Conference, "The Clinical Pharmacology of Salicylates," *Calif. Med., 110,* 410 (1969).

(6) H. S. Seltzer, "Drug-Induced Hypoglycemia," *Diabetes, 21,* 955 (1972).

(7) G. A. Limbeck *et al.,* "Salicylates and Hypoglycemia," *Amer. J. Dis. Child., 109,* 165 (1965).

[For additional information, see *Hypoglycemic Therapy,* p. 422.]

Nonproprietary and Trade Names of Drugs

Acetohexamide—*Dymelor*
Aluminum aspirin—*Available in combination products*
Aspirin—*Available alone or as a fixed combination in many trade name products, especially over-the-counter preparations*
Calcium carbaspirin—*Calurin*
Carbethyl salicylate—*Sal-Ethyl Carbonate*
Chlorpropamide—*Diabinese*

Choline salicylate—*Actasal, Arthropan*
Magnesium salicylate—*Various manufacturers*
Potassium salicylate—*Various manufacturers*
Salicylamide—*Various manufacturers*
Sodium salicylate—*Various manufacturers*
Tolazamide—*Tolinase*
Tolbutamide—*Orinase*

Prepared and evaluated by the Scientific Review Subpanels on Hypoglycemic Agents and Analgesics and reviewed by Practitioner Panel III.

Chlorpropamide—Cortisone

Summary—The hyperglycemic action of cortisone may offset the hypoglycemic effect of chlorpropamide, but the clinical data about the drug interaction are limited and unreliable. To maintain control of diabetes when these drugs are administered concurrently, an upward adjustment of the chlorpropamide dose or a reduction of the cortisone dose may be required. There is a possibility that concurrent administration of chlorpropamide and cortisone may increase the likelihood of precipitating a gastric ulcer, but there are no clinical reports of this effect occurring in humans.

Related Drugs—The following drugs are chemically and pharmacologically related to cortisone and should interact in a similar manner: **betamethasone, dexamethasone, fludrocortisone, fluprednisone, hydrocortisone (cortisol), meprednisone, methylprednisolone, paramethasone, prednisolone, prednisone,** and **triamcinolone.** However, clinical evidence about these drug interactions is lacking.

Acetohexamide, tolazamide, and **tolbutamide** are hypoglycemic sulfonylurea compounds related to chlorpropamide and may interact similarly, although no documentation exists.

Pharmacological Effect and Mechanism—Glucocorticoids increase hepatic glycogenesis and gluconeogenesis, decrease peripheral glucose utilization, and alter levels of enzyme activity involved in carbohydrate metabolism (1). Prolonged exposure to large doses of glucocorticoids may cause a diabetic-like syndrome associated with increased resistance to insulin and a decreased tolerance to glucose (2). Chlorpropamide sensitizes β-pancreatic cells to glucose and the resultant insulin secretion. This action can be demonstrated in both maturity-onset diabetic patients and nondiabetic subjects (3). Chlorpropamide is ineffective in completely pancreatectomized patients and juvenile-onset diabetic patients (2), indicating that it exerts its action in the pancreas. However, at high dose levels, extrapancreatic effects on the inhibition of hepatic glucose output and hepatic uptake of endogenous insulin have also been reported (2, 4).

Evaluation of Clinical Data—In a study (5) evaluating cortisone's effect on the action of chlorpropamide, five adult diabetic patients received a single dose of cortisone (200 mg po) and chlorpropamide (dose not reported) concurrently. The serum glucose levels initially dropped in three patients, but the decrease was maintained in only one subject. The investigators suggested that chlorpropamide, in the amounts given, could not overcome the hyperglycemic action of cortisone.

A potentially serious side effect of chronic, high-dose glucocorticoid therapy is the steroid-induced peptic ulcer. Sulfonylureas may exacerbate preexisting peptic ulcers (1). Therefore, concurrent use of chlorpropamide and cortisone may increase the likelihood of precipitating a gastric ulcer.

■ In diabetic subjects, the requirements for chlorpropamide may be increased when cortisone is used in high doses. Additionally, there is a possibility that concurrent administration of chlorpropamide and cortisone may increase the likelihood of precipitating a gastric ulcer. However, the clinical significance of the chlorpropamide–cortisone interaction has not been established.

Recommendations—To maintain control of diabetes, an upward adjustment of the chlorpropamide dose or a reduction of the cortisone dose may be necessary when these drugs are administered concurrently. Also, the patient should be observed for the development of gastric ulcers.

The diabetogenic effect of cortisone may cause similar problems for patients receiving insulin or phenformin, but concurrent use of either drug with cortisone has not been studied.

References

(1) "Drill's Pharmacology in Medicine," 4th ed., J. R. DiPalma, Ed., McGraw-Hill, New York, N.Y., 1971, pp. 1515, 1542.

(2) "The Pharmacological Basis of Therapeutics," 5th ed., L. S. Goodman and A. Gilman, Eds., Macmillan, New York, NY 10022, 1975, pp. 1481, 1520.

(3) H. D. Briedahl *et al.*, "Insulin and Oral Hypoglycemic Agents I: Physiological and Clinical Aspects," *Drugs, 3,* 79 (1972).

(4) J. M. Feldman and H. E. Lebovitz, "Appraisal of the Extrapancreatic Actions of Sulfonylureas," *Arch. Intern. Med., 123,* 314 (1969).

(5) T. S. Danowski *et al.*, "Cortisone Enhancement of Peripheral Utilization of Glucose and the Effects of Chlorpropamide," *Ann. N.Y. Acad. Sci., 74,* 988 (1959).

[For additional information, see *Hypoglycemic Therapy*, p. 422.]

Nonproprietary and Trade Names of Drugs

Acetohexamide—*Dymelor*
Betamethasone—*Celestone*
Chlorpropamide—*Diabinese*
Cortisone acetate—*Cortone Acetate*
Dexamethasone—*Decadron, Hexadrol*
Fludrocortisone acetate—*Florinef Acetate*
Fluprednisolone—*Alphadrol*
Hydrocortisone—*Various manufacturers*
Insulin—*Iletin*
Meprednisone—*Betapar*

Methylprednisolone—*Medrol*
Paramethasone acetate—*Haldrone*
Phenformin hydrochloride—*DBI, Meltrol*
Prednisolone—*Delta-Cortef, Meticortelone, Sterane*
Prednisone—*Delta-dome, Deltasone, Deltra, Meticorten, Paracort*
Tolazamide—*Tolinase*
Tolbutamide—*Orinase*
Triamcinolone—*Aristocort, Kenacort*

Prepared and evaluated by the Scientific Review Subpanels on Hypoglycemic Agents and Steroids and reviewed by Practitioner Panel IV.

Chlorpropamide—Hydrochlorothiazide

Summary—Many diabetic patients regulated by chlorpropamide or other sulfonylureas exhibit impaired diabetic control when any thiazide diuretic is added to the drug regimen. This effect is usually, but not always, reversible when the diuretic is discontinued, when increased potassium supplementation is used, or when higher doses of the hypoglycemic agent are employed.

Related Drugs—This drug interaction may occur with **acetohexamide** (1), **tolazamide** (1), and **tolbutamide** (1).

All **thiazide diuretics** have the potential for producing kaliuresis and hypokalemia (2), which are probably essential steps in the pathogenesis of the drug interaction. **Benzthiazide** (2), **chlorothiazide** (1), and **trichlormethiazide** (1) have been documented to interact similarly. **Chlorthalidone, metolazone,** and **quinethazone** are structurally related to the thiazide diuretics (2) and should be expected to interact in a similar manner. Potassium-depleting diuretics also are available in many combination products.

Pharmacological Effect and Mechanism—This interaction is manifested clinically by a loss of diabetic control that may result in glycosuria or hyperglycemia. A study in humans (3) indicated that trichlormethiazide-induced hyperglycemia may be due to a decrease in the amount of endogenous insulin released. However, an *in vitro* study on rat pancreatic tissue failed to demonstrate this effect (4).

There is no evidence to suggest that the thiazides inhibit the hypoglycemic effect of exogenously administered insulin. There is impairment of the insulin effect on both muscle (5) and adipose (6, 7) tissues of chlorothiazide-treated animals, even without a striking potassium depletion, although hypokalemia is generally believed to be a contributory factor in the pathogenesis of this drug interaction (8).

Evaluation of Clinical Data—Thiazide diuretics may cause hyperglycemia (1) or exacerbate diabetes mellitus (1, 9–14). However, some studies were only several weeks in duration (11, 12) or did not use pretreatment levels of glucose as a baseline (13, 14).

A study of 101 hypertensive patients receiving ethacrynic acid (100 mg/day po), furosemide (80 mg/day po), or hydrochlorothiazide (50 mg/day po) indicated that these diuretics had little diabetogenic effect in most patients when given for 1 year (10). Only two of 56 patients receiving hydrochlorothiazide developed clinical diabetes. The glucose tolerance test in these patients improved after the withdrawal of the thiazide diuretic, implicating these drugs as the probable causative factor. All patients already diagnosed as being diabetic were excluded from this study.

In a study of 30 nonketotic, maturity-onset diabetic patients (1), treatment with chlorothiazide (500 mg/day po) and trichlormethiazide (4 mg/day po) caused a statistically significant ($p<0.01$) increase in the mean serum glucose levels during a 3–6-month period when compared to pretreatment values. Patients had diabetes, diabetes with hypertension, or diabetes with atherosclerotic heart disease. The oral hypoglycemic drugs used were acetohexamide, chlorpropamide, and tolbutamide. Insulin also was used in some cases. The dose of the oral hypoglycemic agent had to be increased in four patients, tolbutamide had to be replaced with insulin in one patient, and the insulin dose had to be increased in two patients. No problems were encountered by the patients controlled by diet alone. There was no dramatic deterioration of diabetic control in any patient during thiazide therapy. Discontinuation of the thiazide diuretic caused a significant decrease in the serum glucose levels of the

30 patients studied. The improvement was not sufficient to necessitate reduction in the dose of insulin or the sulfonylurea but was adequate to allow a return to tolbutamide control in the patient switched to insulin.

■ Use of a thiazide diuretic may impair control of diabetes in patients treated by diet or with oral hypoglycemic agents or insulin, but only to a limited extent (1). There is no evidence that this drug interaction is progressive if both drugs are continued indefinitely, but often the loss of control is so striking that a prompt revision of the therapeutic program is indicated (12). Moreover, the variables that affect the daily control of diabetes such as dietary indiscretions, emotional stress, and minor infections may often obscure the hyperglycemic effect of thiazides in individual patients (1). It appears that approximately 10% of patients treated with oral hypoglycemic agents requires either an increase in dosage or a change to insulin treatment while being treated by thiazide diuretics (1). This hyperglycemia is usually, but not always, reversed when the thiazide diuretic is discontinued (10, 12). Some diabetic patients, but not all, may respond to increased potassium supplementation and/or higher doses of the hypoglycemic agent (1, 10, 15).

Recommendations—Diabetic patients controlled by diet or with oral hypoglycemic agents or insulin should be monitored closely for hyperglycemia and hypokalemia before and after thiazide or thiazide-like diuretics are initiated. Also, patients who have been maintained on such combination therapy should be observed for symptoms of hypoglycemia when the thiazide-like diuretic is withdrawn from the regimen. Since the development of hypokalemia may be responsible for the pathogenesis of this drug interaction, therapy should be geared to preventing abnormal potassium loss.

If hypokalemia occurs, it can be corrected by: (*a*) ensuring that the patient maintains a potassium-rich and low sodium diet (*e.g.*, bananas, dried dates, fruit juices, and peaches), (*b*) administering oral potassium supplements [liquid forms are preferred over slow-release tablets because the tablets, unlike the liquid, have been reported to cause gastrointestinal (GI) ulceration in a small number of patients with impaired motility of the GI tract (16–18)], or (*c*) administering potassium-sparing diuretics such as spironolactone or triamterene with the potassium-depleting diuretic. Additionally, the dose of the hypoglycemic drug may be increased or insulin therapy may be substituted in sufficient dosage to control the diabetic state.

Most studies, but not all, have shown that furosemide has little effect on the glucose tolerance of diabetic and nondiabetic patients (10, 14, 19, 20). Ethacrynic acid also is less likely to affect glucose tolerance (10, 20). Nevertheless, similar precautions should be exercised with diabetic patients taking ethacrynic acid or furosemide because there is still a possibility that a loss of diabetic control may occur.

References

(1) P. C. Kansal *et al.*, "Thiazide Diuretics and Control of Diabetes Mellitus," *S. Med. J.*, *62*, 1372 (1969).

(2) "The Pharmacological Basis of Therapeutics," 5th ed., L. S. Goodman and A. Gilman, Eds., Macmillan, New York, NY 10022, 1975, p. 829.

(3) S. S. Fajans *et al.*, "Benzothiadiazine Suppression of Insulin Release from Normal and Abnormal Islet Tissue in Man," *J. Clin. Invest.*, *45*, 481 (1966).

(4) W. Malaisse and F. Malaisse-Lagae, "Effect of Thiazides upon Insulin Secretion *In Vitro*," *Arch. Int. Pharmacodyn. Ther.*, *171*, 235 (1968).

(5) C. A. Barnett and J. E. Whitney, "The Effect of Diazoxide and Chlorothiazide on Glucose Uptake In Vitro," *Metabolism*, *15*, 88 (1966).

(6) J. B. Field and S. Mandell, "Effects of Thiazides on Glucose Uptake and Oxidation of Rat Muscle and Adipose Tissue," *Metabolism*, *13*, 959 (1964).

(7) H. P. Settle, Jr., *et al.*, "Toxic Effects of a Chlorothiazide–Diazoxide Combination on Adipose Tissue and Kidneys of Intact Rats," *Diabetologia*, *4*, 136 (1968).

(8) J. W. Conn, "Hypertension, The Potassium Ion and Impaired Carbohydrate Tolerance," *N. Engl. J. Med.*, *273*, 1135 (1965).

(9) J. W. Runyan, Jr., "Influence of Thiazide Diuretics on Carbohydrate Metabolism in Patients with Mild Diabetes," *N. Engl. J. Med.*, *267*, 541 (1962).

(10) E. M. Kohner *et al.*, "Effect of Diuretic Therapy on Glucose Tolerance in Hypertensive Patients," *Lancet*, i, 986 (1971).

(11) N. Samaan *et al.*, "Diabetogenic Action of Benzothiadiazines," *Lancet*, ii, 1244 (1963).

(12) A. D. Shapiro *et al.*, "Effect of Thiazides on Carbohydrate Metabolism in Patients with Hypertension," *N. Engl. J. Med.*, *265*, 1028 (1961).

(13) F. W. Wolf *et al.*, "Drug-Induced Diabetes," *J. Amer. Med. Ass.*, *185*, 568 (1963).

(14) A. Breckenridge *et al.*, "Glucose Tolerance in Hypertensive Patients on Long-Term Diuretic Therapy," *Lancet*, i, 61 (1967).

(15) M. I. Rapoport and H. F. Hurd, "Thiazide-Induced Glucose Intolerance Treated with Potassium," *Arch. Intern. Med.*, *113*, 405 (1964).

(16) M. A. Farquharson-Roberts *et al.*, "Perforation of Small Bowel Due to Slow Release Potassium Chloride (Slow-K)," *Brit. Med. J.*, *3*, 206 (1975).

(17) S. J. Heffernan and J. J. Murphy, "Ulceration of Small Intestine and Slow-Release Potassium Tablets," *Brit. Med. J.*, *2*, 746 (1975).

(18) "Who Needs Slow-Release Potassium Tablets," *Med. Lett.*, *17*, 73 (1975).

(19) W. P. U. Jackson and M. Nellen, "Effect of Frusemide on Carbohydrate Metabolism, Blood-Pressure and Other Modalities: A Comparison with Chlorothiazide," *Brit. Med. J.*, *2*, 333 (1966).

(20) A. Kaldor *et al.*, "Diabetogenic Effect of Oral Diuretics in Asymptomatic Diabetes," *Int. J. Clin. Pharmacol.*, *11*, 232 (1975).

[For additional information, see *Hypoglycemic Therapy*, p. 422.]

Nonproprietary and Trade Names of Drugs

Acetohexamide—*Dymelor*
Bendroflumethiazide—*Naturetin*
Benzthiazide—*Aquatag, Exna*
Chlorothiazide—*Diuril*
Chlorpropamide—*Diabinese*
Chlorthalidone—*Hygroton, Regroton*
Cyclothiazide—*Anhydron*
Ethacrynic acid—*Edecrin*
Flumethiazide—*Rautrax*
Furosemide—*Lasix*
Hydrochlorothiazide—*Esidrix, Hydro-Diuril, Oretic*
Hydroflumethiazide—*Saluron*

Insulin—*Iletin*
Mercaptomerin sodium—*Thiomerin*
Methyclothiazide—*Aquatensen, Enduron*
Metolazone—*Zaroxolyn*
Polythiazide—*Renese*
Quinethazone—*Hydromox*
Spironolactone—*Aldactone*
Tolazamide—*Tolinase*
Tolbutamide—*Orinase*
Triamterene—*Dyrenium*
Trichlormethiazide—*Metahydrin, Naqua*
Various combination products containing a diuretic are available.

Prepared and evaluated by the Scientific Review Subpanels on Hypoglycemic Agents and Diuretics and reviewed by Practitioner Panel V.

Dexamethasone—Phenobarbital

Summary—The systemic effects of administered corticosteroids such as the synthetic steroid dexamethasone and the natural hormone hydrocortisone (cortisol) may be diminished by large doses of barbiturates such as phenobarbital. If these drugs are used concurrently, the patient should be observed for symptoms of decreased corticosteroid effectiveness.

Related Drugs—In addition to dexamethasone and **hydrocortisone, methylprednisolone** (1) and **prednisone** (2) have been shown to interact with phenobarbital in humans. Other corticosteroids such as **betamethasone, cortisone, fludrocortisone, fluprednisolone, meprednisone, paramethasone, prednisolone,** and **triamcinolone** also may be expected to interact with phenobarbital, although there have been no reports documenting such interactions.

Barbital (3) and **pentobarbital** (4) have been shown to interact with corticosteroids. Until more clinical data are available, other **barbiturates** also could be expected to affect corticosteroid metabolism.

Pharmacological Effect and Mechanism—Barbiturates inhibit the physiological production of cortisol through interference with adrenocorticotropin hormone (ACTH) production in rats, particularly in stressful situations (4, 5). The decreased ACTH production could be causally related to the abnormal behavior (*i.e.,* increased "maze running time," increased food intake, and concomitant weight increase) of rats chronically treated with barbital sodium since ACTH can antagonize these effects, possibly through a central mechanism (6). When barbiturates are withdrawn, ACTH-treated rats exhibited increased hyperexcitability and seizures compared with rats treated with a barbiturate only (7).

Barbiturates also enhance the metabolism and degradation of various drugs including corticosteroids. Studies in rats and humans indicated that steroid hormones act as substrates for drug-metabolizing enzymes in liver microsomes (8). Barbiturate administration can cause the induction of hepatic microsomal drug-metabolizing enzymes in rats (8) and has been shown to influence the metabolism of testosterone and cortisol (hydrocortisone) in humans (9, 10).

The net effect of this barbiturate induction is an increase in production of polar metabolites of cortisol of which the major component is 6β-hydroxycortisol (9, 11).

Evaluation of Clinical Data—Five chronic schizophrenic females (who were not receiving any other medication) were given phenobarbital (260–520 mg/day po) (11). Three subjects were later given a single dose of hydrocortisone (300 mg po) with and without phenobarbital. The results showed a highly significant increase ($\sim$ two- to threefold) in the urinary excretion of 6β-hydroxycortisol following administration of phenobarbital.

The effects of phenobarbital therapy (120 mg/day po in four divided doses for 3 weeks) on plasma kinetics of labeled dexamethasone were investigated in 11 asthmatic patients (2). Phenobarbital caused a 44% mean decrease in the serum half-life and an 88% increase in the metabolic clearance rate of dexamethasone when compared with values obtained before phenobarbital treatment in the same group. All other medication had been discontinued 3 weeks prior to the study except in three patients who were receiving prednisone. These three patients had poorly controlled asthma and had been taking prednisone for more than 6 months. Attempts to discontinue prednisone were unsuccessful. After the administration of phenobarbital, the patients showed clinical deterioration, decreased pulmonary function, and a rise in the eosinophil count (indicative of the decreased adrenocorticosteroid effect). Their status improved after discontinuation of phenobarbital. The non-prednisone-dependent patients did not show similar changes after phenobarbital therapy.

■ It is likely that continued administration of phenobarbital and other barbiturates reduces the effectiveness of corticosteroids in steroid-dependent patients with asthma. This effect appears to be dose related (12) and has only been observed with high doses of phenobarbital used in long-term therapy. Although not documented, barbiturates also may decrease the effectiveness of corticosteroids in replacement therapy for adrenal insufficiency (*e.g.,* in Addison's disease).

Recommendations—Phenobarbital and other barbiturates are present in many combination products, but they are probably present in low enough amounts not to effect the metabolism of the corticosteroids if the drugs are taken concurrently (10).

However, if phenobarbital or other barbiturates are administered in high doses (at least 120 mg of phenobarbital/day in adults) to steroid-dependent patients, these patients should be observed for clinical evidence of decreased corticosteroid effectiveness. If a drug interaction occurs, an alternative drug should be considered or the dose of the corticosteroid should be increased. The benzodiazepines may be used as alternatives to barbiturates for antianxiety and sedative effects, but they may cause respiratory depression and should be used with caution in patients with compromised pulmonary function (13).

All patients requiring either physiological replacement or pharmacological doses of glucocorticoids should be assessed clinically for adrenal function and/or pharmacological response to steroids after treatment with barbiturates. Barbiturates should be administered with care to patients with borderline hypoadrenal function, whether of pituitary or primary adrenal origin.

For analogous reasons, the dexamethasone suppression test may give false-positive results (*i.e.*, erroneously categorize patients as nonsuppressible) in patients receiving barbiturates, due to acceleration of hepatic microsomal enzyme activity (8).

References

(1) M. R. Stjernholm and F. H. Katz, "Effects of Diphenylhydantoin, Phenobarbital, and Diazepam on the Metabolism of Methylprednisolone and Its Sodium Succinate," *J. Clin. Endocrinol. Metab.*, *41*, 887 (1975).

(2) S. M. Brooks *et al.*, "Adverse Effects of Phenobarbital on Corticosteroid Metabolism in Patients with Bronchial Asthma," *N. Engl. J. Med.*, *286*, 1125 (1972).

(3) S. Burstein *et al.*, "Metabolism of 2α- and 6β-Hydroxycortisol in Man: Determination of Production Rates of 6β-Hydroxycortisol with and without Phenobarbital Administration," *J. Clin. Endocrinol.*, *27*, 491 (1967).

(4) C. Rerup and P. Hedner, "The Effect of Pentobarbital (Nembutal, Mebumal NFN) on Corticotrophin Release in the Rat," *Acta Endocrinol.*, *39*, 518 (1962).

(5) B. E. Leonard, "The Effect of the Chronic Administration of Barbitone Sodium on Pituitary-Adrenal Function in the Rat," *Biochem. Pharmacol.*, *15*, 263 (1966).

(6) B. E. Leonard, "The Effect of Sodium Barbitone, Alone and Together with ACTH and Amphetamine, on the Behavior of the Rat in the Multiple 'T' Maze," *Int. J. Neuropharmacol.*, *8*, 427 (1969).

(7) C. Torda and H. G. Wolff, "Effects of Various Concentrations of Adrenocorticotrophic Hormone on Electrical Activity of Brain and on Sensitivity to Convulsion-Inducing Agents," *Amer. J. Physiol.*, *168*, 406 (1952).

(8) R. M. Kuntzman *et al.*, "Stimulatory Effect of N-Phenylbarbital (Phetharbital) on Cortisol Hydroxylation in Man," *Biochem. Pharmacol.*, *17*, 565 (1968).

(9) A. L. Southren *et al.*, "Effect of N-Phenylbarbital (Phetharbital) on the Metabolism of Testosterone and Cortisol in Man," *J. Clin. Endocrinol. Metab.*, *29*, 251 (1969).

(10) P. L. Morselli *et al.*, "Metabolism of Exogenous Cortisol in Humans. Influence of Phenobarbital Treatment on Plasma Cortisol Disappearance Rate," *Rev. Eur. Etudes, Clin. Biol.*, *15*, 195 (1970).

(11) S. Burstein and E. L. Klaiber, "Phenobarbital-Induced Increase in 6-β-Hydroxycortisol Excretion: Clue to Its Significance in Human Urine," *J. Clin. Endocrinol.*, *25*, 293 (1965).

(12) C. J. Falliers, "Corticosteroids and Phenobarbital in Asthma," *N. Engl. J. Med.*, *287*, 201 (1972).

(13) "Benzodiazepines in Clinical Practice," D. J. Greenblatt and R. I. Shader, Eds., Raven, New York, NY 10024, 1974, pp. 147–148.

[For additional information, see *Corticosteroid Therapy*, p. 411.]

Nonproprietary and Trade Names of Drugs

Allobarbital—*Diadol*
Amobarbital—*Amytal and various combination products*
Aprobarbital—*Alurate*
Barbital—*Neurondia*
Betamethasone—*Celestone*

Butabarbital sodium—*Butisol Sodium*
Butalbital—*Available in combination products*
Cortisone acetate—*Cortone Acetate*
Dexamethasone—*Decadron, Hexadrol*
Fludrocortisone acetate—*Florinef Acetate*

Fluprednisolone—*Alphadrol*
Hexobarbital—*Sombulex*
Hydrocortisone—*Various manufacturers*
Mephobarbital—*Mebaral, Mebroin*
Meprednisone—*Betapar*
Metharbital—*Gemonil*
Methohexital sodium—*Brevital Sodium*
Methylprednisolone—*Medrol*
Paramethasone acetate—*Haldrone*
Pentobarbital—*Nembutal and various com-
  bination products*

Phenobarbital—*Eskabarb, Luminal*
Prednisolone—*Delta-Cortef, Meticortelone,
  Sterane*
Prednisone—*Delta-dome, Deltasone, Deltra,
  Meticorten, Paracort*
Secobarbital—*Seconal and various combi-
  nation products*
Talbutal—*Lotusate*
Thiopental sodium—*Pentothal Sodium*
Triamcinolone—*Aristocort, Kenacort*

*Prepared and evaluated by the Scientific Review Sub-
panel on Steroids and reviewed by Practitioner Panel V.*

Dexamethasone—Phenytoin*

Summary—Phenytoin impairs the response to dexamethasone in the dexamethasone suppression test. It has not been determined if this effect of phenytoin is
sufficient to impair the therapeutic response to dexamethasone. However, patients should be observed for diminished therapeutic effects of dexamethasone
when these drugs are used concurrently.

Related Drugs—Phenytoin is also known to increase the metabolism of **hydrocortisone
(cortisol)** (1) and **methylprednisolone** (2) in humans. It is likely that other corticosteroids such as **betamethasone, cortisone, fludrocortisone, fluprednisolone, meprednisone,
paramethasone, prednisolone, prednisone,** and **triamcinolone** would interact similarly.
    Although this drug interaction has been reported only with phenytoin, it may also
occur with other hydantoins such as **ethotoin** and **mephenytoin** as well as with other
chemically and pharmacologically similar anticonvulsants such as **primidone.**

Pharmacological Effect and Mechanism—Phenytoin inhibits the suppression of plasma cortisol (hydrocortisone) levels following administration of dexamethasone (dexamethasone suppression test) (3–7). One study (4) in rats indicated that phenytoin
may accelerate hepatic conjugation and biliary excretion of dexamethasone. The study
also eliminated the possibility that phenytoin decreased the gastrointestinal absorption
of dexamethasone. In the same report, urinary levels of total and conjugated steroids
were increased in humans. However, in other human studies measuring the metabolic kinetics of this interaction, phenytoin may have increased dexamethasone
metabolism by enhancing its conversion to unconjugated metabolites of greater
polarity (8, 9).

Evaluation of Clinical Data—In seven patients without Cushing's syndrome, phenytoin treatment (300–400 mg/day po for 2–16 months) resulted in interference in the
plasma cortisol (hydrocortisone) response in the dexamethasone suppression test (3).
This effect was considerable when compared to the results obtained in the absence of
phenytoin therapy in some of the same patients. The effect of phenytoin on the urinary
17-hydroxycorticosteroid–dexamethasone suppression test may not be as great as its
effect on the plasma cortisol–dexamethasone suppression test, but it may be sufficient
to cause confusion in diagnosis.

---
*Phenytoin is the new official name for diphenylhydantoin.

The plasma corticosteroid level following the dexamethasone suppression test (0.5 mg po every 6 hr for eight doses) in nine patients receiving chronic phenytoin therapy (4) was markedly higher than that of control subjects (indicating a lack of suppression of dexamethasone). This effect was not seen when larger doses of dexamethasone (*e.g.*, 8.0 mg/day po for 8 days) were used in the test. Another study (5) showed that the dexamethasone suppression test in patients with primary open angle glaucoma was inhibited by phenytoin pretreatment, although to a smaller degree than in normal patients.

Twenty patients with supratentorial tumors required greater than normally prescribed doses of dexamethasone to control accompanying cerebral edema (10). Eighteen of the 20 patients were receiving phenytoin, which possibly impaired the clinical effectiveness of dexamethasone and necessitated the higher doses.

A 15-year-old patient suffering from systemic lupus erythematosus was switched from prednisone to an "equivalent" dose of dexamethasone (16 mg/day po) (11). The patient also was receiving phenytoin (300 mg/day po). The patient's condition deteriorated when switched to dexamethasone. The patient's temperature increased and anemia and leukopenia occurred. The deterioration was reversed when the patient was switched back to prednisone. The investigators attributed the ineffectiveness of dexamethasone to concurrent administration of phenytoin, but it may have been due to too low a dose of dexamethasone. The effect of increasing the dose of dexamethasone or of administering dexamethasone without phenytoin was not investigated.

■ The effect of phenytoin on dexamethasone suppression tests is well documented and of sufficient magnitude to cause difficulty in interpretation of results. Practitioners evaluating these suppression tests must be aware of which patients are receiving phenytoin. The clinical data describing inhibition of the therapeutic effect of dexamethasone by phenytoin are insufficient to predict the clinical outcome of this interaction.

Recommendations—Dexamethasone suppression tests should be interpreted with caution in patients receiving phenytoin. Drugs other than phenytoin that may act through hepatic enzyme induction such as the barbiturates (see *Dexamethasone–Phenobarbital*, p. 42) also should be considered suspect until more information is available. If the dexamethasone suppression test is used in patients who have been receiving phenytoin (or other enzyme inducers) chronically, a higher dose of dexamethasone (2 mg every 6 hr for six doses) may be useful.

Based on current information, there is no contraindication to concurrent therapy with dexamethasone and phenytoin. However, pending further information, patients receiving both drugs concurrently should be observed for possible diminution of the therapeutic effect of dexamethasone.

References

(1) E. E. Werk *et al.*, "Cortisol Production in Epileptic Patients Treated with Diphenylhydantoin," *Clin. Pharmacol. Ther.*, *12*, 698 (1971).

(2) M. J. Stjernholm and F. H. Katz, "Effects of Diphenylhydantoin, Phenobarbital, and Diazepam on the Metabolism of Methylprednisolone and Its Sodium Succinate," *J. Clin. Endocrinol. Metab.*, *41*, 887 (1975).

(3) E. E. Werk *et al.*, "Interference in the Effect of Dexamethasone by Diphenylhydantoin," *N. Engl. J. Med.*, *281*, 32 (1969).

(4) W. Jubiz *et al.*, "Effect of Diphenylhydantoin on the Metabolism of Dexamethasone. Mechanism of the Abnormal Dexamethasone Suppression in Humans," *N. Engl. J. Med.*, *283*, 11 (1970).

(5) B. Becker *et al.*, "Diphenylhydantoin and Dexamethasone-Induced Changes of Plasma Cortisol: Comparison of Patients with and without Glaucoma," *J. Clin. Endocrinol.*, *32*, 669 (1971).

(6) W. Jubiz *et al.*, "Failure of Dexamethasone Suppression in Patients on Chronic Diphenylhydantoin Therapy," *Clin. Res.*, *17*, 106 (1969).

(7) "Laboratory Test Works in Patients on Medication," *J. Amer. Med. Ass.,* *225*, 1586 (1973).

(8) N. Haque *et al.,* "Studies on Dexamethasone Metabolism in Man: Effect of Diphenylhydantoin," *J. Clin. Endocrinol., 34,* 44 (1972).

(9) N. Haque *et al.,* "Studies on Dexamethasone Metabolism in Man: Effect of Diphenylhydantoin," *Lab. Clin. Med., 76,* 865 (1970).

(10) J. Ranauden *et al.,* "Dose Dependency of Decadron in Patients with Partially Excised Brain Tumors," *J. Neurosurg., 39,* 302 (1973).

(11) J. J. Boylan *et al.,* "Phenytoin Interference with Dexamethasone," letter to the editor, *J. Amer. Med. Ass., 235,* 802 (1976).

[For additional information, see *Corticosteroid Therapy,* p. 411, and *Dexamethasone–Phenobarbital,* p. 42.]

Nonproprietary and Trade Names of Drugs

Betamethasone—*Celestone*
Cortisone acetate—*Cortone Acetate*
Dexamethasone—*Decadron, Hexadrol*
Ethotoin—*Peganone*
Fludrocortisone acetate—*Florinef Acetate*
Fluprednisolone—*Alphadrol*
Hydrocortisone—*Various manufacturers*
Mephenytoin—*Mesantoin*
Meprednisone—*Betapar*

Methylprednisolone—*Medrol*
Paramethasone acetate—*Haldrone*
Phenytoin—*Dilantin*
Prednisolone—*Delta-Cortef, Meticortelone, Sterane*
Prednisone—*Delta-dome, Deltasone, Deltra, Meticorten, Paracort*
Primidone—*Mysoline*
Triamcinolone—*Aristocort, Kenacort*

Prepared and evaluated by the Scientific Review Subpanel on Steroids and reviewed by Practitioner Panel IV.

Diazepam—Alcohol

Summary—Concurrent ingestion of diazepam and alcohol causes an intensification of the central nervous system (CNS) effects of each drug. Contradictory evidence indicates that chlordiazepoxide may antagonize, enhance, or exert no effect on the CNS effects of alcohol. Patients receiving any benzodiazepine compound should be warned to avoid alcohol, since concurrent ingestion could result in an impairment of their ability to drive an automobile or operate hazardous machinery.

Related Drugs—**Chlordiazepoxide** (1) and **nitrazepam** (2) have been reported to interact with alcohol, although reports evaluating the effects of chlordiazepoxide on alcohol are contradictory. Other **benzodiazepines** may interact similarly with alcohol.

Pharmacological Effect and Mechanism—The mechanism of action of the reported drug interaction between diazepam or other benzodiazepines and alcohol is not known. Studies on the absorption, metabolism, and excretion of alcohol and the benzodiazepines showed that these parameters are unaffected by concurrent ingestion (3–7). The most popular theory is that the interaction takes place at the receptor sites in the CNS (4, 5).

Evaluation of Clinical Data—The short-term effects of diazepam and alcohol were determined in 40 healthy subjects (8). Single doses of diazepam (5–10 mg po) and alcohol (0.5–0.8 g/kg po) were given concurrently and the subjects performed various psychomotor tests designed to simulate skills necessary for driving an automobile or operating machinery. The study was double blind with a control group, and the data were analyzed statistically. Neither alcohol nor diazepam significantly affected these psychomotor skills but together these drugs significantly impaired the subject's performance. This effect occurred within 30 min after concurrent ingestion.

The same investigators, using the same trial design, later measured the effects of alcohol on long-term administration of diazepam (9). Diazepam (15 mg/day po) was administered to 20 subjects for 2 weeks, and alcohol (0.5 g/kg po) was given on Days 1 and 14. The long-term administration of diazepam was more deleterious on psychomotor performance than short-term administration. Concurrent ingestion of alcohol produced a more pronounced enhancement after short-term administration of diazepam than after long-term administration. The most significant effects of this drug interaction occurred within 30 min after alcohol ingestion.

Additional studies by the same investigators (2, 10) with the same study design showed that concurrent use of diazepam and alcohol significantly impaired subjects' performances in simulated driving conditions (*e.g.*, monotonous and emergency situations) and that alcohol can enhance the effects of an evening dose of diazepam (10 mg po) when administered 10 hr later in the morning. Other investigators (5) using different test conditions observed similar impairment of psychomotor performance after concurrent ingestion of diazepam (10 mg po) and alcohol (0.74 g/kg po).

The reported effects from concurrent ingestion of chlordiazepoxide and alcohol are conflicting. Chlordiazepoxide has been shown to have no effect or an additive or synergistic effect on the CNS depression induced by alcohol.

The effects of chlordiazepoxide (50 mg po during a 36-hr period) alone and with alcohol (0.5 g/kg po) in 20 healthy subjects were measured in a double-blind controlled study (11). The subjects' ability to drive or control a vehicle was determined, and an objective assessment scale of the emotional, behavioral, and neurological characteristics of each person was utilized. There was no significant evidence of any impairment in the subjects' performances in these tests when chlordiazepoxide was administered alone or with alcohol. Other well-controlled studies reported similar results with different study designs (12–14). These studies utilized healthy subjects, and varying doses of chlordiazepoxide (15–40 mg/day po for up to 4 days) and alcohol (~ 0.81–1.21 g/kg po) were used.

Chlordiazepoxide also has been reported to antagonize the depressant effects of alcohol. This antagonism was found in a controlled study of 80 females scheduled for minor gynecological surgery (6) who were given alcohol (up to 550 ml iv of an 8% solution) as an anesthetic. In these patients, the preanesthetic dose of chlordiazepoxide (100–140 mg im) caused a significant antagonism of the effects of alcohol. When chlordiazepoxide was used, the amount of alcohol needed to induce sleep was much larger than in the control group and the length of time for induction was longer. The investigators also noted that more patients receiving chlordiazepoxide were delirious during the induction phase of the anesthetic and in the postoperative phase than in the control group. Diazepam (30 mg im) also was tested in another group of 62 patients, and no antagonism (or enhancement) was observed.

A similar antagonism also was observed at lower doses of chlordiazepoxide and alcohol (7). Chlordiazepoxide (20 mg/day po) and alcohol (0.33–0.66 g/kg po) were given concurrently to eight healthy subjects. Estimates were made of the subjective mood of these subjects and their objective performance. The results indicated that chlordiazepoxide counteracted the effect of alcohol in most subjective moods and also the objective performance of the subjects.

Chlordiazepoxide also was reported to enhance the impairment of driving skills caused by alcohol (1). In a double-blind controlled study of 40 healthy subjects, chlordiazepoxide (10–25 mg po) alone and with alcohol (0.5–0.8 g/kg po) caused a deleterious effect on the subjects' coordination and reaction times, skills necessary for careful driving. This effect was slightly less than the effects of diazepam (5–10 mg po) and alcohol (0.5–0.8 g/kg po) given concurrently to another group of subjects in the same experiment. The investigators postulated that the difference in results from this study and previous experiments may have been due to the type of psychomotor skills measured in the other studies. Another study (15) of the effects of chlordiazepoxide (10–20 mg po) and alcohol (blood alcohol levels, 80 mg/100 ml) on driving ability also reported that these drugs enhance each other's depressant effects.

The effect of alcohol (0.5 g/kg po) on hypnotic doses of nitrazepam (5–10 mg po) was measured in two controlled studies of healthy subjects (2, 16). In each study, alcohol was ingested 10 hr after an evening dose of nitrazepam. The results showed a significant impairment in psychomotor ability and coordination. This report also suggested that middle-aged and older subjects are more sensitive to the effects of benzodiazepines.

■ Chlordiazepoxide has been reported to antagonize (6, 7), enhance (1, 15), or exert no influence (11–14) on the CNS depressant effects of alcohol. However, there are substantial data to indicate that diazepam (2, 5, 8–10) and nitrazepam (2, 16) enhance the CNS depressant effects of alcohol.

The different results from the numerous experiments on this drug interaction are probably due to the different experimental designs used, the skills measured as test parameters, the doses used, relative potency of each benzodiazepine, and the length of the experiment. Most studies used single doses of the drugs, but cumulative dose studies of a week or more have shown a more pronounced effect (10). One report (14) suggested that the differences in the results of many experiments may be due to the psychomotor skill measured. Chlordiazepoxide and diazepam have been reported to antagonize the effects of alcohol on the measured attention of subjects but can enhance the effects of alcohol on the subjects' reactive and coordinative skills. It has also been suggested (8, 10, 13) that deficiencies in study design such as inadequate practice time, poor choice of subjects, and the failure to eliminate influencing factors such as fatigue or the placebo effect may have influenced the results. Additionally, most studies were done using simulated driving conditions or other artificial environments in an attempt to approximate actual driving conditions. Many investigators (5, 8, 13) question the validity of extrapolating the results acquired from these test environments to the actual conditions of driving or operating machinery.

Recommendations—Patients receiving a benzodiazepine should avoid using alcohol. If patients treated with a benzodiazepine drink alcohol, they should be warned that alcohol may produce greater impairment of their ability to drive an automobile and that it could endanger their safety in operating hazardous machinery. The patient should be aware that this drug interaction can occur 30 min after simultaneous ingestion (8) or even if alcohol is ingested 10 hr after the last benzodiazepine dose (2).

Other CNS depressant drugs such as chloral hydrate (see *Chloral Hydrate–Alcohol*, p. 20), ethchlorvynol (17), glutethimide (18), meprobamate (see *Meprobamate–Alcohol*, p. 145), phenobarbital (see *Phenobarbital–Alcohol*, p. 180), and possibly methaqualone (19) interact with alcohol in a manner similar to diazepam.

References

(1) M. Linnoila, "Effects of Diazepam, Chlordiazepoxide, Thioridazine, Haloperidol, Flupenthixole and Alcohol on Psychomotor Skills Related to Driving," *Ann. Exp. Med. Biol. Fenn., 51,* 125 (1973).

(2) M. Linnoila, "Drug Interaction on Psychomotor Skills Related to Driving: Hypnotics and Alcohol," *Ann. Exp. Med. Biol. Fenn., 51,* 118 (1973).

(3) M. Linnoila *et al.,* "Serum Chlordiazepoxide, Diazepam and Thioridazine Concentrations after the Simultaneous Ingestion of Alcohol or Placebo Drink," *Ann. Clin. Res., 6,* 4 (1974).

(4) P. L. Morselli *et al.,* "Further Observations on the Interaction between Ethanol and Psychotropic Drugs," *Arzneim.-Forsch., 21,* 20 (1971).

(5) J. Morland *et al.,* "Combined Effects of Diazepam and Ethanol on Mental and Psychomotor Functions," *Acta Pharmacol. Toxicol., 34,* 5 (1974).

(6) J. W. Dundee *et al.,* "Alcohol and the Benzodiazepines," *Quart. J. Stud. Alc., 32,* 960 (1971).

(7) L. Goldberg, "Behavioral and Physiological Effects of Alcohol on Man," *Psychosom. Med., 28,* 570 (1966).

(8) M. Linnoila and M. J. Mattila, "Drug Interaction on Psychomotor Skills Related to Driving: Diazepam and Alcohol," *Eur. J. Clin. Pharmacol.,* 5, 186 (1973).

(9) M. Linnoila *et al.,* "Effect of Treatment with Diazepam or Lithium and Alcohol on Psychomotor Skills Related to Driving," *Eur. J. Clin. Pharmacol.,* 7, 337 (1974).

(10) M. Linnoila and S. Hakkinen, "Effects of Diazepam and Codeine, Alone and in Combination with Alcohol, on Simulated Driving," *Clin. Pharmacol. Ther., 15,* 368 (1974).

(11) T. A. Betts *et al.,* "Effects of Four Commonly-Used Tranquillizers on Low-Speed Driving Performance Tests," *Brit. Med. J., 4,* 580 (1972).

(12) A. Hoffer, "Lack of Potentiation by Chlordiazepoxide (Librium) of Depression or Excitation Due to Alcohol," *Can. Med. Ass. J., 87,* 920 (1962).

(13) A. I. Miller *et al.,* "Effects of Combined Chlordiazepoxide and Alcohol in Man," *Quart. J. Stud. Alc., 24,* 9 (1963).

(14) F. W. Hughes *et al.,* "Comparative Effect in Human Subjects of Chlordiazepoxide, Diazepam, and Placebo on Mental and Physical Performance," *Clin. Pharmacol. Ther., 6,* 139 (1965).

(15) P. Kielholz *et al.,* "Tests of Driving Ability for Estimating the Effects of Alcohol, Tranquilizers and Hypnotics," *Deut. Med. Wochenschr., 94,* 301 (1969).

(16) I. Saario *et al.,* "Interaction of Drugs with Alcohol on Human Psychomotor Skills Related to Driving: Effect of Sleep Deprivation or Two Weeks' Treatment with Hypnotics," *J. Clin. Pharmacol., 15,* 52 (1975).

(17) A. Flemenbaum and B. Gunby, "Ethchlorvynol (Placidyl) Abuse and Withdrawal (Review of Clinical Picture and Report of Two Cases)," *Dis. Nerv. Syst., 32,* 188 (1971).

(18) G. P. Mould *et al.,* "Interaction of Glutethimide and Phenobarbitone with Ethanol in Man," *J. Pharm. Pharmacol., 24,* 894 (1972).

(19) D. S. Inaba *et al.,* "Methaqualone Abuse. 'Luding Out'," *J. Amer. Med. Ass., 224,* 1505 (1973).

[For additional information, see *Sedative–Hypnotic Therapy,* p. 442.]

Nonproprietary and Trade Names of Drugs

Alcohol—*Various products and beverages*
Chloral hydrate—*Kessodrate, Noctec, Somnos*
Chlordiazepoxide—*Libritabs*
Chlordiazepoxide hydrochloride—*Librium and various combination products*
Clonazepam—*Clonopin*
Clorazepate dipotassium—*Tranxene*
Diazepam—*Valium*

Ethchlorvynol—*Placidyl*
Flurazepam hydrochloride—*Dalmane*
Glutethimide—*Doriden*
Meprobamate—*Equanil, Meprospan, Miltown, and various combination products*
Methaqualone—*Quaalude, Sopor*
Nitrazepam—*Mogadon*
Oxazepam—*Serax*
Phenobarbital—*Eskabarb, Luminal*

Prepared and evaluated by the Scientific Review Subpanel on Psychotropic Agents and reviewed by Practitioner Panel VI.

Digitalis—Calcium

Summary—An increase in the serum calcium concentration markedly enhances the action of digitalis, whereas calcium chelators which decrease the serum calcium level diminish the effects of the cardiac glycosides. Although there are inconclusive clinical data about this drug interaction, care should be used when rapidly administering intravenous calcium to patients receiving digitalis therapy.

Related Drugs—Cardiac glycosides commonly used in therapy that would be expected to interact similarly include **acetyldigitoxin, deslanoside, digitoxin, digoxin, gitalin, lanatoside C,** and **ouabain.**

Various calcium salts such as the **carbonate, chloride, gluceptate,** and **gluconate** which provide calcium ions are available alone or in combination.

Pharmacological Effect and Mechanism—An increase in the intracellular concentration of calcium ion can activate the contractile mechanism in a cell, and contraction in cardiac muscle has been associated with an enhanced influx of calcium (1). Isotope studies have substantiated the hypothesis that calcium is essentially involved in the inotropic action of the cardiac glycosides (1). The administration of calcium greatly enhances the action of all cardiotonic drugs (2), while calcium chelators counteract or diminish their effects (3). Many actions of digitalis in the heart are similar to those of calcium (3). The cardiac glycosides usually produce a net loss of potassium from the myocardium and since potassium is physiologically antagonistic to calcium, its loss enhances the action of calcium on the contractile elements (3, 4). An increase in calcium reduces the concentration of ouabain necessary to cause blockade of the chronotropic response to vagal stimulation (5).

High doses of calcium administered by intravenous infusion to dogs enhanced the sensitivity of the heart muscle to digitalis-induced arrhythmias (2). The dose of the digitalis glycosides needed to produce these arrhythmias was reduced by approximately one-third in the presence of high doses of calcium.

Cardiac arrhythmias believed to be due to digitalis intoxication were lessened or abolished *via* calcium chelation by the administration of edetate disodium (6). The reduction in serum ionizable calcium induced by the administration of edetate disodium to digitalis-treated subjects is attended by a prompt and consistent reversal of the digitalis-induced shortening of the ejection time index (7).

Evaluation of Clinical Data—The only clinical report of this drug interaction described two deaths that occurred following the intramuscular injection of digitalis and the intravenous injection of calcium gluconate or chloride (8). However, no definite cause and effect relationship was established between these deaths and concurrent use of calcium and digitalis. A lowering of the concentration of calcium in blood has been reported to decrease or abolish cardiac arrhythmias due to digitalis intoxication (6, 7, 9).

■ Although the administration (particularly intravenous) of calcium to patients receiving digitalis may increase the possibility of digitalis-induced arrhythmias, the human data about the significance of this drug interaction are inconclusive. Although a drug interaction occurs in animals, the amount of calcium used in these studies was much greater than the maximum calcium levels expected to be present in humans (2).

Recommendations—If intravenous administration of calcium is necessary in patients receiving digitalis therapy, it is recommended that this procedure be accomplished slowly and with caution. Edetate disodium may be useful for treating the hypercalcemia that may occur during digitalis toxicity (6, 7), but this drug should be used cautiously in patients with hypokalemia and congestive heart failure and should not be given to patients with renal failure (10).

References

(1) W. G. Nayler, "Calcium Exchange in Cardiac Muscle: A Basic Mechanism of Drug Action," *Amer. Heart J., 73,* 379 (1967).

(2) G. T. Nola *et al.,* "Assessment of the Synergistic Relationship between Serum Calcium and Digitalis," *Amer. Heart J., 79,* 499 (1970).

(3) T. R. Sherrod, "The Cardiac Glycosides," *Hosp. Practice, 2,* 56 (1967).

(4) D. T. Mason, "Digitalis Pharmacology and Therapeutics: Recent Advances," *Ann. Intern. Med., 80,* 520 (1974).

(5) N. Toda and T. C. West, "Modification by Sodium and Calcium of the Cardiotoxicity Induced by Ouabain," *J. Pharmacol. Exp. Ther., 154,* 239 (1966).

(6) S. Jick and R. Karsh, "The Effect of Calcium Chelation on Cardiac Arrhythmias and Conduction Disturbances," *Amer. J. Cardiol., 43,* 287 (1959).

(7) S. Cohen *et al.,* "Antagonism of the Contractile Effect of Digitalis by

(8) J. O. Bower and H. A. K. Mengle, "The Additive Effects of Calcium and Digitalis," *J. Amer. Med. Ass., 106,* 1151 (1936).

(9) B. Surawicz *et al.,* "Treatment of Cardiac Arrhythmias with Salts of Ethylenediamine Tetraacetic Acid (EDTA)," *Amer. Heart J., 58,* 493 (1959).

(10) "The Pharmacological Basis of Therapeutics," 5th ed., L. S. Goodman and A. Gilman, Eds., Macmillan, New York, NY 10022, 1975, p. 587.

EDTA in the Normal Human Ventricle," *Amer. Heart J., 69,* 502 (1965).

[For additional information, see *Cardiac Glycoside Therapy,* p. 407.]

Nonproprietary and Trade Names of Drugs

Acetyldigitoxin—*Acylanid*
Calcium carbonate, chloride, gluceptate, and gluconate—*Various manufacturers*
Deslanoside—*Cedilanid-D*
Digitalis—*Various manufacturers*
Digitoxin—*Crystodigin, Digitaline Nativelle, Myodigin, Purodigin*

Digoxin—*Lanoxin*
Gitalin—*Gitaligin*
Lanatoside C—*Cedilanid*
Ouabain—*Various manufacturers*

Prepared and evaluated by the Scientific Review Subpanel on Cardiac Glycosides and reviewed by Practitioner Panel III.

Digitalis—Chlorothiazide

Summary—Patients receiving chlorothiazide and related diuretics may develop electrolyte disturbances (*e.g.,* primarily hypokalemia, but also hypomagnesemia and hypercalcemia) which may enhance the cardiotoxicity of digitalis. Electrolyte values and liver, renal, and cardiac function should be monitored closely to avoid cardiac manifestations of digitalis toxicity (*e.g.,* arrhythmias).

Related Drugs—Digitalis glycosides reported to interact with diuretics are **digitalis leaf** (1–3), **digitoxin** (1, 2), **digoxin** (1, 2, 4), and **lanatoside C** (3). Other cardiac glycosides expected to interact include **acetyldigitoxin, gitalin,** and **ouabain.**

All **potassium-depleting diuretics** can be expected to interact with cardiac glycosides in a similar manner. In addition to **thiazide diuretics,** such interactions have been documented with **chlorthalidone** (3, 5), **ethacrynic acid** (3), **furosemide** (3, 4), and **mercurial diuretics** (1–3). **Metolazone** and **quinethazone** are structurally related to thiazide diuretics, can cause hypokalemia (6), and may be expected to interact with cardiac glycosides. Potassium-depleting diuretics also are available in many combination products.

Pharmacological Effect and Mechanism—The digitalis glycosides enhance contraction in the failing or normal heart and improve cardiac output (7–11). The proposed mechanism of this action is inhibition of the enzyme (sodium–potassium adenosine triphosphatase) that controls the sodium–potassium pump, resulting in the inhibition of potassium and sodium transport across the cell membrane (12). The intracellular sodium level is increased, thereby stimulating sodium–calcium transport and providing a greater quantity of calcium to the contractile apparatus in the myocardium. Excitation–contraction coupling is enhanced, and more forceful myocardial contractions occur (7).

Chlorthalidone, ethacrynic acid, furosemide, mercurial diuretics, and thiazide diuretics may cause hypokalemia which will enhance the cardiotoxic effects of the digitalis glycosides (1–5, 7, 13). Extracellular hypokalemia occurs quite often but intracellular hypokalemia does not occur as frequently (14–16). Extracellular potassium probably competes with digitalis glycosides for binding to the enzyme which controls the sodium–potassium pump (7). If extracellular potassium is decreased, more digitalis is bound to the enzyme, thus inhibiting the pump and causing less potassium to be pumped into the cell. Myocardial contractility increases, and arrhythmias may occur (7, 12).

The theory that hypokalemia induces digitalis toxicity has been questioned by the observation that acute or chronic hypokalemia did not sensitize the dog heart to digitalis (17). However, other investigators (18, 19) stated that these animal results cannot be extrapolated to humans because of the differences in drug administration, physiology between the dog and the human heart, and environmental conditions.

Potassium-depleting diuretics can cause magnesium deficiency. Hypomagnesemia also may inhibit the activity of the sodium–potassium pump, resulting in decreased tissue potassium and possibly digitalis toxicity (20–24). Ethacrynic acid and furosemide may increase calcium excretion while chlorthalidone and thiazide diuretics may decrease calcium excretion (22, 25). Decreased serum calcium levels could decrease the inotropic effect of digitalis (26), and increased serum calcium levels could increase the effect (27).

Evaluation of Clinical Data—In a 12-month study of 88 patients who exhibited 92 episodes of cardiotoxicity attributed to digitalis intoxication, 61 patients (69%) also were receiving thiazide or mercurial diuretics (28). All types of digitalis preparations were employed, but digoxin, gitalin, and lanatoside C were the most commonly used. The major types of rhythm disturbances were premature ventricular contractions, atrioventricular dissociation, first-degree heart block, and bigeminal rhythm. Although the investigators assumed that the cardiotoxicity which occurred was due to electrolyte imbalance, other precipitating factors such as acute myocardial infarction, chronic lung disease with hypoxia, renal insufficiency, and cerebrovascular accidents could not be ruled out.

A prospective study of 60 patients who experienced a toxic reaction to a digitalis glycoside or digitalis leaf preparation indicated that 24 patients (40%) were receiving either mercurial or thiazide diuretics. The investigators considered diuretic therapy to be a contributing or precipitating factor in the digitalis toxicity (1). Most diuretic-treated patients were receiving potassium supplements, and only eight had plasma potassium values below normal. The most common symptoms were cardiac manifestations including premature ventricular contractions, complete atrioventricular block, and atrioventricular dissociation. The more frequent digitalis drugs used were digitalis leaf, digitoxin, and digoxin.

An epidemiological study of 441 patients receiving digoxin showed that 81 patients (18.4%) had side effects attributed to digoxin (4). Potassium depletion due to diuretics (plasma potassium levels, <3.5 mEq/liter) occurred in 13 (16%) of 81 patients who developed toxicity and 13 (3.8%) of the 360 patients who did not. The association of diuretic-induced hypokalemia with digoxin toxicity was statistically significant. The two diuretics most frequently used were furosemide and hydrochlorothiazide. A higher degree of association was noted with furosemide than with hydrochlorothiazide. The use of a mercurial diuretic (mercuhydrin) did not correlate significantly with toxicity; other diuretics such as ethacrynic acid were not given with digoxin often enough for evaluation.

Other retrospective studies (2, 3, 13) also associated diuretic-induced hypokalemia with digitalis toxicity, but a causal relationship was not established.

However, other studies have not associated digitalis toxicity with diuretic therapy or with low plasma potassium levels. In a study of 135 patients who had been taking either digitalis leaf, digitoxin, or digoxin (29), there was no significant difference in the use of diuretics between the patients with and without toxicity. There was also no significant difference in the mean plasma potassium level.

The lack of association was also found in retrospective analysis of the medical records of 1140 courses of digitalis therapy in a general hospital during a 4-year period (30). This analysis resulted in the identification of 191 patients (16.8%) who exhibited signs of digitalis intoxication. There was no increased risk of intoxication in patients undergoing digitalis therapy with plasma potassium values less than 3.5 mEq/liter when compared with normal plasma potassium values.

■ Although a number of investigations indicate that diuretic-induced hypokalemia is associated with digitalis toxicity (1–4, 13, 28), other studies did not show a similar correlation (29, 30). The difference in results may be due to the fact that most studies reporting a drug interaction between digitalis glycosides and potassium-depleting diuretics were either retrospective (2, 13) or epidemiological (4). Therefore, other potential causative factors for hypokalemia [*e.g.,* vomiting, Cushing's disease, cardiac failure, renal dysfunction, and other drugs (31)] could not be ruled out (4, 28). Moreover, the toxic reactions to digitalis could have been caused by factors other than electrolyte disturbances, such as an improper maintenance dose of digitalis glycoside, an excessive loading dose, or the concurrent use of other drugs (13, 30). Additionally, other investigators criticized the differing definition of digitalis intoxication and the variation in patient characteristics in these studies (32). In the only prospective controlled study, no significant difference in diuretic use was found between the patients with digitalis toxicity and those without digitalis toxicity (29).

Another significant factor to consider when evaluating these studies is the inability to determine intracellular potassium levels. The utilization of plasma potassium levels to approximate the intracellular concentration is imprecise because this parameter only reflects 3% of total body potassium. A decrease in the plasma potassium level does not always indicate a proportional decrease in the total body potassium or the intracellular potassium level. Furthermore, the designation of hypokalemia (plasma potassium levels, <3.5 mEq/liter) in patients is arbitrary, and there is little evidence that patients with potassium levels slightly below normal will exhibit digitalis toxicity (14, 33).

Recommendations—Potassium supplements may be considered for all patients taking digitalis glycosides and potassium-depleting diuretics concurrently (31, 33). However, baseline plasma potassium levels should be determined before potassium supplements are given. If low plasma potassium levels are present (<3.5 mEq/liter), dietary supplementation should be considered when feasible (34). Foods with high potassium and low sodium content such as bananas, dried dates, fruit juices, and peaches may be recommended (35). If potassium supplements are necessary, liquid forms are preferred over slow-release tablets because the tablets, unlike the liquid, have been reported to cause gastrointestinal (GI) ulceration in a small number of patients with impaired motility of the GI tract (36–38). Potassium-sparing diuretics such as spironolactone and triamterene also have been recommended as alternative diuretic therapy (31, 33). All patients do not need potassium supplements, and the danger of hyperkalemia occurring should be considered, particularly in patients with renal insufficiency and in patients receiving potassium-sparing diuretics (14, 15, 31, 33).

After the initial determination of the plasma potassium level, the test should be repeated in 1–2-month intervals until the plasma potassium level is within normal limits (3.8–5.0 mEq/liter). Then serum electrolyte determinations should be made every 4–6 months (33). More frequent intervals may be necessary if clinical signs and symptoms indicate the development of digitalis toxicity.

Other baseline tests should be performed to detect and avoid electrolyte imbalance or acidosis. These tests include those for liver and renal function, blood pH and carbon dioxide (pCO_2), and serum chloride levels. An ECG should also be performed periodically to identify cardiac manifestations of digitalis toxicity (7, 14, 15).

The most common early cardiac manifestations of digitalis toxicity are cardiac arrhythmias (3). Although digitalis is known to cause every type of arrhythmia (39), the most common types occurring when digitalis and diuretics are given concurrently are premature ventricular contractions, first-degree heart block, and atrioventricular dissociation (1–4, 28). The treatment for digitalis-induced cardiac arrhythmias depends on factors such as serum electrolyte levels, renal function, acid–base balance, and the presence or absence of atrioventricular block. Digitalis preparations should always be discontinued whenever digitalis intoxication occurs.

When hypokalemia is the cause, intravenous or oral potassium chloride is the treatment of choice when there is no contraindication for its use (*e.g.,* in the presence of conduction disturbances such as atrioventricular block). Other approaches involve use of phenytoin, procainamide, propranolol, or quinidine, depending on the type of arrhythmia. Chelating agents such as cholestyramine resin have also been used with some success, especially with digitoxin (see *Digoxin–Cholestyramine,* p. 62). Cardioversion by direct-current shock is not effective in abolishing digitalis-induced tachyarrhythmias and may aggravate the condition (32, 39).

References

(1) A. A. Tawakkol *et al.,* "A Prospective Study of Digitalis Toxicity in a Large City Hospital," *Med. Ann. D.C., 36,* 402 (1967).

(2) A. Soffer, "The Changing Clinical Picture of Digitalis Intoxication," *Arch. Intern. Med., 107,* 681 (1961).

(3) A. W. Jorgenson and O. H. Sorensen, "Digitalis Intoxication—A Comparative Study on the Incidence of Digitalis Intoxication during the Periods 1950-52 and 1964-66," *Acta Med. Scand., 188,* 179 (1970).

(4) S. Shapiro *et al.,* "The Epidemiology of Digoxin. A Study in Three Boston Hospitals," *J. Chron. Dis., 22,* 361 (1969).

(5) C. Bengtsson *et al.,* "Effect of Different Doses of Chlorthalidone on Blood Pressure, Serum Potassium, and Serum Urate," *Brit. Med. J., 1,* 197 (1975).

(6) "The Pharmacological Basis of Therapeutics," 5th ed., L. S. Goodman and A. Gilman, Eds., Macmillan, New York, NY 10022, 1975, p. 829.

(7) D. T. Mason, "Digitalis Pharmacology and Therapeutics: Recent Advances," *Ann. Intern. Med., 80,* 520 (1974).

(8) D. T. Mason and E. Braunwald, "Digitalis: New Facts about an Old Drug," *Amer. J. Cardiol., 22,* 151 (1968).

(9) D. T. Mason *et al.,* "New Developments in the Understanding of the Actions of the Digitalis Glycosides," *Progr. Cardiov. Dis., 11,* 443 (1969).

(10) R. J. Capone *et al.,* "Digitalis in Mitral Stenosis with Normal Sinus Rhythm: Studies of Left Atrial Contractility and Cardiac Hemodynamics," abstract, *Circulation, 46,* suppl. 2, 75 (1972).

(11) D. T. Mason and E. Braunwald, "Studies on Digitalis. X. Effects of Ouabain on Forearm Vascular Resistance and Venous Tone in Normal Subjects and in Patients in Heart Failure," *J. Clin. Invest., 43,* 532 (1964).

(12) T. W. Smith and E. Haber, "Digitalis," *N. Engl. J. Med., 289,* 945 (1973).

(13) L. S. Dreifus *et al.,* "Digitalis Intolerance," *Geriatrics, 18,* 494 (1963).

(14) P. R. Wilkinson *et al.,* "Total Body and Serum Potassium during Prolonged Thiazide Therapy for Essential Hypertension," *Lancet, i,* 759 (1975).

(15) H. J. Dargie *et al.,* "Total Body Potassium in Long-Term Frusemide Therapy: Is Potassium Supplementation Necessary?" *Brit. Med. J., 4,* 316 (1974).

(16) R. P. S. Edmondson *et al.,* "Leucocyte Electrolytes in Cardiac and Non-Cardiac Patients Receiving Diuretics," *Lancet, i,* 12 (1974).

(17) P. F. Binnion, "Hypokalemia and Digoxin-Induced Arrhythmias," *Lancet, i*, 343 (1975).

(18) P. A. Poole-Wilson *et al.*, "Hypokalemia, Digitalis, and Arrhythmias," *Lancet, i*, 575 (1975).

(19) E. G. Corbett, Jr., "Hypokalemia and Digoxin-Induced Arrhythmias," *Lancet, i*, 742 (1975).

(20) R. H. Seller *et al.*, "Serum and Erythrocytic Magnesium Levels in Congestive Heart Failure. Effects of Hydrochlorothiazide," *Amer. J. Cardiol., 17*, 786 (1966).

(21) R. H. Goldman *et al.*, "The Effect on Myocardial 3H-Digoxin of Magnesium Deficiency," *Proc. Soc. Exp. Biol. Med., 136*, 747 (1971).

(22) "Calcium, Magnesium, and Diuretics," *Brit. Med. J., 1*, 170 (1975).

(23) W. O. Smith *et al.*, "The Influence of Various Diuretic Agents on the Urinary Excretion of Magnesium in Non-Edematous Subjects," *Clin. Res., 7*, 162 (1959).

(24) Y. W. Kim *et al.*, "Serum Magnesium and Cardiac Arrhythmias with Special Reference to Digitalis Intoxication," *Amer. J. Med. Sci., 242*, 127 (1961).

(25) E. Gursel, "Effects of Diuretics on Renal and Intestinal Handling of Calcium," *N.Y. State J. Med., 70*, 399 (1970).

(26) N. Toda and T. C. West, "Modification by Sodium and Calcium of the Cardiotoxicity Induced by Ouabain," *J. Pharmacol. Exp. Ther., 154*, 239 (1966).

(27) C. G. Duarte *et al.*, "Thiazide-Induced Hypercalcemia," *N. Engl. J. Med., 284*, 828 (1971).

(28) P. L. Rodensky and F. Wasserman, "Observations on Digitalis Intoxication," *Arch. Intern. Med., 108*, 171 (1961).

(29) G. A. Beller *et al.*, "Digitalis Intoxication. A Prospective Clinical Study with Serum Level Correlations," *N. Engl. J. Med., 284*, 989 (1971).

(30) R. I. Ogilvie and J. Ruedy, "An Educational Program in Digitalis Therapy," *J. Amer. Med. Ass., 222*, 50 (1972).

(31) "Who Needs Potassium?" *Brit. Med. J., 4*, 307 (1974).

(32) T. W. Smith and E. Haber, "Digitalis," *N. Engl. J. Med., 289*, 1125 (1973).

(33) C. J. Edmonds and B. Jasani, "Total-Body Potassium in Hypertensive Patients during Prolonged Diuretic Therapy," *Lancet, ii*, 8 (1972).

(34) M. C. Bateson and A. F. Lant, "Dietary Potassium and Diuretic Therapy," *Lancet, ii*, 381 (1973).

(35) "Documenta Geigy Scientific Tables," Basel, Switzerland, 1970, p. 498.

(36) M. A. Farquharson-Roberts *et al.*, "Perforation of Small Bowel Due to Slow Release Potassium Chloride (Slow-K)," *Brit. Med. J., 3*, 206 (1975).

(37) S. J. Heffernan and J. J. Murphy, "Ulceration of Small Intestine and Slow-Release Potassium Tablets," *Brit. Med. J., 2*, 746 (1975).

(38) "Who Needs Slow-Release Potassium Tablets," *Med. Lett., 17*, 73 (1975).

(39) K. Y. Chung and J. Thomas, "Arrhythmias Caused by Digitalis Toxicity," *Geriatrics, 20*, 1006 (1965).

[For additional information, see *Cardiac Glycoside Therapy*, p. 407, and *Diuretic Therapy*, p. 414.]

Nonproprietary and Trade Names of Drugs

Acetyldigitoxin—*Acylanid*
Bendroflumethiazide—*Naturetin*
Benzthiazide—*Aquatag, Exna*
Chlorothiazide—*Diuril*
Chlorthalidone—*Hygroton, Regroton*
Cyclothiazide—*Anhydron*
Digitalis leaf—*Various manufacturers*
Digitoxin—*Crystodigin, Digitaline Nativelle, Myodigin, Purodigin*
Digoxin—*Lanoxin*
Ethacrynic acid—*Edecrin*
Flumethiazide—*Rautrax*
Furosemide—*Lasix*
Gitalin—*Gitaligin*
Hydrochlorothiazide—*Esidrix, Hydro-Diuril, Oretic*

Hydroflumethiazide—*Saluron*
Lanatoside C—*Cedilanid*
Mercaptomerin sodium—*Thiomerin*
Metolazone—*Zaroxolyn*
Methyclothiazide—*Aquatensen, Enduron*
Ouabain—*Various manufacturers*
Polythiazide—*Renese*
Quinethazone—*Hydromox*
Spironolactone—*Aldactone*
Triamterene—*Dyrenium*
Trichlormethiazide—*Metahydrin, Naqua*
Various combination products containing a diuretic are available.

Prepared and evaluated by the Scientific Review Subpanels on Cardiac Glycosides and Diuretics and reviewed by Practitioner Panel IV.

Digitalis—Phenytoin*

Summary—Although it has been reported that phenytoin may enhance digitalis-induced bradycardia or may decrease serum digitoxin levels, there is no evidence to indicate that these effects are clinically significant. However, as with all antiarrhythmic agents, it would be prudent to monitor the patient for signs of drug-induced bradycardia and other arrhythmias.

Related Drugs—Related digitalis compounds include **digitalis leaf preparations** and the following cardiac glycosides: **acetyldigitoxin, deslanoside, digitoxin, digoxin, gitalin, lanatoside C,** and **ouabain.** Other hydantoin derivatives are **ethotoin** and **mephenytoin.**

Pharmacological Effect and Mechanism—The primary action of the digitalis glycosides is to increase the force of myocardial contraction in both the failing and healthy heart. This inotropic effect may be related to the ability of digitalis to inhibit sodium–potassium adenosine triphosphatase, the enzyme that acts as the sodium pump for the cardiac muscle cell (1). The degree of inotropic action of the digitalis glycosides increases progressively with increasing doses until disturbances of cardiac rhythm occur (2).

The antiarrhythmic effect of phenytoin is probably due to a prevention of the uptake of sodium into the cardiac muscle cell, stabilizing the stimulatory threshold of the cell (3). This action results in depressed ventricular automaticity and enhanced atrioventricular conduction in the myocardial tissue (4). One report indicated that phenytoin administration increased the dose of acetylstrophanthidin necessary to produce ventricular tachycardia in dogs (5). Furthermore, phenytoin inhibited the dysrhythmia of cardiac tissue due to ouabain in isolated guinea pig atria (6).

Phenytoin markedly decreased the steady-state concentration of digitoxin in the plasma of one patient, suggesting an increase in the rate of elimination of digitoxin (7).

Evaluation of Clinical Data—Most data indicate that intravenous administration of phenytoin increases the dose of digitalis necessary to produce toxicity and that phenytoin is usually effective in the treatment of digitalis-induced arrhythmias in humans (8–10). For example, in 23 patients who had digitalis-induced arrhythmias, 19 responded to phenytoin administration (250 mg iv initially and then 100–300 mg/day po if needed) with abolition or marked suppression of ventricular ectopic foci or with conversion of supraventricular arrhythmias to a regular sinus rhythm (9).

In another study of 14 humans (10), ouabain infusion produced an increase in atrioventricular conduction time, whereas phenytoin administration (5 mg/kg iv) consistently decreased atrioventricular conduction time. In addition, the ouabain-induced increase in atrioventricular conduction time was reversed by phenytoin.

There have been some suggestions that phenytoin (200–300 mg/day po) enhances digitalis-induced bradycardia (11). However, this conclusion was based on the observation of one patient who also had Down's syndrome (mongolism). Since this condition reportedly has caused bradycardia and heart block (12, 13), the bradycardia may have been due to the pathological condition of the patient and not the use of digitalis and phenytoin.

■ Although it has been reported that phenytoin may enhance digitalis-induced bradycardia (11) or decrease serum digitoxin levels (7), there is little indication that these effects are clinically significant. Moreover, most clinical data suggest that parenteral phenytoin is effective in counteracting the disturbances in cardiac rhythm caused by digitalis intoxication.

---

*Phenytoin is the new official name for diphenylhydantoin.

Recommendations—The advantageous effects of phenytoin in prevention of digitalis-induced arrhythmias seem to outweigh any potential adverse effects that may occur during concurrent administration of the drugs. However, as with all antiarrhythmic agents, patients receiving digitalis glycosides and phenytoin concurrently should be monitored closely for signs of drug-induced bradycardia and other arrhythmias.

References

(1) T. W. Smith and E. Haber, "Digitalis," *N. Engl. J. Med.*, *289*, 945 (1973).

(2) T. W. Smith and E. Haber, "Digitalis," *N. Engl. J. Med.*, *289*, 1010 (1973).

(3) J. H. Pincus *et al.*, "Studies on the Mechanism of Action of Diphenyl-hydantoin," *Arch. Neurol.*, *22*, 566 (1970).

(4) A. N. Damato, "Diphenylhydantoin: Pharmacological and Clinical Use," *Progr. Cardiov. Dis.*, *12*, 1 (1969).

(5) R. H. Helfant *et al.*, "Protection from Digitalis Toxicity with the Prophylactic Use of Diphenylhydantoin Sodium," *Circulation*, *36*, 119 (1967).

(6) T. Godfraind *et al.*, "The Action of Diphenylhydantoin upon Drug Binding, Ionic Effects and Inotropic Action of Ouabain," *Arch. Int. Pharmacodyn. Ther.*, *191*, 66 (1973).

(7) H. M. Solomon *et al.*, "Interactions between Digitoxin and Other Drugs *In Vitro* and *In Vivo*," *Ann. N.Y. Acad. Sci.*, *179*, 362 (1971).

(8) F. A. Bashour *et al.*, "Treatment of Digitalis Toxicity by Diphenylhydantoin (Dilantin)," *Dis. Chest*, *53*, 263 (1968).

(9) J. S. Karliner, "Intravenous Diphenylhydantoin Sodium (Dilantin) in Cardiac Arrhythmias," *Dis. Chest*, *51*, 256 (1967).

(10) R. H. Helfant *et al.*, "Effects of Diphenylhydantoin on Atrioventricular Conduction in Man," *Circulation*, *36*, 686 (1967).

(11) N. M. A. Viukari and K. Aho, "Digoxin-Phenytoin Interaction," *Brit. Med. J.*, *2*, 51 (1970).

(12) "The Heart," 2nd ed., J. W. Hurst and R. B. Logue, Eds., McGraw-Hill, New York, N.Y., 1970, p. 655.

(13) "Principles of Internal Medicine," 6th ed., M. W. Wintrobe *et al.*, Eds., McGraw-Hill, New York, N.Y., 1970, pp. 1169–1170.

[For additional information, see *Cardiac Glycoside Therapy*, p. 407.]

Nonproprietary and Trade Names of Drugs

Acetyldigitoxin—*Acylanid*
Deslanoside—*Cedilanid-D*
Digitalis—*Various manufacturers*
Digitoxin—*Crystodigin, Digitaline Nativelle, Myodigin, Purodigin*
Digoxin—*Lanoxin*

Ethotoin—*Peganone*
Gitalin—*Gitaligin*
Lanatoside C—*Cedilanid*
Mephenytoin—*Mesantoin*
Ouabain—*Various manufacturers*
Phenytoin—*Dilantin*

Prepared and evaluated by the Scientific Review Subpanel on Cardiac Glycosides and reviewed by Practitioner Panel VI.

Digitalis—Reserpine

Summary—Several clinical and experimental reports indicate that the concurrent use of cardiac glycosides and rauwolfia alkaloids may increase the likelihood of cardiac arrhythmias due to digitalis. However, the data are unreliable and a causal relationship has not been established. In most cases, these agents could probably be administered concurrently without adverse effects, but the possibility of serious drug-induced arrhythmias should be considered, particularly in patients with atrial fibrillation.

Related Drugs—Cardiac glycosides reported to interact with reserpine include **digitoxin** (1), **digoxin** (2), **lanatoside C** (1), and **ouabain** (1, 3). Other glycosides such as **acetyldigitoxin, deslanoside, digitalis leaf,** and **gitalin** may interact in a similar manner. Whole root preparations and individual alkaloids of **Rauwolfia serpentina** have been implicated in suspected interactions (4). In addition, **alseroxylon, deserpi-**

dine, rescinnamine, syrosingopine, and any combination product containing reserpine may also aggravate digitalis toxicity.

Pharmacological Effect and Mechanism—The arrhythmic action of high doses of digitalis may be attributed to alterations of the refractory period, impulse transmission, and automaticity of cardiac tissues. Alterations in centrally mediated sympathetic activity and changes in vagal tone also may be of considerable importance (5).

Rauwolfia preparations alone have been implicated in provoking arrhythmias (4, 6), but the mechanism of this effect is unknown. Reserpine causes a depletion of myocardial catecholamines (7) and a transient rise in free catecholamines during the early phase of reserpine treatment (5, 8, 9). Although the transient rise in catecholamines theoretically may be responsible for the enhancement of digitalis-induced arrhythmias, animal studies showed that the arrhythmias are unrelated to catecholamine release (7). Digitalis and reserpine also indirectly augment vagal tone. Such enhancement may contribute to an increase in ventricular automaticity during concurrent administration of loading doses of digitalis and reserpine (10).

Although reserpine interferes with the cardiac action of digitalis and other cardiac glycosides to decrease digitalis intoxication in laboratory animals when given as pretreatment (1, 3, 5, 11–15), this interference is probably independent of its norepinephrine-depleting properties (7).

Evaluation of Clinical Data—Reports of suspected digitalis–reserpine interactions are brief and do not establish a definite cause and effect relationship. In one report (16) when therapy was initiated by the concurrent administration of digoxin and reserpine, the observed arrhythmias could have been caused by either agent.

The concurrent administration of a diuretic, a rauwolfia preparation, and digitalis hinders interpretation of another report, although the arrhythmias were present only during intermittent periods of rauwolfia therapy (4). Atrial tachycardia, heart block, ventricular tachycardia, bigeminy, and atrial fibrillation were reported in three patients; these arrhythmias appeared to be associated with the administration of reserpine following loading doses of digitalis. Although it was emphasized by the investigators that these drugs were administered concurrently to a large number of patients, the report did not reveal the incidence of cardiac toxicity due to either agent alone or to concurrent use.

A single-blind study of 30 patients divided into two groups of 15 patients each indicated that the incidence of arrhythmias was greater in the group receiving digitalis preparations and rauwolfia alkaloids (seven out of 15 patients) than in the group receiving rauwolfia alkaloids alone (three out of 15 patients) (6). Discontinuation of the rauwolfia alkaloids in five patients who had received concurrent therapy resulted in a restoration of normal sinus rhythm.

Another study reported that reserpine enhanced the toxicity (ventricular arrhythmias and varying degrees of heart block) of loading doses of acetylstrophanthidin in patients with atrial fibrillation (10).

■ Digitalis preparations and rauwolfia alkaloids may be administered concurrently to hypertensive patients requiring treatment for congestive heart failure, but the incidence of adverse effects clearly attributable to reserpine is unclear. The interaction would result in excessive vagal activity and cardiac slowing, predisposing the myocardium to ventricular arrhythmias. Some results (10) indicate that the risk would be especially high in patients with atrial fibrillation. The vagal influences of these compounds could reduce the ventricular rate to the point where the time for diastolic depolarization and eventual firing of ectopic foci is allowed. In this situation, the release of catecholamines would increase appreciably the risk of cardiac arrhythmias. In addition, the interaction would be detrimental to therapeutic use of digitalis since it would hinder interpretation of the ECG indications of overdigitalization.

Recommendations—Concurrent administration of digitalis preparations and reserpine is not contraindicated. An interaction would be more likely to occur if large parenteral doses (rarely given) of reserpine are administered following or simultaneously with loading doses of digitalis. Also, it would not be prudent to administer these drugs to patients with atrial fibrillation. In most suspected adverse reactions, normal cardiac rhythm was reestablished when either reserpine or both digitalis and reserpine were withheld. However, more vigorous measures such as the administration of potassium and antiarrhythmic drugs might be required (17).

References

(1) B. Levitt and J. Roberts, "The Capacity of Different Digitalis Materials to Induce Ventricular Rhythm Disturbances in the Reserpine-Pretreated Cat," *J. Pharmacol. Exp. Ther.*, *156*, 159 (1967).

(2) F. I. Marcus *et al.*, "The Effect of Reserpine on the Metabolism of Tritiated Digoxin in the Dog and in Man," *J. Pharmacol. Exp. Ther.*, *159*, 314 (1968).

(3) F. R. Ciofalo, "Relationship between Ouabain-Induced Arrhythmia in the Rabbit and Tissue Catecholamines," *Eur. J. Pharmacol.*, *9*, 281 (1970).

(4) B. N. Wilson and N. A. Wimberley, "Production of Premature Ventricular Contractions by Rauwolfia," *J. Amer. Med. Ass.*, *159*, 1363 (1955).

(5) L. D. Boyajy and C. B. Nash, "Influence of Reserpine on Arrhythmias, Inotropic Effects, and Myocardial Potassium Balance Induced by Digitalis Materials," *J. Pharmacol. Exp. Ther.*, *148*, 193 (1965).

(6) C. J. Schreader and M. M. Etzl, "Premature Ventricular Contractions Due to Rauwolfia Therapy," *J. Amer. Med. Ass.*, *162*, 1256 (1956).

(7) J. F. Spann *et al.*, "Studies on Digitalis XIV: Influence of Cardiac Norepinephrine Stores on the Response of Isolated Heart Muscle to Digitalis," *Circ. Res.*, *19*, 326 (1966).

(8) H. L. Dick *et al.*, "Reserpine-Digitalis Toxicity. Case Reports of Cardiac Arrhythmias Occurring during Reserpine-Digitalis Therapy and a Review of the Litreature with Supporting Animal Experiments," *Arch. Intern. Med.*, *109*, 503 (1962).

(9) J. R. DiPalma, "Reserpine Antagonism of Digitalis Heart Block," *Fed. Proc.*, *17*, 364 (1958).

(10) B. Lown *et al.*, "Effect of Digitalis in Patients Receiving Reserpine," *Circulation*, *24*, 1185 (1961).

(11) D. T. Mason, "Clinical Significance of Recent Advances in the Pharmacology of Cardiovascular Drugs," *Conn. Med.*, *32*, 183 (1968).

(12) J. Roberts *et al.*, "Influence of Reserpine and βTM 10 on Digitalis-Induced Ventricular Arrhythmia," *Circ. Res.*, *13*, 149 (1963).

(13) A. G. Phansalkar *et al.*, "A Study of Digoxin, Thyroxine and Reserpine Interrelationship," *Arch. Int. Pharmacodyn. Ther.*, *182*, 44 (1969).

(14) M. Takagi *et al.*, "Tolerance of Reserpinized Dogs to Digitalis," *Amer. J Cardiol.*, *15*, 203 (1965).

(15) G. Fawaz, "Effect of Reserpine and Pronethalol on the Therapeutic and Toxic Actions of Digitalis in the Dog Heart–Lung Preparation," *Brit. J. Pharmacol. Chemother.*, *29*, 302 (1967).

(16) A. Soffer, "Digitalis Intoxication, Reserpine, and Double Tachycardia," *J. Amer. Med. Ass.*, *191*, 777 (1965).

(17) T. W. Smith and E. Haber, "Digitalis," *N. Engl. J. Med.*, *289*, 1125 (1973).

[For additional information, see *Cardiac Glycoside Therapy*, p. 407.]

Nonproprietary and Trade Names of Drugs

Acetyldigitoxin—*Acylanid*
Alseroxylon—*Rautensin, Rauwiloid*
Deslanoside—*Cedilanid-D*
Deserpidine—*Harmonyl*
Digitalis—*Various manufacturers*
Digitoxin—*Crystodigin, Digitaline Nativelle, Myodigin, Purodigin*
Digoxin—*Lanoxin*
Gitalin—*Gitaligin*

Lanatoside C—*Cedilanid*
Ouabain—*Various manufacturers*
Rauwolfia serpentina—*Raudixin and various combination products*
Rescinnamine—*Moderil*
Reserpine—*Reserpoid, Sandril, Serpasil, and various combination products*
Syrosingopine—*Singoserp*

Prepared and evaluated by the Scientific Review Subpanel on Cardiac Glycosides and reviewed by Practitioner Panel I.

Digitoxin—Spironolactone

Summary—Spironolactone protects rats from digitoxin cardiotoxicity but there is no evidence that this protection occurs in humans. Plasma potassium levels should be determined periodically to prevent hyperkalemia, and the patient should be evaluated continually to ensure that the therapeutic effects of digitoxin are not decreased.

Related Drugs—Similar cardiac glycosides are **acetyldigitoxin, deslanoside, digitalis leaf preparations, digitalis, digoxin, gitalin, lanatoside C,** and **ouabain.** Other diuretics that conserve potassium include **amiloride** and **triamterene.**

Pharmacological Effect and Mechanism—The mechanism of action of digitoxin and other cardiac glycosides is not completely understood. It is apparent, however, that the potassium ion plays a role. Increased extracellular potassium levels decrease automaticity and suppress ectopic beats induced by digitalis. Hypokalemia is associated with the appearance of arrhythmias in the presence of even subtherapeutic doses of the glycosides. Hypokalemia occurs frequently, but not always, with administration of potassium-depleting diuretics such as the thiazide diuretics (1).

Spironolactone is considered to be a competitive inhibitor of aldosterone, presumably by competing for renal receptor sites in the distal tubule (2). This competition results in a loss of sodium ions without a concomitant loss of potassium ions. Spironolactone may cause increased potassium levels, particularly in renal disease (2, 3).

Several animal studies demonstrated that spironolactone protects against digitoxin poisoning, suggesting the possibility that spironolactone may cause a reduction in toxicity of digitoxin in humans. However, it appears that this interaction has little or no dependence on the potassium-sparing effects of spironolactone. The available evidence suggests that the protective effect of spironolactone is due to its ability to act as an enzyme-inducing agent in the liver, resulting in a shorter half-life for digitoxin (4, 5). In a further study (6), other potassium-sparing diuretics as well as potassium ion itself did not protect rats against digitoxin toxicity, and several anabolic androgens protected the rat against fatal digitoxin intoxication irrespective of their effects upon electrolyte metabolism.

Evaluation of Clinical Data—Several studies on the treatment of long-standing decompensated heart disease, which is usually complicated by hyperaldosteronism, indicated an improved tolerance to cardiac glycosides (7–9). However, these data are insufficient to determine whether spironolactone exerts the same protective effect relative to digitalis toxicity in the human as in the rat.

■ Although studies indicate that spironolactone protects the rat against digitoxin intoxication (10), there is no evidence to support the possibility of this effect occurring in humans.

Recommendations—Until more clinical data are published, patients receiving digitoxin and spironolactone concurrently should be monitored for possible decreases in digitoxin effect. The development of hyperkalemia also is a potential risk in patients receiving potassium-sparing diuretics and for this reason potassium supplements are contraindicated and plasma potassium levels should be determined periodically (11).

References

(1) H. B. Zimmerman *et al.*, "The Action of Potassium on the Atrioventricular Node in Digitalized Patients," *Dis. Chest*, *43*, 377 (1962).

(2) R. H. Seller *et al.*, "Aldosterone Antagonists in Diuretic Therapy, Their Effect on the Refractory Period," *Arch. Intern. Med.*, *113*, 350 (1964).

(3) C. L. Gantt and R. W. Ecklund, "Significance of Aldosterone Antagonism in the Treatment of Edema and Ascites," *Amer. J. Med., 33,* 490 (1962).

(4) H. Selye *et al.,* "Effect of Spironolactone and Norbolethone on the Toxicity of Digitalis Compounds in the Rat," *Brit. J. Pharmacol., 37,* 485 (1969).

(5) B. Solymoss *et al.,* "Effect of Various Steroids on Microsomal Aliphatic Hydroxylation and N-Dealkylation," *Eur. J. Pharmacol., 10,* 127 (1970).

(6) H. Selye *et al.,* "Prevention of Digitoxin Poisoning by Various Steroids," *J. Pharm. Sci., 58,* 1055 (1969).

(7) A. Tourniaire *et al.,* "Effet de la Spironolactone sur L'Hyperexcitabilite Myocardique des Cardiopathies Decompensees," *Lyon Med., 214,* 1219 (1965).

(8) A. Tourniaire *et al.,* "L'Hyperexcitabilite Myocardique des Cardiopathies Decompensees. Effet de la Spironolactone," *Sem. Hop. Paris, 45,* 1388 (1969).

(9) A. Varenne *et al.,* "Etude de L'Action Clinique d'une Spironolactone sur L'Excitabilite Musculaire et L'Electrocardiogramme," *Gaz. Med. France, 72,* 5869 (1967).

(10) B. Solymoss *et al.,* "Protection by Spironolactone and Oxandrolone against Chronic Digitoxin or Indomethacin Intoxication," *Toxicol. Appl. Pharmacol., 18,* 586 (1971).

(11) J. E. Doherty and J. J. Kane, "Clinical Pharmacology and Therapeutic Use of Digitalis Glycosides," *Drugs, 6,* 182 (1973).

[For additional information, see *Cardiac Glycoside Therapy,* p. 407.]

Nonproprietary and Trade Names of Drugs

Acetyldigitoxin—*Acylanid*
Amiloride—*Colectril*
Deslanoside—*Cedilanid-D*
Digitalis—*Various manufacturers*
Digitoxin—*Crystodigin, Digitaline Nativelle, Myodigin, Purodigin*
Digoxin—*Lanoxin*

Gitalin—*Gitaligin*
Lanatoside C—*Cedilanid*
Ouabain—*Various manufacturers*
Spironolactone—*Aldactone*
Triamterene—*Dyrenium*
Various combination products containing a diuretic are available.

Prepared and evaluated by the Scientific Review Subpanel on Cardiac Glycosides and reviewed by Practitioner Panel II.

Digoxin—Cholestyramine

Summary—Simultaneous use of cholestyramine resin and orally administered digoxin or digitoxin reduces the absorption and physiological disposition of the cardiac glycoside. To minimize the effects of this drug interaction, it would be prudent to administer digoxin or digitoxin 1.5 hr before cholestyramine.

Related Drugs—**Colestipol** (1), an insoluble, nonabsorbable anion-exchange resin not yet commercially available in the United States, also binds **digitoxin** and digoxin in humans (1, 2). **Polyamine-methylene resin** is another anion-exchange resin similar to cholestyramine, but it has not been associated with cardiac glycoside interactions.

Both colestipol and cholestyramine resins are expected to bind other orally administered cardiac glycosides, such as **acetyldigitoxin, deslanoside, digitalis, gitalin,** and **lanatoside C.** However, the clinical significance of such interactions remains to be determined.

Pharmacological Effect and Mechanism—Two proposed mechanisms of interaction between the cardiac glycosides and cholestyramine have arisen from animal (3, 4) and *in vitro* (1, 4–6) experiments. The hypothesis for the first mechanism was derived from the two animal studies and suggests that cholestyramine resin interrupts the enterohepatic circulation of digitoxin or digoxin, resulting in reduced reabsorption and increased fecal excretion of the cardiac glycoside. This mechanism is probably more applicable to digitoxin because it undergoes more enterohepatic circulation in humans (7) than does digoxin (8).

A second mechanism has been postulated from *in vitro* studies. Bile acids and digoxin or digitoxin may compete for common binding sites on the cholestyramine resin (1). The bile acid is strongly attached to the resin (1) whereas the cardiac glycoside is loosely bound and can be washed off by rinsing with a buffer (9). The amount of cardiac glycoside bound is related to the amount of cholestyramine present (6) and may or may not be affected by the presence of bile or duodenal juices (1, 4). The binding is independent of pH and temperature changes (4). Based on this evidence, the theory states that cholestyramine binds the cardiac glycoside in the gastrointestinal (GI) tract, preventing or delaying its absorption (4, 5). Prevention of the absorption of the cardiac glycosides would be more clinically important than a delay in the absorption. Digitoxin may be more tightly bound to cholestyramine than digoxin (6) and less susceptible to displacement by bile.

Evaluation of Clinical Data—Maintenance doses of cholestyramine (16 g/day po) were administered to seven healthy subjects beginning 8 hr after being stabilized with 1.2 mg of ^{3}H-digitoxin (7). The half-life and the cardiac response to digitoxin were used to measure the amount of digitoxin present in the body. Cholestyramine treatment resulted in a reduction in half-life of total serum radioactivity from 11.5 to 6.6 days. In addition, cholestyramine treatment was accompanied by a more rapid return to baseline values of digitoxin-induced changes in the cardiac rhythm (4).

Colestipol was administered (10 g po immediately and 5 g po every 6–8 hr) to one patient with digoxin intoxication and four patients with digitoxin intoxication (1). Two patients with digoxin intoxication and one patient with digitoxin intoxication were treated with only standard supportive measures to obtain the "normal" rate of disappearance of digitalis glycoside from plasma. Clinical signs and symptoms of digitalis intoxication and serum cardiac glycoside levels subsided in a much shorter time in the patients treated with colestipol. Colestipol also shortened the serum half-life of digitoxin from 9.5 days in the controls to an average of 2.5 days and shortened the serum half-life of digoxin from 1.9 days to 16 hr.

Four subjects who were maintained on digoxin (0.25–0.5 mg/day po) had substantially lower serum digoxin levels during concurrent therapy with cholestyramine (4–16 g/day po) than without the resin (10). Two subjects ingested single doses (0.5 mg po) of digoxin and two received long-term administration of digoxin (0.25 mg/day po). In all subjects, the serum levels of digoxin returned to the higher levels attained prior to cholestyramine administration after the resin was discontinued. Another two subjects received digitoxin (0.1 mg/day po) on a long-term basis concurrently with cholestyramine (16 g/day po with 4 g being ingested simultaneously with digitoxin). The serum level of digitoxin gradually fell to substantially (amount not reported) lower levels and increased after cholestyramine administration was discontinued.

In a brief report (2), no significant alteration in serum cardiac glycoside levels occurred when cholestyramine or colestipol was ingested 1.5 hr after digoxin (0.125–0.25 mg po) or digitoxin (0.1–0.2 mg po). Some of the 10 patients received cholestyramine (12 g/day po) for 1 year; others received colestipol (15 g po) or a placebo.

■ These studies indicate that ion-exchange resins such as cholestyramine reduce the serum cardiac glycoside level when given simultaneously. The effect may be greater with digitoxin than digoxin since it undergoes more enterohepatic circulation than digoxin (7, 8). Although there is little clinical documentation, this effect may be beneficial when treating digitalis toxicity, particularly when the toxicity is caused by digitoxin.

Recommendations—Administration of digoxin or digitoxin at least 1.5 hr before cholestyramine will avoid significant GI interference between the two drugs (11). Patients should be instructed about the problem of simultaneous use of the drugs. Without a proper dose schedule for the two medications, the resultant GI binding of digoxin or digitoxin and changes in excretion may lead to fluctuating dosage requirements and suboptimal digoxin or digitoxin activity.

A patient stabilized on digoxin or digitoxin during simultaneous administration of cholestyramine could experience digoxin or digitoxin intoxication if the resin was subsequently discontinued or scheduled at a different time. Efficacy of therapy should be monitored through use of serum digitoxin or digoxin levels and by observation of clinical signs and symptoms.

References

(1) G. Bazzano and G. S. Bazzano, "Digitalis Intoxication. Treatment with a New Steroid-Binding Resin," *J. Amer. Med. Ass.*, *220*, 828 (1972).

(2) G. Bazzano and G. S. Bazzano, "Effect of Digitalis-Binding Resins on Cardiac Glycoside Plasma Levels," *Clin. Res.*, *20*, 24 (1972).

(3) W. G. Thompson, "Effect of Cholestyramine on Absorption of ³H Digoxin in Rats," *Dig. Dis.*, *18*, 851 (1973).

(4) J. H. Caldwell and N. J. Greenberger, "Interruption of the Enterohepatic Circulation of Digitoxin by Cholestyramine. I. Protection against Lethal Digitoxin Intoxication," *J. Clin. Invest.*, *50*, 2626 (1971).

(5) J. H. Caldwell and N. J. Greenberger, "Cholestyramine Enhances Digitalis Excretion and Protects against Lethal Intoxication," *J. Clin. Invest.*, *49*, 16A (1970).

(6) R. Saral and J. L. Spratt, "Alteration of Oral Digitoxin Toxicity and Its *In Vitro* Binding by Cholestyramine," *Arch. Int. Pharmacodyn. Ther.*, *167*, 10 (1967).

(7) J. H. Caldwell *et al.*, "Interruption of the Enterohepatic Circulation of Digitoxin by Cholestyramine. II. Effect on Metabolic Disposition of Tritium-Labeled Digitoxin and Cardiac Systolic Intervals in Man," *J. Clin. Invest.*, *50*, 2638 (1971).

(8) J. E. Doherty *et al.*, "Tritiated Digoxin. XIV. Enterohepatic Circulation, Absorption and Excretion Studies in Human Volunteers," *Circulation*, *42*, 867 (1970).

(9) D. G. Gallo *et al.*, "The Interaction between Cholestyramine and Drugs," *Proc. Soc. Exp. Biol. Med.*, *120*, 60 (1965).

(10) T. W. Smith, in "New Approaches to the Management of Digitalis Intoxication," in "Symposium on Digitalis," Ole Storstein, Ed., Gyldendal Norsk Forlag, Oslo, Norway, 1974, p. 312.

(11) J. T. Bigger, Jr., and H. C. Strauss, "Digitalis Toxicity: Drug Interactions Promoting Toxicity and the Management of Toxicity," *Sem. Drug Treat.*, *2* (2), 147 (1972).

[For additional information, see *Cardiac Glycoside Therapy*, p. 407.]

Nonproprietary and Trade Names of Drugs

Acetyldigitoxin—*Acylanid*
Cholestyramine resin—*Cuemid, Questran*
Colestipol hydrochloride—*Colestid*
Deslanoside—*Cedilanid-D*
Digitalis—*Various manufacturers*
Digitoxin—*Crystodigin, Digitaline Nativelle, Myodigin, Purodigin*

Digoxin—*Lanoxin*
Gitalin—*Gitaligin*
Lanatoside C—*Cedilanid*
Polyamine-methylene resin—*Resinat*

Prepared and evaluated by the Scientific Review Subpanel on Cardiac Glycosides and reviewed by Practitioner Panel III.

Digoxin—Propantheline

Summary—Concurrent use of propantheline with slow-dissolving tablets of digoxin may cause increased serum digoxin levels. This interaction can be avoided by using only those digoxin tablets that are fast dissolving by USP standards. However, the practitioner should be alert for signs of digitalis toxicity in any patient receiving digoxin tablets and propantheline concurrently.

Related Drugs—Although no documentation exists, other anticholinergic agents, such as **anisotropine, belladonna alkaloids, dicyclomine, glycopyrrolate, hexocyclium, isopropamide, methantheline, methscopolamine, oxyphencyclimine, oxyphenonium, pipenzolate, piperidolate,** and **tridihexethyl,** would be expected to interact with digoxin tablets.

Digitoxin is more completely absorbed from the gastrointestinal (GI) tract than digoxin (1), although it probably undergoes more enterohepatic circulation in humans (2). There is no documentation of a drug interaction occurring between propantheline and digitoxin and it is doubtful that one will occur. Other drugs related to digoxin include **acetyldigitoxin, deslanoside, digitalis, gitalin, lanatoside C,** and **ouabain.**

Pharmacological Effect and Mechanism—Propantheline decreases the tone, amplitude, and frequency of peristaltic contractions. It inhibits GI motility by relaxing smooth muscles, prolongs the GI transit time of ingested material, and allows for more complete absorption (3). Physiological absorption of digoxin from digoxin tablets demonstrating a "slow *in vitro* dissolution rate" but not that from tablets having a "fast *in vitro* dissolution rate" is affected by the anticholinergic effects of propantheline which serve to prolong the intestinal transit time. The extended transit time appears to permit greater release of digoxin into the GI lumen, thereby promoting more complete absorption and higher serum digoxin levels (4). Subsequently, the serum digoxin level becomes elevated, reflecting the greater degree of bioavailability and GI absorption.

Variation in the bioavailability and in the percentage of absorption of digoxin (5–7) occurs among various digoxin products and also among different lots of tablets prepared by the same manufacturer (8–12). These slow-dissolving tablets of digoxin may release less than 40% of the cardiac glycoside, whereas tablet formulations with desirable dissolution characteristics release 50–75% of the labeled amount of digoxin (5, 6). Since 80–100% of digoxin is absorbed from solution (5, 7), the bioavailability and serum digoxin level achieved from the latter dosage form are expected to be less susceptible to the GI effects of propantheline than solid dosage forms.

Another proposed mechanism (13) for the digoxin–propantheline interaction is based on the fact that 6–7% of digoxin is eliminated by the biliary tract (14) *via* enterohepatic circulation. Propantheline retards biliary flow which could result in the accumulation of digoxin with a subsequent increase in the serum digoxin level due to decreased biliary excretion.

Evaluation of Clinical Data—The effects of oral propantheline on the absorption of digoxin from tablets and liquid dosage forms were studied *in vivo* (4). Nine of 13 elderly females with cerebrovascular accidents receiving maintenance digoxin therapy showed a 30% increase in serum digoxin levels after 10 days of concurrent propantheline administration (15 mg po three times daily). Although the daily intake of digoxin was not stated, the mean serum digoxin level was 1.02 ng/ml during treatment with digoxin tablets alone and 1.33 ng/ml when propantheline was administered concurrently ($p<0.01$). Serum digoxin levels were unchanged in three patients and declined in another. All patients had normal serum electrolyte values and renal function tests throughout the study.

Baseline serum digoxin levels were obtained after the administration of digoxin (0.5 mg po) in tablet and liquid dosage forms in eight healthy subjects after fasting overnight (4). Initially, four subjects received digoxin (0.5 mg) in tablet form with water and four subjects received digoxin (0.5 mg) in liquid form with a small amount of water. A week later, the same subjects received propantheline (30 mg po) 30 min prior to taking digoxin as before. Serum digoxin levels were elevated when compared to baseline values in the subjects receiving digoxin in tablet form; however, propantheline did not induce any obvious change in the serum digoxin levels in the subjects who received the liquid digoxin preparation.

A subsequent report (15) by the same investigators showed that propantheline significantly elevated serum digoxin levels in eight patients who received a slow-dissolving brand of digoxin while exerting a minimal change with a fast-dissolving brand of digoxin. The patients received single doses of digoxin (25 mg/day po) without propantheline and with propantheline (10 mg po three times daily). All eight subjects received each treatment program for 10 days. The mean serum digoxin levels ($p<0.01$) were as follows: for slow-dissolving tablets, digoxin alone = 0.96 ng/ml, and digoxin with propantheline = 1.35 ng/ml; for fast-dissolving tablets, digoxin alone = 1.69 ng/ml, and digoxin with propantheline = 1.75 ng/ml.

■ If digoxin tablets that exhibit relatively slow release rates are given concurrently with propantheline, the resultant decrease in GI motility caused by propantheline may cause an increase in the amount of digoxin absorbed. However, this interaction does not occur in those patients who are receiving either the liquid preparations of digoxin or the tablet preparations that release their ingredients quickly. Therefore, this effect may be significant only in those patients who begin taking propantheline or any other anticholinergic drug while being maintained on tablets that exhibit comparatively slow release rates of digoxin.

Recommendations—This interaction can best be prevented by the use of liquid digoxin formulations or those digoxin tablet formulations that dissolve rapidly by USP standards. However, the practitioner should be alert for signs of toxicity due to digoxin whenever propantheline is given concurrently. The most dangerous sign is cardiac arrhythmia, but the patient may also exhibit GI symptoms such as nausea, vomiting, or anorexia; acute fatigue or muscle weakness; headaches; ocular disturbances such as hazy vision; or psychic disturbances (3).

Discontinuation of propantheline in a patient being concurrently maintained on slow-dissolving digoxin tablets may require upward adjustment in the digoxin dosage to achieve comparable serum digoxin levels.

References

(1) T. W. Smith and E. Haber, "Digitalis," *N. Engl. J. Med., 289,* 1063 (1973).

(2) J. E. Doherty *et al.,* "Tritiated Digoxin. XIV. Enterohepatic Circulation, Absorption and Excretion Studies in Human Volunteers," *Circulation, 42,* 867 (1970).

(3) "The Pharmacological Basis of Therapeutics," 5th ed., L. S. Goodman and A. Gilman, Eds., Macmillan, New York, NY 10022, 1975, pp. 514–532.

(4) V. Manninen *et al.,* "Altered Absorption of Digoxin in Patients Given Propantheline and Metoclopramide," *Lancet, i,* 398 (1973).

(5) J. G. Wagner *et al.,* "Equivalence Lack in Digoxin Plasma Levels," *J. Amer. Med. Ass., 224,* 199 (1973).

(6) D. H. Huffman and D. L. Azarnoff, "Absorption of Orally Given Digoxin Preparations," *J. Amer. Med. Ass., 222,* 957 (1972).

(7) J. E. Doherty, "The Clinical Pharmacology of Digitalis Glycosides: A Review," *Amer. J. Med. Sci., 255,* 382 (1968).

(8) J. Lindenbaum *et al.,* "Variation in Biologic Availability of Digoxin from Four Preparations," *N. Engl. J. Med., 285,* 1344 (1971).

(9) M. J. Stewart and E. Simpson, "New Formulation of Lanoxin: Expected Plasma Levels of Digoxin," *Lancet, ii*, 541 (1972).

(10) B. Whiting *et al.*, "New Formulation of Digoxin," *Lancet, ii*, 922 (1972).

(11) V. Manninen *et al.*, "New Formulation of Digoxin," *Lancet, ii*, 922 (1972).

(12) J. Lindenbaum *et al.*, "Correlation of Digoxin-Tablet Dissolution-Rate with Biological Availability," *Lancet, i*, 1215 (1973).

(13) W. G. Thompson, "Altered Absorption of Digoxin in Patients Given Propantheline and Metoclopramide," *Lancet, i*, 783 (1973).

(14) J. E. Doherty *et al.*, "New Information Regarding Digitalis Metabolism," *Chest, 59*, 433 (1971).

(15) V. Manninen *et al.*, "Effect of Propantheline and Metoclopramide on Absorption of Digoxin," *Lancet, i*, 1118 (1973).

[For additional information, see *Cardiac Glycoside Therapy*, p. 407.]

Nonproprietary and Trade Names of Drugs

Acetyldigitoxin—*Acylanid*
Anisotropine methylbromide—*Valpin*
Deslanoside—*Cedilanid-D*
Dicyclomine hydrochloride—*Bentyl and various combination products*
Digitalis—*Various manufacturers*
Digitoxin—*Crystodigin, Digitaline Nativelle, Myodigin, Purodigin*
Digoxin—*Lanoxin*
Gitalin—*Gitaligin*
Glycopyrrolate—*Robinul, Robinul Forte*
Hexocyclium methylsulfate—*Tral*

Isopropamide iodide—*Darbid*
Lanatoside C—*Cedilanid*
Methantheline bromide—*Banthine*
Methscopolamine bromide—*Pamine*
Ouabain—*Various manufacturers*
Oxyphencyclimine hydrochloride—*Daricon*
Oxyphenonium bromide—*Antrenyl Bromide*
Pipenzolate bromide—*Piptal*
Piperidolate hydrochloride—*Dactil*
Propantheline bromide—*Pro-Banthine*
Tridihexethyl chloride—*Pathilon*

Prepared and evaluated by the Scientific Review Subpanel on Cardiac Glycosides and reviewed by Practitioner Panel VI.

Ephedrine—Reserpine

Summary—Although pretreatment with reserpine theoretically may antagonize the cardiovascular response to subsequently administered ephedrine, there is little clinical evidence to support this theory. Nevertheless, patients receiving reserpine who are unresponsive to therapeutic doses of ephedrine should be switched to direct-acting sympathomimetics (such as levarterenol or phenylephrine) if a vasopressor drug is indicated.

Related Drugs—Other sympathomimetic agents related to ephedrine that interact with reserpine in animals include the **amphetamines, methylphenidate,** and **tyramine** (1). **Phenylpropanolamine** acts similarly to ephedrine and theoretically could interact with reserpine. Although all reported interactions were with reserpine, other rauwolfia derivatives, **alseroxylon, deserpidine, rescinnamine,** and **syrosingopine,** would also be expected to interact with ephedrine.

Pharmacological Effect and Mechanism—Sympathomimetics like ephedrine and related compounds (*e.g.*, amphetamine, metaraminol, and phenylpropanolamine) stimulate the adrenergic receptor site directly and indirectly by promoting the release of norepinephrine from its storage vesicles in the sympathetic nerve endings (2).

This "mixed" activity varies with the type of sympathomimetic and the dose of the drug used (3). Additionally, the ability of reserpine to antagonize the sympathomimetic drug is dependent on the type of activity (direct or indirect) that predominates.

Reserpine depletes the peripheral vascular adrenergic nerve endings of catecholamines and reduces their intraneuronal storage. When reserpine is given before ephedrine, it may antagonize the indirect action of ephedrine, resulting in a decreased cardiovascular response to this sympathomimetic (4). Investigations in animals have shown that the pressor response and cardiac-stimulating effects of ephedrine may be reduced but not abolished by reserpine pretreatment (5–7), which illustrates the direct- and indirect-stimulating properties of ephedrine.

Evaluation of Clinical Data—Clinical data concerning this problem are limited and difficult to assess. Ephedrine (16 mg im) was ineffective in an 18-month-old child who had accidentally ingested reserpine (~6.5 mg) (8). However, in another report, an adequate pressor response was obtained with normal adult therapeutic doses of ephedrine (10–25 mg iv) (9).

One case was reported in which a patient's blood pressure fell from a systolic level of 180 to 80 mm Hg during surgery (10). The hypotension was corrected with ephedrine (25 mg iv). This patient had been taking reserpine for 4 years which was withheld for 10 days prior to surgery. Another patient in this series became hypotensive during surgery and did not respond to intravenous ephedrine. This patient was maintained on levarterenol for 30 min and then placed on ephedrine with satisfactory results. This positive response to ephedrine was most likely secondary to the replenishing of the nerve ending stores with norepinephrine (levarterenol) during the infusion.

Several clinical observations (10–13) reporting severe hypotension during surgery in patients receiving reserpine led to the belief that the reserpine-induced depletion of nerve ending transmitter stores could have catastrophic effects during periods of stress. It was subsequently recommended that reserpine therapy be discontinued 2 weeks prior to elective surgery. The attenuated response to ephedrine was utilized for assessing the degree of norepinephrine depletion in patients receiving reserpine prior to anesthesia (14). However, another study (15) could not duplicate the results of the "ephedrine test."

Subsequent animal (16–18) and clinical (19) studies showed that reserpine therapy does not necessarily predispose the subject to circulatory collapse during stressful conditions. Consequently, the 2-week withdrawal period prior to surgery is not generally necessary. If hypotension does occur, it can be treated by using a direct-acting vasopressor (*e.g.*, levarterenol or phenylephrine) in preference to one that is dependent on norepinephrine release for its effects.

■ Although an interaction between ephedrine and reserpine is well documented in animals, there is little clinical evidence that this drug interaction occurs in humans. Moreover, other causative factors such as the dual action of ephedrine, high doses of ephedrine or reserpine, and the presence of other drugs were not ruled out in the reported studies.

Recommendations—If ephedrine fails to elicit a pressor response in a patient known to be receiving reserpine, a change to an agent such as levarterenol, methoxamine, or phenylephrine that stimulates adrenergic receptors directly is indicated. Metaraminol, a mixed-acting sympathomimetic, has been used successfully as a vasopressor in reserpine-treated patients (13). If an alternative pressor drug is administered, smaller doses may be satisfactory since the vasculature in reserpine-treated patients is often more sensitive to the pressor action of direct-acting sympathomimetic drugs (13).

References

(1) J. H. Burn and M. J. Rand, "The Action of Sympathomimetic Amines in Animals Treated with Reserpine," *J. Physiol.*, *144*, 314 (1958).

(2) J. M. Sneddon and P. Turner, "Ephedrine Mydriasis in Hypertension and the Response to Treatment," *Clin. Pharmacol. Ther.*, *10*, 64 (1969).

(3) J. Axelrod and R. Weinshilboum, "Catecholamines," *N. Engl. J. Med.*, *287*, 237 (1972).

(4) U. Trendelenburg, "Supersensitivity and Subsensitivity to Sympathomimetic Amines," *Pharmacol. Rev.*, *15*, 225 (1963).

(5) J. I. Moore and N. C. Moran, "Cardiac Contractile Force Responses to Ephedrine and Other Sympathomimetic Amines in Dogs after Pretreatment with Reserpine," *J. Pharmacol. Exp. Ther.*, *136*, 89 (1962).

(6) R. A. Maxwell *et al.*, "A Differential Effect of Reserpine on Pressor Amine Activity and Its Relationship to Other Agents Producing This Effect," *J. Pharmacol. Exp. Ther.*, *125*, 178 (1959).

(7) U. Trendelenburg *et al.*, "Modification by Reserpine of the Response of the Atrial Pacemaker to Sympathomimetic Amines," *J. Pharmacol. Exp. Ther.*, *141*, 301 (1963).

(8) T. Phillips, "Overdose of Reserpine," letter to the editor, *Brit. Med. J.*, *2*, 969 (1955).

(9) R. H. Noce *et al.*, "Reserpine (Serpasil) in the Management of the Mentally Ill," *J. Amer. Med. Ass.*, *158*, 11 (1955).

(10) C. H. Ziegler and J. B. Lovette, "Operative Complications after Therapy with Reserpine and Reserpine Compounds," *J. Amer. Med. Ass.*, *176*, 916 (1961).

(11) C. S. Coakley *et al.*, "Circulatory Responses during Anesthesia of Patients on Rauwolfia Therapy," *J. Amer. Med. Ass.*, *161*, 1143 (1956).

(12) M. Minuck, "Reaction to Drugs during Surgery and Anaesthesia," *Can. Med. Ass. J.*, *82*, 1008 (1960).

(13) A. A. Smessaert and R. G. Hicks, "Problems Caused by Rauwolfia Drugs during Anesthesia and Surgery," *N.Y. State J. Med.*, *61*, 2399 (1961).

(14) D. L. Crandell, "The Anesthetic Hazards in Patients on Antihypertensive Therapy," *J. Amer. Med. Ass.*, *179*, 495 (1962).

(15) W. Hamelberg and P. P. Bosomworth, "Evaluation of Ephedrine Test," *J. Amer. Med. Ass.*, *183*, 782 (1963).

(16) M. H. Alper *et al.*, "Pharmacology of Reserpine and Its Implications for Anesthesia," *Anesthesiology*, *24*, 524 (1963).

(17) E. E. Bagwell *et al.*, "Influence of Reserpine on Cardiovascular and Sympatho-Adrenal Responses to Ether Anesthesia in the Dog," *Anesthesiology*, *25*, 15 (1964).

(18) E. E. Bagwell *et al.*, "Influence of Reserpine on Cardiovascular and Sympatho-Adrenal Responses to Cyclopropane Anesthesia in the Dog," *Anesthesiology*, *25*, 148 (1964).

(19) W. M. Munson and J. A. Jenicek, "Effect of Anesthetic Agents on Patients Receiving Reserpine Therapy," *Anesthesiology*, *23*, 741 (1962).

[For additional information, see *Adrenergic Therapy*, p. 332.]

Nonproprietary and Trade Names of Drugs

Alseroxylon—*Rautensin, Rauwiloid*
Amphetamine complex—*Biphetamine*
Amphetamine sulfate—*Benzedrine*
Deserpidine—*Harmonyl*
Dextroamphetamine sulfate—*Dexedrine and various combination products*
Ephedrine hydrochloride and sulfate— *Various manufacturers*
Methamphetamine hydrochloride—*Desoxyn, Norodin Hydrochloride, Syndrox*
Methylphenidate hydrochloride—*Ritalin Hydrochloride*

Phenylpropanolamine hydrochloride— *Various combination products*
Rauwolfia serpentina—*Raudixin and various combination products*
Rescinnamine—*Moderil*
Reserpine—*Reserpoid, Sandril, Serpasil, and various combination products*
Syrosingopine—*Singoserp*
Tyramine—*Various foods and beverages*

Prepared and evaluated by the Scientific Review Subpanel on Autonomic Agents and reviewed by Practitioner Panel I.

Ether—Neomycin

Summary—Depression of neuromuscular transmission can be produced independently with ether or neomycin. When used concurrently, these drugs may produce enhanced respiratory depression or prolonged neuromuscular blockade. Adequate precautions should be taken to avoid any harmful consequences due to concurrent use.

Related Drugs—Inhalation anesthetic agents such as **cyclopropane** (1, 2), **halothane** (3), **methoxyflurane** (3), and **nitrous oxide** (3) have also been reported to interact with neomycin and related drugs. Although not documented, **chloroform, enflurane, ethyl chloride, fluroxene, halopropane, trichloroethylene,** and **trichloromonofluoromethane** may interact in a similar manner.

Aminoglycoside antibiotics such as **kanamycin** (3) and **streptomycin** (3) are known to interact with ether and related agents. **Colistin** (4), **dihydrostreptomycin** (4), **gentamicin** (4), and **viomycin** (4) have been shown to have neuromuscular blocking activity similar to neomycin and may interact similarly with ether.

Pharmacological Effect and Mechanism—Muscle response to both direct and indirect electrical stimulation is profoundly affected by ether (5), which indicates that ether has a neuromuscular blocking action at both junctional (end plate) and nonjunctional (muscle) sites. *In vitro* studies indicated that the primary neuromuscular blocking action of anesthetics like ether is due to their ability to depress depolarization at the junctional (end plate) site and that the depolarization must be depressed by about 50% before the neuromuscular blockade occurs (6).

The prime action of neomycin appears to be at the neuromuscular junction (end plate) rather than at nonjunctional (muscle) sites. Neomycin has been shown to antagonize end-plate depolarization by acetylcholine and can prevent potassium from producing an increase in frequency of miniature end-plate potentials (7). Neomycin neuromuscular blockade is directly related to dose and probably results from a combination of the reduced sensitivity of the postjunctional membrane and interference with transmitter release (8).

Evaluation of Clinical Data—Paralysis resulting from the parenteral administration of antibiotics was restricted to laboratory observations until respiratory arrest was reported in four patients following the intraperitoneal administration of neomycin (9).

Subsequent reports of respiratory arrest (1, 10, 11) as well as prolonged neuromuscular blockade (12) established a causal relationship between neomycin administration and ether anesthesia. Neomycin (1 g ip) administered during surgery reduced minute volume ventilation in 66% of patients studied, while 500 mg produced similar respiratory depression in 33% of anesthetized patients regardless of the anesthetic agent or technique (13).

No neuromuscular blocking effects were reported in another study of 18 patients given neomycin (1 g ip) during surgery, followed by 500 mg every 6 hr through an indwelling catheter (14). A review of reported complications, however, implicates a dose of as little as 500 mg in children and 1–5 g in adults, levels well within the recommended therapeutic range for intraperitoneal neomycin.

Neomycin respiratory depression is dependent upon the blood level of neomycin achieved and does not occur if a neomycin–dextran complex (neolymphin) is used instead of neomycin, presumably because lower serum levels of neomycin are attained (13).

■ Large doses of neomycin or related antibiotics alone in children or debilitated patients may produce respiratory depression. In the presence of ether or other inhalation anesthetic agents, smaller intraperitoneal doses of the antibiotic may produce respiratory arrest or prolonged neuromuscular blockade. All reported respiratory complications followed intraperitoneal neomycin administration, reflecting the high absorption from peritoneal surfaces. There are no reports of respiratory depression after oral or intramuscular administration of neomycin. Anesthetic–neomycin neuromuscular blockade can be greatly increased and prolonged by the concurrent use of neuromuscular blocking drugs such as pancuronium, succinylcholine, or tubocurarine during anesthesia (see *Tubocurarine–Neomycin*, p. 254).

Recommendations—Intraperitoneal antibiotic therapy has been widespread and frequent in the treatment of bacterial peritonitis. Both surgeon and anesthesiologist must be prepared to treat the neuromuscular and respiratory depression that will frequently be produced, particularly if muscle relaxant drugs were also used during anesthesia (see *Tubocurarine–Neomycin*, p. 254). Perhaps a satisfactory compromise would be the insertion of an intraperitoneal catheter at the time of surgery and the administration of antibiotic drugs later when the effects of the anesthetic drugs are no longer evident at the neuromuscular junction. However, this technique is very hazardous and patients treated in this manner should be monitored closely for symptoms of neuromuscular blockade following administration of the antibiotic.

If neuromuscular blockade and respiratory depression are encountered, the intravenous use of neostigmine (0.2–2.5 mg), calcium (1 g), and possibly sodium bicarbonate (dose not reported), either alone or concurrently, may be helpful in reversing the blockade (3, 15) in some, but not all, patients. The administration of analeptic agents (*e.g.*, doxapram and nikethamide) is of no value (3). The wisest and probably safest procedure is to administer supportive care and ventilatory assistance while monitoring the status of the neuromuscular function. This procedure should be continued until the neuromuscular blockade has passed. Secondary circulatory collapse also may occur (3) and vital signs should be monitored closely. If circulation is depressed, volume replacement should be instituted.

Other antibiotics such as bacitracin, clindamycin (16), polymyxin (4), and tetracyclines (4) are neuromuscular blocking agents and may interact with ether. Therefore, similar precautions should be taken when these antibiotics are administered with ether and related anesthetics.

References

(1) B. M. Webber, "Respiratory Arrest following Intraperitoneal Administration of Neomycin," *AMA Arch. Surg.*, *75*, 174 (1957).

(2) W. P. G. Jones, "Calcium Treatment for Ineffective Respiration Resulting from Administration of Neomycin," *J. Amer. Med. Ass.*, *170*, 943 (1959).

(3) C. B. Pittinger *et al.*, "Antibiotic-Induced Paralysis," *Anesth. Analg.*, *49*, 487 (1970).

(4) C. Pittinger and R. Adamson, "Antibiotic Blockade of Neuromuscular Function," *Ann. Rev. Pharmacol.*, *12*, 169 (1972).

(5) P. B. Sabawala and J. B. Dillon, "Action of Volatile Anesthetics on Human Muscle Preparations," *Anesthesiology*, *19*, 587 (1958).

(6) B. E. Waud and D. R. Waud, "Comparison of the Effects of General Anesthetics on the End-plate of Skeletal Muscle," *Anesthesiology*, *43*, 540 (1975).

(7) D. Elmqvist and J.-O. Josefsson, "The Nature of the Neuromuscular Block Produced by Neomycine," *Acta Physiol. Scand.*, *54*, 105 (1962).

(8) A. P. Corrado *et al.*, "Neuro-muscular Blockade by Neomycin Potentiation by Ether Anesthesia and d-Tubocurarine and Antagonism by Calcium and Prostigmine," *Arch. Int. Pharmacodyn. Ther.*, *121*, 380 (1959).

(9) J. E. Pridgen, "Respiratory Arrest Thought to be Due to Intraperitoneal Neomycin," *Surgery*, *40*, 571 (1956).

(10) Case Report 190, *ASA Newsletter*, *21*, 38 (1957).

(11) Case Report 203, *ASA Newsletter*, *22*, 33 (1958).

(12) C. B. Pittinger *et al.*, "The Neuromuscular Blocking Action of Neomycin: A Concern of the Anesthesiologist," *Anesth. Analg.*, *37*, 276 (1958).

(13) P. Markalous, "Respiration and the Intraperitoneal Application of Neomycin and Neolymphin," *Anaesthesia, 17*, 427 (1962).

(14) W. E. Schatten, "Intraperitoneal Antibiotic Administration in the Treatment of Acute Bacterial Peritonitis," *Surg. Gynecol. Obstet., 102*, 339 (1956).

(15) V. F. Stanley *et al.*, "Neomycin-Curare Neuromuscular Block and Reversal in Cats," *Anesthesiology, 31*, 228 (1969).

(16) R. P. Fodgall and R. D. Miller, "Prolongation of a Pancuronium-Induced Neuromuscular Blockade by Clindamycin," *Anesthesiology, 41*, 407 (1974).

[For additional information, see *Anesthetic Therapy*, p. 345.]

Nonproprietary and Trade Names of Drugs

Bacitracin—*Various manufacturers*
Chloroform—*Various manufacturers*
Chlortetracycline hydrochloride—*Aureomycin*
Clindamycin hydrochloride—*Cleocin Hydrochloride*
Colistin sulfate—*Coly-Mycin S*
Cyclopropane—*Various manufacturers*
Demeclocycline—*Declomycin*
Dihydrostreptomycin sulfate—*Various manufacturers*
Doxycycline monohydrate—*Doxychel, Doxy-II Monohydrate, Vibramycin Monohydrate*
Enflurane—*Ethrane*
Ether—*Various manufacturers*
Ethyl chloride—*Various manufacturers*
Fluroxene—*Fluromar*
Gentamicin sulfate—*Garamycin*
Halopropane—*Tebron*
Halothane—*Fluothane*
Kanamycin sulfate—*Kantrex*
Methacycline hydrochloride—*Rondomycin*
Methoxyflurane—*Penthrane*
Minocycline hydrochloride—*Minocin, Vectrin*

Neomycin sulfate—*Mycifradin Sulfate, Myciguent, Neobiotic*
Nitrous oxide—*Various manufacturers*
Oxytetracycline—*Dalimycin, Terramycin*
Oxytetracycline hydrochloride—*Oxy-Kesso-Tetra, Oxy-Tetrachel, Terramycin Hydrochloride*
Polymyxin B sulfate—*Various manufacturers*
Streptomycin sulfate—*Various manufacturers*
Tetracycline—*Achromycin, Panmycin, Panmycin KM, Sumycin, Tetracyn, Tetrex-S*
Tetracycline hydrochloride—*Achromycin, Bristacycline, Cyclopar, Panmycin, Robitet, Steclin, Sumycin, Tetracyn*
Tetracycline phosphate complex—*Tetrex*
Trichloroethylene—*Trilene*
Trichloromonofluoromethane—*Various manufacturers*
Viomycin sulfate—*Vinactone Sulfate, Viocin Sulfate*

Prepared and evaluated by the Scientific Review Subpanel on Anesthetics and reviewed by Practitioner Panel VI.

Ferrous Sulfate—Ascorbic Acid

Summary—Concurrent administration of sufficient amounts (>200 mg po) of ascorbic acid increases the absorption of elemental iron in the gastrointestinal (GI) tract. Since iron alone is usually absorbed sufficiently to correct deficiencies in body stores, concurrent therapy is not recommended for routine treatment of uncomplicated iron deficiency states.

Related Drugs—The absorption of other iron salts such as the **fumarate, gluconate,** and **lactate** also may be enhanced to varying degrees when administered with appropriate amounts of ascorbic acid.

Pharmacological Effect and Mechanism—Inorganic iron is used in the prevention and treatment of microcytic, hypochromic anemias and other iron deficiency states. Maximal absorption of iron occurs primarily in the proximal portion of the small intestine. Iron from the diet must be converted to the more soluble ferrous form to be absorbed (1, 2). Most commercial iron preparations are in the ferrous form.

Animal studies indicated that a variable amount of the iron retained in the duodenal and jejunal area is transferred to the plasma iron-binding protein transferrin. The remainder of retained iron then stays within the mucosal cell in the form of ferritin. In iron deficiency, most iron is transferred to the plasma, while in the presence of normal iron stores or iron "overload," much of the iron remains in the intestinal mucosal cell as ferritin and is eventually lost when the cell is shed from the intestinal wall. Iron loss is enhanced in overload and diminished in periods of iron deficiency (3).

The absorption of iron can be influenced by other endogenous factors. Increased erythropoietic activity increases iron absorption (4). Slower GI motility and transit time or increased secretions of either gastric or pancreatic juices also influence the quantity of iron absorbed from the GI tract (4, 5).

Exogenous factors such as food also affect iron absorption. Ascorbic acid, as part of the foodstuff or ingested independently, is thought to increase the absorption of iron by virtue of its ability to lower pH (and thus increase the solubility of iron), to reduce the ferric ion to the more soluble ferrous ion, and to combine with the iron molecule to form an unstable metal complex, which acts as an iron "donor" by releasing its metal to the gut wall for absorption (1).

Evaluation of Clinical Data—Forty-one nonanemic subjects and one patient with pernicious anemia were given elemental iron (30 mg po in solution) every morning for 10 days following an overnight fast (6). Two iron solutions were prepared, one labeled with radioactive ^{55}Fe and the other with radioactive ^{59}Fe, and were given on alternate days. Ascorbic acid (50–500 mg po) also was given with the iron solution every other day. Two weeks after the last iron dose, blood samples were drawn and the levels of ^{55}Fe and ^{59}Fe in the red blood cell mass were measured and compared. In each case, patients served as their own controls. The results indicated that serum levels of the radioactive iron incorporated into hemoglobin after concurrent administration of ascorbic acid (>200 mg) were at least 1.33 (mean value) times the serum levels of radioactive iron achieved without ascorbic acid or with low doses (<200 mg) of ascorbic acid. In those patients receiving 500 mg of ascorbic acid, serum iron levels were 1.48 (mean value) times those achieved without ascorbic acid administration. The increases in serum iron levels were statistically significant.

In another study (7), 40 patients (mean hemoglobin level, >11 g/100 ml) picked randomly from a medical ward were given 200 mg of ferrous sulfate (containing 65 mg of elemental iron) on Day 1 and then were given ferrous sulfate concurrently with 50 and 1000 mg of ascorbic acid on subsequent days at least 4 days apart. Each morning, baseline serum iron levels were determined at 8 a.m. (the same time at which the drugs were administered) and then hourly until noon. There was no significant difference in the serum iron levels of the patients after ferrous sulfate alone or with 50 mg of ascorbic acid. However, there was a statistically significant increase of 19.5 μg/100 ml (mean value) in the serum iron levels of the subjects after the 1000-mg dose of ascorbic acid was given concurrently with ferrous sulfate. Moreover, the mean absorption curve of iron was higher by an average of 24 μg/100 ml.

In a third study (8), 10 anemic children and infants (mean hemoglobin level, 5.1 g/100 ml) were given ferric ammonium citrate solution (equivalent to 20–25 mg/ kg of elemental iron) and 500–750 mg of ascorbic acid in divided doses. Another 10 patients (mean hemoglobin level, 4.2 g/100 ml) received the same dose of iron but received multivitamins (containing approximately 36 mg of ascorbic acid) instead of the larger dose of ascorbic acid. Hemoglobin levels were used as a parameter to measure iron absorption. Children treated with iron and ascorbic acid (500–750 mg) reached the desired level of 11 g/100 ml in 21 days compared to 29 days for the children receiving iron and multivitamins.

■ Ascorbic acid, in doses of at least 200 mg po, may increase the serum iron levels in some patients when the two drugs are administered concurrently. However, it is difficult to determine if such an increase is due to the presence of ascorbic acid or to other endogenous or exogenous variables that also influence iron absorption (1, 5). Because most individuals are able to absorb orally ingested iron adequately without concurrent administration of ascorbic acid, there is little therapeutic indication for combining these two drugs. Although concurrent therapy may correct iron deficiency anemia in children (8), there are no clinical data indicating that concurrent therapy is any more effective than iron administration alone.

Recommendations—Since the absorption of iron salts alone has been shown to be adequate in most humans, there is little justification for concurrent use of ascorbic acid in the treatment of uncomplicated iron deficiency states. However, concurrent administration of ascorbic acid and iron may be useful in patients who have difficulty in absorbing adequate quantities of iron (*e.g.*, infants and young children with severe anemia). Concurrent therapy, particularly if ascorbic acid is given in doses greater than 400 mg/day, should not be used in pregnant women because of the potential danger of conditioning the fetus to increased requirements of ascorbic acid (9). Furthermore, the wide variation in amounts of ascorbic acid (200–1000 mg) reported to enhance iron absorption makes the use of combinations of these agents in fixed dose ratios undesirable.

References

(1) W. Forth and W. Rummel, "Iron Absorption," *Physiol. Rev.*, *53*, 724 (1973).

(2) "The Pharmacological Basis of Therapeutics," 5th ed., L. S. Goodman and A. Gilman, Eds., Macmillan, New York, NY 10022, 1975, pp. 1309–1320.

(3) R. W. Charlton *et al.*, "The Role of the Intestinal Mucosa in Iron Absorption," *J. Clin. Invest.*, *44*, 543 (1965).

(4) A. J. Giorgio, "Current Concepts of Iron Metabolism and the Iron Deficiency Anemias," *Med. Clin. N. Amer.*, *54*, 1399 (1970).

(5) T. H. Bothwell *et al.*, "Iron Absorption I: Factors Influencing Absorption," *J. Lab. Clin. Med.*, *51*, 24 (1958).

(6) H. Brise and L. Hallberg, "Effect of Ascorbic Acid on Iron Absorption," *Acta Med. Scand.*, *171*, suppl., 51 (1962).

(7) P. C. Lee *et al.*, "Large and Small Doses of Ascorbic Acid in the Absorption of Ferrous Iron," *Can. Med. Ass. J.*, *97*, 181 (1967).

(8) M. K. Gorten and J. E. Bradley, "The Treatment of Nutritional Anemia in Infancy and Childhood with Oral Iron and Ascorbic Acid," *J. Pediat.*, *45*, 1 (1954).

(9) W. A. Cochrane, "Overnutrition in Prenatal and Neonatal Life: A Problem?" *Can. Med. Ass. J.*, *93*, 893 (1965).

[For additional information, see *Vitamin Therapy*, p. 449.]

Nonproprietary and Trade Names of Drugs

Ascorbic acid—*Available alone and in combination with many iron salts*
Ferrocholinate—*Chel-Iron, Ferrolip*

Ferrous fumarate, gluconate, lactate, and sulfate—*Various manufacturers, available alone or as a fixed combination*

Prepared and evaluated by the Scientific Review Subpanel on Vitamins and reviewed by Practitioner Panel I.

Gallamine Triethiodide—Diazepam

Summary—In anesthetized patients, the intravenous administration of diazepam may increase the intensity and prolong the duration of the neuromuscular block-ade produced by gallamine triethiodide. Clinical reports concerning this inter-action are conflicting. Until more information is available, close monitoring for unusual increases in the intensity and the duration of respiratory depression is indicated in anesthetized patients receiving these two drugs concurrently.

Related Drugs—Other benzodiazepines such as **chlordiazepoxide, clonazepam, cloraze-pate, flurazepam, nitrazepam,** and **oxazepam** might be expected to interact similarly with gallamine triethiodide and other nondepolarizing neuromuscular blocking agents such as **pancuronium** and **tubocurarine,** as well as depolarizing neuromuscular block-ing agents such as **decamethonium** and **succinylcholine.** However, there is no docu-mentation to support this suggestion.

Pharmacological Effect and Mechanism—Gallamine triethiodide and other non-depolarizing neuromuscular blocking agents produce skeletal muscle relaxation by combining with the receptor site at the neuromuscular junction and blocking the action of the neurotransmitter acetylcholine (1).

Diazepam produces skeletal muscle relaxation in both animals and humans (2) by its inhibitory effect on polysynaptic reflexes in the spinal cord and/or supraspinal structures such as the reticular facilatory system (3). Diazepam may also exert a peripheral action at the neuromuscular junction involving direct muscle depression (4). This peripheral effect was demonstrable only at very high concentrations of diazepam and did not account for the other observed actions.

There are insufficient data to explain the possible mechanism for the gallamine triethiodide–diazepam interaction.

Evaluation of Clinical Data—Neuromuscular transmission was studied by recording the force of thumb adduction following the electrical stimulation of the ulnar nerve (5). Diazepam (0.15–0.20 mg/kg iv) in four anesthetized patients following gallamine triethiodide administration (40–60 mg iv) increased the intensity and duration of the neuromuscular blockade produced by a second dose of gallamine triethiodide adminis-tered 78–123 min following the control dose of the muscle relaxant.

The same type of experimental model (thumb adduction following ulnar nerve stimulation) was used in a study of five anesthetized patients (4). Diazepam (0.3–0.6 mg/kg iv), injected while the myoneural junction was recovering from the effect of gallamine triethiodide (20 mg/m²), did not alter the recovery rate of the neuromuscular blockade.

■ Although intravenous diazepam has been reported to intensify and prolong the duration of neuromuscular blockade produced by gallamine triethiodide, the clinical evidence is conflicting. The discrepancy in the two studies may be due to the methodology employed. One study (5) used the same patients as controls while the other (4) employed a control group different from the experimental group. Thus, the results of the study using the same patients as controls could actually represent enhancement of neuromuscular blockade by a second dose of tubocurarine or gallamine triethiodide. The incidence and clinical significance of this drug interaction, therefore, are yet to be determined.

Recommendations—Until further clinical evidence is available, anesthetized patients should be monitored closely for signs of any unusual increases in the intensity or duration of the respiratory depression caused by gallamine triethiodide.

References

(1) "The Pharmacological Basis of Thera-peutics," 5th ed., L. S. Goodman and A. Gilman, Eds., Macmillan, New York, NY 10022, 1975, pp. 578–580.

(2) G. Zbinden and L. O. Randall, "Phar-macology of Benzodiazepines: Labora-tory and Clinical Correlations," *Advan. Pharmacol.*, 5, 213 (1967).

(3) S. H. Ngai *et al.*, "Effect of Diazepam and Other Central Nervous System De-pressants on Spinal Reflexes in Cats: A Study of Site of Action," *J. Pharmacol. Exp. Ther.*, *153*, 344 (1966).

(4) K. Dretchen *et al.*, "The Interaction of Diazepam with Myoneural Blocking Agents," *Anesthesiology*, *34*, 463 (1971).

(5) S. A. Feldman and B. E. Crawley, "Interactions of Diazepam with the Muscle-Relaxant Drugs," *Brit. Med. J.*, *2*, 336 (1970).

[For additional information, see *Muscle Relaxant Therapy*, p. 435.]

Nonproprietary and Trade Names of Drugs

Chlordiazepoxide—*Libritabs*
Chlordiazepoxide hydrochloride—*Librium and various combination products*
Clonazepam—*Clonopin*
Clorazepate dipotassium—*Tranxene*
Decamethonium bromide—*Syncurine*
Diazepam—*Valium*
Flurazepam hydrochloride—*Dalmane*
Gallamine triethiodide—*Flaxedil*
Metocurine (dimethyl tubocurarine) chloride—*Mecostrin*

Metocurine (dimethyl tubocurarine) iodide—*Metubine*
Nitrazepam—*Mogadon*
Óxazepam—*Serax*
Pancuronium bromide—*Pavulon*
Succinylcholine chloride—*Anectine, Quelicin Chloride*
Tubocurarine chloride—*Tubarine*

Prepared and evaluated by the Scientific Review Subpanel on Muscle Relaxants and reviewed by Practitioner Panel VI.

Gentamicin—Carbenicillin

Summary—Gentamicin, when administered concurrently with carbenicillin, has been reported to be more effective than either drug alone against certain sus-ceptible organisms. However, the activity of gentamicin appears to be dimin-ished significantly by carbenicillin when mixed *in vitro* for prolonged periods prior to administration. Therefore, carbenicillin and gentamicin should not be mixed in the same solution and should be administered parenterally at different time intervals.

Related Drugs—**Colistimethate** and aminoglycosides such as **kanamycin, neomycin, streptomycin,** and **tobramycin** may interact similarly with carbenicillin. Penicillins such as **ampicillin** and **penicillin G,** mixed *in vitro* with gentamicin, also cause the loss of gentamicin antimicrobial activity (1, 2).

Pharmacological Effect and Mechanism—Beneficial therapeutic effects of concur-rent gentamicin and carbenicillin administration were reported for infections due to *Pseudomonas aeruginosa* and *Proteus mirabilis*. However, the therapeutic effect of these drugs against *Klebsiella* and *Escherichia coli* has been poor (3). Concurrent use apparently prevents the emergence of mutant strains resistant to either agent alone (4).

In vitro evidence suggests physicochemical incompatibility of gentamicin and carbenicillin dependent upon time of exposure, temperature, and carbenicillin concen-tration (1, 5–7).

Evaluation of Clinical Data—The beneficial therapeutic effect of concurrent parenteral administration of gentamicin and carbenicillin has been reported, and such
therapy has been encouraged based on clinical experience (3, 6, 8). Other studies
suggested that concurrent use of gentamicin and carbenicillin results in inactivation
of gentamicin (5, 6), probably by a physical incompatibility occurring when the
antibiotics are mixed in the same intravenous solution (6, 7).

■ Clinical experience indicates that beneficial therapeutic effects are achieved by the
concurrent administration of gentamicin and carbenicillin in the treatment of *Pseudomonas* infections. The *in vitro* inactivation of gentamicin by carbenicillin is not a
contraindication to the concurrent use of these antibiotics in the treatment of sepsis
provided they are not mixed together in the same infusion fluid.

Recommendations—Prolonged contact of gentamicin and carbenicillin in the same
infusion fluid should be avoided. If concurrent administration can only be accomplished intravenously, gentamicin and carbenicillin should be physically separated by
using separate infusion fluids and given at different intervals about 1–2 hr apart.

References

(1) L. Riff and G. G. Jackson, "Gentamicin
    plus Carbenicillin," *Lancet, i,* 592
    (1971).
(2) B. Lynn, "Carbenicillin plus Genta-
    micin," *Lancet, i,* 653 (1971).
(3) C. B. Smith *et al.,* "Use of Gentamicin
    in Combinations with Other Antibi-
    otics," *J. Infec. Dis., 119,* 370 (1969).
(4) A. W. Nunnery *et al.,* "Carbenicillin:
    in-vivo Synergism and Combined Ther-
    apy," *J. Infec. Dis., 122,* S78 (1970).

(5) J. E. McLaughlin and D. S. Reeves,
    "Clinical and Laboratory Evidence for
    the Inactivation of Gentamicin by
    Carbenicillin," *Lancet, i,* 261 (1971).
(6) S. Eykyn *et al.,* "Gentamicin plus Car-
    benicillin," *Lancet, i,* 545 (1971).
(7) M. E. Levison and D. Kaye, "Carbeni-
    cillin plus Gentamicin," *Lancet, ii,* 45
    (1971).
(8) J. Klastersky, "Carbenicillin plus
    Gentamicin," *Lancet, i,* 653 (1971).

[For additional information, see *Anti-Infective Therapy,* p. 388.]

Nonproprietary and Trade Names of Drugs

Ampicillin—*Alpen, Amcill, Omnipen,*
  Penbritin, Polycillin, Principen, Totacillin
Carbenicillin disodium—*Geopen, Pyopen*
Colistimethate sodium—*Coly-Mycin M*
Gentamicin sulfate—*Garamycin*
Kanamycin sulfate—*Kantrex*
Neomycin sulfate—*Mycifradin Sulfate,*
  Myciguent, Neobiotic
Penicillin G benzathine—*Bicillin, Permapen*

Penicillin G potassium—*Dramcillin,*
  G-Recillin, Hyasorb, Kesso-Pen,
  Palocillin S-10, Pedacillin, Pentids,
  Pfizerpen, Sugracillin
Penicillin G procaine—*Crysticillin AS,*
  Diurnal-Penicillin, Duracillin A.S.,
  Pentids-P, Pfizerpen-AS, Wycillin
Streptomycin sulfate—*Various*
  manufacturers
Tobramycin sulfate—*Nebcin*

*Prepared and evaluated by the Scientific Review Subpanel
on Anti-Infectives and reviewed by Practitioner Panel VI.*

Griseofulvin—Phenobarbital

Summary—The serum levels of orally administered griseofulvin may be lowered
to clinically ineffective levels by concurrent administration of phenobarbital.
Substitution of an alternative agent for phenobarbital or an increase in the dose
(preferably by increasing the number of divided doses) of griseofulvin may be
necessary.

Related Drugs—Phenobarbital does not appear to interact with other antifungal
agents; however, other **barbiturates** may similarly affect griseofulvin.

Pharmacological Effect and Mechanism—The only effect shown by concurrent oral administration of griseofulvin and phenobarbital is a reduction in clinical effectiveness of griseofulvin; reduced serum griseofulvin levels have been reported after phenobarbital administration (1–4).

The mechanism for this interaction is controversial. Several early studies in rats (2) and humans (3, 4) and subsequent review articles suggested that the mechanism was a phenobarbital-induced increase in the metabolism of griseofulvin.

However, in another study (1), no reduction in serum levels was found when griseofulvin was administered intravenously. Therefore, these investigators suggested that the mechanism was phenobarbital interference with griseofulvin absorption rather than an increase in griseofulvin metabolism. There are two theories offered for the reduction in absorption: (a) phenobarbital may decrease the degree of dispersion of the drug from the tablet granules, thereby reducing the surface area available for dissolution, or (b) phenobarbital may decrease the transit time in that section of the intestine from which griseofulvin is maximally absorbed by stimulating bile secretion which, in turn, stimulates peristalsis.

If it is true that phenobarbital decreases the gastrointestinal absorption of griseofulvin, there should be an increase in the amount of free griseofulvin in the feces, a fact not reported in any study.

Evaluation of Clinical Data—A reduction in serum griseofulvin levels occurred in four males and four females after oral phenobarbital administration (3). Each subject received a total of 210 mg po of phenobarbital over approximately 60 hr prior to a single dose of griseofulvin (500 mg po). Serum levels were then determined for the next 26 hr. No data were given for chronic treatment with griseofulvin.

A female (age 38) failed to respond to griseofulvin in another report (4), although the invading microorganism was griseofulvin sensitive. The failure was attributed to phenobarbital because the patient was receiving this drug (120 mg/day po) for the control of petit mal seizures.

Six healthy males were given both intravenous (300 mg) and oral (500 mg) microcrystalline griseofulvin. When phenobarbital (90 mg/day po) was given for 3–4 days prior to a single dose of griseofulvin, a reduction in serum levels of the antifungal agent was noted after oral administration, but not after intravenous administration.

■ Griseofulvin given at normal oral doses may be less effective or ineffective if the patient is receiving phenobarbital concurrently. The incidence and degree of lowering of serum levels as a function of the dose of both agents have not been well established.

Recommendations—When possible, phenobarbital should be avoided during griseofulvin therapy and some other nonbarbiturate sedative–hypnotic should be used. When concurrent administration of griseofulvin and phenobarbital is required (e.g., in some convulsive disorders and/or severe fungal infections) and there is indication of poor clinical effect, serum griseofulvin levels should be monitored. The dosage of griseofulvin may also have to be increased, preferably in divided doses to allow more time for drug absorption during transit through the upper intestinal tract.

References

(1) S. Riegelman et al., "Griseofulvin–Phenobarbital Interaction in Man," J. Amer. Med. Ass., 213, 426 (1970).

(2) D. Busfield et al., "An Effect of Phenobarbitone on Griseofulvin Metabolism in the Rat," Brit. J. Pharmacol., 22, 137 (1964).

(3) D. Busfield et al., "An Effect of Phenobarbitone on Blood-Levels of Griseofulvin in Man," Lancet, ii, 1042 (1963).

(4) E. Lorenc, "A New Factor in Griseofulvin Treatment Failures," Mo. Med., 64, 32 (1967).

[For additional information, see Anti-Infective Therapy, p. 388.]

Nonproprietary and Trade Names of Drugs

Allobarbital—*Diadol*
Amobarbital—*Amytal and various combination products*
Aprobarbital—*Alurate*
Barbital—*Neurondia*
Butabarbital sodium—*Butisol Sodium*
Butalbital—*Available in combination products*
Griseofulvin—*Fulvicin U/F, Grifulvin V, Grisactin, Gris-PEG*
Hexobarbital—*Sombulex*

Mephobarbital—*Mebaral, Mebroin*
Metharbital—*Gemonil*
Methohexital sodium—*Brevital Sodium*
Pentobarbital—*Nembutal and various combination products*
Phenobarbital—*Eskabarb, Luminal*
Secobarbital—*Seconal and various combination products*
Talbutal—*Lotusate*
Thiopental sodium—*Pentothal Sodium*

Prepared and evaluated by the Scientific Review Subpanel on Anti-Infectives and reviewed by Practitioner Panel IV.

Guanethidine—Alcohol

Summary—Alcohol may enhance the antihypertensive effects of guanethidine. Patients treated with guanethidine should be cautioned that they may experience symptoms of postural hypotension and syncope and that these symptoms may worsen if alcoholic beverages are ingested.

Related Drugs—**Bethanidine** and **debrisoquin** are chemically and pharmacologically related to guanethidine and could be expected to interact with alcohol in a similar manner.

Pharmacological Effect and Mechanism—Guanethidine interferes with the storage and release of catecholamines from postganglionic sympathetic nerve fibers producing adrenergic neuron blockade (1). The reduction of vasomotor tone and the impairment of reflex adaptation on changing from a supine or sitting position to a standing position can lead to orthostatic hypotension and syncope. Such episodes are not restricted to the dose adjustment period but occur characteristically on arising from a prone position and during periods of muscular exercise or exertion.

Alcohol exerts profound vasodilator effects (2, 3), primarily on cutaneous vessels, and blood flow through the skeletal muscular bed is either unchanged or decreased (4, 5). The mechanism of action of the vascular effects of alcohol is yet to be determined. Alcohol is not a direct peripheral vasodilator and is assumed to act through central inhibition of sympathetic tone and depression of the medullary vasomotor center (6). However, the fact that alcohol, directly and indirectly through its acetaldehyde metabolite, causes catecholamine release might explain the different cardiovascular responses observed under various experimental conditions (7–9).

In addition, there is evidence that alcohol has a direct depressant effect on the myocardium (10, 11). As little as 60 ml of whiskey caused a statistically significant decrease in the stroke volume and therefore lowered the cardiac output of chronic alcoholics and of patients with cardiac disease of varying etiology (12). A progressive drop in cardiac output and arterial pressure was demonstrated (13) in eight patients with stable coronary heart disease after the ingestion of 0.5 g/kg of 100% alcohol diluted with water over 2 min. In contrast, results from studies conducted with healthy volunteers are not uniform but generally show a heart rate-dependent reflex increase in cardiac output and, especially with higher blood alcohol levels (120 mg/ 100 ml), a decrease in peripheral resistance (14, 15).

Evaluation of Clinical Data—No specific studies have been conducted concerning the guanethidine–alcohol interaction. However, the occurrence of hypotensive episodes induced by alcohol in patients treated with guanethidine has been frequent enough to warrant numerous comments (1, 16, 17) and inclusion of a warning in the manufacturer's drug package insert. A typical setting for an attack of postural hypotension is the cocktail party where people remain standing, frequently in a warm room (18). Other instances in which postural hypotension occurs are after physical exercise, after rising quickly from a sitting or prone position, and after showers or baths (1). Syncope occurs when the initial symptoms of dizziness or weakness are ignored. The "coopera- tion" of a patient by squatting at cocktail parties when hypotension occurs has been suggested (19). One report cautioned that hypotensive symptoms are experienced after ingestion of alcohol, but a small amount of alcohol (*e.g.,* a cocktail) before dinner is usually well tolerated and, in fact, may aid in preventing the usual evening upswing in blood pressure of patients treated with guanethidine (20).

■ There are no reports that indicate the actual frequency and seriousness of hypo- tensive episodes attributed to concurrent use of guanethidine and alcohol. However, hypertensive patients receiving guanethidine who would be especially prone to experi- ence symptoms of hypotension and syncope after ingestion of alcohol are assumed to have the following characteristics: (*a*) those whose cardiovascular reflex adaptation is compromised or marginal, (*b*) those who also suffer from hypertensive or coronary heart disease, (*c*) those whose vascular system shows arteriosclerotic or arteriolar degeneration, and (*d*) those who consume large quantities of alcohol.

Recommendations—Patients receiving guanethidine for treatment of hypertension, particularly those with myocardial insufficiency, should be instructed that concurrent alcohol ingestion may impair blood pressure control and may produce fainting spells and blackouts. The postural or orthostatic component of the syndrome should be emphasized. The patient should be advised that such episodes occur characteristically while standing, after rising rapidly from a sitting or prone position, or after physical exercise. When experiencing such episodes or when any related signs of weakness or dizziness occur, the patient must sit down or lie down immediately.

References

(1) "The Pharmacological Basis of Thera- peutics," 5th ed., L. S. Goodman and A. Gilman, Eds., Macmillan, New York, NY 10022, 1975, pp. 553–556.

(2) E. Cook and G. Brown, "The Vaso- dilating Effects of Ethyl Alcohol on the Peripheral Arteries," *Proc. Mayo Clin., 7,* 449 (1932).

(3) R. Docter and R. Perkins, "The Effects of Ethyl Alcohol on Autonomic and Muscular Responses in Humans," *Quart. J. Stud. Alc., 22,* 374 (1960).

(4) E. Fewings *et al.,* "The Effects of Ethyl Alcohol on the Blood Vessels of the Hand and Forearm in Man," *Brit. J. Pharmacol. Chemother., 27,* 93 (1966).

(5) J. Gillespie, "Vasodilator Properties of Alcohol," *Brit. Med. J., 2,* 274 (1967).

(6) P. Naitok, in "Biology of Alcoholism," vol. 2, B. Kissin and H. Begleiter, Eds., Plenum, New York, N.Y., 1972, pp. 367–427.

(7) A. Anton, "Ethanol and Urinary Cate- cholamines in Man," *Clin. Pharmacol. Ther., 6,* 462 (1965).

(8) V. E. Davis *et al.,* "Ethanol-Induced Alterations of Norepinephrine Metab- olism in Man," *J. Lab. Clin. Med., 69,* 787 (1967).

(9) J. Nakano and A. Prancan, "Effects of Adrenergic Blockade on Cardiovascu- lar Responses to Ethanol and Acetal- dehyde," *Arch. Int. Pharmacodyn. Ther., 196,* 259 (1972).

(10) A. Gimena *et al.,* "Effects of Ethanol on Cellular Membrane Potentials and Contractility of Isolated Rat Atrium," *Amer. J. Physiol., 203,* 194 (1962).

(11) T. Regan *et al.*, "The Acute Metabolic
and Hemodynamic Responses of the
Left Ventricle to Ethanol," *J. Clin.
Invest.*, 45, 270 (1966).
(12) L. Gould *et al.*, "Cardiac Effects of a
Cocktail," *J. Amer. Med. Ass.*, 218,
1799 (1971).
(13) N. Conway, "Haemodynamic Effects of
Ethyl Alcohol in Patients with Coronary Heart Disease," *Brit. Heart J.*,
30, 638 (1968).
(14) D. Riff *et al.*, "Acute Hemodynamic
Effects of Ethanol on Normal Human
Volunteers," *Amer. Heart J.*, 78, 592
(1969).
(15) R. Juchems and R. Klobe, "Hemodynamic Effects of Ethyl Alcohol in
Man," *Amer. Heart J.*, 78, 133 (1969).

(16) O. Bienvenu, "Essential Hypertension," *Med. Clin. N. Amer.*, 51, 967
(1967).
(17) F. H. Meyer *et al.*, "Review of Medical Pharmacology," Lange Medical
Publications, Los Altos, Calif., 1968,
p. 116.
(18) N. Moser and A. Goldman, "Hypertensive Vascular Disease: Diagnosis
and Treatment," Lippincott, Philadelphia, Pa., 1967, p. 246.
(19) G. Pickering, "High Blood Pressure,"
2nd ed., Grune and Stratton, New
York, N.Y., 1968, p. 405.
(20) E. Freis, "Guanethidine," *Progr.
Cardiov. Dis.*, 8, 183 (1965).

[For additional information, see *Antihypertensive Therapy*, p. 381.]

Nonproprietary and Trade Names of Drugs

Alcohol—*Various products and beverages*   Debrisoquin sulfate—*Declinax*
Bethanidine sulfate*—*Esbatal*   Guanethidine sulfate—*Ismelin Sulfate*

---

* Not yet commercially available in the United States.

*Prepared and evaluated by the Scientific Review Subpanel on
Antihypertensive Agents and reviewed by Practitioner Panel II.*

Guanethidine—Chlorpromazine

Summary—Chlorpromazine may reverse the antihypertensive effects of guanethidine and their concurrent use should be avoided. If these drugs must be
given together, the patient should be monitored closely for possible reversal of
guanethidine's antihypertensive effect.

Related Drugs—In rats, chlorpromazine was more effective than other phenothiazines
in reducing the uptake of norepinephrine in the nerve cell (1) and may interact with
guanethidine to a greater degree than other phenothiazines. Nevertheless, all **phenothiazines** may be able to reverse the antihypertensive activity of guanethidine.

  Bethanidine and **debrisoquin** are chemically and pharmacologically related to
guanethidine and can be expected to interact with phenothiazines in a similar manner.

Pharmacological Effect and Mechanism—For guanethidine to exert its pharmacological effects, the drug must be taken into the postganglionic adrenergic neuron by
a relatively nonspecific amine transport system. Once within the adrenergic neuron,
guanethidine prevents the release of norepinephrine and depletes norepinephrine
stores. The result is a decreased pressor response to adrenergic neuronal activity (2).
The same transport system also is responsible for the reuptake of norepinephrine and
other pharmacologically related agents. Some results (3, 4) showed that chlorpromazine, which is structurally similar to the tricyclic antidepressant imipramine, can

reverse the antihypertensive effects of guanethidine apparently by blocking the uptake of guanethidine at its site of action.

Chlorpromazine also exhibits α-adrenergic receptor blocking effects (5) which are manifested as decreased standing or sitting blood pressure (6). Although there is a possibility of additive hypotensive effects occurring after concurrent administration of guanethidine and chlorpromazine, this effect has not been reported in clinical practice.

Evaluation of Clinical Data—Chlorpromazine reversed the antihypertensive effects of guanethidine (60–150 mg/day po) in four patients diagnosed as having moderate to severe essential hypertension (3). After stabilization of antihypertensive therapy, each patient received chlorpromazine (100–400 mg/day po) concurrently with guanethidine. Both chlorpromazine and guanethidine were continued for at least 12 days. Then chlorpromazine was discontinued and guanethidine was continued at the same dose as originally determined. Chlorpromazine was reintroduced in two cases. In each case, chlorpromazine partially reversed the antihypertensive effects of guanethidine. The reversal occurred within a few days (actual number not reported) to more than 1 week after chlorpromazine was initiated. Additionally, in three of the six tests given to these two patients, a statistically significant rebound increase in blood pressure to levels above those attained with guanethidine alone occurred during the chlorpromazine withdrawal phase.

Two severely hypertensive patients stabilized on maintenance doses of guanethidine (80 mg/day po) were given chlorpromazine (200–300 mg/day po) (4). In the first patient, the addition of chlorpromazine caused the standing diastolic pressure to rise from 94±3.1 to 112±4.6 mm Hg, while in the second patient, the average diastolic pressure rose from 105±2.5 to 127±1.9 mm Hg.

A single dose of prochlorperazine (25 mg/day po) had no effect on hypotension induced by guanethidine (30–40 mg/day po) in five patients with essential hypertension (7). The conflicting results may be due to the fact that the observation period was very short (8 hr) and may have been insufficient for prochlorperazine to produce a significant change in the concentration of guanethidine at its site of action.

■ Although the data are limited, chlorpromazine may cause a clinically significant reversal of the antihypertensive effect of guanethidine. The fact that the phenothiazine tranquilizers are structurally similar to the tricyclic antidepressants, a group of drugs well documented to reverse the antihypertensive effect of guanethidine (see *Guanethidine–Desipramine*, p. 83), also lends support to the significance of this interaction.

On a milligram to milligram basis, chlorpromazine may be a less potent antagonist of guanethidine than are the tricyclic antidepressants (8). However, doses of the phenothiazines may be relatively higher than those of the tricyclic antidepressants and therefore may significantly antagonize the antihypertensive activity of guanethidine.

Recommendations—Until the extent of antagonism of the antihypertensive activity of guanethidine by phenothiazines is determined, all guanethidine-treated hypertensive patients receiving chlorpromazine or other phenothiazines should be monitored closely for a possible reversal of guanethidine's antihypertensive effect. Methyldopa does not rely on the same transport mechanism as guanethidine for pharmacological response and may be an appropriate alternative antihypertensive (2).

Other psychotropic drugs with similar therapeutic indications are not safe alternatives to chlorpromazine. The butyrophenones (*e.g.*, haloperidol) and the thioxanthenes (*e.g.*, thiothixene) cause a similar antagonism of guanethidine, although it is not as significant (3). Molindone is a new psychotropic agent structurally unrelated to the butyrophenones, phenothiazines, and thioxanthenes (9). Since the effects of this drug on guanethidine have not been examined, concurrent therapy of molindone with guanethidine should be monitored closely.

References

(1) D. Tuck *et al.*, "Drug Interactions: Effect of Chlorpromazine on the Uptake of Monoamines into Adrenergic Neurons in Man," *Lancet, ii*, 492 (1972).

(2) J. R. Mitchell *et al.*, "Guanethidine and Related Agents III. Antagonism by Drugs Which Inhibit the Norepinephrine Pump in Man," *J. Clin. Invest.*, *49*, 1596 (1970).

(3) D. S. Janowsky *et al.*, "Antagonism of Guanethidine by Chlorpromazine," *Amer. J. Psychiat.*, *130*, 808 (1973).

(4) W. E. Fann *et al.*, "Chlorpromazine Reversal of the Antihypertensive Action of Guanethidine," *Lancet, ii*, 436 (1971).

(5) W. R. Martin *et al.*, "Chlorpromazine III. The Effects of Chlorpromazine and Chlorpromazine Sulfoxide on Vascular Responses to *L*-Epinephrine and Levarterenol," *J. Pharmacol. Exp. Ther.*, *130* 37 (1960).

(6) B. Korol *et al.*, "Effects of Chronic Chlorpromazine Administration on Systemic Arterial Pressure in Schizophrenic Patients: Relationship of Body Position to Blood Pressure," *Clin. Pharmacol. Ther.*, *6*, 587 (1965).

(7) K. F. Ober and R. I. H. Wang, "Drug Interactions with Guanethidine," *Clin. Pharmacol. Ther.*, *14*, 190 (1973).

(8) C. A. Stone *et al.*, "Antagonism of Certain Effects of Catecholamine-Depleting Agents by Antidepressant and Related Drugs," *J. Pharmacol. Exp. Ther.*, *144*, 196 (1964).

(9) F. J. Ayd, "A Critical Evaluation of Molindone: A New Indole Derivative Neuroleptic," *Dis. Nerv. Syst.*, *35*, 447 (1974).

[For additional information, see *Antihypertensive Therapy*, p. 381.]

Nonproprietary and Trade Names of Drugs

Acetophenazine maleate—*Tindal*
Bethanidine sulfate*—*Esbatal*
Butaperazine maleate—*Repoise Maleate*
Carphenazine maleate—*Proketazine*
Chlorpromazine—*Chlor-PZ, Promapar, Thorazine*
Debrisoquin sulfate—*Declinax*
Fluphenazine enanthate—*Prolixin Enanthate*
Fluphenazine hydrochloride—*Permitil, Prolixin*
Guanethidine sulfate—*Ismelin Sulfate*
Haloperidol—*Haldol*
Mesoridazine—*Serentil*

Methyldopa—*Aldomet*
Molindone hydrochloride—*Moban*
Perphenazine—*Trilafon and various combination products*
Piperacetazine—*Quide*
Prochlorperazine—*Compazine and various combination products*
Promazine hydrochloride—*Sparine*
Thiopropazate hydrochloride—*Dartal*
Thiothixene—*Navane*
Thioridazine hydrochloride—*Mellaril*
Trifluoperazine hydrochloride—*Stelazine*
Triflupromazine hydrochloride—*Vesprin*

* Not yet commercially available in the United States.

Prepared and evaluated by the Scientific Review Subpanel on Antihypertensive Agents and reviewed by Practitioner Panel IV.

Guanethidine—Desipramine

Summary—The antihypertensive effect of guanethidine can be antagonized by concurrent administration of desipramine and these drugs should not be used together. If guanethidine must be used concurrently with a tricyclic antidepressant, doxepin, at doses of less than 100 mg/day po, appears not to block guanethidine's antihypertensive effect and may be a useful alternative when concurrent therapy with guanethidine and a tricyclic antidepressant is indicated. Other possibilities are to increase the dose of guanethidine or to use an alternative antihypertensive agent that is not significantly affected by the tricyclic antidepressants (*e.g.,* methyldopa).

Related Drugs—Some evidence suggests that **amitriptyline** (1), **imipramine** (2), **nortriptyline** (3), and **protriptyline** (3), agents chemically and pharmacologically related to desipramine, may antagonize the antihypertensive effect of guanethidine and other related guanidinium hypotensive agents such as **bethanidine** (3) and **debrisoquin** (3). **Doxepin,** in doses of less than 100 mg/day po, appears to have little influence on the activity of guanethidine (4, 5).

Pharmacological Effect and Mechanism—Guanethidine is transported to its site of action within adrenergic neurons by a transport system also responsible for the uptake of norepinephrine and several indirect-acting sympathomimetic amines such as ephedrine and the amphetamines (6). Accumulation of guanethidine within the adrenergic neuron is necessary for its antihypertensive effect (3). It has been suggested that desipramine and related compounds inhibit the uptake of guanethidine into the neuron terminal, thereby preventing its accumulation at these sites (3).

Evaluation of Clinical Data—In a controlled study (3) of 13 hypertensive patients, desipramine and protriptyline produced a significant reversal of the antihypertensive effects of guanethidine in every patient studied. Desipramine also antagonized the antihypertensive effects of bethanidine and debrisoquin but had no effect on the action of methyldopa. The dosages of desipramine (50–150 mg/day po) and protriptyline (20 mg/day po) that produced this effect were well within the recommended dosage ranges. The antagonism of guanethidine was not immediate but required 1 or 2 days before maximum antagonism was seen. Following discontinuation of desipramine, the antihypertensive action of guanethidine did not reappear for 5–7 days. The slowly developed antagonism is consistent with the suggestion that the antidepressant blocks further uptake of guanethidine into the neuron (3). The rate at which the antihypertensive effect of guanethidine decreases depends on the concentration of the drug already in the neuron. Imipramine (75 mg/day po) also was reported to antagonize the antihypertensive effect and certain side effects of guanethidine (dose not reported) in three hypertensive patients (2).

Initiation of amitriptyline therapy (75 mg/day po) in a patient whose hypertension was adequately controlled with guanethidine (75 mg/day po), methyldopa (750 mg/day po), and trichlormethiazide (8 mg/day po) resulted in a reversal of the effects of guanethidine (1). The reversal occurred 5 days after the initiation of amitriptyline therapy. It was necessary to increase the dosage of guanethidine to 300 mg/day to obtain the same antihypertensive effect. After amitriptyline therapy was discontinued, 18 days elapsed before the antagonism was overcome. The antagonism produced by amitriptyline appears to be slower in onset and more prolonged in duration than that seen with desipramine and protriptyline, thus making the potential problem more difficult to recognize. Desipramine and protriptyline have been shown to be more potent than amitriptyline as inhibitors of the system that transports guanethidine to its site of action in the sympathetic neuron (7). The difference in potency may explain the more rapid block of guanethidine's effect produced by these drugs (1).

One report (6) indicated that imipramine (150 mg po) did not antagonize the effect of guanethidine since such an effect was not noted within a 12-hr period. In another report (8), a single dose of amitriptyline (50 mg po) did not decrease the antihypertensive effect of guanethidine in five hypertensive patients during an 8-hr observation period. The short observation period may explain the failure to note an altered effect in either report since there was probably insufficient time for imipramine or amitriptyline to produce a significant change in the concentration of guanethidine at its site of action.

The development of unresponsive cardiac standstill in a patient receiving guanethidine (125 mg/day po) and imipramine (75 mg/day po) also was described (9). However, the mechanism for this effect is not known.

Although the antidepressant, doxepin, is similar in many ways to the other tricyclic antidepressants, it does not block the effects of guanethidine when administered in doses of less than 100 mg (4, 5). At a dosage range of 100–300 mg/day, doxepin produced a significant antagonism of the hypotensive effect of guanethidine (4, 5). However, the antagonism was less marked than that noted with desipramine.

■ Although the reported studies of this interaction have not involved a large number of patients and some short-term studies have shown no drug interaction occurring, it appears that the hypotensive effect of guanethidine is antagonized when desipramine or another tricyclic antidepressant is given concurrently. However, doxepin, in doses of less than 100 mg/day po, does not appear to be antagonistic to the effects of guanethidine (5). At doxepin doses of 100–300 mg, significant antagonism of guanethidine's antihypertensive effect does occur (4, 5).

Recommendations—Generally, concurrent administration of tricyclic antidepressants and guanethidine should be avoided. If it is necessary to administer a tricyclic antidepressant to a patient receiving guanethidine, doxepin (particularly <100 mg/day po) would probably be the best choice since the available evidence indicates that it is less likely to alter the effects of guanethidine (5).

An alternative antihypertensive drug may be used. The use of methyldopa plus a diuretic, instead of guanethidine, may provide better control of the hypertension than guanethidine. Desipramine and imipramine antagonized the antihypertensive effects of methyldopa in cats (10, 11), but this antagonism has not occurred in humans (3).

Another possibility is to increase the guanethidine dose to overcome the antagonism. High doses of guanethidine (300 mg/day) have been successful in overcoming the antagonism produced by the tricyclic antidepressants (1). When guanethidine is given concurrently with desipramine or another agent which has been shown to alter its effect, the therapy should be monitored closely for a minimum of 7 days with the recognition that the guanethidine dose may have to be increased.

References

(1) J. F. Meyer et al., "Insidious and Prolonged Antagonism of Guanethidine by Amitriptyline," J. Amer. Med. Ass., 213, 1487 (1970).

(2) A. W. D. Leishman et al., "Antagonism of Guanethidine by Imipramine," letter to the editor, Lancet, i, 112 (1963).

(3) J. R. Mitchell et al., "Guanethidine and Related Agents III. Antagonism by Drugs which Inhibit the Norepinephrine Pump in Man," J. Clin. Invest., 49, 1596 (1970). [Preliminary communication: J. R. Mitchell et al., "Antagonism of the Antihypertensive Action of Guanethidine Sulfate by Desipramine Hydrochloride," J. Amer. Med. Ass., 202, 973 (1967).]

(4) J. A. Oates et al., "Effect of Doxepin on the Norepinephrine Pump," Psychosomatics, 10, 12 (1969).

(5) W. E. Fann et al., "Doxepin: Effects on Transport of Biogenic Amines in Man," Psychopharmacologia, 22, 111 (1971).

(6) O. D. Gulati et al., "Antagonism of Adrenergic Neuron Blockade in Hypertensive Subjects," Clin. Pharmacol. Ther., 7, 510 (1966).

(7) C. A. Stone et al., "Antagonism of Certain Effects of Catecholamine-Depleting Agents by Antidepressant and Related Drugs," J. Pharmacol. Exp. Ther., 144, 196 (1964).

(8) K. F. Ober and R. I. H. Wang, "Drug Interactions with Guanethidine," Clin. Pharmacol. Ther., 14, 190 (1973).

(9) R. B. Williams and C. Sherter, "Cardiac Complications of Tricyclic Antidepressant Therapy," Ann. Intern. Med., 74, 395 (1971).

(10) H. W. Van Spanning and P. A. van Zwieten, "The Interaction between Alpha Methyl Dopa and Tricyclic Antidepressants," Int. J. Pharmacol. Biopharm., 11, 65 (1975).

(11) P. A. van Zwieten et al., "Interaction between Centrally Acting Hypotensive Drugs and Tricyclic Antidepressants," Arch. Int. Pharmacodyn. Ther., 214, 12 (1975).

[For additional information, see Antihypertensive Therapy, p. 381.]

Nonproprietary and Trade Names of Drugs

Amitriptyline hydrochloride—*Elavil Hydrochloride and various combination products*
Bethanidine sulfate*—*Estabal*
Debrisoquin sulfate—*Declinax*
Desipramine hydrochloride—*Norpramin, Pertofrane*
Doxepin hydrochloride—*Adapin, Sinequan*

Guanethidine sulfate—*Ismelin Sulfate*
Imipramine hydrochloride—*Presamine, Tofranil, Tofranil PM*
Nortriptyline hydrochloride—*Aventyl Hydrochloride*
Protriptyline hydrochloride—*Vivactil Hydrochloride*

* Not yet commercially available in the United States.

Prepared and evaluated by the Scientific Review Subpanel on Antihypertensive Agents and reviewed by Practitioner Panel V.

Guanethidine—Dextroamphetamine

Summary—The antihypertensive action of guanethidine may be blocked by dextroamphetamine and related compounds; therefore, concurrent use of these drugs should be avoided.

Related Drugs—**Bethanidine** and **debrisoquin** are chemically and pharmacologically related to guanethidine and may also interact with dextroamphetamine. **Methamphetamine** (1) has also been reported to block the antihypertensive effects of guanethidine. **Ephedrine** (2) and **methylphenidate** (1) are chemically and pharmacologically related to the **amphetamines** and have been shown to interact to a lesser extent with guanethidine. **Phenylpropanolamine** also is related chemically and pharmacologically to the amphetamines and has antagonized the effects of bethanidine (3).

Pharmacological Effect and Mechanism—The mechanism by which guanethidine elicits an antihypertensive effect is related primarily to its ability to block the release of norepinephrine from the sympathetic nerve endings. This blockade is dependent apparently on the active transport of guanethidine into the nerve terminal. There is also a latent depletion of norepinephrine similar to that observed with reserpine, but this effect is probably of secondary importance. The guanethidine-induced neuronal blockade effectively reduces sympathetic tone in the peripheral vasculature and heart, resulting in a decrease in blood pressure that is more pronounced in the upright position (4, 5).

The amphetamines and similarly acting drugs are dependent primarily on the release of norepinephrine from sympathetic nerve endings for their peripheral action (5). Consequently, in the presence of guanethidine, their activity is impaired. However, there is evidence that these drugs also have a strong affinity for the same site within the nerve ending as occupied by guanethidine (6). This affinity is sufficiently great to displace guanethidine if it is present or to inhibit its uptake into the nerve ending when guanethidine is administered following amphetamine (6–10). This antagonism existed not only in an acute experimental situation but also when guanethidine was administered daily for periods up to 12 days. In the latter case, amphetamine reversed the antihypertensive effects of guanethidine (7). The rapid onset of amphetamine-induced reversal suggests a direct effect on vasoconstrictor receptors in addition to competition for the transport mechanism (2).

Evaluation of Clinical Data—A cold pressor test (used to measure susceptibility to hypertension) was administered to five hypertensive subjects prior to and following treatment with guanethidine (1). Guanethidine (25–35 mg/day po) was administered until a maximum reduction in pressure was obtained (usually 2 weeks). A cold pressor test performed at this time was negative. Dextroamphetamine (10 mg po) or methamphetamine (50 mg im) then was administered, and the cold pressor test was repeated at intervals. Six hours after drug administration, both drugs had effectively antagonized the guanethidine-induced blockade of the cold pressor test and reduced the antihypertensive effects of guanethidine. Methylphenidate (20 mg po) produced a similar, but less pronounced, antagonism of the effects of guanethidine at 6 hr. At 2 hr, ephedrine partially reversed the effects of guanethidine in five patients. At 6 hr, there was no antagonism of guanethidine by ephedrine, although the blood pressure was somewhat elevated.

In another study (2), five adults with essential hypertension received guanethidine (15–20 mg/day po) during the entire study. A single dose of dextroamphetamine (10 mg po) resulted in a rapid and uniform rise in blood pressure. This rise was attributed to a direct vasoconstrictor effect of dextroamphetamine rather than a blockade of guanethidine's action.

A case of ventricular tachycardia due to decreased blood pressure was associated with concurrent administration of guanethidine (25 mg/day po) and methylphenidate (10 mg/day po) (11). When guanethidine and methylphenidate were discontinued and antiarrhythmic drugs were administered, sinus rhythm returned. Since other causative factors were not ruled out, this association was not established definitely.

■ Dextroamphetamine, methamphetamine, and, to a lesser extent, ephedrine and methylphenidate appear to cause a clinically significant antagonism of the antihypertensive effects of guanethidine. This drug interaction seems to occur rapidly.

Recommendations—Dextroamphetamine and related compounds should not be used concurrently with guanethidine. If dextroamphetamine must be used, a drug such as clonidine or methyldopa (alone or in combination with a thiazide diuretic) whose antihypertensive action has not been reported to be altered by concurrent administration of dextroamphetamine should be used instead of guanethidine. However, since there are no data indicating that a drug interaction does *not* occur, patients receiving the alternative antihypertensive drugs and dextroamphetamine concurrently should have their blood pressure monitored closely. Additionally, because guanethidine exerts its antihypertensive effects for several days after it is discontinued (12), patient response to an alternative antihypertensive drug may be enhanced for the first few days after the drugs have been changed.

References

(1) O. D. Gulati *et al.*, "Antagonism of Adrenergic Neuron Blockade in Hypertensive Subjects," *Clin. Pharmacol. Ther.*, 7, 510 (1966).

(2) K. F. Ober and R. I. H. Wang, "Drug Interactions with Guanethidine," *Clin. Pharmacol. Ther.*, 14, 190 (1973).

(3) J. R. Misage and R. H. McDonald, "Antagonism of Hypotensive Action of Bethanidine by 'Common Cold' Remedy," *Brit. Med. J.*, 4, 347 (1970).

(4) A. L. A. Boura and A. F. Green, "Adrenergic Neurone Blocking Agents," *Ann. Rev. Pharmacol.*, 5, 183 (1965).

(5) A. Giachetti *et al.*, "Mechanism of Action of Adrenergic Neuronal Blocking Drugs," *Pharmacologist*, 9, 235 (1967).

(6) M. D. Day and M. J. Rand, "Evidence for a Competitive Antagonism of Guanethidine by Dexamphetamine," *Brit. J. Pharmacol.*, 20, 17 (1963).

(7) M. D. Day, "Effect of Sympathomimetic Amines on the Blocking Action of Guanethidine, Bretylium and Xylocholine," *Brit. J. Pharmacol.*, 18, 421 (1962).

(8) M. D. Day and M. J. Rand, "Antagonism of Guanethidine by Dexamphetamine and Other Related Sympathomimetic Amines," *J. Pharm. Pharmacol.*, 14, 541 (1962).

(9) M. J. Follenfant and R. D. Robson, "The Antagonism of Adrenergic Neurone Blockade by Amphetamine and Dexamphetamine in the Rat and Guinea-Pig," *Brit. J. Pharmacol.*, *38*, 792 (1970).

(10) O. T. Flegin *et al.*, "The Mechanism of the Reversal of the Effect of Guanethidine by Amphetamines in Cat and Man," *Brit. J. Pharmacol.*, *39*, 253P (1970).

(11) B. S. Deshmankar and J. A. Lewis, "Ventricular Tachycardia Associated with the Administration of Methylphenidate during Guanethidine Therapy," *Can. Med. Ass. J.*, *97*, 1166 (1967).

(12) "The Pharmacological Basis of Therapeutics," 5th ed., L. S. Goodman and A. Gilman, Eds., Macmillan, New York, NY 10022, 1975, pp. 556–557.

[For additional information, see *Antihypertensive Therapy*, p. 381; *Guanethidine–Desipramine*, p. 83; and *Phenylephrine–Guanethidine*, p. 186.]

Nonproprietary and Trade Names of Drugs

Amphetamine complex—*Biphetamine*
Amphetamine sulfate—*Benzedrine*
Bethanidine sulfate *—*Esbatal*
Debrisoquin sulfate—*Declinax*
Dextroamphetamine sulfate—*Dexedrine and various combination products*
Ephedrine hydrochloride and sulfate—*Various manufacturers*

Guanethidine sulfate—*Ismelin Sulfate*
Methamphetamine hydrochloride—*Desoxyn, Norodin Hydrochloride, Syndrox*
Methylphenidate hydrochloride—*Ritalin Hydrochloride*
Phenylpropanolamine hydrochloride—*Various combination products*

* Not yet commercially available in the United States.

Prepared and evaluated by the Scientific Review Subpanel on Antihypertensive Agents and reviewed by Practitioner Panel III.

Guanethidine—Hydrochlorothiazide

Summary—Clinical studies indicate that concurrent administration of guanethidine and hydrochlorothiazide is therapeutically useful in the treatment of hypertension. Thiazides enhance the antihypertensive action of guanethidine, allowing the dose of guanethidine to be reduced and decreasing the incidence of adverse reactions, particularly orthostatic and exercise-associated hypotension. Hydrochlorothiazide also is useful in eliminating sodium retention, edema, and the eventual resistance to guanethidine's antihypertensive effect associated with its long-term administration.

Related Drugs—Although the only documentation of this drug interaction involves hydrochlorothiazide, other **thiazide diuretics** may produce a comparable effect on the hypotensive action of guanethidine. **Chlorthalidone, metolazone,** and **quinethazone** are structurally related to thiazide diuretics (1) and should be expected to interact with guanethidine also. Thiazide diuretics are available in many combination products.

Bethanidine and **debrisoquin** are chemically and pharmacologically related to guanethidine and may be expected to interact with hydrochlorothiazide.

Pharmacological Effect and Mechanism—When administered alone, guanethidine effectively reduces the standing systolic and diastolic pressures. In the supine position, there is no significant change in the systolic pressure and only a moderate fall in the diastolic pressure. However, the use of hydrochlorothiazide and lower doses of guanethidine produces a significant fall in both supine and standing systolic and diastolic pressures (2).

The mechanism by which thiazide diuretics lower blood pressure has not been firmly established. Earlier studies suggested that the antihypertensive effect of thiazides was caused by a decrease in cardiac output due to volume reduction and by direct relaxation of peripheral vascular smooth muscle (1, 3). This evidence was based partially on studies with diazoxide, a thiazide derivative that acts primarily on pre-capillary resistance vessels rather than on postcapillary capacitance vessels (1, 4). Thiazide diuretics were believed to have a similar, but smaller and more gradual, effect (1). Current evidence, however, suggests that thiazides have only an indirect effect on peripheral vascular resistance, which develops gradually as sodium depletion or volume reduction alters vascular reactivity and diminishes the effectiveness of sympathetic reflexes (5).

Guanethidine produces its antihypertensive action by interfering with the release of norepinephrine in the peripheral terminals of sympathetic nerves (6, 7). There is also a latent depletion of norepinephrine similar to that observed with reserpine, but this effect is probably of secondary importance. The guanethidine-induced neuronal blockade results in decreased peripheral resistance, venous pooling, and reduced cardiac output. The normal compensatory venous constriction that occurs in the standing position is controlled by the carotid sinus reflex which utilizes norepinephrine as the transmitter that activates the vascular receptors. The activation of the vascular receptors leads to an increase in vascular tone. Reduction of the tissue stores of norepinephrine by guanethidine interferes with this action. Under clinical conditions, the transition from a supine to a standing position on arising may enhance orthostatic hypotension with resulting dizziness and weakness and, in some instances, fainting and collapse. Lower doses of guanethidine used concurrently with thiazides permit a satisfactory reduction in blood pressure with less impairment of the venoconstrictive reflex (2).

Chronic use of guanethidine also is associated with sodium retention, edema, and a progressive resistance to its antihypertensive effect which cannot be controlled by increasing the dose. The addition of a thiazide reduces these effects (8).

Evaluation of Clinical Data—Significant clinical documentation indicates that hydro-chlorothiazide augments the antihypertensive effect of guanethidine (8–12). Reduction in the dose of guanethidine decreases the incidence of adverse reactions and permits smoother control of the blood pressure, particularly when patients are in the supine position.

■ There is substantial clinical evidence that the concurrent use of a thiazide diuretic and guanethidine allows a reduction in the guanethidine dose which decreases the adverse reactions to guanethidine, particularly orthostatic hypotension.

Recommendations—In the treatment of moderate to severe hypertension, it is recom-mended that advantage be taken of the enhanced effect of a thiazide diuretic on the antihypertensive action of guanethidine. A reduction in the dose of guanethidine and monitoring of the patient's plasma potassium level may be necessary with the addition of a thiazide diuretic.

Other diuretics (*e.g.*, ethacrynic acid, furosemide, the mercurial diuretics, and spironolactone) have antihypertensive properties, but it is unclear if this effect is due to fluid depletion or to decreased vascular resistance. Triamterene, a potassium-sparing diuretic, does not have an antihypertensive effect (1).

References

(1) "The Pharmacological Basis of Thera-peutics," 5th ed., L. S. Goodman and A. Gilman, Eds., Macmillan, New York, NY 10022, 1975, pp. 712–729, 830.

(2) R. F. Maronde *et al.*, "Comparison of Guanethidine and Guanethidine Plus a Thiazide Diuretic," *Amer. J. Med. Sci., 242,* 228 (1961).

(3) J. Conway and H. Palmero, "The Vascular Effect of the Thiazide Diuretics," *Arch. Intern. Med.*, *111*, 203 (1963).

(4) A. A. Rubin *et al.*, "Acute Circulatory Effects of Diazoxide and Sodium Nitrite," *J. Pharmacol. Exp. Ther.*, *140*, 46 (1963).

(5) R. C. Tarazi, "Diuretic Drugs: Mechanisms of Antihypertensive Action," in "Hypertension: Mechanisms and Management; The Twenty-Sixth Hahnemann Symposium," G. Onesti *et al.*, Eds., Grune and Stratton, New York, N.Y., 1973.

(6) D. W. Richardson *et al.*, "Circulatory Effects of Guanethidine. Clinical, Renal, and Cardiac Responses to Treatment with a Novel Antihypertensive Drug," *Circulation*, *22*, 184 (1960).

(7) R. A. Maxwell *et al.*, "Pharmacology of [2-(Octahydro-1-Azocinyl)-Ethyl]-Guanidine Sulfate (Su-5864)," *J. Pharmacol. Exp. Ther.*, *128*, 22 (1960).

(8) G. Blanshard and W. Essigman, "Guanethidine and Hydrochlorothiazide in the Treatment of Hypertension," *Lancet*, *ii*, 334 (1961).

(9) F. B. Schultz, "The Use of Guanethidine in Private Practice," *J. Med. Ass. State Ala.*, *31*(6), 177 (1961).

(10) A. N. Brest and J. H. Moyer, Symposium on Guanethidine (Ismelin), Memphis, Tenn., April 22, 1960.

(11) R. V. Ford, "Treatment of Hypertension with Guanethidine and Hydrochlorothiazide," *Geriatrics*, *16*, 577 (1961).

(12) M. S. Klapper and L. Richard, "Guanethidine in Hypertension," *S. Med. J.*, *55*, 75 (1962).

[For additional information, see *Antihypertensive Therapy*, p. 381.]

Nonproprietary and Trade Names of Drugs

Bendroflumethiazide—*Naturetin*
Benzthiazide—*Aquatag, Exna*
Bethanidine sulfate*—*Estabal*
Chlorothiazide—*Diuril*
Chlorthalidone—*Hygroton, Regroton*
Cyclothiazide—*Anhydron*
Debrisoquin sulfate—*Declinax*
Ethacrynic acid—*Edecrin*
Flumethiazide—*Rautrax*
Furosemide—*Lasix*
Guanethidine sulfate—*Ismelin Sulfate*
Hydrochlorothiazide—*Esidrix, HydroDiuril, Oretic*

Hydroflumethiazide—*Saluron*
Mercaptomerin sodium—*Thiomerin*
Methyclothiazide—*Aquatensen, Enduron*
Metolazone—*Zaroxolyn*
Polythiazide—*Renese*
Quinethazone—*Hydromox*
Spironolactone—*Aldactone*
Triamterene—*Dyrenium*
Trichlormethiazide—*Metahydrin, Naqua*
Various combination products containing a diuretic are available.

* Not yet commercially available in the United States.

Prepared and evaluated by the Scientific Review Subpanel on Antihypertensive Agents and reviewed by Practitioner Panel VI.

Halothane—Epinephrine

Summary—The parenteral, primarily intravenous, administration of epinephrine during halothane anesthesia may lead to serious ventricular arrhythmias including ventricular fibrillation. Intravenous administration of epinephrine concurrently with halothane is strongly discouraged but subcutaneous or intramuscular administration can be safe, provided appropriate precautions are taken.

Related Drugs—**Levarterenol (norepinephrine)** has been shown to interact with halothane and other general anesthetics in a manner similar to epinephrine (1). **Isoproterenol** causes similar effects on the heart (2) and, although not documented, would probably interact similarly with halothane. Although **amphetamine, ephedrine, mephentermine, metaraminol, methoxamine,** and **phenylephrine** do not exert direct effects on the heart (1), they do affect the heart indirectly by releasing norepinephrine and may produce arrhythmias (2). Arrhythmias have been observed occasionally in animals and humans treated with indirect sympathomimetics and general anesthetics (2).

Other general anesthetics reduce the arrhythmia-producing dose of epinephrine. In decreasing order of liability to induce this response in animals (2), these general anesthetics are: **trichloroethylene** (3), **ethyl chloride** (2), **trichloromonofluoromethane** (4), **cyclopropane** (5), **chloroform** (2), **methoxyflurane** (2), **fluroxene** (2, 4), and **enflurane** (6). However, the order is based on animal studies; clinical data demonstrate that the order may be different in humans (2). Other general anesthetics include **ether, halopropane,** and **nitrous oxide.**

Pharmacological Effect and Mechanism—Cardiac arrhythmias follow the administration of many sympathomimetics if sufficiently large doses are used. In varying degrees, cyclopropane and halogenated hydrocarbon anesthetics reduce the dose at which sympathomimetics elicit arrhythmias (6–9). Although the exact mechanism for the development of anesthetic-induced arrhythmias is unknown, cyclopropane and halothane produce conduction changes which increase impulse reentry into the myocardial tissue. Additionally, studies in dogs indicated that blood pressure and heart rate also influence the anesthetic's ability to precipitate arrhythmias (10).

Anesthetic-associated sympathomimetic-induced arrhythmias are probably mediated by β-adrenergic receptors since these arrhythmias are prevented by β-adrenergic blocking agents (2). The α-adrenergic blocking agents occasionally demonstrate an antiarrhythmic effect that is likely due to prevention of an increase in blood pressure resulting from the sympathomimetic. Elevation of arterial blood pressure reduces the dose of catecholamine necessary to induce ectopic ventricular rhythms in animals receiving cyclopropane (5, 11).

Cardiac arrhythmias during cyclopropane anesthesia also can be elicited by hypercapnia and/or hypoxia (3, 12), apparently through the stimulation of the release of endogenous catecholamines.

Evaluation of Clinical Data—There are numerous reports that discuss the occurrence of cardiac arrhythmias after concurrent use of epinephrine and certain general anesthetics. Most early reports were cases of cardiac arrhythmias and cardiac arrests following the inhalation of cyclopropane, halothane, or trichloroethylene (13).

A study of 51 patients during halothane anesthesia demonstrated that intravenous administration of epinephrine or levarterenol in infusion rates of greater than 10 μg/min could precipitate serious ventricular arrhythmias (14). Patients who were hypertensive and had arteriosclerotic cardiac disease were more likely than others to develop these arrhythmias.

One hundred patients undergoing oral surgery were anesthetized with halothane and were given submucosal injections of epinephrine (5–20 μg) (15). Cardiac arrhythmias attributed to halothane alone occurred in 13% of the patients before epinephrine injection. Epinephrine was considered the cause of the arrhythmias in another 11% of the patients who developed arrhythmias after epinephrine injection.

Twenty-nine patients undergoing oral surgical procedures during halothane anesthesia were given epinephrine (0.4 or 0.8 mg sc) (16). Arrhythmias developed in 40% of the patients (two of five) who received 0.8 mg of epinephrine and in 8.3% of the patients (two of 24) who received 0.4 mg of epinephrine.

The effects of epinephrine administered concurrently with cyclopropane, halothane, nitrous oxide, or trichloroethylene were studied in three experiments with 270 patients (3, 17, 18). Epinephrine administered subcutaneously in doses of 0.1 mg or less during 10 min or 0.3 mg or less during 60 min did not cause any arrhythmias when halothane, nitrous oxide, or trichloroethylene was used concurrently. Arrhythmias occurred in 30% of the patients receiving a similar dose of epinephrine concurrently with cyclopropane. In subsequent trials, one-half of the previous dose of epinephrine was given concurrently with cyclopropane, and no arrhythmias were produced (19). More recent investigations in adults (20) and children (6, 21–23) demonstrated that halothane can be used safely with low topical doses of epinephrine.

■ It appears that the early reports of arrhythmias and fatalities associated with the concurrent use of epinephrine with selected general anesthetics were due to the administration of too large a dose of epinephrine at too rapid a rate (2). The possible contributing role of elevations in blood pressure, hypoxia, and respiratory acidosis is often difficult to assess but these conditions could be possible causative or aggravating factors (11, 12).

Recommendations—Intravenous use of epinephrine during surgery with halothane and related general anesthetics should be strongly discouraged. In those rare situations during surgery when intravenous epinephrine is necessary, nitrous oxide anesthesia supplemented with ether, muscle relaxants, or narcotics should be used instead of the halogenated anesthetics (7, 17).

Epinephrine can be used safely subcutaneously provided the following precautions are observed: (a) the patient is adequately ventilated to prevent hypoxia or respiratory acidosis (3, 7, 17, 18); (b) the total dose of epinephrine in the average adult does not exceed 100 μg (10 ml of a 1:100,000 solution) in any 10-min period or 300 μg (30 ml of a 1:300,000 solution) during 1 hr (3, 7, 14); (c) the concentration of epinephrine used is not greater than 1:100,000 (3, 7, 17) (the concentration of epinephrine is not important if the total dose of epinephrine administered is monitored closely); (d) the dose does not exceed 3.5 μg/kg in infants, 2.5 μg/kg in children up to 2 years of age (21), or 1.45 μg/kg in children over 2 years of age (23); (e) a minimum effective concentration of halogenated anesthetic is maintained (16); (f) the drugs are not used concurrently in patients with hypertension or other cardiovascular disorders (16); and (g) the cardiac rhythm is continuously monitored during and after the injection (16). Since cyclopropane has been shown to increase endogenous catecholamine levels (24), it is recommended that the dose of epinephrine be reduced by 20% (a 1:120,000 solution) when used concurrently with cyclopropane (19).

If arrhythmias occur after the administration of epinephrine, lidocaine or propranolol is the drug of choice depending on the type of arrhythmias (25). Lidocaine may be preferred when multiple or unknown types of arrhythmias occur because of the possible undesirable effects associated with the β-adrenergic blockade of propranolol (e.g., reduction in contractility) (15, 26).

When administration of a sympathetic bronchodilator is necessary in patients receiving halogenated anesthetics, the use of an agent with greater specificity than isoproterenol for the β-2-adrenergic receptors of bronchial smooth muscle (such as terbutaline) is indicated (1).

References

(1) "The Pharmacological Basis of Therapeutics," 5th ed., L. S. Goodman and A. Gilman, Eds., Macmillan, New York, NY 10022, 1975, pp. 368–481, 497, 502.

(2) R. L. Katz and R. A. Epstein, "The Interaction of Anesthetic Agents and Adrenergic Drugs to Produce Cardiac Arrhythmias," *Anesthesiology*, *29*, 763 (1968).

(3) R. S. Matteo *et al.*, "The Injection of Epinephrine during General Anesthesia with Halogenated Hydrocarbons and Cyclopropane in Man. 1. Trichlorethylene," *Anesthesiology*, *23*, 360 (1962).

(4) T. A. Joas and W. C. Stevens, "Comparison of the Arrhythmic Doses of Epinephrine during Forane, Halothane, and Fluroxene Anesthesia in Dogs," *Anesthesiology*, *35*, 48 (1971).

(5) R. L. Katz, "Effects of Alpha and Beta Adrenergic Blocking Agents on Cyclopropane–Catecholamine Cardiac Arrhythmias," *Anesthesiology*, *26*, 289 (1965).

(6) L. S. Reisner and P. Lippman, "Ventricular Arrhythmias after Epinephrine Injection in Enflurane and Halothane Anesthesia," *Anesth. Analg.*, *54*, 468 (1975).

(7) M. Johnstone, "Adrenaline and Nor-adrenaline during Anaesthesia," *Anaesthesia, 8,* 32 (1953).

(8) W. J. Meek *et al.,* "The Effects of Ether, Chloroform and Cyclopropane on Cardiac Automaticity," *J. Pharmacol. Exp. Ther., 61,* 240 (1937).

(9) L. E. Morris *et al.,* "Epinephrine Induced Cardiac Irregularities in the Dog during Anesthesia with Trichloroethylene, Cyclopropane, Ethyl Chloride and Chloroform," *Anesthesiology, 14,* 153 (1953).

(10) J. Zink *et al.,* "Halothane–Epinephrine-Induced Cardiac Arrhythmias and the Role of Heart Rate," *Anesthesiology, 43,* 548 (1975).

(11) G. K. Moe *et al.,* "The Role of Arterial Pressure in the Induction of Idioventricular Rhythms under Cyclopropane Anesthesia," *J. Pharmacol. Exp. Ther., 94,* 319 (1948).

(12) H. L. Price *et al.,* "Cyclopropane Anesthesia, II. Epinephrine and Norepinephrine in Initiation of Ventricular Arrhythmias by Carbon Dioxide Inhalation," *Anesthesiology, 19,* 619 (1958).

(13) R. L. Katz and G. J. Katz, "Surgical Infiltration of Pressor Drugs and Their Interaction with Volatile Anaesthetics," *Brit. J. Anaesth., 38,* 712 (1966).

(14) N. Andersen and S. H. Johansen, "Incidence of Catechol-Amine-Induced Arrhythmias during Halothane Anesthesia," *Anesthesiology, 24,* 51 (1963).

(15) A. M. Forbes, "Halothane, Adrenaline and Cardiac Arrest," *Anaesthesia, 21,* 22 (1966).

(16) W. I. Hirshom *et al.,* "Arrhythmias Produced by Combinations of Halothane and Small Amounts of Vasopressor," *Brit. J. Oral Surg., 2,* 131 (1964–65).

(17) R. L. Katz *et al.,* "The Injection of Epinephrine during General Anesthesia with Halogenated Hydrocarbons and Cyclopropane in Man. 2. Halothane," *Anesthesiology, 23,* 597 (1962).

(18) R. S. Matteo *et al.,* "The Injection of Epinephrine during General Anesthesia with Halogenated Hydrocarbons and Cyclopropane in Man. 3. Cyclopropane," *Anesthesiology, 24,* 327 (1963).

(19) R. L. Katz, "Epinephrine and PLV-2: Cardiac Rhythm and Local Vasoconstrictor Effects," *Anesthesiology, 26,* 619 (1965).

(20) J. G. Brock-Utne, "Adrenaline Infiltration during Halothane Anaesthesia," *Brit. J. Anaesth., 44,* 234 (1972).

(21) W. A. Wallbank, "Cardiac Effects of Halothane and Adrenaline in Hare-Lip and Cleft-Palate Surgery," *Brit. J. Anaesth., 42,* 548 (1970).

(22) J. H. Lee *et al.,* "Use of Topical Epinephrine in Tonsillectomy and Adenoidectomy with Halothane Anesthesia," *Anesth. Analg., 51,* 64 (1972).

(23) A. P. Melgrave, "The Use of Epinephrine in the Presence of Halothane in Children," *Can. Anaesth. Soc. J., 17,* 256 (1970).

(24) H. L. Price *et al.,* "Sympatho-Adrenal Responses to General Anesthesia in Man and Their Relation to Hemodynamics," *Anesthesiology, 20,* 563 (1959).

(25) D. T. Mason *et al.,* "Antiarrhythmic Agents I: Mechanisms of Action and Clinical Pharmacology," *Drugs, 5,* 261 (1973).

(26) E. Ikezono *et al.,* "Effects of Propranolol on Epinephrine-Induced Arrhythmias during Halothane Anesthesia in Man and Cats," *Anesth. Analg., 48,* 598 (1969).

[For additional information, see *Adrenergic Therapy,* p. 332.]

Nonproprietary and Trade Names of Drugs

Amphetamine complex—*Biphetamine*
Amphetamine sulfate—*Benzedrine*
Chloroform—*Various manufacturers*
Cyclopropane—*Various manufacturers*
Enflurane—*Ethrane*
Ephedrine—*Various manufacturers*
Epinephrine hydrochloride—*Adrenalin Hydrochloride*
Ether—*Various manufacturers*
Ethyl chloride—*Various manufacturers*
Fluroxene—*Fluromar*
Halopropane—*Tebron*
Halothane—*Fluothane*
Isoproterenol hydrochloride—*Isuprel Hydrochloride*

Levarterenol bitartrate—*Levophed Bitartrate*
Mephentermine—*Wyamine*
Metaraminol bitartrate—*Aramine*
Methoxamine hydrochloride—*Vasoxyl*
Methoxyflurane—*Penthrane*
Nitrous oxide—*Various manufacturers*
Phenylephrine hydrochloride—*Neo-Synephrine Hydrochloride and various combination products*
Trichloroethylene—*Trilene*
Trichloromonofluoromethane—*Various manufacturers*

Prepared and evaluated by the Scientific Review Subpanel on Anesthetics and reviewed by Practitioner Panel I.

Heparin—Dextran

Summary—Limited data suggest that dextran may enhance the anticoagulant action of heparin when administered concurrently. Although the data are inadequate to document the clinical significance of this interaction, baseline laboratory measurements of anticoagulant activity should be obtained upon initiation of concurrent therapy as well as at frequent intervals during such therapy.

Related Drugs—There are no commercially available drugs chemically related to either dextran or heparin.

Pharmacological Effect and Mechanism—Dextran alone has no significant effect on coagulation when used in dosages recommended by the manufacturer. Dosages exceeding the manufacturer's recommendation may cause a prolongation of bleeding time (1). The use of dextran in a patient receiving heparin may possibly cause excessive bleeding (2, 3). The major pharmacological effect of heparin is its antithrombin action (4). Dextran has many effects upon hemostasis including hemodilution (3), reduction in viscosity (3), alteration of cell suspensions (3), prevention or reversal of erythrocyte aggregation (5), inhibition of platelet agglutination (5), and alteration of the sol-gel transformation from fibrinogen to fibrin (3). It has been demonstrated in dogs and in humans that heparin and dextran have independent effects which prolong coagulation time and decrease clot strength or elasticity (3).

Evaluation of Clinical Data—The concurrent use of heparin and dextran 40 (low-molecular weight dextran) has been reported in many case studies (6–13) with no mention of untoward effects or of any observed drug interaction. One review of dextrans stated that concurrent administration of dextran and heparin may result in excessive bleeding (2). It was recommended that the dosage of heparin be reduced by one-half to one-third when given with dextran.

The only original clinical data supporting the alleged drug interaction was from a study of one male subject (3). This subject received 5000 units of heparin as a control and on the next day 1% of body weight (91 kg) of dextran 75 followed by 5000 units of intravenous heparin sodium. The data (not analyzed statistically) showed differences between the heparin–dextran infusion and heparin alone. The coagulation time was prolonged, and clot strength was reduced especially at 4–6 hr after the heparin–dextran infusion.

In a related study (14), the effects of the concurrent use of dextran and warfarin in 98 vascular operative procedures were measured. The results showed a lower incidence of arterial thrombosis after the use of the two agents compared to the use of dextran alone. Only one case of hemorrhage was reported. However, no attempt was made to extrapolate these results to the effects of concurrent heparin–dextran administration.

■ Most clinical reports of concurrent heparin–dextran administration do not suggest any drug interaction, although no effort was made in these reports to study such effects. The one report (3) indicating that a significant drug interaction occurs lacked proper controls and statistical analysis. Without additional data, the clinical significance of the purported interaction is questionable.

Recommendations—The data are too inconclusive to recommend anything other than procedures to obtain baseline data (Lee–White clotting time, activated prothrombin time, or thrombin time) and to repeat these measurements several hours after concurrent therapy is initiated and at frequent intervals until stable anticoagulation is achieved.

References

(1) "Physicians' Desk Reference," 29th ed., Medical Economics, Inc., Oradell, NJ 07649, 1975, p. 1183.

(2) M. Atik, "Dextrans, Their Use in Surgery and Medicine with Emphasis on the Low Molecular Weight Fractions," *Anesthesiology*, *27*, 425 (1966).

(3) W. L. Bloom and S. S. Brewer, Jr., "The Independent Yet Synergistic Effects of Heparin and Dextran," *Acta Chir. Scand.*, *387*, suppl., 53 (1968).

(4) "The Pharmacological Basis of Therapeutics," 5th ed., L. S. Goodman and A. Gilman, Eds., Macmillan, New York, NY 10022, 1975, p. 1353.

(5) Package insert, Rheomacrodex, Pharmacia Laboratories Inc., Piscataway, NJ 08854, June 1975.

(6) C. M. Evarts, "Diagnosis and Treatment of Fat Embolism," *J. Amer. Med. Ass.*, *194*, 899 (1965).

(7) J. C. B. Serjeant, "Mesenteric Embolus Treated with Low-Molecular-Weight Dextran," *Lancet*, *i*, 139 (1965).

(8) W. J. Daniel *et al.*, "Treatment of Mesenteric Embolism with Dextran 40," *Lancet*, *i*, 567 (1966).

(9) R. J. Gregory, "The Rapid Lowering of Hematocrit by Exchange Transfusion of Rheomacrodex Dextran 40," *Acta Med. Scand.*, *189*, 551 (1971).

(10) M. Giromini *et al.*, "Anurie Provoquee par la Perfusion de Dextran de Faible Poids Moleculaire," *Presse Med.*, *75*, 2561 (1967).

(11) R. Burgos-Calderon and J. E. Figueroa, "Acute Oliguric Renal Failure Associated with Low-Molecular-Weight Dextran," *Bol. Asoc. Med. P.R.*, *64*, 1 (1972).

(12) A. M. Munster, "Low Molecular Weight Dextran in the Treatment of Phlegmasia Caerulea Dolens," *Med. J. Aust.*, *1*, 851 (1965).

(13) J. J. Bergan *et al.*, "Low Molecular Weight Dextran in Treatment of Severe Ischemia," *Arch. Surg.*, *91*, 338 (1965).

(14) T. H. Kluge *et al.*, "Thrombosis Prophylaxis with Dextran and Warfarin in Vascular Operations," *Surg. Gynecol. Obstet.*, *135*, 941 (1972).

[For additional information, see *Anticoagulant Therapy*, p. 358.]

Nonproprietary and Trade Names of Drugs

Dextran 40—*Gentran 40, LMD 10%, Rheomacrodex, Rheotan*

Dextran 75—*Dextran 6%, Gentran 75, Macrodex*
Heparin sodium—*Various manufacturers*

Prepared and evaluated by the Scientific Review Subpanel on Anticoagulants and reviewed by Practitioner Panel I.

Hexobarbital—Propranolol

Summary—Propranolol increases the acute central nervous system (CNS) toxicity of ether, hexobarbital, morphine, and urethan in mice. Since no adverse drug interactions with propranolol and CNS depressants have been reported in humans, no additional precautions are necessary when these drugs are administered concurrently.

Related Drugs—The sedation produced by **pentobarbital** has been enhanced by propranolol in mice (1). There is no documentation that other **barbiturates** interact with propranolol.

Pharmacological Effect and Mechanism—The administration of propranolol to animals previously treated with hexobarbital increased the acute toxicity of the barbiturate (2). It is suggested that the enhanced effect of propranolol and CNS depressants in mice is due to central rather than peripheral effects (3). Upon oral administration, propranolol is hydroxylated at the C-4 position, resulting in a minor metabolite that is also pharmacologically active. It is believed that this occurs in the liver since 4-hydroxypropranolol is not produced after intravenous administration (3, 4). Naphthoxylactic acid is the major metabolite identified in the urine (4, 5). The naphthyl group of the β-adrenergic blockers is responsible for the CNS depressant effect. Animal studies have shown that β-blockers without the naphthyl moiety produce stimulation rather than the depression seen with propranolol (2).

Evaluation of Clinical Data—There are no clinical reports of toxic effects between propranolol and hexobarbital or other barbiturates, although doses of propranolol up to 4000 mg/day have been employed in the treatment of hypertension in the United Kingdom (6).

■ Based on this lack of clinical data, it appears that this drug interaction is not clinically significant.

Recommendations—The concurrent administration of barbiturates and propranolol need not be avoided and no additional precautions are necessary when these drugs are administered together.

References

(1) K. P. Singh *et al.*, "Effects of Propranolol (a Beta Adrenergic Blocking Agent) on Some Central Nervous System Parameters," *Indian J. Med. Res.*, *59*, 786 (1971).

(2) W. Murmann *et al.*, "Central Nervous System Effects of Four β-Adrenergic Receptor Blocking Agents," *J. Pharm. Pharmacol.*, *18*, 317 (1966).

(3) W. Murmann *et al.*, "Effects of Hexobarbitone, Ether, Morphine and Urethane upon the Acute Toxicity of Propranolol and D-(—)-INPEA," *J. Pharm. Pharmacol.*, *18*, 692 (1966).

(4) A. Hayes and R. G. Cooper, "Studies on the Absorption, Distribution and Excretion of Propranolol in Rat, Dog and Monkey," *J. Pharmacol. Exp. Ther.*, *176*, 302 (1971).

(5) J. W. Paterson *et al.*, "The Pharmacodynamics and Metabolism of Propranolol in Man," *Pharmacol. Clin.*, *2*, 127 (1970).

(6) B. N. C. Prichard and P. M. S. Gillam, "Treatment of Hypertension with Propranolol," *Brit. Med. J.*, *1*, 7 (1969).

[For additional information, see *Antiarrhythmia Therapy*, p. 350.]

Nonproprietary and Trade Names of Drugs

Allobarbital—*Diadol*
Amobarbital—*Amytal and various combination products*
Aprobarbital—*Alurate*
Barbital—*Neurondia*
Butabarbital sodium—*Butisol Sodium*
Butalbital—*Available in combination products*
Hexobarbital—*Sombulex*
Mephobarbital—*Mebaral, Mebroin*

Metharbital—*Geminol*
Methohexital sodium—*Brevital Sodium*
Pentobarbital—*Nembutal and various combination products*
Phenobarbital—*Eskabarb, Luminal*
Propranolol hydrochloride—*Inderal*
Secobarbital—*Seconal and various combination products*
Talbutal—*Lotusate*
Thiopental sodium—*Pentothal Sodium*

Prepared and evaluated by the Scientific Review Subpanel on Sedative–Hypnotics and reviewed by Practitioner Panel VI.

Imipramine—Ethinyl Estradiol

Summary—Ethinyl estradiol may increase the number of toxic reactions to imipramine, but the clinical evidence for this drug interaction is limited and unreliable. Patients receiving these drugs concurrently should be observed closely for unexpected imipramine-induced adverse reactions. If adverse reactions occur, the dose of either imipramine or ethinyl estradiol should be reduced or one drug should be discontinued.

Related Drugs—In addition to ethinyl estradiol, **conjugated estrogens** have been reported to interact with imipramine (1). Although not documented, this drug interaction may occur between other **estrogenic substances** and other **tricyclic antidepressants.**

Ethinyl estradiol and related compounds are common ingredients in many oral contraceptives.

Pharmacological Effect and Mechanism—The exact mechanism of this reported drug interaction is unclear. Estrogens may inhibit the N-oxidation and the demethylation of imipramine causing accumulation of imipramine in the brain and other tissues (2), but this theory has not been critically evaluated. However, other steroids such as norethindrone (a progesterone derivative) produced similar effects with imipramine in mice (3). Additionally, ethinyl estradiol inhibited the metabolism of ethylmorphine and hexobarbital in rats (4).

Evaluation of Clinical Data—Thirty women (20–45 years of age) diagnosed as having primary depression were divided into four groups (5, 6). Ten patients received a placebo, 10 patients received imipramine and a placebo, five patients received imipramine and ethinyl estradiol (50 μg/day po), and five patients received imipramine and estradiol (25 μg/day po). The imipramine dose was 150 mg/day po. The patients were given ethinyl estradiol for 2 weeks and imipramine for 6 weeks.

In the first 2 weeks, the imipramine dose had to be reduced to 75 mg in four of the five women receiving 50 μg of ethinyl estradiol because of side effects including severe lethargy, hypotension, and coarse tremor.

Other side effects observed in the group receiving ethinyl estradiol (25 or 50 μg/day po) were urinary retention (one patient) and drowsiness (the majority of patients). Hypotension was prevalent only in the group receiving 50 μg of ethinyl estradiol. The investigators concluded that ethinyl estradiol increased the toxicity of tricyclic antidepressants and that these drugs probably could not be used concurrently for any therapeutic benefit.

Another report concerned a 32-year-old woman who had been taking conjugated estrogens (2.5 mg/day po) and imipramine (100 mg/day po) for at least 3 years (1). A review of her visits during this period indicated that she had almost always complained of lethargy and showed signs of depersonalization and an occasional tremor. Two years after she had begun this therapy, the patient increased her dosage of estrogen to 5 mg and then to 7.5 mg to get more energy, resulting in a hospital admission for extreme lethargy, nausea, constant headaches, and low blood pressure. The patient continued to manifest these symptoms until estrogen therapy was discontinued. The symptoms decreased significantly and did not recur when lower doses of conjugated estrogens (0.625 mg/day po) were initiated later.

■ Little reliable information supports the theory that exogenously administered estrogens affect a patient's response to imipramine. The initial starting dose of imipramine (150 mg/day po) used in the unpublished study (6) may have been responsible for the adverse effects reported. Also, there are no data on the effects of estrogen alone in the patients studied and this drug may have caused some of the reported adverse effects. Additionally, although the subjects studied had been diagnosed as suffering from primary depression, they also had a variety of other mental and psychological disorders and all patients were members of a correctional institution. Therefore, they may not have been a representative sample.

Recommendations—If imipramine and estrogens must be used concurrently, the patient should be observed closely for any unexpected toxicities caused by imipramine. If toxic symptoms do occur, the dose of imipramine or estrogen should be reduced or one drug should be discontinued.

References

(1) R. C. Khurana, "Estrogen-Imipramine Interaction," letter to the editor, *J. Amer. Med. Ass., 222,* 702 (1972).

(2) S. M. Somani and R. C. Khurana, "Mechanism of Estrogen-Imipramine Interaction," letter to the editor, *J. Amer. Med. Ass., 223,* 560 (1973).

(3) G. D. Bellward *et al.,* "The Effects of Pretreatment of Mice with Norethindrone on the Metabolism of 14C-Imipramine by the Liver Microsomal Drug-Metabolizing Enzymes," *Can. J. Physiol. Pharmacol., 52,* 28 (1974).

(4) T. P. Tephly and G. J. Mannering, "Inhibition of Drug Metabolism V. Inhibition of Drug Metabolism by Steroids," *Mol. Pharmacol., 4,* 10 (1968).

(5) "Estrogen May Well Affect Response to Antidepressant," *J. Amer. Med. Ass., 219,* 143 (1972).

(6) A. J. Prange *et al.,* "The Effect of Estrogen on Imipramine Response in Depressed Women," presented at the 5th World Congress on Psychiatry, Mexico City, Mexico, November 1971.

[For additional information, see *Antipsychotic Therapy,* p. 397.]

Nonproprietary and Trade Names of Drugs

Amitriptyline hydrochloride—*Elavil Hydrochloride and various combination products*
Benzestrol—*Chemestrogen*
Chlorotrianisene—*TACE*
Conjugated estrogens—*Premarin*
Desipramine hydrochloride—*Norpramin, Pertofrane*
Dienestrol—*DV, Synestrol*
Doxepin hydrochloride—*Adapin, Sinequan*
Esterified estrogens—*Amnestrogen, Evex, Menest, SK-Estrogens*
Estradiol—*Aquadiol, Progynon*
Estradiol benzoate—*Progynon Benzoate*
Estradiol cypionate—*Depo-Estradiol Cypionate*
Estradiol dipropionate—*Ovocylin Dipropionate*
Estradiol valerate—*Delestrogen, Duratrad, Estate*
Estrone—*Estrusol, Glyestrin, Menformon (A), Theelin, Wynestron*

Estrone piperazine sulfate—*Ogen*
Estrone potassium sulfate—*Femspan, Spanestrin P, Theelin R-P*
Estrone sodium sulfate—*Morestin*
Ethinyl estradiol—*Demulen, Estinyl, Feminone, Lynoral, Norlestrin, Oracon, Ovral, Palonyl*
Hexestrol—*Available under generic name*
Imipramine hydrochloride—*Presamine, Tofranil, Tofranil PM*
Mestranol—*Enovid, Norinyl, Ortho-Novum, Ovulen*
Methallenestril—*Vallestril*
Nortriptyline hydrochloride—*Aventyl Hydrochloride*
Promethestrol dipropionate—*Meprane Dipropionate*
Protriptyline hydrochloride—*Vivactil Hydrochloride*

Prepared and evaluated by the Scientific Review Subpanel on Psychotropic Agents and reviewed by Practitioner Panel VI.

Imipramine—Reserpine

Summary—Although concurrent administration of imipramine and reserpine may be effective in treating imipramine-refractory endogenous depression, the potential hazards associated with excessive central nervous system (CNS) stimulation (*e.g.*, hyperexcitability and resultant mania) produced by these drugs indicate that their concurrent use should be limited to selected patients under carefully controlled conditions.

Related Drugs—**Desipramine** is the only drug related to imipramine reported to interact with reserpine (1). However, **amitriptyline, doxepin, nortriptyline,** and **protriptyline** are chemically and pharmacologically related to imipramine and also may interact with reserpine.

Although not documented, **alseroxylon, deserpidine, rescinnamine,** and **syrosingopine** are structurally and pharmacologically related to reserpine and may interact similarly. Reserpine and related alkaloids are present in low doses in several combination antihypertensive products.

Pharmacological Effect and Mechanism—Reserpine causes a specific central depression (characterized as tranquilization) and depression of the sympathetic nervous system, centrally and peripherally, and has been employed as an antipsychotic and antihypertensive agent. Its neuronal activity may be related to its ability to reduce the amount of 5-hydroxytryptamine (serotonin) and norepinephrine stored in nerve endings where these chemicals act as neurotransmitters. The amine-depleting action of reserpine appears to be intraneuronal as the amines are converted to their inactive deaminated metabolites by monoamine oxidase before being released. The onset of action of reserpine is slow, possibly because of the prolonged time course of this amine depletion or its limited permeability into neuronal tissue (2).

Imipramine is classified as an antidepressant, but it also exerts anticholinergic and antihistaminic activity. Its effect on the depressed patient has been described as a depression of inhibitory functions in the brain rather than as the euphoric stimulation produced by the monoamine oxidase inhibitors (3). The mechanism by which imipramine is thought to induce its behavioral effects is through blockade of neuronal uptake of released norepinephrine, allowing the neurotransmitter to persist longer at its receptor sites (4).

Imipramine and related drugs antagonize the autonomic and behavioral effects of reserpine in animals (4–6). Animals exhibit excitation and arousal after receiving both drugs rather than the usual tranquilization induced by reserpine alone.

Evaluation of Clinical Data—Although reserpine may induce a psychic depressive reaction, administration of reserpine during desipramine therapy (average dose, 75 mg/day) produced a "stimulating" (*e.g.*, reserpine reversal) effect in seven depressed patients (1). After initial hyperexcitability and a manic reaction, patients improved dramatically after 2 days of reserpine administration. The interaction was not noted unless high doses of reserpine (7–10 mg/day po) were employed.

In another study (7), concurrent administration of reserpine (7.5–10 mg/day po) and imipramine (up to 300 mg/day po) for 2 days was effective in treating endogenous depression (14 out of 15 patients) after a short initial manic phase. In six of these patients, the improvement was maintained after reserpine was discontinued. All 15 patients had been refractory to imipramine therapy prior to the use of reserpine. However, all patients experienced a cutaneous vasodilation due to this concurrent therapy and some patients suffered from diarrhea as a result of increased intestinal peristalsis.

In a study (8) involving 10 patients unresponsive to imipramine (225 mg/day po), the addition of reserpine (10 mg/day po) did not produce observable objective improvement, but it did cause a severe manic reaction in one patient.

■ The addition of high doses of reserpine (7–10 mg) to the drug regimen of imipramine-treated patients may result in some improvement in the patient's response to imipramine. However, the clinical data are not conclusive. The two studies (1, 7) that reported this effect were not well controlled and used a small number of patients. A third study (8), better controlled but also with a small number of patients, failed to confirm these earlier findings. Moreover, concurrent administration of imipramine and reserpine has resulted in some undesirable side effects, such as diarrhea, precipitation of a manic reaction, and cutaneous vasodilation (1, 7).

Recommendations—Despite possible benefits of concurrent imipramine–reserpine therapy in patients refractory to imipramine alone, this therapy should be attempted only in severely depressed patients unresponsive to other antidepressant drugs. Patients receiving these drugs should be observed closely for symptoms of excessive CNS stimulation (*e.g.*, hyperexcitability and possibly mania).

Reserpine has caused severe depression (9) in doses lower (0.6–4 mg/day po) than the dose reported to enhance the effects of imipramine (7–10 mg/day po), and it has been recommended that this drug be avoided in depressed patients (10). However, no added depression was observed in several studies of concurrent therapy when higher doses of reserpine were used (1, 7, 8).

References

(1) W. Poldinger, "Combined Administration of Desipramine and Reserpine or Tetrabenazine in Depressed Patients," *Psychopharmacologia, 4*, 308 (1963).

(2) M. H. Alper *et al.*, "Pharmacology of Reserpine and Its Implications for Anesthesia," *Anesthesiology, 24,* 524 (1963).

(3) D. O. Lewis, "Pharmacodynamics of Depression and Its Relation to Therapy," *Brit. J. Clin. Pract., 28,* 21 (1974).

(4) S. Garattini and A. Jori, "Interactions between Imipramine-like Drugs and Reserpine on Body Temperature," in Proc. 1st Int. Symp., Milan, 1966, Int. Cong. Series No. 122, Excerpta Medica Foundation, p. 89.

(5) M. Osborne, "Interaction of Imipramine with Sympathomimetic Amines and Reserpine," *Arch. Int. Pharmacodyn. Ther., 138,* 492 (1962).

(6) F. Sulser *et al.*, "The Action of Desmethylimipramine in Counteracting Sedation and Cholinergic Effects of Reserpine-like Drugs," *J. Pharmacol. Exp. Ther., 144,* 321 (1964).

(7) L. Haskovec and K. Rysanek, "The Action of Reserpine in Imipramine-Resistant Depressive Patient: A Clinical and Biochemical Study," *Psychopharmacologia, 11,* 18 (1967).

(8) M. W. P. Carney *et al.*, "Effects of Imipramine and Reserpine in Depression," *Psychopharmacologia, 14,* 349 (1969).

(9) J. C. Muller *et al.*, "Depression and Anxiety Occurring during Rauwolfia Therapy," *J. Amer. Med. Ass., 159,* 836 (1955).

(10) "Drugs That Cause Depression," *Med. Lett., 14,* 34 (1972).

[For additional information, see *Antidepressant Therapy*, p. 373.]

Nonproprietary and Trade Names of Drugs

Alseroxylon—*Rautensin, Rauwiloid*
Amitriptyline hydrochloride—*Elavil Hydrochloride and various combination products*
Deserpidine—*Harmonyl*
Desipramine hydrochloride—*Norpramin, Pertofrane*
Doxepin hydrochloride—*Adapin, Sinequan*
Imipramine hydrochloride—*Presamine, Tofranil, Tofranil PM*

Nortriptyline hydrochloride—*Aventyl Hydrochloride*
Protriptyline hydrochloride—*Vivactil Hydrochloride*
Rauwolfia serpentina—*Raudixin and various combination products*
Rescinnamine—*Moderil*
Reserpine—*Reserpoid, Sandril, Serpasil, and various combination products*
Syrosingopine—*Singoserp*

Prepared and evaluated by the Scientific Review Subpanel on Psychotropic Agents and reviewed by Practitioner Panel V.

Imipramine—Thyroid

Summary—Liothyronine and other thyroid products may enhance the clinical effectiveness of imipramine and other tricyclic antidepressants. However, extensive confirmatory evidence is lacking and negative results have been reported. Patients who fail to respond to imipramine or other tricyclic antidepressants should be examined for hypothyroidism which should be corrected if found. The addition of liothyronine (25 μg/day po) to the tricyclic drug regimen might be considered in carefully selected patients if the patient is refractory to tricyclic antidepressants alone.

Related Drugs—**Amitriptyline** (1, 2) and **protriptyline** (2) also have been shown to interact with thyroid preparations. Other tricyclic antidepressants (*e.g.*, **desipramine, doxepin,** and **nortriptyline**) may interact in the same way.

All thyroid compounds should be expected to interact with the tricyclic antidepressants in a similar manner. **Liothyronine (triiodothyronine)** has been used in most studies because its activity is easy to control and it is relatively safe (3).

Pharmacological Effect and Mechanism—Results from animal studies are consistent with the clinical observation that liothyronine enhances the antidepressant activity of imipramine. Several mechanisms have been proposed, but they remain speculative and controversial (4).

Evaluation of Clinical Data—The original observation of an imipramine–thyroid interaction was reported after paroxysmal atrial tachycardia occurred in a patient receiving imipramine and thyroxine concurrently (5). This observation suggested that the toxicity of imipramine may be increased by concurrent administration of thyroid hormone.

There have been a number of controlled studies demonstrating the clinical effectiveness of concurrent imipramine (or other tricyclic antidepressants) and thyroid therapy. In one double-blind controlled study (6), imipramine (150 mg/day po) was administered to 20 euthyroid patients with retarded depression. Beginning on Day 5, 10 patients were given liothyronine (25 μg/day po) while the remaining 10 patients received a placebo. Imipramine and liothyronine produced a more rapid improvement in retarded depressed patients than did imipramine alone. Females appeared to be more responsive than males, and there was no significant difference in side effects between the tested patients and the control group.

In a 28-day double-blind controlled study, the same investigators (7) observed the effect of concurrent administration in 20 patients with severe primary depression. On the fifth day of imipramine therapy (150 mg/day po), patients received liothyronine (25 μg/day po) or a placebo. A significant improvement in the onset and efficacy of imipramine resulted when liothyronine was given concurrently compared to the control group. No significant differences in side effects were found between the two groups.

To determine if thyroid preparations enhance the effectiveness of tricyclic antidepressant therapy (2), 25 retarded depressed patients who had been refractory or who had responded inadequately to tricyclic antidepressant therapy were given liothyronine (25 μg/day po) concurrently with a tricyclic antidepressant. The study was single blind. Twenty-three patients received imipramine (150 mg/day po), one received amitriptyline (150 mg/day po), and another received protriptyline (40 mg/day po). Fourteen patients (including the patients taking amitriptyline and protriptyline) responded favorably and nine improved temporarily or not at all. Improvement was rapid, occurring in as little as a few hours up to 5.5 days. Four of eight patients who were followed for more than 10 months relapsed 5–8 months after initiation of therapy. The investigators classified the type of depression each patient had and concluded that these drugs were ineffective in schizo-affective disorders and of limited use in neurotic depression, but were useful in retarded depression.

Other studies showed that females react more favorably to concurrent therapy than males (8) and that amitriptyline interacts similarly with liothyronine (1). Thyroid-stimulating hormone and liothyronine produce the same effect but the dosage of thyroid-stimulating hormone is more difficult to control (9).

The effects of concurrent imipramine and liothyronine were evaluated in a double-blind controlled study of 49 patients with primary depression (10). Liothyronine failed to enhance the antidepressant effect of imipramine in these patients.

■ There is considerable clinical evidence that a patient's thyroid state affects the response to tricyclic antidepressant drugs (6–8). The addition of liothyronine (25 μg/day) may prevent the relatively long lag time that occurs before the clinical effectiveness of tricyclic antidepressants is observed. However, extensive confirmatory studies are lacking and negative results also have been reported (10). Side effects due to concurrent administration have been rare (1, 7).

Recommendations—Patients who fail to respond to imipramine or other tricyclic antidepressants should be examined for hypothyroidism, which should be corrected if found. The addition of liothyronine (25 μg/day po) to the tricyclic drug regimen might be considered if there is a particular need for a rapid response or if the patient is refractory to tricyclic antidepressants alone. The dose of liothyronine should be increased cautiously in patients with cardiovascular disease, particularly if initially hypothyroid, because of the risk of coronary occlusive changes (11, 12).

References

(1) D. Wheatley, "Potentiation of Amitriptyline by Thyroid Hormone," *Arch. Gen. Psychiat.*, *26*, 229 (1972).

(2) B. V. Earle, "Thyroid Hormone and Tricyclic Antidepressants in Resistant Depressions," *Amer. J. Psychiat.*, *126*, 1667 (1970).

(3) A. J. Prange, Jr., *et al.*, "Acceleration of Imipramine Antidepressant Activity by Thyroid Hormone," Scientific Proceeding in Summary Form. Paper presented at 124th Annual Meeting of American Psychiatric Association, May 15, 1968.

(4) "The Thyroid Axis, Drugs, and Behavior," A. J. Prange, Ed., Raven, New York, NY 10024, 1974, p. 43.

(5) A. J. Prange, Jr., "Paroxysmal Auricular Tachycardia Apparently Resulting from Combined Thyroid–Imipramine Treatment," *Amer. J. Psychiat.*, *119*, 994 (1963).

(6) A. J. Prange, Jr., *et al.*, "Enhancement of Imipramine Antidepressant Activity by Thyroid Hormone," *Amer. J. Psychiat.*, *126*, 457 (1969).

(7) I. C. Wilson *et al.*, "Thyroid-Hormone Enhancement of Imipramine in Nonretarded Depressions," *N. Engl. J. Med.*, *282*, 1063 (1970).

(8) A. Coppen *et al.*, "The Comparative Antidepressant Value of L-Tryptophan and Imipramine with and without Attempted Potentiation by Triiodothyronine," Presented to the Collegium International Neuro-Psychopharmacologicum, Prague, Czechoslovakia, August 1970.

(9) A. J. Prange, Jr., *et al.*, "Enhancement of Imipramine by Thyroid Stimulating Hormone: Clinical and Theoretical Implications," *Amer. J. Psychiat.*, *127*, 191 (1970).

(10) J. P. Feighner *et al.*, "Hormonal Potentiation of Imipramine and ECT in Primary Depression," *Amer. J. Psychiat.*, *128*, 50 (1972).

(11) N. Shafer, "Caution in Thyroid Therapy," letter to the editor, *N. Engl. J. Med.*, *283*, 211 (1970).

(12) I. C. Wilson, "Caution in Thyroid Therapy," letter to the editor, *N. Engl. J. Med.*, *283*, 211 (1970).

[For additional information, see *Antidepressant Therapy*, p. 373.]

Nonproprietary and Trade Names of Drugs

Amitriptyline hydrochloride—*Elavil Hydrochloride and various combination products*
Desipramine hydrochloride—*Norpramin, Pertofrane*
Dextrothyroxine sodium—*Choloxin*
Doxepin hydrochloride—*Adapin, Sinequan*
Imipramine hydrochloride—*Presamine, Tofranil, Tofranil PM*
Levothyroxine sodium—*Letter, Synthroid*

Liothyronine sodium—*Cytomel*
Liotrix—*Euthroid, Thyrolar*
Nortriptyline hydrochloride—*Aventyl Hydrochloride*
Protriptyline hydrochloride—*Vivactil Hydrochloride*
Thyroglobulin—*Proloid*
Thyroid—*Thyrar*
Thyroxine fraction—*Various manufacturers*

Prepared and evaluated by the Scientific Review Subpanel on Psychotropic Agents and reviewed by Practitioner Panel I.

Imipramine—Tranylcypromine

Summary—Severe interactions have been reported when tricyclic antidepressant drugs (*e.g.,* imipramine) have been given concurrently with a monoamine oxidase inhibitor (*e.g.,* tranylcypromine). Symptoms of the interaction include hyperpyrexia, excitability, muscular rigidity, fluctuations in blood pressure, and coma which can, in rare instances, progress to death. Concurrent use of these drugs should be attempted only in carefully selected and closely supervised patients who have not responded to any conventional treatment for depression.

Related Drugs—At the time this interaction was first reported, the most widely used drugs in the two antidepressant categories were imipramine and tranylcypromine; therefore, most reports concern these agents. Other monoamine oxidase inhibitors less often involved are **isocarboxazid** (1), **pargyline** (1), and **phenelzine** (1).

Other tricyclic antidepressants less often implicated are **amitriptyline** (1) and **desipramine** (1). Although not documented, **doxepin, nortriptyline,** and **protriptyline** can be expected to interact with tranylcypromine in a manner similar to imipramine. There is no evidence that concurrent administration of imipramine and tranylcypromine is likely to be more dangerous than other tricyclic antidepressants taken concurrently with other monoamine oxidase inhibitors.

Pharmacological Effect and Mechanism—Two possible mechanisms for this interaction have been discussed (2): (*a*) the monoamine oxidase inhibitor may enhance the effect of the tricyclic antidepressant indirectly through inhibition of microsomal enzymes, and (*b*) the tricyclic antidepressant may sensitize adrenergic receptors to amines which then accumulate extraneuronally as a result of monoamine oxidase inhibition. Animal experiments to test these hypotheses have yielded conflicting results and offer little clarification into the possible morbidity underlying concurrent tricyclic antidepressant and monoamine oxidase inhibitor therapy. The studies have often employed doses grossly in excess (sometimes toxic) of therapeutic equivalents used in humans. A syndrome of hyperpyrexia, restlessness, and death in rabbits was produced when amitriptyline was given intravenously after 3 days of pretreatment with an experimental monoamine oxidase inhibitor (3). In a similar way, massive parenteral doses of a monoamine oxidase inhibitor produced fatalities when followed by imipramine (4). The additive effects of either drug in both studies cannot be assessed;

greater quantities of the same drug may, and do, enhance mortality rates. Moreover, other studies (5) obtained varying effects depending on species or reported differing results with various tricyclic antidepressants.

There have been some suggestions that monoamine oxidase inhibitors may interfere with the metabolism of the tricyclic antidepressants, but this theory was not supported in a study of eight patients who were receiving amitriptyline and isocarboxazid concurrently (6).

Evaluation of Clinical Data—The clinical data are inconclusive and the possible enhanced effects of tricyclic antidepressant and monoamine oxidase inhibitor therapy in producing the reported morbidity are obscure. An extensive review (1) of published literature and unpublished information both from the Food and Drug Administration and all manufacturers of these compounds revealed 25 anecdotal cases of interactions of drugs in these two categories. Four of these reports probably concern the same patients. Furthermore, the information is difficult to evaluate: drugs had been taken in excess (overdose) in six cases; other drugs with known central nervous system (CNS) effects were taken in eight other instances; and the tricyclic drug had been given parenterally in four cases. In the remaining seven instances, a syndrome of sweating, tremors, restlessness, and hyperpyrexia was reported when both drugs were taken orally in normal dosages; all of these patients recovered after experiencing these symptoms.

Thus, the clinical pictures are consistent with documented reports of side effects resulting with the individual use of either drug. Either agent when used at full doses may, in rare instances, give rise to these CNS effects (1). Moreover, the underlying medical status of the patients in these reports is not known.

Based on the cases reported, it appears that the interaction is more likely to occur if excessive doses of either drug are used and if the tricyclic antidepressant is given parenterally after a period of enzyme inhibition induced by monoamine oxidase inhibitors.

There are also numerous reports (1, 7–16) providing clinical information that support the safe and effective concurrent use of these two types of drugs to treat depression refractory to single drug treatment. In such instances, the drugs were given concurrently and there were no acute adverse symptoms, although an increase of minor symptoms such as dry mouth, constipation, fatigue, and weight gain may occur (9).

■ There is inconclusive evidence that concurrent tricyclic antidepressant and monoamine oxidase inhibitor therapy is dangerous if used for carefully selected patients in therapeutic doses under close medical supervision.

Recommendations—If patients are monitored closely, concurrent therapy with imipramine and tranylcypromine may be used safely in selected patients who have not responded to any conventional drug treatment for depression. It is not possible to recommend any particular tricyclic antidepressant and monoamine oxidase inhibitor that can be regarded with certainty as free from risk since the clinical and animal data are conflicting.

To ensure proper patient selection, the criteria to be used include adequate clinical diagnosis excluding neurotic-characterological or schizophrenic depressions, careful physical examinations excluding those individuals who would present a medical risk, and careful screening of patients for those who will strictly adhere to the dietary precautions.

The possible adverse effects of this drug interaction, although infrequent, are potentially serious, even fatal. Treatment of symptoms has generally been supportive, including use of α-adrenergic blocking agents (e.g., phentolamine) to control hypertension and tepid sponging for hyperpyrexia (1, 17).

References

(1) M. Schuckit *et al.*, "Tricyclic Antidepressants and Monoamine Oxidase Inhibitors. Combination Therapy in the Treatment of Depression," *Arch. Gen. Psychiat.*, *24*, 509 (1971).

(2) F. Sjoqvist, "Psychotropic Drugs (2). Interaction between Monoamine Oxidase (MAO) Inhibitors and Other Substances," *Proc. Roy. Soc. Med.*, *58*, 967 (1965).

(3) M. Nymark and I. M. Nielsen, "Reactions Due to the Combination of Monoamineoxidase Inhibitors with Thymoleptics, Pethidine, or Methylamphetamine," *Lancet*, *ii*, 524 (1963).

(4) A. H. Loveless and D. R. Maxwell, "A Comparison of the Effects of Imipramine, Trimipramine and Some Other Drugs in Rabbits Treated with a Monoamine Oxidase Inhibitor," *Brit. J. Pharmacol.*, *25*, 158 (1965).

(5) P. Guilmot and G. Rucquoy, "Dangers in the Too Rapid Substitution of Imipramine for a Monoamine Oxidase Inhibitor and in the Combination of Nialamide–Isoniazid–Barbiturates at High Doses in Psychiatric Therapy," *Acta Neurol. Belg.*, *67*, 159 (1967).

(6) J. Snowdon and R. Braithwaite, "Combined Antidepressant Medication," *Brit. J. Psychiat.*, *125*, 610 (1974).

(7) D. R. Gander, "Treatment of Depressive Illnesses with Combined Antidepressants," *Lancet*, *ii*, 107 (1965).

(8) W. Sargant *et al.*, "New Treatment of Some Chronic Tension States," *Brit. Med. J.*, *1*, 322 (1966).

(9) "Combining the Antidepressant Drugs," editorial, *Lancet*, *ii*, 118 (1965).

(10) D. R. Gander, in "Antidepressant Drugs: Proceedings of First International Symposium," Excerpta Medica International Congress Series No. 122, S. Garattini and M. N. G. Dukes, Eds., 1967, pp. 886–918.

(11) W. Sargant, "Antidepressant Drugs," *Brit. Med. J.*, *1*, 1495 (1965).

(12) W. Sargant, "Psychotropic Drugs," *Brit. Med. J.*, *3*, 861 (1967).

(13) W. Sargant, "Combining the Antidepressant Drugs," *Brit. Med. J.*, *1*, 251 (1965).

(14) P. Dally, "Chemotherapy of Psychiatric Disorders," Plenum, New York, N.Y., 1967.

(15) D. Kelly *et al.*, "Treatment of Phobic States with Antidepressants. A Retrospective Study of 246 Patients," *Brit. J. Psychiat.*, *116*, 387 (1970).

(16) F. Winston, "Combined Antidepressant Therapy," *Brit. J. Psychiat.*, *118*, 301 (1971).

(17) A. V. Simmons *et al.*, "Case of Self-Poisoning with Multiple Antidepressant Drugs," *Lancet*, *i*, 214 (1970).

[For additional information, see *Antidepressant Therapy*, p. 373.]

Nonproprietary and Trade Names of Drugs

Amitriptyline hydrochloride—*Elavil Hydrochloride and various combination products*
Desipramine hydrochloride—*Norpramin, Pertofrane*
Doxepin hydrochloride—*Adapin, Sinequan*
Imipramine hydrochloride—*Presamine, Tofranil, Tofranil PM*
Isocarboxazid—*Marplan*

Nortriptyline hydrochloride—*Aventyl Hydrochloride*
Pargyline hydrochloride—*Eutonyl and various combination products*
Phenelzine sulfate—*Nardil*
Protriptyline hydrochloride—*Vivactil Hydrochloride*
Tranylcypromine—*Parnate*

Prepared and evaluated by the Scientific Review Subpanel on Psychotropic Agents and reviewed by Practitioner Panel II.

Indomethacin—Aspirin

Summary—Aspirin may decrease the serum levels of indomethacin when these drugs are administered concurrently. However, the clinical outcome of this drug interaction has not been established. Until more clinical data about the drug interaction are available, it is prudent to observe the patient closely for a possible decrease in the therapeutic effectiveness of indomethacin.

Related Drugs—Since aspirin is the acetyl derivative of salicylic acid, it is possible that other **salicylates** may interfere with the absorption of indomethacin (1).

Pharmacological Effect and Mechanism—The mechanism of this reported drug interaction is unclear. An early theory suggested that aspirin impaired the gastrointestinal absorption of indomethacin, causing a decrease in the serum level and urinary excretion of indomethacin and a rise in its fecal excretion (1). The proposed mechanism was not substantiated by later investigations in animals (2) and in humans (3).

A preliminary report of a study in humans indicated that intravenous administration of radioactive indomethacin concurrently with oral doses of aspirin resulted in decreased renal clearance of indomethacin, although no change in its serum levels occurred (4). In the same study, concurrent administration of oral doses of indomethacin and aspirin resulted in decreased renal clearance and decreased serum levels of indomethacin. It was concluded from these results that aspirin increases the nonrenal clearance of indomethacin and decreases its renal clearance. The decreased serum indomethacin levels after oral administration of indomethacin and aspirin were attributed to decreased bioavailability of indomethacin.

Preliminary radiotracer studies in rats determined that intravenous use of salicylic acid increases the biliary elimination of indomethacin and decreases serum and urinary levels of indomethacin (2). However, it is questionable whether these same mechanisms would occur in humans where there is little enterohepatic circulation of indomethacin (5).

Indomethacin and aspirin inhibited edema induced by carrageenan, an irritating substance, but concurrent use did not produce an expected additive effect (6). Similar results were found in rats (7) when one dose of aspirin (1–3 mg/kg po) was given prior to or 1 day after indomethacin (0.5 mg/kg po). Abatement of the anti-inflammatory activity of a single dose of indomethacin lasted for 2 weeks. However, the same investigators also reported that concurrent daily administration of the drugs for 2 weeks did not result in any apparent antagonism (7, 8).

Evaluation of Clinical Data—In a study of eight patients with rheumatoid arthritis (1), the concurrent administration of aspirin (1.8–3.6 g/day po for 4 days) and a single dose of indomethacin (100 mg po) resulted in lower (by 20–25%) serum indomethacin levels (determined by radioisotope tracer techniques) than in a control group of seven patients who received indomethacin alone. However, the clinical effects of the decreased serum indomethacin levels were not measured, so the therapeutic significance of this drug interaction is unknown.

One large cooperative study of 136 patients with rheumatoid arthritis failed to show any difference in frequency, extent, and rate of change of symptoms between the indomethacin–aspirin group and the placebo–aspirin group (9). During the 3-month period, each patient in both groups was permitted to take aspirin as needed. The indomethacin-treated group received daily incremental indomethacin doses of 50 mg until side effects developed or until the 200-mg/day level was reached. The liberal intake of aspirin (quantity not reported) and its influence on the absorption of indomethacin were thought to have contributed to the clinical results. Nevertheless, the pharmacological effects of aspirin itself may have been adequate to compensate for the loss of indomethacin activity from the indomethacin–aspirin interaction.

A study of eight healthy adults and 33 patients with rheumatoid arthritis showed no significant differences in the serum indomethacin levels after concurrent administration of buffered aspirin compared to indomethacin alone (3). The eight healthy adults received one dose of indomethacin (50 mg po) with buffered aspirin (3.6 g po) and without aspirin. The 33 arthritic patients received indomethacin (150 mg/day po) for 6 days with buffered aspirin (3.6–5 g po) given the last 3 days.

Another study compared the clinical effects of aspirin or indomethacin alone with the concurrent use of these drugs (10). Twenty rheumatoid arthritic patients were given indomethacin (100 mg/day po) with or without aspirin (4 g/day po). Evaluation of the clinical indexes of inflammation showed no significant difference between the treatment groups.

■ The therapeutic significance of the indomethacin–aspirin interaction has not been clearly established. In one controlled clinical study reporting a drug interaction (1), the patient sample size was small and the test method used to measure the effect of salicylates on serum indomethacin levels is considered unreliable by some investigators (3). Moreover, the correlation between clinical effect and serum indomethacin levels is uncertain (3) and other studies indicated that no drug interaction occurs (3, 10). Since no study has measured the long-term effects of concurrent use of indomethacin and aspirin, the possibility that chronic aspirin administration may affect the long-term therapeutic response to indomethacin cannot be ignored.

Recommendations—Until well-controlled studies determine the long-term effects of concurrent use of these drugs, possible interference by aspirin, particularly in large doses, should be considered in those arthritic patients who are unresponsive to indomethacin therapy. One study (3) reported that buffered aspirin (3.6 g/day po) does not interact with indomethacin, but it is still prudent to observe the patient receiving such aspirin formulations closely for possible interference with the therapeutic effectiveness of indomethacin.

Although rectal administration of indomethacin has been recommended to prevent this drug interaction (11), the results of one study showed that decreased serum indomethacin levels also occurred after concurrent administration of aspirin orally and indomethacin rectally (12).

References

(1) R. Jeremy and J. Towson, "Interaction between Aspirin and Indomethacin in the Treatment of Rheumatoid Arthritis," *Med. J. Aust.*, *2*, 127 (1970).

(2) D. W. Yesair *et al.*, "Comparative Effects of Salicylic Acid, Phenylbutazone, Probenecid and Other Anions on the Metabolism, Distribution and Excretion of Indomethacin in Rats," *Biochem. Pharmacol.*, *19*, 1591 (1970).

(3) G. D. Champion *et al.*, "The Effect of Aspirin on Serum Indomethacin," *Clin. Pharmacol. Ther.*, *13*, 239 (1972).

(4) B. W. Lei *et al.*, "The Influence of Aspirin on the Absorption and Disposition of Indomethacin," abstract, *Clin. Pharmacol. Ther.*, *19*, 110 (1976).

(5) D. E. Duggan *et al.*, "The Metabolism of Indomethacin in Man," *J. Pharmacol. Exp. Ther.*, *181*, 563 (1972).

(6) Z. E. Mielens *et al.*, "Interaction of Aspirin with Non-Steroidal Anti-Inflammatory Drugs in Rats," *J. Pharm. Pharmacol.*, *20*, 567 (1968).

(7) C. G. Van Arman and G. W. Nuss, "Pharmacological Interaction of Indomethacin with Other Anti-Inflammatory Drugs," *Pharmacologist*, *12*, 202 (1970).

(8) "One Drug May Be Better than Two," *Amer. Drug.*, *162*, 31 (1970).

(9) The Cooperating Clinics Committee of the American Rheumatism Association, "A Three-Month Trial of Indomethacin in Rheumatoid Arthritis, with Special Reference to Analysis and Inference," *Clin. Pharmacol. Ther.*, *8*, 11 (1967).

(10) P. M. Brooks *et al.*, "Indomethacin–Aspirin Interaction: A Clinical Appraisal," *Brit. Med. J.*, *3*, 69 (1975).

(11) B. Lindquist *et al.*, "Effect of Concurrent Administration of Aspirin and Indomethacin on Serum Concentrations," *Clin. Pharmacol. Ther.*, *15*, 247 (1974).

(12) E. Kaldestad *et al.*, "Interaction of Indomethacin and Acetylsalicylic Acid as Shown by Serum Concentrations of Indomethacin and Salicylate," *Eur. J. Clin. Pharmacol.*, *9*, 199 (1975).

[For additional information, see *Analgesic Therapy (Nonnarcotic)*, p. 341.]

Nonproprietary and Trade Names of Drugs

Aluminum aspirin—*Available in
  combination products*
Aspirin—*Available alone or as a fixed
  combination in many trade name products,
  especially over-the-counter preparations*
Calcium carbaspirin—*Calurin*
Carbethyl salicylate—*Sal-Ethyl Carbonate*

Choline salicylate—*Actasal, Arthropan*
Indomethacin—*Indocin*
Magnesium salicylate—*Various
  manufacturers*
Potassium salicylate—*Various
  manufacturers*
Sodium salicylate—*Various manufacturers*

*Prepared and evaluated by the Scientific Review Subpanel
on Analgesics and reviewed by Practitioner Panel IV.*

Indomethacin—Probenecid

Summary—Concurrent administration of probenecid causes an approximately twofold increase in serum indomethacin levels. The mechanism of this interaction is competition between indomethacin and probenecid at the renal tubular excretion site. This increase may result in enhanced clinical effectiveness of indomethacin but also may result in increased toxic reactions. Concurrent administration should be considered only in selected patients who can be observed closely for any signs of a toxic reaction to indomethacin.

Related Drugs—**Sulfinpyrazone** is a uricosuric drug pharmacologically related to probenecid. Although there is no documentation, this drug could also interact with indomethacin.

Pharmacological Effect and Mechanism—Excretion rates of indomethacin in humans range from 50 to 90% of the administered dose in 24 hr. About two-thirds of the drug and its metabolites (conjugated and free) is excreted by the kidneys (1–3). Probenecid is excreted by a mechanism (4) which competes with the tubular secretion of weak organic acids (such as indomethacin), resulting in decreased excretion of probenecid.

Indomethacin is 90% bound to plasma proteins and probenecid is 85–90% bound. Probenecid theoretically may displace indomethacin from its binding site but there are no data to support this possibility (5).

Evaluation of Clinical Data—The excretion rate of radiolabeled indomethacin and renal function were determined in six patients, three normal and three suffering from gout (6). The patients then were given probenecid (4.0 g po) for 1 day, probenecid (2.0 g po) with indomethacin (100 mg po) on the next day, and finally probenecid (2.0 g po) for 1 additional day. The baseline urinary excretion of radioactivity when indomethacin was given alone amounted to 30–49% in a 48-hr period. In contrast, it fell to 14–39% in the presence of probenecid. Because of the lowered excretion rate, the serum radioactivity levels were about 50% higher during probenecid administration. The indomethacin half-life (determined from labeled drug levels) was prolonged from a mean of 10.1 hr when given alone to a mean of 17.6 hr when given with probenecid.

In the same study, clearance determinations in another group of six healthy persons confirmed the mechanism of tubular secretion of indomethacin and marked inhibition of its excretion in the presence of probenecid. The reverse effect, namely the possible decrease of probenecid excretion resulting from indomethacin administration, was not studied. The uricosuric effect of probenecid was measured in the gouty patients and remained unaltered in the presence of indomethacin.

Three groups of patients with sero-positive rheumatoid arthritis were studied to determine the effect of the addition of probenecid to oral and rectal drug regimens of indomethacin (7). In group I, 12 patients who had received indomethacin (50 mg/day po) for at least 2 months were given probenecid (1 g/day po) for 1 week. In group II, 10 patients who had been taking indomethacin (50 mg po three times daily for at least 2 months) received probenecid (500 mg po twice daily for 2 weeks). The clinical effectiveness of indomethacin (*e.g.*, duration of morning stiffness, articular index of joint tenderness, and grip strength measurement) was evaluated during this 2-week period. In group III, six patients given indomethacin (100 mg) rectally at night were studied 2 days before and 2 days after probenecid (500 mg po) was administered. Clinical effectiveness of indomethacin also was assessed in these patients.

The results, determined by spectrophotometric analysis, showed that concurrent probenecid–indomethacin administration approximately doubled the serum indomethacin level. This increase occurred with both oral and rectal administrations of indomethacin. The improvement in the morning stiffness, joint tenderness, and grip strength indexes during probenecid administration indicated that the increased serum indomethacin levels were associated with increased drug effectiveness. Two patients in group I and two patients in group II manifested side effects from indomethacin (*e.g.*, headaches and lightheadedness); discontinuation of indomethacin was necessary for the two patients in group I.

In a brief report of nine patients with rheumatic diseases, the peak serum indomethacin levels (dose, 150 mg/day po) were doubled when probenecid (dose not reported) was given concurrently (8). However, the investigators did not study the clinical effects of this twofold increase in the serum indomethacin levels.

■ The fact that probenecid increases serum indomethacin levels seems clearly established. However, since the reported studies were done on a short-term basis and there is considerable variability of serum indomethacin levels between individuals (9), it is difficult to predict the long-term clinical or toxic effects of concurrent use after chronic administration.

Recommendations—Further studies of the long-term effects of chronic concurrent use of indomethacin and probenecid are needed before the beneficial effects of this drug interaction are established. Because the high incidence of clinical toxicity of indomethacin is dose related, any patient receiving these drugs concurrently should be observed closely for symptoms of toxic reactions to indomethacin [*e.g.*, gastrointestinal side effects, headache, dizziness, lightheadedness, and mental confusion (10–12)]. Moreover, the indomethacin dose should be reduced to yield the lowest effective serum level.

Because indomethacin is primarily metabolized in the liver (5) and excreted mainly through the kidney (1–3), concurrent administration should be used with even greater caution in patients with hepatic or renal impairment.

References

(1) R. E. Harman *et al.*, "The Metabolites of Indomethacin, A New Anti-Inflammatory Drug," *J. Pharmacol. Exp. Ther.*, *143*, 215 (1964).

(2) H. B. Hucker *et al.*, "Studies on the Absorption, Distribution and Excretion of Indomethacin in Various Species," *J. Pharmacol. Exp. Ther.*, *153*, 237 (1966).

(3) D. E. Duggan *et al.*, "The Metabolism of Indomethacin in Man," *J. Pharmacol. Exp. Ther.*, *181*, 563 (1972).

(4) I. M. Weiner *et al.*, "On the Mechanism of Action of Probenecid on Renal Tubular Secretion," *Bull. Johns Hopkins Hosp.*, *106*, 333 (1960).

(5) "The Pharmacological Basis of Therapeutics," 5th ed., L. S. Goodman and A. Gilman, Eds., Macmillan, New York, NY 10022, 1975, pp. 342, 863.

(6) M. D. Skeith et al., "The Renal Excretion of Indomethacin and Its Inhibition by Probenecid," Clin. Pharmacol. Ther., 9, 89 (1968).

(7) P. M. Brooks et al., "The Clinical Significance of the Indomethacin-Probenecid Interaction," Brit. J. Clin. Pharmacol., 1, 287 (1974).

(8) W. Emori et al., "The Pharmacokinetics of Indomethacin in Serum," Clin. Pharmacol. Ther., 14, 134 (1973).

(9) G. D. Champion et al., "The Effect of Aspirin on Serum Indomethacin," Clin. Pharmacol. Ther., 13, 239 (1972).

(10) The Cooperating Clinics Committee of the American Rheumatism Association, "A Three-Month Trial of Indomethacin in Rheumatoid Arthritis, with Special Reference to Analysis and Inference," Clin. Pharmacol. Ther., 8, 11 (1967).

(11) G. L. Bach, "Adverse Reactions of Antirheumatic Drugs," Int. J. Clin. Pharmacol., 7, 198 (1973).

(12) W. M. O'Brien, "Indomethacin: A Survey of Clinical Trials," Clin. Pharmacol. Ther., 9, 94 (1968).

[For additional information, see *Analgesic Therapy (Nonnarcotic)*, p. 341.]

Nonproprietary and Trade Names of Drugs

Indomethacin—*Indocin*   Sulfinpyrazone—*Anturane*
Probenecid—*Benemid*

Prepared and evaluated by the Scientific Review Subpanel on Analgesics and reviewed by Practitioner Panel V.

Insulin—Phenelzine

Summary—Administration of monoamine oxidase inhibitors (*e.g.*, phenelzine) to diabetic patients receiving insulin may increase the occurrence of symptoms of hypoglycemia. Reduction of the insulin dose may be necessary in patients receiving insulin and phenelzine concurrently.

Related Drugs—Monoamine oxidase inhibitors such as **mebanazine** (1), **pargyline** (2, 3), and **tranylcypromine** (4–8) have been shown to enhance the hypoglycemic activity of insulin in animals. **Isocarboxazid** has been shown to interact with insulin in humans (9).

Pharmacological Effect and Mechanism—Enhancement of the hypoglycemic action of insulin by the administration of monoamine oxidase inhibitors is well documented in animals (2, 3, 5–7, 10, 11) and in humans (1, 9, 12–14). Several theories have been proposed to explain this enhancement, but the exact mechanism of this interaction remains undetermined. It was postulated (4, 15) that the monoamine oxidase inhibitor-induced enhancement of the hypoglycemic effect is due to partial failure of the compensatory function of the adrenergic nervous system, perhaps through replacement of the adrenergic transmitter by a "false neurotransmitter," octopamine (4). Octopamine, unlike the adrenergic transmitter, does not have adrenergic effects and will not induce compensatory hyperglycemia (7).

Conflicting data indicate that tranylcypromine stimulates (5, 16) and impairs (8, 17) *in vitro* insulin release from the pancreas. Additionally, inhibition of gluconeogenesis *via* insulin release or by a direct mechanism involving inhibition of transaminase reactions (18) also may contribute to the enhancement of the hypoglycemic effect.

Evaluation of Clinical Data—Spontaneous hypoglycemic episodes were reported in a 68-year-old female diabetic patient receiving insulin (48 units/day) during treatment with mebanazine (15–25 mg/day po), a hydrazine monoamine oxidase inhibitor (1). These episodes persisted until the insulin dose was reduced progressively by 30%. In the majority of 35 patients who had both diabetes (maturity onset) and depression and who were receiving chlorpropamide, insulin, or tolbutamide, chronic treatment with mebanazine (10–15 mg/day po) significantly improved their glucose tolerance curves (12). Patients refractory to chlorpropamide (dose not reported) and tolbutamide (dose not reported) became responsive to oral hypoglycemic agents after mebanazine administration.

Concurrent administration of mebanazine (20 mg/day po) or phenelzine (45 mg/day po) enhanced the hypoglycemic effect of insulin in patients suffering from depression. In diabetic patients poorly controlled with sulfonylureas, mebanazine improved the glucose tolerance test (13).

■ Based on the published evidence, potentially serious symptoms of hypoglycemia may result when a monoamine oxidase inhibitor is administered to a diabetic patient receiving insulin. In socially isolated and nonhospitalized diabetic patients, such concurrent therapy could induce a prolonged or even fatal hypoglycemic state.

Recommendations—Since monoamine oxidase inhibitors may enhance the hypoglycemic action of insulin in animals and in human diabetic patients, concurrent administration of monoamine oxidase inhibitors and insulin to diabetic subjects may be potentially dangerous. Such concurrent administration would call for close clinical evaluation of the serum glucose level and a possible reduction in the insulin dose.

The sulfonylureas chlorpropamide (12) and tolbutamide (12) have also been reported to interact with monoamine oxidase inhibitors. Although not documented, the other sulfonylureas (acetohexamide and tolazamide) should be expected to interact also. Therefore, similar precautions should be taken when these drugs are administered concurrently with monoamine oxidase inhibitors.

References

(1) A. J. Cooper and K. M. G. Keddie, "Hypotensive Collapse and Hypoglycaemia after Mebanazine—A Monoamine-Oxidase Inhibitor," *Lancet, ii,* 1133 (1964).

(2) L. A. Frohman, "Stimulation of Insulin Secretion in Rats by Pargyline and Mebanazine," *Diabetes, 20,* 266 (1971).

(3) W. Z. Potter *et al.*, "Possible Role of Hydrazine Group in Hypoglycemia Associated with the Use of Certain Monoamine-Oxidase Inhibitors (MAOI's)," *Diabetes, 18,* 538 (1969).

(4) I. J. Kopin *et al.*, "'False Neurochemical Transmitters' and the Mechanism of Sympathetic Blockade by Monoamine Oxidase Inhibitors," *J. Pharmacol. Exp. Ther., 147,* 186 (1965).

(5) R. Bressler *et al.*, "Tranylcypromine: A Potent Insulin Secretagogue and Hypoglycemic Agent," *Diabetes, 17,* 617 (1968).

(6) A. J. Cooper and G. Ashcroft, "Potentiation of Insulin Hypoglycaemia by M.A.O.I. Antidepressant Drugs," *Lancet, i,* 407 (1966).

(7) A. M. Barrett, "The Mode of Action of Insulin Potentiation by Mebanazine," *J. Pharm. Pharmacol., 22,* 291 (1970).

(8) H. Aleyassine and S. H. Lee, "Inhibition by Hydrazine, Phenelzine and Pargyline of Insulin Release from Rat Pancreas," *Endocrinology, 89,* 125 (1971).

(9) H. M. van Praag and B. Leijnse, "The Influence of Some Antidepressives of the Hydrazine Type on the Glucose Metabolism in Depressed Patients," *Clin. Chim. Acta, 8,* 466 (1963).

(10) P. I. Adnitt, "Monoamineoxidase Inhibition and Insulin Sensitivity," *J. Endocrinol., 42,* 417 (1968).

(11) A. M. Barrett, "Modification of the Hypoglycaemic Response to Tolbutamide and Insulin by Mebanazine—An Inhibitor of Monoamine Oxidase," *J. Pharm. Pharmacol., 17,* 19 (1965).

(12) L. Wickstrom and K. Pettersson, "Treatment of Diabetics with Monoamine-Oxidase Inhibitors," *Lancet, ii,* 995 (1964).

(13) P. I. Adnitt, "Hypoglycemic Action of Monoamineoxidase Inhibitors (MAOI's)," *Diabetes*, *17*, 628 (1968).

(14) J. Weiss *et al.*, "Effects of Iproniazid and Similar Compounds on the Gastrointestinal Tract," *Ann. N.Y. Acad. Sci.*, *80*, 854 (1959).

(15) A. J. Cooper and G. Ashcroft, "Modification of Insulin and Sulfonylurea Hypoglycemia by Monoamine-Oxidase Inhibitor Drugs," editorial, *Diabetes*, *16*, 272 (1967).

(16) R. E. Hernandez *et al.*, "In Vitro Insulinogenic Effect of Two Monoamine-Oxidase Inhibitors," *Diabetes*, *18*, 417 (1969).

(17) H. Aleyassine and S. H. Lee, "Inhibition of Insulin Release by Substrates and Inhibitors of Monoamine Oxidase," *Amer. J. Physiol.*, *222*, 565 (1972).

(18) L. Triner *et al.*, "The Effect of Some Monoamine Oxidase Inhibitors on Gluconeogenesis," *Life Sci.*, *8*, 1281 (1969).

[For additional information, see *Hypoglycemic Therapy*, p. 422.]

Nonproprietary and Trade Names of Drugs

Acetohexamide—*Dymelor*
Chlorpropamide—*Diabinese*
Insulin—*Iletin*
Isocarboxazid—*Marplan*
Mebanazine*—*Actomol*
Pargyline hydrochloride—*Eutonyl and various combination products*

Phenelzine sulfate—*Nardil*
Tolazamide—*Tolinase*
Tolbutamide—*Orinase*
Tranylcypromine—*Parnate*

* Not yet commercially available in the United States.

Prepared and evaluated by the Scientific Review Subpanels on Hypoglycemic Agents and Psychotropic Agents and reviewed by Practitioner Panel III.

Insulin—Phenytoin*

Summary—Diabetic patients receiving phenytoin should be monitored closely for unexpected elevations of serum glucose levels and symptoms of hyperglycemia (*e.g.,* ataxia, coma, drowsiness, lethargy, hypotension, polydipsia, and polyuria). If such symptoms occur, a reduction in the dosage of phenytoin should be attempted.

Related Drugs—*In vitro* studies showed that **mephenytoin** is equivalent to phenytoin in its inhibition of insulin secretion (1). Other hydantoin analogs such as **ethotoin** have not been tested.

Pharmacological Effect and Mechanism—Phenytoin inhibits both basal insulin secretion and insulin secretion that occurs after stimulation by hyperglycemia, tolbutamide, or methacholine (1, 2). *In vitro* studies (1) indicated that phenytoin may diminish release of insulin and cause hyperglycemia by stimulating the sodium–potassium adenosine triphosphatase pump, causing decreased intracellular sodium and depressed excitability of the pancreatic cells.

Results of another animal study suggested a stimulation of the hypothalamus and sympathoadrenal system, thus inhibiting insulin release (3), but there is little direct evidence to support this.

---

* Phenytoin is the new official name for diphenylhydantoin.

Evaluation of Clinical Data—There have been at least 12 reported cases of hyperglycemia occurring with the oral and parenteral administration of large doses of phenytoin (4–12). In some instances, the dosage of phenytoin was in the toxic range (5–8). The hyperglycemia definitely appeared to be dose related and was usually reversible when phenytoin was discontinued or reduced. The symptoms of hyperglycemia were ataxia, drowsiness, lethargy, and psychosis (5–9). The other cases involved patients who experienced fatal, hyperosmolar, nonketotic coma in which phenytoin was considered a contributory factor. However, other drugs also were given and a causal relationship between coma and phenytoin administration was not established.

Despite 12 cases of phenytoin-induced hyperglycemia, no clinical data indicate that phenytoin blocks the hypoglycemic effects of exogenously administered insulin. In one case when these drugs were used concurrently (4), a patient developed hyperglycemia (serum glucose level, 1260 mg/100 ml) 3 hr after phenytoin administration (200 mg iv). Subsequent administration of insulin (200 units iv and 200 units im) did not lower the serum glucose levels to normal. However, no speculation was made about a possible interaction because the patient's lack of response to insulin might have been due to concomitant renal failure.

■ Phenytoin alone may inhibit endogenous insulin secretion resulting in clinically significant symptoms of hyperglycemia (*e.g.,* ataxia, coma, drowsiness, lethargy, hypotension, polydipsia, and polyuria). There is no evidence that phenytoin antagonizes exogenously administered insulin.

Recommendations—Phenytoin may inhibit endogenous insulin secretion and may cause clinically significant symptoms of hyperglycemia (*e.g.,* ataxia, coma, drowsiness, lethargy, hypotension, polydipsia, and polyuria) in diabetic patients. If such symptoms occur, a discontinuation of phenytoin or a reduction in its dose should be attempted.

Since sulfonylurea hypoglycemic drugs (*e.g.,* acetohexamide, chlorpropamide, tolazamide, and tolbutamide) act by stimulation of the pancreatic β-cells to release insulin (13), their action theoretically may be affected by phenytoin also. Therefore, adjustments in their dosage may be necessary whenever phenytoin is added to or withdrawn from the drug regimen of a sulfonylurea-treated patient.

References

(1) J. S. Kizer *et al.,* "The In Vitro Inhibition of Insulin Secretion by Diphenylhydantoin," *J. Clin. Invest.,* *49,* 1942 (1970).

(2) S. R. Levin *et al.,* "Inhibition of Insulin Secretion by Diphenylhydantoin in the Isolated Perfused Pancreas," *J. Clin. Endocrinol. Metab.,* *30,* 400 (1970).

(3) N. R. Bilton *et al.,* "Effects of Convulsions and Anticonvulsants on Blood Sugar in Rabbits," *Epilepsia,* *6,* 243 (1965).

(4) E. M. Goldberg and S. S. Sanbar, "Hyperglycemic, Nonketotic Coma following Administration of Dilantin (Diphenylhydantoin)," *Diabetes,* *18,* 101 (1969).

(5) J. P. Klein, "Diphenylhydantoin Intoxication Associated with Hyperglycemia," *J. Pediat.,* *69,* 463 (1966).

(6) J. R. Dahl, "Diphenylhydantoin Toxic Psychosis with Associated Hyperglycemia," *Calif. Med.,* *107,* 345 (1967).

(7) D. M. Said *et al.,* "Hyperglycemia Associated with Diphenylhydantoin (Dilantin) Intoxication," *Med. Ann. D. C.,* *37,* 170 (1968).

(8) B. H. Peters and N. A. Samaan, "Hyperglycemia with Relative Hypoinsulinemia in Diphenylhydantoin Toxicity," *N. Engl. J. Med.,* *281,* 91 (1969).

(9) B. L. Fariss and C. L. Lutcher, "Diphenylhydantoin-Induced Hyperglycemia and Impaired Insulin Release. Effect of Dosage," *Diabetes,* *20,* 177 (1971).

(10) E. M. Goldberg and S. S. Sanbar, "Hyperglycemic Hyperosmolar Coma following Administration of Dilantin (Diphenylhydantoin)," *Diabetes,* *18,* suppl. 1, 356 (1969).

(11) J. E. Gerich *et al.,* "Clinical and Metabolic Characteristics of Hyperosmolar Nonketotic Coma," *Diabetes,* *20,* 228 (1971).

(12) T. Treasure and P. A. Toseland, "Hyperglycaemia Due to Phenytoin Toxicity," *Arch. Dis. Child.*, *46*, 563 (1971).

(13) R. S. Yalow *et al.*, "Comparison of Plasma Insulin Levels following Administration of Tolbutamide and Glucose," *Diabetes*, *9*, 356 (1960).

[For additional information, see *Hypoglycemic Therapy*, p. 422.]

Nonproprietary and Trade Names of Drugs

Acetohexamide—*Dymelor*
Chlorpropamide—*Diabinese*
Ethotoin—*Peganone*
Insulin—*Iletin*

Mephenytoin—*Mesantoin*
Phenytoin—*Dilantin*
Tolazamide—*Tolinase*
Tolbutamide—*Orinase*

Prepared and evaluated by the Scientific Review Subpanels on Hypoglycemic Agents and Anticonvulsants and reviewed by Practitioner Panel I.

Insulin—Propranolol

Summary—The interference of propranolol with carbohydrate metabolism poses risks of hypoglycemia and possibly hyperglycemia in diabetic patients or in patients predisposed to diabetes. Consequently, adjustment in the dosage of insulin may be necessary to prevent hypoglycemic or hyperglycemic episodes when these drugs are given concurrently. Serum glucose levels should be determined frequently in patients receiving these drugs since propranolol may block the symptoms of hypoglycemia.

Related Drugs—Propranolol is currently the only β-adrenergic blocking agent approved for use in the United States. Because the interference of carbohydrate metabolism by propranolol may be independent of its β-adrenergic blocking effect (1–3), the effect of other β-adrenergic blockers cannot be predicted.

Pharmacological Effect and Mechanism—It is unclear how propranolol affects the physiological response to exogenous and endogenous insulin, although it is known that propranolol influences certain aspects of carbohydrate metabolism. Propranolol has been shown to inhibit skeletal muscle glycogenolysis (4–6), and since glycogenolysis normally leads to decreased glucose utilization (7), this inhibition may contribute indirectly to hypoglycemia by permitting the continued peripheral utilization of glucose. Furthermore, propranolol also inhibits the rebound of glucose levels in nondiabetic individuals following insulin administration (8). This action may be due to propranolol-induced suppression of lipolysis (8, 9).

Additionally, propranolol interferes with the stimulation of insulin release from pancreatic β-cells caused by both epinephrine (1) and tolbutamide (2, 10). This interference may be attributed either to propranolol-induced blockade of the β-adrenergic receptors in the pancreatic β-cells (1, 10) or to augmentation of epinephrine's a-adrenergic suppression of insulin release (11).

The result of these actions in humans has usually been hypoglycemia (12–15), although a hyperglycemic response to propranolol has been reported (16, 17).

Evaluation of Clinical Data—There are many reports describing cases of severe hypoglycemic episodes in patients receiving propranolol. One report (12) cited two cases of recurrent, severe hypoglycemia in patients treated with propranolol. The discontinuation of propranolol was associated in each case with the cessation of the hypoglycemic episodes. A nondiabetic 9-year-old female, given nothing by mouth for 20 hr prior to minor plastic surgery, suffered a hypoglycemic seizure (serum glucose level, 12 mg%) after receiving propranolol (13). This observation was verified by fasting the patient for 24 hr and then administering propranolol (2 mg iv). The serum glucose level dropped from 65 to 34 mg% in 95 min. A 71-year-old patient taking propranolol (40 mg four times daily) over 4 years for angina developed hypoglycemia (serum glucose level, 38 mg%) after anterior myocardial infarction (14). Symptoms of severe hypoglycemia were reported in two children receiving propranolol (for the cyanosis associated with tetralogy of Fallot) following the restriction of food intake for 16–24 hr (15).

Hyperosmolar nonketotic diabetic coma recurred in a 46-year-old male hypertensive patient maintained for 1 year on propranolol (240 mg/day po) and hydralazine (200 mg/day po) (16). In a more complete discussion of the case (17), extensive metabolic studies of the patient indicated that the severe hyperglycemia (serum glucose level, 1130 mg%) was most likely the result of ineffective physiological utilization of dietary fats and carbohydrates caused by the inhibition of lipolysis and/or impairment of insulin secretion by propranolol. However, a possible contributing factor may have been reflex sympathomimetic discharge following the administration of hydralazine.

In one case of functional insulinoma, propranolol (80 mg/day po) suppressed insulin release in response to oral glucose and intravenous arginine and prevented hypoglycemia (11).

■ The interference of propranolol with carbohydrate metabolism poses definite risks of hypoglycemia and possibly hyperglycemia in diabetic subjects and other susceptible patients. The risk is further complicated by propranolol's blockade of both the warning symptoms of hypoglycemia (*e.g.*, palpitation or tachycardia and sweating) and the compensatory protective reaction (17, 18) to this metabolic imbalance.

However, the metabolic blockade also has proven useful for preventing ketoacidosis in diabetic children who had demonstrated a propensity for repeated, frequent, and severe episodes of this metabolic dysfunction (9) and in treating a functional insulinoma (11). Propranolol also has proved useful in modifying the adverse cardiovascular effects induced by hypoglycemia (*e.g.*, tachycardia, increased cardiac output, and widened pulse pressure) (19).

Recommendations—The use of propranolol in diabetic patients or in patients predisposed to diabetes can result in a disturbance of carbohydrate metabolism and should be avoided. If insulin and propranolol must be given concurrently, periodic serum glucose levels should be determined to adjust (probably reduce) the insulin dosage if necessary.

Because propranolol affects carbohydrate metabolism, similar precautions would be applicable to concurrent use of the oral hypoglycemics (*e.g.*, sulfonylureas and phenformin).

References

(1) D. Porte, Jr., "A Receptor Mechanism for the Inhibition of Insulin Release by Epinephrine in Man," *J. Clin. Invest., 46*, 86 (1967).

(2) F. Massara *et al.,* "Depressed Tolbutamide-Induced Insulin Response in Subjects Treated with Propranolol," *Diabetologia, 7,* 287 (1971).

(3) J. L. Beck *et al.,* "The Hypoglycemic Effect of Propranolol," *Horm. Metab. Res., 2,* 277 (1970).

(4) R. A. Salvador *et al.,* "Inhibition by Butoxamine, Propranolol and MJ1999 of the Glycogenolytic Action of the Catecholamines in the Rat," *Biochem. Pharmacol., 16,* 2037 (1967).

(5) J. H. Brown et al., "Oral Effectiveness of Beta Adrenergic Antagonists in Preventing Epinephrine-Induced Metabolic Responses," J. Pharmacol. Exp. Ther., 163, 25 (1968).

(6) E. A. Abramson and R. A. Arky, "Role of Beta-Adrenergic Receptors in Counterregulation to Insulin-Induced Hypoglycemia," Diabetes, 17, 141 (1968).

(7) H. T. Narahara et al., "Carbohydrate Metabolism and Its Disorders," vol. 1, F. Dickens et al., Eds., Academic, New York, N.Y., 1968, pp. 375–395.

(8) E. A. Abramson et al., "Effects of Propranolol on the Hormonal and Metabolic Responses to Insulin-Induced Hypoglycaemia," Lancet, ii, 1386 (1966).

(9) L. Baker et al., "Beta Adrenergic Blockade and Juvenile Diabetes: Acute Studies and Long-Term Therapeutic Trial," J. Pediat., 75, 19 (1969).

(10) O. De Divitiis et al., "Tolbutamide and Propranolol," Lancet, i, 749 (1968).

(11) I. Blum et al., "Prevention of Hypoglycemic Attacks by Propranolol in a Patient Suffering from Insulinoma," Diabetes, 24, 535 (1975).

(12) M. N. Kotler et al., "Hypoglycaemia Precipitated by Propranolol," Lancet, ii, 1389 (1966).

(13) T. F. Mackintosh, "Propranolol and Hypoglycaemia," letter to the editor, Lancet, i, 104 (1967).

(14) R. Wray and S. B. J. Sutcliffe, "Propranolol-Induced Hypoglycaemia and Myocardial Infarction," letter to the editor, Brit. Med. J., 2, 592 (1972).

(15) J. T. McBride et al., "Hypoglycemia Associated with Propranolol," Pediatrics, 51, 1085 (1973).

(16) S. Podolsky, "Recurrent Hyperosmolar Non-Ketotic Diabetic Coma (HNC) Caused by Propranolol Therapy," Clin. Res., 19, 354 (1971).

(17) S. Podolsky and C. G. Pattavina, "Hyperosmolar Nonketotic Diabetic Coma: A Complication of Propranolol Therapy," Metabolism, 22, 685 (1973).

(18) "Propranolol—New Uses," Med. Lett., 15, 49 (1973).

(19) R. H. Lloyd-Mostyn and S. Oram, "Modification by Propranolol of Cardiovascular Effects of Induced Hypoglycaemia," Lancet, i, 1213 (1975).

[For additional information, see Hypoglycemic Therapy, p. 422.]

Nonproprietary and Trade Names of Drugs

Acetohexamide—Dymelor
Chlorpropamide—Diabinese
Insulin—Iletin
Phenformin hydrochloride—DBI, Meltrol

Propranolol hydrochloride—Inderal
Tolazamide—Tolinase
Tolbutamide—Orinase

Prepared and evaluated by the Scientific Review Subpanels on Hypoglycemic Agents and Antiarrhythmic Agents and reviewed by Practitioner Panel II.

Isoniazid—Aluminum Hydroxide

Summary—The simultaneous administration of large doses of aluminum hydroxide may delay or decrease the absorption of isoniazid and may decrease the peak serum levels of the anti-infective. Although the clinical effects of this drug interaction are not known, it is prudent to administer isoniazid at least 1 hr prior to antacid administration.

Related Drugs—The one study of this interaction used aluminum hydroxide and an **aluminum–magnesium compound** (magaldrate) (1). Although not documented, other **aluminum-containing antacids** might influence the absorption of isoniazid.

Pharmacological Effect and Mechanism—Aluminum hydroxide is capable of delaying gastric emptying (2). Since isoniazid is absorbed primarily from the intestine (3), a delay in gastric emptying results in delayed isoniazid absorption and decreased peak serum isoniazid levels (1).

Another possible mechanism is the formation of insoluble metallic complexes between aluminum hydroxide and isoniazid. *In vitro* studies showed that ferrous and magnesium ions complex with isoniazid in alkaline media (4). However, other *in vitro* observations (1) indicate that this mechanism is unlikely.

Evaluation of Clinical Data—The data pertaining to this interaction are limited to one study (1) of 11 patients receiving isoniazid (100–300 mg/day po) for tuberculosis. The patients ingested 45 ml of water or antacid at 6, 7, and 8 a.m. with the third dose being followed by isoniazid and 120 ml of water. In addition to the blood sample taken just before 8 a.m., samples were obtained 1, 2, 4, and 6 hr after isoniazid administration. Each patient was restudied in a similar manner with water or antacid at least 2 days after the first study.

When aluminum hydroxide gel was employed as the antacid, there was a statistically significant ($p<0.05$) decrease in the 1-hr and peak concentrations of isoniazid as well as in the areas under the plasma concentration–time curves in the majority of patients. However, the response was not as pronounced or as consistent when magaldrate (an aluminum–magnesium hydroxide gel) was used as the antacid, suggesting that there can be considerable variability depending on the particular antacid employed. [Magaldrate and calcium or magnesium ions have less pronounced effects on gastric emptying than aluminum ions (5).] The effect of the aluminum-containing antacids on isoniazid levels was not as great as might have been anticipated on the basis of animal studies (1).

There was no evidence of reduced clinical effectiveness of isoniazid in these patients when aluminum hydroxide and isoniazid were given simultaneously, and the peak serum level of isoniazid obtained after concurrent use of these drugs (4 μg/ml) was still much higher than the minimum inhibitory concentration of isoniazid (0.2 μg/ml) (6).

■ Aluminum hydroxide delays absorption and decreases the 1-hr and peak serum levels of isoniazid in some patients (1). The clinical significance of this drug interaction cannot be assessed from the limited data available; additional data from long-term studies of concurrent therapy are needed.

There are no reports of reduced clinical effectiveness resulting from the drug interaction, and the decrease in the 1-hr and peak serum isoniazid levels observed (1), although statistically significant, did not fall below the minimum inhibitory concentration for isoniazid. No differentiation was made between slow inactivators of isoniazid (persons who would exhibit high serum levels of isoniazid) and rapid inactivators (persons who would exhibit low serum levels). No attempt was made to screen out drugs or disease states that might have influenced the results. Some patients, for example, were receiving aminosalicylic acid concurrently, a drug known to slow isoniazid metabolism and to cause an increase in serum isoniazid levels (7). Moreover, the dose of antacid employed (135 ml over 2 hr) is four times greater than a normal dose [usually 30 ml every 4–6 hr (8)].

Recommendations—Although it has not been demonstrated that the concurrent use of aluminum hydroxide decreases the clinical effectiveness of isoniazid, a delay or decrease in isoniazid absorption is likely when an aluminum-containing antacid is given simultaneously. Isoniazid should be given at least 1 hr prior to the administration of an antacid to minimize the risk of an interaction. Since isoniazid is often administered as a single daily dose (9), this recommendation presents no difficulty in using an antacid for a gastrointestinal (GI) condition. Isoniazid is generally well tolerated but it can cause GI reactions (10). In such cases, administration of smaller divided doses of isoniazid or simultaneous administration of food may be useful alternatives.

References

(1) A. Hurwitz and D. L. Schlozman, "Effects of Antacids on Gastrointestinal Absorption of Isoniazid in Rat and Man," *Amer. Rev. Resp. Dis.*, *109*, 41 (1974).

(2) M. Hava and A. Hurwitz, "The Relaxing Effect of Aluminum and Lanthanum on Rat and Human Gastric Smooth Muscle In Vitro," *Eur. J. Pharmacol.*, *22*, 156 (1973).

(3) "Drill's Pharmacology in Medicine," 4th ed., J. R. DiPalma, Ed., McGraw-Hill, New York, N.Y., 1971, p. 1719.

(4) E. D. Weinberg, "The Mutual Effects of Antimicrobial Compounds and Metallic Cations," *Bacteriol. Rev.*, *21*, 46 (1957).

(5) A. Hurwitz and M. B. Sheehan, "The Effects of Antacids on the Absorption of Orally Administered Pentobarbital in the Rat," *J. Pharmacol. Exp. Ther.*, *179*, 124 (1971).

(6) "Antibiotics and Chemotherapy," 2nd ed., L. P. Garrod and F. O'Grady, Eds., E. S. Livingston, London, England, 1968, p. 392.

(7) A. Hanngren *et al.*, "Inactivation of Isoniazid (INH) in Swedish Tuberculosis Patients before and during Treatment with Para-Aminosalicylic Acid (PAS)," *Scand. J. Resp. Dis.*, *51*, 61 (1970).

(8) "Physicians' Desk Reference," 29th ed., Medical Economics, Inc., Oradell, NJ 07649, 1975, p. 1277.

(9) L. D. Hudson and J. A. Sbarbaro, "Twice Weekly Tuberculosis Chemotherapy," *J. Amer. Med. Ass.*, *223*, 139 (1973).

(10) K. Varis *et al.*, "The Effect of Some Antituberculosis Drugs upon the Upper Gastrointestinal Tract: An Experiment with Para-Aminosalicylic Acid, Isoniazid and Streptomycin," *Scand. J. Gastroenterol.*, *6*, 589 (1971).

[For additional information, see *Anti-Infective Therapy*, p. 388.]

Nonproprietary and Trade Names of Drugs

Aluminum-, calcium-, or magnesium-containing products—*Aludrox, Alzinox, Amphojel, A-M-T, Camalox, Creamalin, Dicarbosil, DiGel, Ducon, Gaviscon, Gelusil, Gelusil-M, Kolantyl Gel, Kudrox, Maalox, Malcogel, Mylanta, Oxaine-M, Phosphaljel, Robalate, Rolaids, Titralac, Trisogel, Tums, WinGel*

Isoniazid—*Various manufacturers*

Prepared and evaluated by the Scientific Review Subpanel on Anti-Infectives and reviewed by Practitioner Panel I.

Isoniazid—Pyridoxine

Summary—Although some experimental evidence indicates that pyridoxine may interfere with the activity of isoniazid, concurrent administration does not appear to alter the clinical effectiveness of isoniazid in eradicating tubercle bacilli in humans. Consequently, pyridoxine should not be withheld when indicated in patients receiving isoniazid.

Related Drugs—There are no chemically and pharmacologically related drugs.

Pharmacological Effect and Mechanism—The mechanism by which isoniazid eradicates tubercle bacilli remains uncertain, but the following mechanisms have been proposed: (*a*) an effect on the cell wall lipid content, (*b*) an inhibition of DNA synthesis with cessation of RNA synthesis, and (*c*) an inhibition of some step in cell glycolysis (1). It is suspected that either combination with an enzyme or reaction with a pigment precursor in the presence of appropriate substances produces some or all of these alterations (2).

In vitro and *in vivo* studies (3–6) showed that pyridoxine has the capacity to neutralize or antagonize the activity of isoniazid against *Mycobacterium tuberculosis.* The mechanism by which this antagonism occurs is uncertain; however, formation of extracellular isoniazid complexes or formation of ineffective metabolites such as pyridoxal isonicotinoyl hydrazone has received consideration (5).

The results of *in vitro* studies demonstrating the neutralization of isoniazid activity by concurrent pyridoxine administration are difficult to compare and correlate because of study design. Nutrients and broths supporting experimental bacterial growth were dissimilar in all instances with regard to composition and content of metallic ions, nitrogen, asparagine, and glutamine salts (5). In addition, more inhibition of isoniazid activity by pyridoxine occurred at the *in vitro* minimum inhibitory concentration of isoniazid (0.025 μg/ml). This inhibition capacity diminished precipitously as isoniazid concentrations rose above 0.08 μg/ml (3). Usual human serum concentrations of isoniazid range between 0.2 and 0.8 μg/ml (1).

In vivo studies in mice indicated that the administration of relatively high dosages of isoniazid (24 mg/kg po) concurrently with pyridoxine did not diminish the antitubercular effects of isoniazid (7). Subsequent studies in mice, using large doses of isoniazid (24 mg/kg po) administered concurrently with large doses of pyridoxine ($\sim$ 7 mg/kg po), demonstrated a substantial impairment of isoniazid activity. This effect began a month after the initiation of concurrent therapy. No antagonism could be demonstrated when smaller doses ($\sim$ 3 mg/kg po) of pyridoxine were administered with smaller doses of isoniazid (6 mg/kg po) (4). The clinically effective dose of isoniazid in humans is reported to be 3–5 mg/kg (1).

Evaluation of Clinical Data—There have been several reports relative to peripheral neuropathies resulting from isoniazid-induced deficiency of pyridoxine (8, 9). Patients classified as slow inactivators of isoniazid are especially prone to these neuropathies (10). This action is thought to be caused by competition between isoniazid and pyridoxine for the enzyme apotryptophanase (8, 11–13). Several investigators recommend that pyridoxine, in doses of 50–100 mg/day, be given prophylactically to patients treated with isoniazid (1, 8).

■ Although several studies demonstrated that interference with isoniazid activity can occur with concurrent pyridoxine administration *in vitro* and in mice (3–6), this effect was not observed in animals at dosages normally used and at serum levels of isoniazid routinely achieved in humans (3). Additionally, there are no clinical reports of failure of isoniazid therapy due to pyridoxine-induced interference.

Recommendations—Concurrent administration of pyridoxine and isoniazid does not reduce the effectiveness of isoniazid in eradicating tubercle bacilli. Pyridoxine therapy should not be withheld when indicated in patients developing peripheral neuropathies while receiving isoniazid.

References

(1) "The Pharmacological Basis of Therapeutics," 5th ed., L. S. Goodman and A. Gilman, Eds., Macmillan, New York, NY 10022, 1975, p. 1325.

(2) J. Youatt, "A Review of the Action of Isoniazid," *Amer. Rev. Resp. Dis.*, *99*, 729 (1969).

(3) H. Pope, "The Neutralization of Isoniazid Activity in Mycobacterium Tuberculosis by Certain Metabolites," *Amer. Rev. Tuberc.*, *73*, 735 (1956).

(4) R. McCune *et al.*, "The Delayed Appearance of Isoniazid Antagonism by Pyridoxine In Vivo," *Amer. Rev. Tuberc.*, *76*, 1100 (1957).

(5) W. H. Beggs and J. W. Jenne, "Mechanism for the Pyridoxal Neutralization of Isoniazid Action on *Mycobacterium tuberculosis*," *J. Bacteriol.*, *94*, 793 (1967).

(6) I. U. Boone *et al.*, "Effect of Pyridoxal on Uptake of C14-Activity from Labeled Isoniazid by Mycobacterium Tuberculosis," *Amer. Rev. Tuberc.*, *76*, 568 (1957).

(7) O. Wasz-Hockert *et al.*, "Concurrent Administration of Pyridoxine and Isoniazid," *Amer. Rev. Tuberc.*, *74*, 471 (1956).

(8) J. M. Robson and F. M. Sullivan, "Antituberculosis Drugs," *Pharmacol. Rev.*, *15*, 169 (1963).

(9) P. R. McCurdy and R. F. Donohoe, "Pyridoxine-Responsive Anemia Conditioned by Isonicotinic Acid Hydrazide," *Blood*, *27*, 352 (1966).

(10) S. Devadetta, "Isoniazid-Induced Encephalopathy," *Lancet*, i, 440 (1965).

(11) R. R. Ross, "Use of Pyridoxine Hydrochloride to Prevent Isoniazid Toxicity," *J. Amer. Med. Ass.*, *168*, 273 (1958).

(12) H. C. Lichstein, "Mechanism of Competitive Action of Isonicotinic Acid Hydrazide and Vitamin B_6," *Proc. Soc. Exp. Biol. Med.*, *85*, 389 (1955).

(13) L. Levy, "Mechanism of Drug-Induced Vitamin B_6 Deficiency," *Ann. N.Y. Acad. Sci.*, *166*, 184 (1969).

[For additional information, see *Anti-Infective Therapy*, p. 388.]

Nonproprietary and Trade Names of Drugs

Isoniazid—*Various manufacturers*

Pyridoxine—*Available in combination with other vitamins*

Prepared and evaluated by the Scientific Review Subpanel on Anti-Infectives and reviewed by Practitioner Panel II.

Kanamycin—Ethacrynic Acid

Summary—Concurrent administration of kanamycin and ethacrynic acid, both potentially ototoxic, causes an increased incidence of ototoxicity, particularly in patients with decreased renal function. Because the outcome of this drug interaction has been either permanent or transient hearing loss, concurrent use of these drugs should be avoided whenever possible.

Related Drugs—Although literature documentation and clinical experience pertain principally to kanamycin and ethacrynic acid, similar reports with the other aminoglycoside antibiotics **gentamicin** (1), **neomycin** (2), **streptomycin** (3–5), and **tobramycin** (6) have appeared. **Amikacin** has not been reported to cause deafness but ototoxicity was attributed to its administration (1 g/day po) (7, 8). **Furosemide**, although not structurally related to ethacrynic acid, has also been reported to cause transient (9, 10) and permanent (11) deafness.

Pharmacological Effect and Mechanism—In the presence of impaired renal function (specific degree not established), the concurrent administration of aminoglycoside antibiotics (in doses generally recommended for patients with impaired renal function) and ethacrynic acid (intravenously in manufacturer-recommended doses) has resulted in hearing losses of varying degrees (12). Hearing loss caused by aminoglycoside antibiotics and ethacrynic acid also has been reported in two patients in the absence of significant azotemia (1).

The mechanisms responsible for the ototoxicity of these agents are unknown. However, the results of one study (13) suggest that high levels of kanamycin in the endolymph may be responsible for its ototoxicity and that kanamycin inhibits adenosine triphosphatase in the stria vascularis of the cochlea. Ethacrynic acid also is a potent inhibitor of adenosine triphosphatase (14) and may augment the inhibition induced by kanamycin. The inhibition of adenosine triphosphatase may be responsible for the changes in the composition of the endolymph seen after ethacrynic acid administration (15).

Evaluation of Clinical Data—The ototoxicity of the aminoglycoside antibiotics, including kanamycin, is well established and occurs on a dose-related basis, particularly in patients with renal dysfunction (12). The ototoxicity of intravenously administered ethacrynic acid (2 mg/kg every 6 hr) was first noted by a single case of acute transient hearing loss (16) and then confirmed in a report of five cases of acute transient hearing loss (3). In all of these patients, poor renal function was noted. These patients received ethacrynic acid doses of 150–300 mg/day po or 50–400 mg/day iv. Additional reports since confirmed that there is a definite cause and effect relationship between decreased renal function and increased ototoxicity, with permanent deafness occurring in some cases (4, 5, 17).

One report described a patient who received kanamycin (1 g), cephalothin (4 g), and corticosteroids (unknown amounts) while having good renal function during the first 30 hr of treatment (17). The patient's renal function deteriorated, and 100 mg of ethacrynic acid in 100 ml of normal saline was administered intravenously over 3–5 min. The patient became totally deaf before the completion of the injection. Partial hearing returned over the next 2 hr, but death due to an unrelated cause prevented further evaluation. Two additional cases were reported (4); however, details in both cases are lacking. One case was a personal communication with the Food and Drug Administration, and the other involved the additional use of streptomycin and irrigations of neomycin.

A report (5) of permanent hearing losses due to kanamycin (500–1000 mg im) included four instances in which the use of ethacrynic acid (50–150 mg iv) was implicated as a contributing factor to the deafness. Two of these cases involved only kanamycin and ethacrynic acid. In one of these cases, the drugs were administered 2 hr apart to a patient with impaired renal function, with bilateral hearing loss occurring in 30 min. The other case involved a hearing loss at 13 days after therapy in which kanamycin was given on Days 1 and 5 with ethacrynic acid on Day 2. This patient also had impaired renal function.

The occurrence of a neurosensory hearing loss was reported (1) following the intravenous administration of standard doses of ethacrynic acid to two nonuremic patients receiving concurrent aminoglycoside antibiotic therapy. The hearing loss was total but transient in one patient and total but permanent in the other.

■ Either transient or permanent hearing loss may result from the concurrent use of ethacrynic acid intravenously with the aminoglycoside antibiotics (*e.g.*, kanamycin). This problem is most likely to occur in patients with impaired renal function, but there is some evidence (1) that this also may be a significant problem in patients with normal renal function.

Although hearing loss has occurred primarily after intravenous administration of ethacrynic acid and the parenteral administration of kanamycin, it has also been associated with the oral administration of these drugs (3, 18).

Recommendations—The concurrent use of these drugs should be avoided whenever possible. If kanamycin and ethacrynic acid must be used together, the patient's renal status should be determined before treatment and regularly checked during treatment. The dose of the antibiotic should be reduced to the minimum effective level. Hearing should be evaluated before and during concurrent use by using audiograms and vestibular tests (19).

References

(1) W. D. Meriwether *et al.*, "Deafness following Standard Intravenous Dose of Ethacrynic Acid," *J. Amer. Med. Ass.*, *216*, 795 (1971).

(2) G. J. Matz *et al.*, "Ototoxicity of Ethacrynic Acid," *Arch. Otolaryng.*, *90*, 60 (1969).

(3) W. J. Schneider and E. L. Becker, "Acute Transient Hearing Loss after Ethacrynic Acid Therapy," *Arch. Intern. Med.*, *177*, 715 (1966).

(4) R. H. Mathog and W. J. Klein, Jr., "Ototoxicity of Ethacrynic Acid and Aminoglycoside Antibiotics in Uremia," *N. Engl. J. Med.*, *280*, 1223 (1969).

(5) A. H. Johnson and C. A. Hamilton, "Kanamycin Ototoxicity—Possible Potentiation by Other Drugs," *S. Med. J.*, *63*, 511 (1970).

(6) A. M. Geddes *et al.*, "Clinical and Laboratory Studies with Tobramycin," *Chemotherapy*, *20*, 245 (1974).

(7) F. P. Tally *et al.*, "Amikacin Therapy for Severe Gram-Negative Sepsis," *Ann. Intern. Med.*, *83*, 484 (1975).

(8) R. D. Meyer, "Amikacin Therapy for Serious Gram-Negative Bacillary Infections," *Ann. Intern. Med.*, *83*, 790 (1975).

(9) D. S. David and P. Hitzig, "Diuretics and Ototoxicity," *N. Engl. J. Med.*, *284*, 1328 (1971).

(10) G. H. Schwartz *et al.*, "Ototoxicity Induced by Furosemide," *N. Engl. J. Med.*, *282*, 1413 (1970).

(11) R. H. Lloyd-Mostyn and I. J. Lord, "Ototoxicity of Intravenous Furosemide," *Lancet*, *ii*, 1156 (1971).

(12) "Drug Induced Deafness," *J. Amer. Med. Ass.*, *224*, 515 (1973).

(13) T. Iinuma *et al.*, "Possible Effects of Various Ototoxic Drugs upon the ATP-Hydrolyzing System in the Stria Vascularis and Spinal Ligament of the Guinea Pig," *Laryngoscope*, *77*, 159 (1967).

(14) J. B. Hook and H. E. Williamson, "Lack of Correlation between Natriuretic Activity and Inhibition of Renal Na-K-Activated ATPase," *Proc. Soc. Exp. Biol. Med.*, *120*, 358 (1965).

(15) E. S. Cohn *et al.*, "Ethacrynic Acid Effect on the Composition of Cochlear Fluids," *Science*, *171*, 910 (1971).

(16) J. F. Maher and G. E. Schreiner, "Studies on Ethacrynic Acid in Patients with Refractory Edema," *Ann. Intern. Med.*, *62*, 15 (1965).

(17) P. S. Ng *et al.*, "Deafness after Ethacrynic Acid," *Lancet*, *i*, 673 (1969).

(18) C. M. Kunin *et al.*, "Absorption of Orally Administered Neomycin and Kanamycin," *N. Engl. J. Med.*, *262*, 380 (1960).

(19) G. J. Matz and R. F. Naunton, "Ototoxic Drugs and Poor Renal Function," *J. Amer. Med. Ass.*, *206*, 2119 (1968).

[For additional information, see *Anti-Infective Therapy*, p. 388.]

Nonproprietary and Trade Names of Drugs

Amikacin sulfate—*Amikin*
Ethacrynic acid—*Edecrin*
Furosemide—*Lasix*
Gentamicin sulfate—*Garamycin*
Kanamycin sulfate—*Kantrex*

Neomycin sulfate—*Mycifradin Sulfate, Myciguent, Neobiotic*
Streptomycin sulfate—*Various manufacturers*
Tobramycin sulfate—*Nebcin*

Prepared and evaluated by the Scientific Review Subpanel on Anti-Infectives and reviewed by Practitioner Panel V.

Levodopa—Chlorpromazine

Summary—Although the clinical effects of concurrent use of these drugs are unpredictable, levodopa and chlorpromazine may block the effects of each other when these drugs are administered together. In instances where no alternative drugs are available and both drugs must be used, the patient should be observed closely for a deterioration of levodopa's antiparkinsonian effect or a decrease in the therapeutic effect of chlorpromazine.

Related Drugs—Other **phenothiazines** would be expected to behave similarly to chlorpromazine.

Pharmacological Effect and Mechanism—Phenothiazines accelerate dopamine production, inhibit dopamine reuptake, and block striatal dopamine receptors (1). The extrapyramidal side effects of the phenothiazines result from a blockade of the dopamine receptor in the basal ganglia and substantia nigra (2). Extrapyramidal symptoms occurring early during phenothiazine treatment include dystonia, akathesia, and pseudoparkinsonism. These symptoms are reversible upon discontinuation of the phenothiazine and may be treated effectively with antiparkinsonian drugs (3). In contrast, persistent dyskinesias (tardive dyskinesias) usually appear after at least 1 year of phenothiazine treatment. Persistent dyskinesias are often irreversible and do not respond to treatment with antiparkinsonian drugs (3).

Levodopa and chlorpromazine can be mutually antagonistic when used concurrently, resulting in a loss of either the antiparkinsonian effect of levodopa (4–6) or the antipsychotic effect of phenothiazines (7, 8). The mechanisms responsible for these effects are not understood but may involve an antagonism between phenothiazines and dopamine at the striatal dopamine receptors.

Evaluation of Clinical Data—In one study (9), levodopa (2 mg/kg iv) reversed chlorpromazine-induced extrapyramidal symptoms in 20 patients. However, in two other studies (7, 8), orally administered levodopa was found to be ineffective in treating phenothiazine-induced extrapyramidal reactions. All of the patients in one study (7) showed a marked deterioration in behavior after the administration of levodopa (1.4–2.6 g/day po) indicating that levodopa also may antagonize the antipsychotic action of phenothiazines. Other studies reported that chlorpromazine may block the adverse and therapeutic actions of levodopa (4, 5).

■ Although the clinical outcome of the concurrent use of these drugs cannot be predicted, some clinical evidence indicates that these drugs may antagonize the therapeutic effects of each other (4, 5, 7).

Recommendations—Because the effect of levodopa and chlorpromazine on each other is unpredictable, patients receiving these drugs concurrently should be observed closely for a deterioration of levodopa's antiparkinsonian effect or for a decrease in the therapeutic effect of chlorpromazine.

References

(1) A. D. Korczyn, "Pathophysiology of Drug-Induced Dyskinesias," *Neuropharmacology, 11* (5), 601 (1972).

(2) "Clinical Handbook of Psychopharmacology," A. DiMascio and R. I. Shader, Eds., Science House, New York, N.Y., 1970, pp. 233–240.

(3) "Psychopharmacological Treatment, Theory and Practice," H. C. B. Denber, Ed., Dekker, New York, NY 10016, 1975, pp. 82–89.

(4) R. C. Duvoisin, "Diphenidol for Levodopa Induced Nausea and Vomiting," *J. Amer. Med. Ass., 221,* 1408 (1972).

(5) J. B. Campbell, "Long-Term Treatment of Parkinson's Disease with Levodopa," *Neurology, 20,* 18 (1970).

(6) R. Jenkins, "Laevo-dopa for Parkinsonism," *Brit. Med. J., 2,* 361 (1970).

(7) J. A. Yaryura-Tobias, "Action of L-Dopa in Drug Induced Extrapyramidalism," *Dis. Nerv. Syst., 31,* 60 (1970).

(8) P. Fleming *et al.,* "Levodopa in Drug-Induced Extrapyramidal Disorders," *Lancet, ii,* 1186 (1970).

(9) A. Bruno and S. C. Bruno, "Effects of L-Dopa on Pharmacological Parkinsonism," *Acta Psychiat. Scand., 42,* 264 (1966).

[For additional information, see *Adrenergic Therapy,* p. 332.]

Nonproprietary and Trade Names of Drugs

Acetophenazine maleate—*Tindal*
Butaperazine maleate—*Repoise Maleate*
Carbidopa–levodopa—*Sinemet*
Carphenazine maleate—*Proketazine*
Chlorpromazine—*Chlor-PZ, Promapar, Thorazine*
Fluphenazine enanthate—*Prolixin Enanthate*
Fluphenazine hydrochloride—*Permitil, Prolixin*
Levodopa—*Dopar, Larodopa*

Mesoridazine—*Serentil*
Perphenazine—*Trilafon and various combination products*
Piperacetazine—*Quide*
Prochlorperazine—*Compazine and various combination products*
Promazine hydrochloride—*Sparine*
Thiopropazate hydrochloride—*Dartal*
Thioridazine hydrochloride—*Mellaril*
Trifluoperazine hydrochloride—*Stelazine*
Triflupromazine hydrochloride—*Vesprin*

Prepared and evaluated by the Scientific Review Subpanel on Autonomic Agents and reviewed by Practitioner Panel V.

Levodopa—Diazepam

Summary—Diazepam may block the therapeutic effect of levodopa when given concurrently to selected parkinsonian patients. However, there are insufficient clinical data to recommend avoiding concurrent use. If deterioration of the therapeutic effect of levodopa occurs in a diazepam-treated patient, diazepam should be considered a possible causative factor.

Related Drugs—The effect of other **benzodiazepines** on levodopa's therapeutic action is not clear. **Chlordiazepoxide** has been reported to antagonize (1, 2) and exert no effect (3) on levodopa. **Nitrazepam** may interact with levodopa, but this drug interaction has not been observed consistently (3). **Flurazepam** (4) and **oxazepam** (3) have been used concurrently with levodopa without causing any loss in antiparkinsonian activity.

Pharmacological Effect and Mechanism—The precise mechanism of action of levodopa is unclear. The most widely accepted theory is that levodopa increases the level of dopamine and thus the activation of the dopamine receptors in the extrapyramidal centers in the brain (primarily in the caudate nucleus and the substantia nigra).

Although there is no direct evidence to support this hypothesis (5), depletion of striatal dopamine is considered to be the most significant biochemical abnormality of parkinsonism and is at least partially responsible for the symptoms of the disease, particularly hypokinesia (6). Levodopa is administered to return the dopamine levels to normal and is converted to dopamine both peripherally and in the central nervous system (CNS) by dopa decarboxylase. Dopamine is then passed along the neuronal axons to the neostriatum where it is released and acts as a chemical transmitter, probably with an inhibitory action (7). Since dopamine cannot enter the CNS, the amount of dopamine formed in the brain is dependent on the amount of levodopa that crosses the blood–brain barrier before it is converted to dopamine by peripheral decarboxylation (6).

The mechanism of the reported interaction between levodopa and the benzodiazepines is not known. Benzodiazepines increase the acetylcholine content in the whole rat brain (8), and parkinsonian patients are known to be very sensitive to the CNS effects of acetylcholine (9, 10). Because the cholinergic and dopaminergic mechanisms in the extrapyramidal centers of the brain appear to be antagonistic (9), the increase in acetylcholine produced by the benzodiazepines may antagonize the dopamine-mediated response to levodopa.

Evaluation of Clinical Data—Eight patients were observed (3) after concurrent administration of normal therapeutic doses of levodopa and a benzodiazepine. The study was double blind, and observations were continued for an average of 31 weeks (range, 3–40 weeks). The patients were given one of the following benzodiazepines (doses not reported except for diazepam): chlordiazepoxide, diazepam, nitrazepam, or oxazepam. Three patients treated with chlordiazepoxide, one patient treated with nitrazepam, and one patient treated with oxazepam showed no signs of unresponsiveness to levodopa. One patient receiving diazepam (5 mg/day po) and the two patients receiving nitrazepam exhibited signs of deterioration of the parkinsonian state. Three additional periods of nitrazepam therapy in the two patients previously taking nitrazepam did not cause similar symptoms.

Another report (6) reviewed patients' responses to levodopa after 12 months of therapy; three patients showed a reversible deterioration in the parkinsonian state when they were given diazepam (5 mg/day po) in addition to levodopa (2.5–3.5 g/day po). [One author of this report also observed another 10 patients that responded similarly when these drugs were given concurrently (personal communication, B. S. Gilligan, Melbourne, Australia).]

A 77-year-old female who had been receiving levodopa (2 g/day po) for 3 months regressed to her original parkinsonian state within 24 hr after chlordiazepoxide (30 mg/day po) was initiated (1). Thirty-six hours after chlordiazepoxide was discontinued her parkinsonian symptoms resolved. The investigator also referred to observing two other patients who had been refractory to levodopa and were taking chlordiazepoxide alone or concurrently with levodopa at the time. No additional details about these patients were given.

Three patients who were unresponsive to levodopa (doses not reported) had received chlordiazepoxide (doses not reported) concurrently (2). The patients' responses to levodopa improved when chlordiazepoxide was discontinued. Although the unresponsiveness to levodopa was attributed to the concurrent administration of chlordiazepoxide, no other information was provided about the patients and a causal relationship cannot be established.

■ The condition of at least nine patients in three separate published reports (1, 3, 6) and 10 patients in an unpublished report (personal communication, B. S. Gilligan, Melbourne, Australia), stabilized on levodopa, deteriorated to the original parkinsonian state when a benzodiazepine was added to the drug regimen. In another report, three patients receiving chlordiazepoxide were unresponsive to levodopa therapy until chlordiazepoxide was removed from the drug regimen (2). Nevertheless, this evidence is insufficient to predict the therapeutic significance of this drug interaction. In the only controlled study (3), five of eight patients exhibited no adverse reaction after benzodiazepine therapy was initiated. Two other patients were rechallenged with a benzodiazepine (nitrazepam), and they suffered no additional problems. Of the 19 remaining cases reported, other factors such as a known variation in a patient's response to levodopa even after stabilization on the drug (11), the long time period usually required for stabilization on levodopa (12), and the high incidence of toxicity from levodopa itself (13) had not been ruled out satisfactorily as possible causes.

Recommendations—Despite reports of a potential interaction between levodopa and diazepam (and other benzodiazepines), the clinical data about this drug interaction are insufficient to recommend that concurrent use of these drugs be avoided. Diazepam and especially flurazepam have been recommended by some investigators as drugs of choice for treating moderately severe insomnia (a condition unaffected by levodopa) in parkinsonian patients (4). However, concurrent administration of a benzodiazepine should be considered a possible causative factor if the condition of a patient stabilized on levodopa deteriorates.

References

(1) L. Mackie, "Drug Antagonism," *Brit. Med. J.*, *2*, 651 (1971).

(2) G. A. Schwartz and S. Fahn, "Newer Medical Treatments in Parkinsonism," *Med. Clin. N. Amer.*, *54*, 773 (1970).

(3) K. R. Hunter *et al.*, "Use of Levodopa with Other Drugs," *Lancet*, *ii*, 1283 (1970).

(4) A. Kales *et al.*, "Sleep in Patients with Parkinson's Disease and Normal Subjects Prior to and following Levodopa Administration," *Clin. Pharmacol. Ther.*, *12*, 397 (1971).

(5) T. N. Chase, "Cerebrospinal Fluid Monoamine Metabolites and Peripheral Decarboxylase Inhibitors in Parkinsonism," *Neurology*, *20*, 36 (1970).

(6) R. N. Brogden *et al.*, "Levodopa: A Review of Its Pharmacological Properties and Therapeutic Use with Particular Reference to Parkinsonism," *Drugs*, *2*, 262 (1971).

(7) H. McLennan and D. H. York, "The Action of Dopamine on Neurones of the Caudate Nucleus," *J. Physiol.*, *189*, 393 (1967).

(8) E. F. Domino and A. E. Wilson, "Psychotropic Drug Influences on Brain Acetylcholine Utilization," *Psychopharmacologia*, *25*, 291 (1972).

(9) H. Klawans *et al.*, "Theoretical Implications of the Use of L-Dopa in Parkinsonism," *Acta Neurol. Scand.*, *46*, 409 (1970).

(10) M. I. Weintraub and M. H. Van Woert, "Reversal by Levodopa of Cholinergic Hypersensitivity in Parkinson's Disease," *N. Engl. J. Med.*, *284*, 412 (1971).

(11) "Levodopa and Related Drugs," *Med. Lett.*, *15*, 21 (1973).

(12) J. Wodak *et al.*, "Review of 12 Months' Treatment with L-Dopa in Parkinson's Disease, with Remarks on Unusual Side Effects," *Med. J. Aust.*, *2*, 1277 (1972).

(13) J. P. Morgan and J. R. Bianchine, "The Clinical Pharmacology of Levodopa," *Rat. Drug Ther.*, *5*, 4 (1971).

[For additional information, see *Adrenergic Therapy*, p. 332.]

Nonproprietary and Trade Names of Drugs

Carbidopa–levodopa—*Sinemet*
Chlordiazepoxide—*Libritabs*
Chlordiazepoxide hydrochloride—*Librium* *and various combination products*
Clonazepam—*Clonopin*
Clorazepate dipotassium—*Tranxene*

Diazepam—*Valium*
Flurazepam hydrochloride—*Dalmane*
Levodopa—*Dopar, Larodopa*
Nitrazepam—*Mogadon*
Oxazepam—*Serax*

Prepared and evaluated by the Scientific Review Subpanel on Autonomic Agents and reviewed by Practitioner Panel IV.

Levodopa—Methyldopa

Summary—Concurrent use of levodopa and methyldopa may enhance the effects of either drug. Although the clinical data are inconclusive, this enhancement may be manifested as adverse effects of either agent. However, in carefully controlled doses and in closely monitored patients, concurrent therapy has been used safely to treat hypertension in selected parkinsonian patients.

Related Drugs—There are no related drugs in current clinical practice.

Pharmacological Effect and Mechanism—Since parkinsonian patients have reduced dopamine concentrations in the extrapyramidal centers of the brain (*e.g.,* the caudate nucleus and the substantia nigra) (1, 2), the success of levodopa therapy is primarily based upon raising the level of dopamine in these extrapyramidal centers through the decarboxylation of levodopa (3). Large doses of levodopa are needed to overcome rapid extracerebral decarboxylation to obtain adequate dopamine levels in the central nervous system (CNS) tissue (3).

Several mechanisms have been proposed to explain the antihypertensive action of methyldopa. The most generally accepted theory is that α-methylnorepinephrine, a metabolite of methyldopa, produces the antihypertensive effect through its actions on the CNS and, to a lesser extent, on the peripheral vasculature (4).

Methyldopa may enhance the antiparkinsonian effects of levodopa by preventing its extracerebral decarboxylation (5, 6), leaving more active form available for transport into the CNS (7). Conversely, methyldopa's central inhibition of dopa decarboxylase may reduce cerebral dopamine, resulting in a parkinsonian-type syndrome (8, 9).

Evaluation of Clinical Data—Eight parkinsonian patients (six hypertensive and two normotensive) were treated with methyldopa (dose not reported) after being stabilized on levodopa (10). All hypertensive patients treated with both drugs experienced improvement of parkinsonian symptoms. The normotensive patients attained comparable antiparkinsonian effects at doses of levodopa that were 50% lower when administered with methyldopa compared to levodopa alone. In another group of patients, the average dose of levodopa was 3.24 g/day po, while the average dose for patients receiving concurrent therapy was 0.96 g/day po. The decreased levodopa dose was associated with a decrease in involuntary movements. The effects of concurrent therapy were not compared with a simple reduction in the levodopa dose.

Twenty-seven of 87 patients receiving methyldopa (125–500 mg/day po) and levodopa (1.5–7 g/day po) concurrently had better clinical improvement (based on the observations of the investigator) than when receiving levodopa alone (11). The effects of concurrent use of methyldopa and levodopa were studied for 2 years. The dose of methyldopa given concurrently to 46 patients was limited by adverse effects such as dyskinesia, vomiting, and grogginess. The adverse effects observed with concurrent therapy were the same types observed with levodopa alone. In some of the 27 patients showing improvement with these drugs, a reduction in the dose of levodopa (up to 30%) was possible. Benefits of concurrent therapy appeared maximal in those patients in whom higher doses of levodopa alone had previously caused nausea, vomiting, or anorexia. A few patients exhibited grogginess and dizziness that could be related to methyldopa itself. No hypotensive episodes occurred at the dosage given. It was also noted that: (a) side effects such as dyskinesia that occurred with levodopa alone recurred when methyldopa was added to a lower levodopa dosage schedule, (b) those patients unresponsive to levodopa, despite high serum levodopa levels, showed no improvement when methyldopa was added, and (c) the addition of methyldopa did not appear to change the general prognosis of the disease (11).

The hypotensive effect of the concurrent use of levodopa and methyldopa was studied for several days (exact time not stated) in 18 patients with parkinsonism (12). A greater fall (statistically significant) in the standing blood pressure was produced when these drugs were given together than when either drug was given alone (although no severe hypotensive episodes occurred). The mean dose of levodopa was 1.5±0.5 g/day po and the dose of methyldopa was 250 mg/day po. No corresponding increase in the effectiveness of levodopa was observed but this could have been due to the short period of the study. The investigators concluded that methyldopa may be used safely in hypertensive patients receiving levodopa if blood pressure and dosage adjustments are monitored closely.

■ Several reports (10–12) indicate that concurrent use of levodopa and methyldopa may enhance the effects of either drug. These studies indicate that this enhancement could result in increased therapeutic effectiveness or in adverse effects depending on individual patient response, the dose of either drug used, or the dose ratio of the drugs.

Recommendations—Concurrent administration of methyldopa and levodopa may be used safely to control hypertension in parkinsonian patients but this use should be restricted to closely monitored patients receiving carefully controlled doses. The occurrence of side effects such as vomiting and grogginess induced by either drug (11) may require a dose reduction or discontinuation of methyldopa. Although methyldopa has been used to reduce the maintenance dose of levodopa in normotensive patients (10, 11), any therapeutic benefit derived from such therapy remains to be proven and such concurrent therapy should not be used.

References

(1) A. Barbeau, "Some Biochemical Disorders in Parkinson's Disease—A Review," *J. Neurosurg.*, *24*, 162 (1966).

(2) O. Hornykiewicz, "Dopamine (3-Hydroxytyramine) and Brain Function," *Pharmacol. Rev.*, *18*, 925 (1966).

(3) K. F. Gey and A. Pletscher, "Distribution and Metabolism of DL-3,4-Dihydroxy[2-14C]phenylalanine in Rat Tissues," *Biochem. J.*, *92*, 300 (1964).

(4) "The Pharmacological Basis of Therapeutics," 5th ed., L. S. Goodman and A. Gilman, Eds., Macmillan, New York, NY 10022, 1975, pp. 707–708.

(5) W. G. Clark and R. S. Pogrund, "Inhibition of DOPA Decarboxylase In Vitro and In Vivo," *Circ. Res.*, *9*, 721 (1961).

(6) S. E. Smith, "The Pharmacological Actions of 3,4-Dihydroxyphenyl-α-methylalanine (α-Methyldopa), an Inhibitor of 5-Hydroxytryptophan Decarboxylase," *Brit. J. Pharmacol.*, *15*, 319 (1960).

(7) A. Pletscher and G. Bartholini, "Selective Rise in Brain Dopamine by Inhibition of Extracerebral Levodopa Decarboxylation," *Clin. Pharmacol. Ther.*, *12*, 344 (1971).

(8) M. J. T. Peaston, "Parkinsonism Associated with Alpha-Methyldopa Therapy," *Brit. Med. J.*, *2*, 168 (1964).

(9) R. A. Vaidya *et al.*, "Galactorrhea and Parkinson-like Syndrome: An Adverse Effect of α-Methyldopa," *Metabolism*, *19*, 1068 (1970).

(10) J. Fermaglich and D. S. O'Doherty, "Second Generation of L-Dopa Therapy," *Neurology*, *21*, 408 (1971).

(11) R. J. Mones, "Evaluation of Alpha Methyl Dopa and Alpha Methyl Dopa Hydrazine with L-Dopa Therapy," *N.Y. State J. Med.*, *74*, 47 (1974).

(12) F. B. Gibberd and E. Small, "Interaction between Levodopa and Methyldopa," *Brit. Med. J.*, *2*, 90 (1973).

[For additional information, see *Adrenergic Therapy*, p. 332.]

Nonproprietary and Trade Names of Drugs

Levodopa—*Dopar, Larodopa*   Methyldopa—*Aldomet*

Prepared and evaluated by the Scientific Review Subpanel on Autonomic Agents and reviewed by Practitioner Panel VI.

Levodopa—Phenelzine

Summary—Levodopa (50 mg or more) causes a significant rise in blood pressure and related harmful symptoms when given to a patient receiving a monoamine oxidase inhibitor such as phenelzine. The hypertensive reaction is blocked when carbidopa, a peripheral decarboxylase inhibitor, is added to the treatment regimen. Concurrent administration of levodopa and monoamine oxidase inhibitors should be avoided and alternative drugs (such as the tricyclic antidepressants) should be used. If a monoamine oxidase inhibitor must be used, a carbidopa–levodopa combination product should be used instead of levodopa.

Related Drugs—Other monoamine oxidase inhibitors that have been reported to interact with levodopa include **isocarboxazid** (1), **pargyline** (2), and **tranylcypromine** (1).

There are no drugs chemically and pharmacologically related to levodopa commercially available in the United States. However, broad bean pods contain dopa in quantities sufficient to precipitate a hypertensive response in patients treated with phenelzine (3).

Pharmacological Effect and Mechanism—The precise mechanism of action of levodopa has not been defined. The major theory is that levodopa increases the level of dopamine in the central nervous system and thus activates the dopamine receptors in the extrapyramidal system in the brain. Since it is thought that reduction in the level of dopamine in the extrapyramidal system is the primary cause of the symptoms of parkinsonism, administration of levodopa would correct this deficiency and return the patient's neurological deficits toward normal (4). Because dopamine does not cross the blood–brain barrier, levodopa must be given. The amount of dopamine formed in the brain is dependent upon the amount of levodopa that crosses the blood–brain barrier before peripheral decarboxylation (5). However, there is no direct evidence to support this hypothesis (6).

Phenelzine, like other monoamine oxidase inhibitors, increases the levels of dopamine in the peripheral tissues and in the brain. Levodopa also increases the levels of dopamine, and a marked enhancement of spontaneous motor activity was reported following levodopa administration in rats treated with monoamine oxidase inhibitors (7). The concurrent administration of carbidopa, a peripheral decarboxylase inhibitor, with levodopa suppresses the hypertensive reaction caused by monoamine oxidase inhibitors, indicating that the hypertensive reaction is peripherally mediated (8).

Evaluation of Clinical Data—The clinical evidence of this drug interaction consists of a few case reports and some clinical studies that described a rise in blood pressure after concurrent administration of levodopa and monoamine oxidase inhibitors. One patient (9) pretreated with a monoamine oxidase inhibitor (dose not reported) experienced a systolic blood pressure rise of 100 mm Hg within 0.5 hr after levodopa administration (50 mg/day po). Another patient's blood pressure rose from approximately 140–160 to 180 mm Hg within 1 hr after administration of levodopa (50 mg/day po) (1). The patient had been receiving phenelzine (45 mg/day po) for 10 days prior to levodopa administration. The monoamine oxidase inhibitor was discontinued and 3 weeks later, single doses of levodopa (up to 500 mg) produced no effect on the patient's blood pressure. This increase in blood pressure also occurred in a normal subject (2) receiving pargyline (50 mg/day po). The blood pressure rose from 120/80 to 204/104 mm Hg within 1 hr after levodopa administration (600 mg/day po). Phentolamine administration (5–15 mg iv) prevented any further rise in blood pressure. The patient also experienced symptoms of throbbing in the head and neck, pounding in the chest, and some cardiac dysrhythmias.

A rise in blood pressure, flushing, and palpitations were reported in four of five healthy young subjects receiving levodopa (75–100 mg/day po) and nialamide (25 mg/day po) for 10 days (10). The symptoms occurred after the ninth day of concurrent therapy in three subjects and on the tenth day in the other subject.

Three patients treated with phenelzine (45–60 mg/day po for 3 weeks) experienced a transitory elevation of blood pressure shortly after levodopa administration (50 mg/day) (11).

In four patients treated with tranylcypromine (30 mg/day po), the administration of carbidopa (300–400 mg/day po) blocked the hypertensive response to a challenge dose of levodopa (125 mg po). These same patients exhibited a significant increase in blood pressure when levodopa (50–200 mg po) was administered alone (8).

■ The evidence indicates that levodopa may cause a significant rise in blood pressure in patients receiving a monoamine oxidase inhibitor. The drug interaction causes potentially harmful symptoms and may occur within 1 hr after levodopa administration. The dose of levodopa used to elicit this response was 50 mg/day, much lower than the therapeutic dose range of levodopa (1–8 g/day po) (12). However, this hypertensive response did not occur when patients also were given carbidopa, a dopa decarboxylase inhibitor (8).

Recommendations—Levodopa and monoamine oxidase inhibitors should not be used concurrently. Tricyclic antidepressants apparently have been used successfully when given concurrently with levodopa and may even improve the response to levodopa (13). Therefore, these drugs may be considered as alternatives to monoamine oxidase inhibitors, although they should be used cautiously due to their cardiotoxic side effects (13).

Since the effects of monoamine oxidase inhibition usually last at least 2 weeks after the drug is discontinued (3), it was suggested (1) that levodopa not be administered until at least 4 weeks after monoamine oxidase inhibitor therapy is discontinued.

Phentolamine (5–15 mg iv) has been used successfully to treat hypertensive episodes resulting from concurrent levodopa and pargyline therapy (2).

If a monoamine oxidase inhibitor must be used concurrently with levodopa, a carbidopa–levodopa combination product should be used instead of levodopa.

References

(1) K. R. Hunter *et al.*, "Monoamine Oxidase Inhibitors and L-Dopa," *Brit. Med. J., 3,* 388 (1970).

(2) J. V. Hodge, "Use of Monoamine-Oxidase Inhibitors," *Lancet, i,* 764 (1965).

(3) F. S. Sjoqvist, "Psychotropic Drugs (2): Interaction between Monoamine Oxidase (MAO) Inhibitors and Other Substances," *Proc. Roy. Soc. Med., 58,* 967 (1965).

(4) R. N. Brogden *et al.*, "Levodopa: A Review of Its Pharmacological Properties and Therapeutic Use with Particular Reference to Parkinsonism," *Drugs, 2,* 262 (1971).

(5) H. McLennan and D. H. York, "The Action of Dopamine on Neurones of the Caudate Nucleus," *J. Physiol., 189,* 393 (1967).

(6) T. N. Chase, "Cerebrospinal Fluid Monoamine Metabolites and Peripheral Decarboxylase Inhibitors in Parkinsonism," *Neurology, 20,* 36 (1970).

(7) O. Hornykiewicz, "Dopamine (3-Hydroxytyramine) and Brain Function," *Pharmacol. Rev., 18,* 925 (1966).

(8) P. F. Teychenne *et al.*, "Interactions of Levodopa with Inhibitors of Monoamine Oxidase and L-Aromatic Amino Acid Decarboxylase," *Clin. Pharmacol. Ther., 18,* 273 (1975).

(9) P. L. McGeer *et al.*, "Drug-Induced Extrapyramidal Reactions. Treatment with Diphenhydramine Hydrochloride and Dihydroxyphenylalanine," *J. Amer. Med. Ass., 177,* 665 (1961).

(10) D. G. Friend *et al.*, "The Action of L-Dihydroxyphenylalanine in Patients Receiving Nialamide," *Clin. Pharmacol. Ther., 6,* 362 (1965).

(11) J. J. Schildkraut *et al.*, "Biochemical and Pressor Effects of Oral D,L-Dihydroxyphenylalanine in Patients Pretreated with Antidepressant Drugs," *Ann. N.Y. Acad. Sci., 107,* 1005 (1963).

(12) "Physicians' Desk Reference," 29th ed., Medical Economics, Inc., Oradell, NJ 07649, 1975, p. 1242.

(13) K. R. Hunter *et al.*, "Use of Levodopa with Other Drugs," *Lancet, ii,* 1283 (1970).

[For additional information, see *Adrenergic Therapy*, p. 332; *Antidepressant Therapy*, p. 373; *Imipramine–Tranylcypromine*, p. 103; *Meperidine–Phenelzine*, p. 142; and *Phenylpropanolamine–Tranylcypromine*, p. 188.]

Nonproprietary and Trade Names of Drugs

Carbidopa–levodopa—*Sinemet*
Isocarboxazid—*Marplan*
Levodopa—*Dopar, Larodopa*
Pargyline hydrochloride—*Eutonyl and various combination products*

Phenelzine sulfate—*Nardil*
Tranylcypromine—*Parnate*

Prepared and evaluated by the Scientific Review Subpanel on Autonomic Agents and reviewed by Practitioner Panel I.

Levodopa—Pyridoxine

Summary—Pyridoxine (vitamin B_6), in doses of 5 mg or more daily, may reduce or abolish the beneficial effects of levodopa in parkinsonism. Patients receiving levodopa therapy should avoid multiple-vitamin preparations and other preparations containing 5 mg or more of pyridoxine. The concurrent use of carbidopa, a peripheral dopa decarboxylase inhibitor, prevents the levodopa-inhibiting effects of pyridoxine and the carbidopa–levodopa combination product is recommended for patients who are receiving pyridoxine supplementation.

Related Drugs—There are no drugs commercially available that are chemically and pharmacologically similar to levodopa and pyridoxine.

Pharmacological Effect and Mechanism—The parkinsonian syndrome of rigidity, akinesia, and tremor has been associated with histological lesions of the substantia nigra and with a depression of the dopamine content of the caudate nucleus (1). Dopamine is suggested to be a neurotransmitter in a neuron system extending from the substantia nigra to the corpus striatum (2). Levodopa rather than dopamine is used because levodopa crosses the blood–brain barrier more readily than dopamine and is rapidly converted to the latter compound (3). Levodopa is metabolized to dopamine by L-aromatic amino acid decarboxylase (dopa decarboxylase) which requires pyridoxal phosphate as a coenzyme. This reaction takes place in the brain as well as in peripheral tissues. To provide substantial amounts of dopamine at appropriate sites in the corpus striatum, large doses of levodopa must be administered to compensate for the peripheral decarboxylation.

Although large doses of levodopa often produce involuntary choreiform movements which are reversed by pyridoxine, the concurrent administration of pyridoxine and levodopa usually results in lower serum levodopa levels and increased parkinsonian symptoms (4). Several mechanisms have been proposed to explain the effect of pyridoxine on levodopa's metabolism. Pyridoxine may alter levodopa's metabolism by Schiff-base formation (5), by increased transamination of levodopa (6), or by acceleration of peripheral nonenzymatic conversion of levodopa to dopamine (4, 7). Although the data are insufficient to permit a definite conclusion, current information favors an acceleration, by pyridoxine, of the peripheral decarboxylation of levodopa, probably in the gastrointestinal tract (8, 9).

Evaluation of Clinical Data—Pyridoxine was administered to 25 patients who had been treated with levodopa (dose not reported) for 1 month or more (4). Initially, doses of 750–1000 mg po of pyridoxine were administered daily. Partial reversal of the levodopa effect was evident within 24 hr and complete reversal occurred after 3–4 days of pyridoxine administration. After cessation of pyridoxine, the levodopa effect gradually returned but 7–10 days or more was required for complete restoration of the therapeutic effect. Smaller doses (50–100 mg/day po) also greatly reduced or abolished the levodopa effect. Doses of 20–60 mg/day po appreciably reversed the levodopa effect but did not completely abolish it. An increase in the symptoms of parkinsonism occurred in eight out of 10 patients receiving doses of 5–10 mg.

In a study of 45 patients (10), 16 patients developed psychiatric manifestations during levodopa therapy (up to 8 g/day po), and four of the patients also received pyridoxine (12.5–24 mg/day po). Buccolingual dyskinesias were present in the four patients treated with pyridoxine and general dyskinesias were observed in three of these patients. Although it was implied that pyridoxine administration reduced the dyskinesias, this effect was probably due to a reduction in the dose of levodopa rather than pyridoxine administration.

The administration of carbidopa, a peripheral dopa decarboxylase inhibitor, has been shown to prevent the reversal of the therapeutic effect of levodopa by pyridoxine (9, 11). Pyridoxine not only failed to decrease the clinical response to levodopa but actually enhanced it. Pyridoxine's enhancement of the clinical effect of levodopa in these studies is presumed to be due to the increased activity of dopa decarboxylase in the corpus striatum produced by pyridoxine in the presence of complete inhibition of extracerebral dopa decarboxylase. The concurrent administration of carbidopa, levodopa, and pyridoxine may result in an improved therapeutic response in the treatment of parkinsonism, but the clinical value has yet to be determined.

Small doses of pyridoxine (10–25 mg/day po) may be useful in abolishing some of the side effects of levodopa. In one patient (12), pyridoxine (10 mg iv) reversed levodopa-induced torsion dystonia without decreasing the effectiveness of levodopa.

■ The evidence clearly indicates that pyridoxine inhibits the pharmacological effects of levodopa. The degree of inhibition is dose related and can occur with pyridoxine doses as small as 5 mg. This inhibition has been used as an alternative to decreasing the dose of levodopa in certain patients experiencing some of the unpleasant side effects of levodopa. However, this approach has limited therapeutic usefulness. The concurrent administration of the dopa decarboxylase inhibitor, carbidopa, prevents this inhibition.

Recommendations—Patients receiving levodopa therapy should avoid multiple-vitamin preparations, antinauseant products, and other preparations containing more than the recommended daily dietary allowance (13) of 2 mg of pyridoxine. Excessive ingestion of foods high in pyridoxine (*e.g.*, fortified breakfast cereals) probably should be avoided by patients taking levodopa.

There are probably exceptions to this recommendation, *i.e.*, patients who also have conditions rendering them relatively pyridoxine deficient, *e.g.*, diabetes mellitus, chronic alcoholism, malnutrition, and malignancies (14). Patients taking isoniazid (15) and cycloserine (16) for tuberculosis and penicillamine (17) for Wilson's disease, cystinuria, and heavy metal intoxication may require pyridoxine supplementation.

Concurrent use of carbidopa prevents the inhibitory effect of pyridoxine on levodopa (9, 11) and is recommended for use in patients receiving pyridoxine supplementation.

References

(1) O. Hornykiewicz, "Dopamine (3-Hydroxytyramine) and Brain Function," *Pharmacol. Rev., 18*, 925 (1966).

(2) N. E. Anden *et al.*, "Demonstration and Mapping Out of Nigra-Neostriatal Dopamine Neurons," *Life Sci., 3*, 523 (1964).

(3) K. F. Gey and A. Pletscher, "Distribution and Metabolism of DL-3,4-Dihydroxy [2-14C]phenylalanine in Rat Tissues," *Biochem. J., 92*, 300 (1964).

(4) R. C. Duvoisin *et al.*, "Pyridoxine Reversal of L-Dopa Effects in Parkinsonism," *Trans. Amer. Neurol. Ass., 94*, 81 (1969).

(5) D. F. Evereo, "L-Dopa as a Vitamin B6 Antagonist," *Lancet, i*, 914 (1971).

(6) T. L. Sourkes *et al.*, "Determination of Catecholamines and Catecholamino Acids by Differential Spectrophotofluorimetry," *Meth. Med. Res., 9*, 147 (1961).

(7) G. C. Cotzias, "Metabolic Modification of Some Neurologic Disorders," *J. Amer. Med. Ass., 210*, 1255 (1969).

(8) A. S. Leon *et al.*, "Pyridoxine Antagonism of Levodopa in Parkinsonism," *J. Amer. Med. Ass., 218*, 1924 (1971).

(9) H. Mars, "Levodopa, Carbidopa, and Pyridoxine in Parkinson Disease," *Arch. Neurol., 30*, 444 (1974).

(10) G. G. Celesia and A. N. Barr, "Psychosis and Other Psychiatric Manifestations of Levodopa Therapy," *Arch. Neurol., 23*, 193 (1970).

(11) M. D. Yahr *et al.*, "Pyridoxine, Levodopa and L-α-Methyldopa Hydrazine Regimen in Parkinsonism," *J. Amer. Med. Ass., 216*, 2141 (1971).

(12) H. D. Jameson, "Pyridoxine for Levodopa-Induced Dystonia," *J. Amer. Med. Ass., 211*, 1700 (1970).

(13) "Recommended Dietary Allowances: A Report of the Food and Nutritional Board of the National Research Coun-

cil," 7th ed., Publication No. 1694, National Academy of Sciences, Washington, D. C., 1968, pp. 43–46.

(14) S. A. Friedman, "Levodopa and Pyridoxine Deficient States," *J. Amer. Med. Ass.*, *214*, 1563 (1970).

(15) S. A. Friedman, "Death following Massive Ingestion of Isoniazid," *Amer. Rev. Resp. Dis.*, *100*, 859 (1969).

(16) K. R. Boucot *et al.*, "Chemotherapy of Pulmonary Tuberculosis in Adults: The Choice of Drugs in Relation to Drug Susceptibility. A Statement of the Committee on Therapy," *Amer. Rev. Resp. Dis.*, *92*, 508 (1965).

(17) I. A. Jaffe, "Antivitamin B_6 Effect of D-Penicillamine," *Ann. N.Y. Acad. Sci.*, *166*, 57 (1969).

[For additional information, see *Adrenergic Therapy*, p. 332.]

Nonproprietary and Trade Names of Drugs

Carbidopa–levodopa—*Sinemet*
Levodopa—*Dopar, Larodopa*
Pyridoxine—*Frequently marketed in combination with other vitamins*

Pyridoxine hydrochloride—*Hexa-Betalin, Hexacrest, Hexavibex*

Prepared and evaluated by the Scientific Review Subpanel on Autonomic Agents and reviewed by Practitioner Panel I.

Lincomycin—Erythromycin

Summary—Erythromycin, because of its greater affinity for the 50 S ribosomal unit of the bacterial cell, theoretically can antagonize the activity of lincomycin by blocking access to the ribosomal binding site. However, this hypothesis lacks supporting data. Nevertheless, the likelihood of cross-interference when these drugs are administered concurrently or consecutively should discourage such use.

Related Drugs—Antibiotics that bind the 50 S ribosomal unit of the bacterial cell (**chloramphenicol** and **oleandomycin**) have the potential for interfering with the activity of lincomycin or its structural analog **clindamycin.**

Pharmacological Effect and Mechanism—Lincomycin and erythromycin are used primarily in the treatment of Gram-positive infections and less frequently for the treatment of *Bacteroides* infections (1). Although the activities of these antibiotics are similar, some differences do exist. Unlike erythromycin, lincomycin is not effective against *Neisseria gonorrhoeae, Mycoplasma pneumoniae, Treponema pallidum,* and group D *Streptococcus* (1). Both antibiotics interfere with protein synthesis in bacterial ribosomes. Lincomycin, like chloramphenicol, interferes with the ribosomal transport of the coding material, messenger RNA, and with the attachment to the ribosomes. Erythromycin interferes with the translocation of the amino acid-carrying substance, transfer RNA, from one ribosomal unit to another (2). Chloramphenicol, erythromycin, and lincomycin bind to the 50 S portion of the ribosomal unit (3). Since only one antibiotic molecule can combine with the 50 S ribosomal unit (4, 5), the presence of more than one antibiotic results in a competition for the binding site. Since erythromycin has a greater affinity for the 50 S ribosomal unit than lincomycin, erythromycin could block the effects of lincomycin by displacing it from the binding site or by preventing binding altogether (2–4, 6–8).

Evaluation of Clinical Data—Although several clinical and microbiological studies (7–15) demonstrated that cross-resistance to lincomycin and erythromycin can develop in many different species of bacteria, no direct clinical interaction between these drugs has been reported. Cross-resistance is believed to be due to the fact that part of the attachment site on the ribosomal subunit can be shared by both lincomycin and erythromycin, and mutations in this common part maintain sensitivity, whereas mutations in the unique parts lead to resistance (16).

It is not surprising that clinical reports clearly demonstrating a cross-interference between these drugs do not exist, since the choice of an antibiotic in rational therapy is dictated by the results of sensitivity testing. Even when therapy is instituted in the absence of culture data, concurrent lincomycin–erythromycin therapy is rare. Except for a few specific instances, *i.e.*, in biliary, genito-urinary, or gastrointestinal tract infections, in patients with penicillin hypersensitivity, or when the site of infection is unknown (1), these antibiotics are not the drugs of choice in the treatment of infections and, therefore, the probability of the reporting of a broad-based interaction is small. Additionally, the tendency of microorganisms to develop cross-resistance to lincomycin and erythromycin may mask the clinical observations of an interaction.

A good example may be the report of *Streptococcus pneumoniae* isolated from pus in the pleural cavity of a 63-year-old male (17). Sensitivity data initially showed the organism to be sensitive to both erythromycin and lincomycin. Treatment with erythromycin (250 mg po four times daily) was initiated. There was little clinical improvement after 11 days and injection of lincomycin (500 mg) into the pleural cavity on alternate days was started. Eleven days later both antibiotics were stopped when a second pleural aspirate revealed the organism to be highly resistant to both lincomycin and erythromycin. The patient was subsequently treated successfully with ampicillin. Whether this demonstrated a case of inhibition of lincomycin activity by erythromycin as suggested (11) or a case of cross-resistance has not been established.

■ Since clinical reports concerning a lincomycin–erythromycin interaction are lacking, it is not possible to evaluate fully the therapeutic significance of this phenomenon. However, it appears that the interaction is not significant in terms of patient management. Nevertheless, the practitioner should be aware of this potential interaction and the possibility of developing cross-resistant strains of bacteria.

Recommendations—Although there are insufficient data to conclude that an interaction occurs between lincomycin and erythromycin, the possibility of the development of cross-interference at the receptor site would offset any therapeutic advantage, if there is any, of such therapy. Therefore, concurrent use of these drugs should be avoided.

References

(1) R. Quintiliani, "Current Concepts in Therapy: General Concepts in the Use of Antibiotics in Adults," *S. Med. J.*, *66*, 940 (1973).

(2) K. Igarashi *et al.*, "Comparative Studies on the Mechanism of Action of Lincomycin, Streptomycin and Erythromycin," *Biochem. Biophys. Res. Commun.*, *37*, 499 (1969).

(3) L. Weinstein, "Modes of Action of Antibiotics on Bacteria and Man," *N.Y. State J. Med.*, *72*, 2166 (1972).

(4) E. R. Garrett *et al.*, "Kinetics and Mechanisms of Action of Drugs on Microorganisms XI: Effect of Erythromycin and Its Supposed Antagonism with Lincomycin on the Microbial Growth of *Escherichia coli*," *J. Pharm. Sci.*, *59*, 1448 (1970).

(5) J. C. H. Mao, "The Stoichiometry of Erythromycin Binding to Ribosomal Particles of *Staphylococcus aureus*," *Biochem. Pharmacol.*, *16*, 2441 (1967).

(6) F. N. Chang and B. Weisblum, "The Specificity of Lincomycin Binding to Ribosomes," *Biochemistry*, *6*, 836 (1967).

(7) S. A. Kabins, "Interactions among Antibiotics and Other Drugs," *J. Amer. Med. Ass.*, *219*, 206 (1972).

(8) B. Weisblum, "Pneumococcus Resistant to Erythromycin and Lincomycin," *Lancet*, *i*, 843 (1967).

(9) J. Desmyter and G. Reybrouck, "Lincomycin Sensitivity of Erythromycin-Resistant Staphylococci," *Chemotherapia*, *9*, 183 (1964–65).

(10) K. Sprunt *et al.*, "Cross Resistance between Lincomycin and Erythromycin
in Viridans Streptococci," *Pediatrics*,
46, 84 (1970).

(11) M. Barber and P. M. Waterworth,
"Antibacterial Activity of Lincomycin
and Pristinamycin: A Comparison with
Erythromycin," *Brit. Med. J.*, *2*, 603
(1964).

(12) E. Sanders *et al.*, "Group A Beta-
Hemolytic Streptococci Resistant to
Erythromycin and Lincomycin," *N.
Engl. J. Med.*, *278*, 538 (1968).

(13) J. W. Kislak, "Type 6 Pneumococcus
Resistant to Erythromycin and Lincomycin," *N. Engl. J. Med.*, *276*, 852
(1967).

(14) J. Desmyter, "Lincomycin Resistance
of Erythromycin Resistant Cocci,"
N. Engl. J. Med., *278*, 967 (1968).

(15) J. M. S. Dixon *et al.*, "Resistance of
Group A Beta-Hemolytic Streptococci
to Lincomycin and Erythromycin,"
Antimicrob. Ag. Chemother., *1*, 333
(1972).

(16) D. Apirion, "Three Genes that Affect
Escherichia coli Ribosomes," *J. Mol.
Biol.*, *30*, 255 (1967).

(17) J. M. S. Dixon *et al.*, "Pneumococcus
Resistant to Erythromycin and Lincomycin," letter to the editor, *Lancet*,
i, 573 (1967).

[For additional information, see *Anti-Infective Therapy*, p. 388.]

Nonproprietary and Trade Names of Drugs

Chloramphenicol—*Amphicol, Chloromycetin,
Mychel*
Clindamycin hydrochloride—*Cleocin
Hydrochloride*
Erythromycin—*E-Mycin, Erythrocin,
Ilotycin*
Erythromycin estolate—*Ilosone*
Erythromycin ethylsuccinate—*Erythrocin
Ethyl Succinate, Pediamycin*

Erythromycin gluceptate—*Ilotycin
Gluceptate*
Erythromycin stearate—*Bristamycin,
Erythrocin Stearate, Ethril*
Lincomycin hydrochloride—*Lincocin*
Oleandomycin phosphate—*Various
manufacturers*

*Prepared and evaluated by the Scientific Review Subpanel
on Anti-Infectives and reviewed by Practitioner Panel III.*

Lincomycin—Kaolin

Summary—Kaolin reduces the gastrointestinal (GI) absorption of lincomycin by
as much as 90% when administered simultaneously. This interaction is clinically significant because there is a relatively high incidence of diarrhea among
patients receiving lincomycin therapy and many antidiarrheal products used to
control the drug-induced diarrhea contain kaolin as the active ingredient. Kaolin-
containing antidiarrheals should be avoided or taken at least 2 hr before
lincomycin.

Related Drugs—**Clindamycin** is produced by 7-chloro substitution of the 7-(R)-hydroxy
group of the parent compound lincomycin. This antibiotic has essentially the same
activity spectrum as lincomycin but, unlike lincomycin, the presence of food in the
GI tract has little or no effect on the absorption of clindamycin following oral administration (1). There is no published information concerning the possible interaction
of clindamycin with kaolin. However, since clindamycin is structurally related to
lincomycin, it seems possible that such an interaction may occur.

Pharmacological Effect and Mechanism—Lincomycin is an antibiotic produced by
Streptomyces lincolnenis and is active against Gram-positive organisms (2). It is

highly effective against most types of *Bacteroides* and other anaerobes. However, it has little activity against Gram-negative bacilli, *Hemophilus influenzae, Neisseria gonorrhoeae,* and enterococci. Diarrhea was reported to occur in up to 20% of patients receiving lincomycin (3). Lincomycin also causes pseudomembranous colitis which is potentially fatal (4). Lincomycin suppresses bacterial protein formation by inhibiting peptide bond synthesis. This inhibition results from lincomycin's ability to bind the 50 S ribosomal subunit of the bacterial cell (5, 6).

Kaolin is a native, hydrated aluminum silicate usually available in powdered or aqueous suspension form. It is commonly used in the treatment of diarrhea and dysentery. Kaolin adsorbs irritating and toxic materials from the intestinal tract and forms a protective demulcent coating on the intestinal mucosa.

The mechanism by which kaolin interferes with the absorption of lincomycin from the GI tract is unknown. The simple physical coating action of kaolin on the intestinal mucosa and kaolin's adsorbent property may interfere with the GI absorption of lincomycin. Lincomycin is rapidly but only partially absorbed from the GI tract under normal conditions. The presence of food in the GI tract markedly inhibits (by as much as 67%) the absorption of lincomycin following its oral administration (7). A kaolin-containing product reduced significantly the GI bioavailability of lincomycin (8).

Evaluation of Clinical Data—One kaolin-containing product had a profound effect on the absorption of lincomycin from the GI tract (9, 10). In this well-controlled four-way crossover study with eight normal adult subjects, when lincomycin (single 0.5-g oral dose) was administered simultaneously with a product containing kaolin, the resulting serum antibiotic levels were approximately one-tenth of the levels obtained when the antibiotic was administered alone after fasting. Moreover, if the kaolin product was administered 2 hr prior to an oral dose of lincomycin, the serum antibiotic levels obtained were approximately equal to those seen in the fasted subjects.

■ The interaction between lincomycin and kaolin is clinically important and results in as much as a 90% reduction in the bioavailability of orally administered lincomycin. In view of the relatively high incidence of GI disturbances (*i.e.,* diarrhea in 20% of lincomycin-treated patients) that occurs in patients receiving lincomycin, such undesirable concurrent therapy may occur rather frequently.

Recommendations—If antidiarrheal therapy is indicated during treatment with lincomycin, consideration should be given to selecting some form of diarrhea control other than products containing kaolin. When a kaolin-containing product must be used, it should be given at least 2 hr before lincomycin. If this schedule proves impractical, lincomycin may be administered by injection or a nondiarrhea-producing antibiotic should be substituted.

References

(1) J. G. Wagner *et al.,* "Absorption, Excretion and Half-Life of Clinimycin in Normal Adult Males," *Amer. J. Med. Sci., 256,* 25 (1968).

(2) K. Kaplan *et al.,* "Microbiological, Pharmacological and Clinical Studies of Lincomycin," *Amer. J. Med. Sci., 250,* 137 (1965).

(3) A. M. Geddes *et al.,* "Lincomycin Hydrochloride: Clinical and Laboratory Studies," *Brit. Med. J., 2,* 670 (1964).

(4) A. M. Geddes, "Lincomycin and Clindamycin Colitis," *Brit. Med. J., 4,* 591 (1974).

(5) J. J. Josten and P. M. Allen, "The Mode of Action of Lincomycin," *Biochem. Biophys. Res. Commun., 14,* 241 (1964).

(6) F. N. Chang *et al.,* "Lincomycin, an Inhibitor of Aminoacyl SRNA Binding to Ribosomes," *Proc. Nat. Acad. Sci. USA, 55,* 431 (1966).

(7) C. E. McCall *et al.*, "Lincomycin: Activity *In Vitro* and Absorption and Excretion in Normal Young Men," *Amer. J. Med. Sci.*, *254*, 144 (1967).

(8) J. G. Wagner, "Aspects of Pharmacokinetics and Biopharmaceutics in Relation to Drug Activity," *Amer. J. Pharm.*, *141*, 5 (1969).

(9) J. G. Wagner, "Design and Data Analysis of Biopharmaceutical Studies in Man," *Can. J. Pharm. Sci.*, *1*, 55 (1966).

(10) J. G. Wagner, "Pharmacokinetics: (1) Definitions, Modeling and Reasons for Measuring Blood Levels and Urinary Excretion, *Drug Intel.*, *2*, 38 (1968).

[For additional information, see *Anti-Infective Therapy*, p. 388.]

Nonproprietary and Trade Names of Drugs

Clindamycin hydrochloride—*Cleocin Hydrochloride*

Kaolin-containing products—*Donnagel, Donnagel-PG, Kao-Con, Kaopectate, Parepectolin, Pargel*
Lincomycin hydrochloride—*Lincocin*

Prepared and evaluated by the Scientific Review Subpanel on Anti-Infectives and reviewed by Practitioner Panel IV.

Lithium Carbonate—Chlorothiazide

Summary—Chlorothiazide and other thiazide diuretics enhance the cardiotoxic and neurotoxic effects of lithium and these drugs should not be administered concurrently. In those rare instances when these drugs must be given together, the patient should be observed closely for signs and symptoms of lithium toxicity. Close monitoring of serum electrolytes and maintenance of adequate fluid, potassium, and sodium intake also are necessary.

Related Drugs—In addition to chlorothiazide, **bendroflumethiazide** and **hydroflumethiazide** similarly affect sodium and potassium renal excretion and decrease (1) or do not increase (2) lithium excretion. Therefore, any **thiazide diuretic** that promotes or enhances the excretion of both sodium and potassium also could be expected to interact with lithium. **Chlorthalidone, metolazone,** and **quinethazone** are structurally similar to the thiazides and may be expected to interact with lithium also.

Pharmacological Effect and Mechanism—Chlorothiazide causes diuresis by inhibiting renal tubular absorption of sodium and increasing the urinary excretion of chloride, sodium, and water. Chlorothiazide also increases the urinary excretion of potassium (3).

Chlorothiazide may increase lithium-induced intracellular depletion of potassium and may cause myocardial irritability and premature ventricular contractions (4). Chlorothiazide also may temporarily deplete intracellular sodium, enabling more lithium to enter the nerve cell. However, unless sodium intake is restricted, intracellular sodium levels remain depleted for only a few days. Compensatory increases in sodium reabsorption in the proximal renal tubule then return the intracellular sodium level to normal.

Since lithium is primarily reabsorbed with sodium in the proximal renal tubule (which is not significantly affected by the thiazide diuretics) and very little in the distal renal tubule (where the thiazide diuretics exert their main action), long-term thiazide administration may lead to an increase in the reabsorption of lithium and a subsequent decrease in lithium clearance. Increased reabsorption may occur even if sodium excretion is unaltered (1, 2, 5, 6). The higher concentrations of lithium could cause lithium toxicity (7, 8).

Evaluation of Clinical Data—Renal clearance of lithium was studied after long-term administration of bendroflumethiazide (2.5 mg/day po) or hydroflumethiazide (25 mg/day po) in 22 patients with edema (2). Lithium clearance was determined at intervals of 2 months before, during, and after thiazide treatment. During the examination period, each patient took a single dose of lithium carbonate (600 mg po) and the concentration of lithium in the urine was measured. The group as a whole had a statistically significant decrease (24%) in the renal clearance of lithium from the beginning of thiazide therapy until the diuretic was discontinued. Creatinine clearance tests indicated that renal function in these patients was normal.

A patient with lithium-induced diabetes insipidus was treated with chlorothiazide (500 mg/day po) intermittently for more than 6 months (9). Chlorothiazide administration resulted in a marked decrease in urine output but also caused the serum lithium level to rise from an average of approximately 1.3 mEq/liter to more than 2 mEq/liter each time chlorothiazide was initiated. In each instance, the lithium dosage was decreased to reduce observed clinical signs of lithium toxicity.

Two patients previously stabilized on lithium carbonate (1200 mg/day po for 21 days) were given chlorothiazide (1 g/day po) concurrently for 2 and 3 days, respectively (10). The patients also had been maintained on a stable sodium dietary intake during this period and were well hydrated. The daily urinary excretion of lithium in each patient gradually decreased, and the daily serum level gradually increased (by 12 and 14%, respectively) when these drugs were given together. The study was terminated when one patient showed clinical signs of lithium toxicity including severe tremors. [Severe tremors are usually not considered a dangerous but rather an inconvenient and relatively harmless adverse reaction which may occur at anytime during lithium therapy and in the absence of thiazides (7, 8).]

Lithium toxicity was described in a newborn infant whose mother had taken lithium carbonate (600–1200 mg/day po) throughout her pregnancy and chlorthalidone (50 mg po) every third day during the last 4 months of her pregnancy (11). Although chlorthalidone was considered a possible causative factor, there was insufficient evidence to indicate that this diuretic was responsible for the lithium toxicity. There are many other factors in the last trimester of pregnancy (such as low sodium intake) which may have caused lithium toxicity in the newborn (12).

■ The clinical significance of the reported interaction between lithium carbonate and chlorothiazide is difficult to determine because there are not enough controlled studies measuring the clinical outcome of concurrent, long-term use of these drugs. Limited data indicate that chlorothiazide and other thiazide diuretics increase serum lithium levels and may lead to symptoms of lithium toxicity.

Recommendations—Chlorothiazide and other thiazide diuretics should not be given concurrently with lithium because of the difficulty in correcting potential lithium poisoning and the severity of some of the toxic symptoms (8). In the rare situations where these drugs must be given together, the patient should be observed closely for signs and symptoms of the neurotoxic (*e.g.*, ataxia, confusion, and mental disorientation) or cardiotoxic (*e.g.*, ECG changes) effects of lithium. Close monitoring of serum electrolytes and maintenance of adequate fluid, potassium, and sodium intake also are necessary. Interpretation of serum lithium levels should take into account this drug interaction. It is less desirable, although possible, to reduce the serum lithium level below the therapeutic range for the treatment of acute mania or as a prophylaxis against manic depressive occurrence. Chlorothiazide should not be given concurrently with lithium carbonate to any patient who is pregnant (12).

There is no specific antidote for lithium poisoning. Osmotic diuresis, alkalinization of the urine, and restoration of serum electrolytes are some measures that have been used successfully (1, 8, 13).

Any diuretic (*e.g.,* ethacrynic acid, furosemide, or mercurial diuretic) that promotes the excretion of potassium and sodium may also increase the possibility of lithium toxicity. Furosemide (13) was considered the causative factor in a report of lithium toxicity in a patient stabilized on lithium (900 mg/day po). The potassium-sparing diuretics, spironolactone and triamterene, did not affect serum lithium levels in a small group of patients (10) and may be safer diuretics to use concurrently with lithium.

References

(1) K. Thomsen and M. Schou, "Renal Lithium Excretion in Man," *Amer. J. Physiol., 215,* 823 (1968).

(2) V. Petersen *et al.,* "Effect of Prolonged Thiazide Treatment on Renal Lithium Clearance," *Brit. Med. J., 3,* 143 (1974).

(3) "AMA Drug Evaluations," 2nd ed., American Medical Association, Chicago, Ill., 1973, pp. 69–73.

(4) R. D. Keynes and R. C. Swan, "The Permeability of Frog Muscle Fibres to Lithium Ions," *J. Physiol., 147,* 626 (1959).

(5) R. G. Demers and G. R. Heninger, "Sodium Intake and Lithium Treatment in Mania," *Amer. J. Psychiat., 128,* 100 (1971).

(6) I. Singer and D. Rotenberg, "Mechanisms of Lithium Action," *N. Engl. J. Med., 289,* 254 (1973).

(7) M. Schou *et al.,* "Pharmacological and Clinical Problems of Lithium Prophylaxis," *Brit. J. Psychiat., 116,* 615 (1970).

(8) B. Shopsin and S. Gershon, "Pharma-cology-Toxicology of the Lithium Ion," in "Lithium: Its Role in Psychiatric Research and Treatment," S. Gershon and B. Shopsin, Eds., Plenum, New York, N.Y., 1973, p. 107.

(9) S. T. Levy *et al.,* "Lithium-Induced Diabetes Insipidus: Manic Symptoms, Brain and Electrolyte Correlates, and Chlorothiazide Treatment," *Amer. J. Psychol., 130,* 1014 (1973).

(10) L. Barr *et al.,* "Recent Advances in the Psychobiology of the Depressive Illnesses," Williams, Katz, and Shield, Eds., DHEW Publication, 1972, p. 49.

(11) W. W. Tannessan and G. G. Hertz, "Toxic Effects of Lithium in Newborn Infants: A Commentary," letter to the editor, *J. Pediat., 81,* 804 (1972).

(12) M. R. Weinstein *et al.,* "Lithium Ion Toxicity and Pregnancy," letter to the editor, *J. Amer. Med. Ass., 214,* 1325 (1970).

(13) H. I. Hurtig and W. L. Dyson, "Lithium Toxicity Enhanced by Diuresis," *N. Engl. J. Med., 290,* 748 (1974).

[For additional information, see *Antipsychotic Therapy,* p. 397.]

Nonproprietary and Trade Names of Drugs

Bendroflumethiazide—*Naturetin*
Benzthiazide—*Aquatag, Exna*
Chlorothiazide—*Diuril*
Chlorthalidone—*Hygroton, Regroton*
Cyclothiazide—*Anhydron*
Ethacrynic acid—*Edecrin*
Flumethiazide—*Rautrax*
Furosemide—*Lasix*
Hydrochlorothiazide—*Esidrix, HydroDiuril, Oretic*
Hydroflumethiazide—*Saluron*
Lithium carbonate—*Eskalith, Lithane, Lithonate*

Mercaptomerin sodium—*Thiomerin*
Methyclothiazide—*Aquatensen, Enduron*
Metolazone—*Zaroxolyn*
Polythiazide—*Renese*
Quinethazone—*Hydromox*
Spironolactone—*Aldactone*
Triamterene—*Dyrenium*
Trichlormethiazide—*Metahydrin, Naqua*
Various combination products containing a diuretic are available.

Prepared and evaluated by the Scientific Review Subpanel on Psychotropic Agents and reviewed by Practitioner Panel IV.

Lithium Carbonate—Potassium Iodide

Summary—The concurrent administration of lithium carbonate and potassium iodide or other iodine-containing compounds may enhance the hypothyroid and goitrogenic effects of either drug. If feasible, baseline thyroid status should be determined for all patients prior to initiation of lithium therapy and at periodic intervals to detect changes in the thyroid–pituitary response. If a hypothyroid state develops, stabilization of the patient's thyroid state with synthetic thyroid preparations (*e.g.,* levothyroxine or liothyronine) should be achieved and potassium iodide or other iodine-containing drugs should be discontinued.

Related Drugs—A possible interaction of lithium carbonate and **isopropamide iodide** has been reported (1). Although literature documentation is lacking, lithium carbonate theoretically could interact with **calcium iodate, calcium iodide, hydriodic acid, iodinated glycerol,** and **sodium iodide.** All over-the-counter and radiographic products containing iodine may also enhance lithium's antithyroid effects.

Pharmacological Effect and Mechanism—Administration of exogenous iodine (from several days to several weeks) to either animals or humans inhibits thyroid hormone synthesis (2). This effect usually does not lead to hypothyroidism as thyroid iodine transport declines with continued excess iodine administration. This decline allows intrathyroidal iodine concentrations to fall below the level necessary to inhibit thyroxine production (3). In some instances, however, chronic iodine administration for months or years has led to hypothyroidism with formation of goiter (4).

After the administration of lithium carbonate, lithium accumulates in the thyroid gland against a concentration gradient (5, 6) and is capable of blocking thyroidal release of liothyronine and thyroxine (7). It has been proposed that the lithium ion may directly inhibit the thyroid-stimulating hormone activation of adenyl cyclase in the thyroid. Since adenyl cyclase is necessary for cyclic adenosine 3',5'-monophosphate (cyclic AMP) production which mediates the release of thyroxine, inhibition of this enzyme by lithium ion would prevent the acute release of thyroid hormone and lead to hypothyroidism (8). Therefore, concurrent use of lithium and iodine-containing compounds may produce hypothyroid states greater than that produced by either drug alone.

Evaluation of Clinical Data—Clinical hypothyroidism was noted in a patient receiving lithium carbonate for more than 2 years as prophylaxis against recurrence of mania and depression (9). The serum lithium level was maintained at 0.6–0.8 mEq/liter. Cessation of lithium therapy resolved the hypothyroid state, but it recurred with the administration of potassium iodide (500 mg po three times daily). When potassium iodide therapy was discontinued, the patient became euthyroid. In a second patient (9), hypothyroidism developed after 3 weeks of lithium carbonate therapy (serum level, 0.5 mEq/liter). When potassium iodide (500 mg po three times daily) was added, the hypothyroidism became more pronounced, as indicated by laboratory tests and clinical signs. All abnormalities were resolved promptly (within 2 weeks) following withdrawal of lithium carbonate and potassium iodide.

These reports complement previously cited observations by the same investigators (10). In one outpatient, hypothyroidism appeared during treatment with either lithium carbonate (1 g/day po) or potassium iodide (1.5 g/day po); each drug was given for 3 weeks. In a second patient, a large goiter appeared 3 weeks after initiating lithium carbonate (750 mg/day po) therapy. The patient was also ingesting several iodine-containing vitamins daily. The goiter disappeared when both lithium carbonate and the vitamins were discontinued. No attempt was made to isolate the cause of the goiter by stopping vitamin therapy first and noting the effect on the size of the goiter.

A patient stabilized on lithium carbonate (900 mg/day po) had a combination product containing haloperidol and isopropamide iodide added to his drug regimen (1). At the same time, the lithium dose was increased to 1800 mg/day po. Clinical and laboratory signs of hypothyroidism were detected about 1 month after the increase in the lithium dose and the addition of the haloperidol–isopropamide iodide combination product. The dose of lithium was then decreased to 600 mg/day po and the haloperidol–isopropamide iodide combination product was discontinued. Levothyroxine (0.05 mg/day po) reversed all signs and symptoms of hypothyroidism in 2 weeks. After the patient was euthyroid, levothyroxine was discontinued. However, a few weeks later signs of hypothyroidism reappeared and levothyroxine administration (0.05 mg/day po) was begun again. It was suggested (11) that the iodine (1 mg/day po) in isopropamide iodide may have enhanced the ability of lithium to induce hypothyroidism, although the increased dose of lithium or the existence of a preexisting defect in the patient's thyroid response may have been the causative factor.

In a retrospective analysis (12) of an earlier case report (13) of myxedema, it was suggested that the combination of lithium carbonate (390 mg/day po) and iodine (140 mg/day po) may have induced the myxedema.

■ Although the data are limited, short-term (acute) and long-term (chronic) lithium administration may result in hypothyroidism, production of goiter, or both, and the concurrent use of iodine-containing preparations could enhance these antithyroid effects. Neither lithium nor iodine ingestion generally results in thyroid pathology, but either or both of these agents may reveal an underlying thyroid defect (14).

Recommendations—Patients taking lithium carbonate should avoid taking over-the-counter and/or prescription iodine-containing preparations. If feasible, thyroid status should be determined prior to initiating lithium carbonate therapy by measuring serum liothyronine, thyroxine, thyroid-stimulating hormone, and antithyroglobulin antibody levels. Periodic determinations of these parameters should be performed to detect changes in the thyroid–pituitary response (14).

The appearance of goiter or detection of abnormal chemical thyroid tests is not an indication to discontinue lithium therapy. Determination of any underlying defect and stabilization of thyroid status with appropriate drugs (*e.g.,* levothyroxine or liothyronine) and discontinuation of any iodine-containing drugs would be the most appropriate action (14).

References

(1) E. D. Luby *et al.,* "Lithium-Carbonate-Induced Myxedema," *J. Amer. Med. Ass., 218,* 1298 (1971).

(2) J. Wolff and I. L. Chaikoff, "Plasma Inorganic Iodide as a Homeostatic Regulator of Thyroid Function," *J. Biol. Chem., 174,* 555 (1948).

(3) L. E. Braverman and S. H. Ingbar, "Changes in Thyroidal Function during Adaptation to Large Doses of Iodide," *J. Clin. Invest., 42,* 1216 (1963).

(4) J. Paris *et al.,* "Iodide Goiter," *J. Clin. Endocrinol. Metab., 20,* 57 (1960).

(5) B. Shopsin *et al.,* "Lithium-Induced Thyroid Disturbance: Case Report and Review," *Compr. Psychiat., 10,* 215 (1969).

(6) S. C. Berens *et al.,* "Lithium Concentration by the Thyroid," *Endocrinology, 87,* 1085 (1970).

(7) S. C. Berens *et al.,* "Antithyroid Effects of Lithium," *J. Clin. Invest., 49,* 1357 (1970).

(8) I. Singer and D. Rotenberg, "Mechanisms of Lithium Action," *N. Engl. J. Med., 289,* 254 (1973).

(9) B. Shopsin *et al.,* "Iodine and Lithium-Induced Hypothyroidism," *Amer. J. Med., 55,* 695 (1973).

(10) B. Shopsin and S. Gershon, "Pharmacology-Toxicology of the Lithium Ion," in "Lithium: Its Role in Psychiatric Research and Treatment," S. Gershon and B. Shopsin, Eds., Plenum, New York, N.Y., 1973, p. 126.

(11) J. D. Wiener, "Lithium Carbonate-Induced Myxedema," letter to the editor, *J. Amer. Med. Ass.*, *220*, 587 (1972).

(12) J. V. Jorgensen *et al.*, "Possible Synergism between Iodine and Lithium Carbonate," letter to the editor, *J. Amer. Med. Ass.*, *223*, 192 (1973).

(13) M. E. Morgan and W. R. Trotter, "Two Cases of Myxoedema Attributed to Iodide Administration," *Lancet*, *ii*, 1335 (1953).

(14) B. Shopsin *et al.*, "Triiodothyronine and Thyroid-Stimulating Hormone Response to Thyrotropin-Releasing Hormone: Newer Aspects of Lithium-Induced Thyroid Disturbance in Man," in "The Thyroid Axis, Drugs, and Behavior," A. J. Prange, Ed., Raven, New York, NY 10024, 1974, p. 177.

[For additional information, see *Antipsychotic Therapy*, p. 397.]

Nonproprietary and Trade Names of Drugs

Calcium iodate—*Calcidin*
Calcium iodide—*Calcidrine, Iophed*
Hydriodic acid—*Various manufacturers*
Iodinated glycerol—*Organidin*
Isopropamide iodide—*Darbid*
Levothyroxine sodium—*Letter, Synthroid*
Liothyronine sodium—*Cytomel*
Liotrix—*Euthroid, Thyrolar*
Lithium carbonate—*Eskalith, Lithane, Lithonate*

Potassium iodide—*Various manufacturers and combination products*
Sodium iodide—*Various manufacturers and combination products*
Thyroglobulin—*Proloid*
Thyroid—*Thyrar*
Thyroxine fraction—*Various manufacturers*

Prepared and evaluated by the Scientific Review Subpanel on Psychotropic Agents and reviewed by Practitioner Panel VI.

Meperidine—Phenelzine

Summary—Concurrent administration of meperidine and phenelzine or other monoamine oxidase inhibitors may result in excitatory and depressant effects on the central nervous system (CNS) leading to deep coma and death. Concurrent use of these drugs should be avoided. If a narcotic analgesic must be used in patients receiving monoamine oxidase inhibitors, morphine is preferable to meperidine. The patient's response to small doses of the narcotic analgesic should be determined prior to the initiation of therapeutic doses.

Related Drugs—In addition to phenelzine, other monoamine oxidase inhibitors reported to interact with meperidine include **pargyline** (1–3) and **tranylcypromine** (1–3). Other agents that specifically inhibit monoamine oxidase, *e.g.*, **isocarboxazid,** may interact with meperidine in a similar fashion.

Dextromethorphan, the *d*-isomer of the codeine analog of levorphanol having antitussive but no analgesic activity, is available in nonprescription products and has interacted with phenelzine resulting in a fatality (4). **Nalorphine hydrobromide** reportedly enhanced the depression caused by a combination injection of meperidine-levallorphan in a patient receiving phenelzine (5).

All other narcotic analgesics should be used with caution in the presence of monoamine oxidase inhibitors.

Pharmacological Effect and Mechanism—Patients treated concurrently with meperidine and monoamine oxidase inhibitors have experienced rigidity, hyperpyrexia, excitement, hypotension, nystagmus with fixed dilated pupils, labored respiration, and deep coma. Three fatalities have been confirmed as a result of this drug interaction

(6). The symptoms of hyperpyrexia and excitement suggest CNS stimulation. Animal studies indicate that this CNS effect occurred with meperidine only in the presence of increased levels of cerebral 5-hydroxytryptamine (serotonin) (7–9). Since the administration of 5-hydroxytryptophan, the precursor of 5-hydroxytryptamine, produces excitatory symptoms indistinguishable from those of the meperidine–monoamine oxidase inhibitor interaction, it has been suggested that meperidine blocks the central 5-hydroxytryptamine uptake mechanism and that this blockade is responsible for the CNS stimulation (10).

The depressant effects of the meperidine–monoamine oxidase inhibitor interaction were suggested to be similar to those of acute meperidine poisoning in humans (11). The symptoms of hypotension, fixed dilated pupils, rigidity, depressed respiration, and deep coma seem to verify this observation. A mechanism proposed to account for these symptoms relates to the ability of monoamine oxidase inhibitors to reduce the rate of biotransformation of meperidine to inactive products, thus allowing for the subsequent accumulation of toxic levels of the drug. Animal studies demonstrated the inhibitory actions of monoamine oxidase inhibitors on the hepatic microsomal drug-metabolizing enzymes, resulting in a reduction of the rate of meperidine demethylation and hydrolysis to normeperidine and meperidinic acid (12, 13). This mechanism is not likely a major contributing factor since the onset of the toxic reactions in humans occurs within too short a time to allow for significant accumulation of meperidine.

Evaluation of Clinical Data—Few patients are reported to have experienced this drug interaction, although concurrent use of meperidine and monoamine oxidase inhibitors was relatively common before the interaction was described (14). A characteristic of the interaction is the extreme rapidity with which toxicity occurs. Hypotension, rigidity, and unconsciousness have occurred within minutes after meperidine administration (100 mg im) in the presence of phenelzine (dose not reported) (15). Three fatalities have been confirmed as a result of this drug interaction (6).

Other narcotic analgesics were implicated in interactions with monoamine oxidase inhibitors (16), but no documentation supports the involvement of these drugs. In fact, severe head and retrosternal pain caused by tranylcypromine (20–40 mg/day po) was alleviated by morphine administration (20 mg, route not reported) with no observable toxicities in five patients (17). No ill effects were reported (1) after the administration of morphine (11 mg im) to a patient receiving oral phenelzine (dose not reported), although a severe interaction resulting in death occurred after two injections of meperidine (totaling 150 mg) were given 7.5 hr apart, starting 2 hr after morphine treatment. The lack of adverse effects from morphine in patients treated with monoamine oxidase inhibitors who had previously reacted to meperidine has also been reported (2).

Another study (18) reported the effects of meperidine (5–40 mg im) and morphine (0.5–4 mg im) in 15 patients each of whom had been receiving an average daily dose of 20 mg of iproniazid, isocarboxazid, phenelzine, or tranylcypromine for 3–8 weeks. Each treatment consisted of four successive injections of increasing doses of either meperidine or morphine given at 45-min intervals over 3 hr. Each patient received both drugs on different days in a crossover design. All patients reacted normally to both drugs, with no sign of any interaction manifestations. The number of patients studied was insufficient to determine the percentage of patients likely to react abnormally to either drug or to determine differences in reactions to meperidine and morphine. Also, the doses of meperidine used (5, 10, 20, and 40 mg) were significantly smaller than the 100-mg doses implicated in the interactions with monoamine oxidase inhibitors. The investigator indicated that only a small number of patients at risk are likely to react abnormally to concurrent administration of meperidine and monoamine oxidase inhibitors.

■ The clinical evidence indicates that a small number of patients treated with mono-amine oxidase inhibitors will probably experience reactions to meperidine. The inter-action is unpredictable and insidious in that life-threatening situations can occur with extreme rapidity due to effects within the CNS.

Recommendations—Meperidine should not be administered concurrently with mono-amine oxidase inhibitors, and other narcotic analgesics should be used with extreme caution. If narcotic analgesics are needed, morphine would be preferable to meperi-dine in these patients. Patients treated with monoamine oxidase inhibitors in which narcotic analgesics cannot be avoided should be tested for responses to small doses of the analgesic prior to the administration of therapeutic doses.

References

(1) H. Palmer, "Potentiation of Pethi-dine," *Brit. Med. J., 2,* 944 (1960).

(2) J. C. Shee, "Dangerous Potentiation of Pethidine by Iproniazid, and Its Treatment," *Brit. Med. J., 2,* 507 (1960).

(3) P. H. Denton *et al.,* "Dangers of Monoamine Oxidase Inhibitors," *Brit. Med. J., 2,* 1752 (1962).

(4) N. Rivers and B. Horner, "Possible Lethal Reaction between Nardil and Dextromethorphan," *Can. Med. Ass. J., 103,* 85 (1970).

(5) D. Cocks and A. Passmore-Rowe, "Dangers of Monoamine Oxidase In-hibitors," *Brit. Med. J., 2,* 1545 (1962).

(6) D. R. Landon and M. D. Milne, "Dan-gers of Monoamine Oxidase Inhibi-tors," *Brit. Med. J., 2,* 1752 (1962).

(7) S. N. C. Gong and K. J. Rogers, "Role of Brain Monoamines in the Fatal Hyperthermia Induced by Pethidine or Imipramine in Rabbits Pretreated with Pargyline," *Brit. J. Pharmacol., 42,* 646 (1971).

(8) K. J. Rogers, "Role of Brain Mono-amines in the Interaction between Pethidine and Tranylcypromine," *Eur. J. Pharmacol., 14,* 86 (1971).

(9) J. G. Sinclair, "The Effects of Meperi-dine and Morphine in Rabbits Pre-treated with Phenelzine," *Toxicol. Appl. Pharmacol., 22,* 231 (1972).

(10) A. Carlsson and M. Lindqvist, "Cen-tral and Peripheral Monoaminergic Membrane-Pump Blockade by Some Addictive Analgesics and Antihista-mines," *J. Pharm. Pharmacol., 21,* 460 (1969).

(11) G. Brownlee and G. W. Williams, "Potentiation of Amphetamine and Pethidine by Monoamineoxidase In-hibitors," *Lancet, i,* 699 (1963).

(12) B. Clark, "The In Vitro Inhibition of the N-Demethylation of Pethidine by Phenelzine (Phenethylhydrazine)," *Biochem. Pharmacol., 16,* 2369 (1967).

(13) N. R. Eade and K. W. Renton, "Effect of Monoamine Oxidase Inhibitors on the N-Demethylation and Hydrolysis of Meperidine," *Biochem. Pharmacol., 19,* 2243 (1970).

(14) N. R. Eade and K. W. Renton, "The Effect of Phenelzine and Tranylcypro-mine on the Degradation of Meperi-dine," *J. Pharmacol. Exp. Ther., 173,* 31 (1970).

(15) N. C. R. W. Reid and D. Jones, "Pethi-dine and Phenelzine," *Brit. Med. J., 1,* 408 (1962).

(16) L. I. Goldberg, "Monoamine Oxidase Inhibitors: Adverse Reactions and Possible Mechanisms," *J. Amer. Med. Ass., 190,* 456 (1964).

(17) D. D. Brown and D. H. Waldron, "An Unusual Reaction to Tranylcypro-mine," *Practitioner, 189,* 83 (1962).

(18) C. D. G. Evans-Prosser, "The Use of Pethidine and Morphine in the Pres-ence of Monoamine Oxidase Inhibi-tors," *Brit. J. Anaesth., 40,* 279 (1968).

[For additional information, see *Analgesic Therapy (Nonnarcotic),* p. 341.]

Nonproprietary and Trade Names of Drugs

Dextromethorphan hydrobromide—*Various manufacturers and combination products*
Isocarboxazid—*Marplan*
Meperidine hydrochloride—*Demerol Hydrochloride*
Nalorphine hydrobromide—*Lethidrone, Norfin*

Nalorphine hydrochloride—*Nalline Hydrochloride*
Pargyline hydrochloride—*Eutonyl and various combination products*
Phenelzine sulfate—*Nardil*
Tranylcypromine—*Parnate*

Prepared and evaluated by the Scientific Review Subpanels on Analge-sics and Psychotropic Agents and reviewed by Practitioner Panel VI.

Meprobamate—Alcohol

Summary—Concurrent ingestion of meprobamate and alcohol can lead to an enhancement of their central nervous system (CNS) depressant effects. The manifestations of this interaction are usually mild or insignificant if alcohol intake does not exceed one or two drinks (90–120 ml of 100-proof whiskey) and meprobamate is taken in a single dose of 200–400 mg. However, because more pronounced and possibly dangerous effects (impairment of driving ability) have been observed when meprobamate was administered to some patients on a chronic basis, patients taking meprobamate should avoid alcohol and should use care when driving an automobile or operating hazardous machinery.

Related Drugs—Propanediol derivatives such as **carisoprodol, chlormezanone, chlorphenesin, methocarbamol,** and **tybamate** are chemically and pharmacologically related to meprobamate and may interact with alcohol in a similar manner. Meprobamate also is available in combination products.

Pharmacological Effect and Mechanism—The effects of this interaction may be described as enhanced CNS depression produced by two agents having sedative–hypnotic properties. The half-life of meprobamate is prolonged significantly when alcohol is administered concurrently for a short period (1). However, the blood clearance of meprobamate is accelerated in persons subjected to a 1-month period of chronic ingestion of excessive amounts of alcohol (2). These findings are interpreted to indicate microsomal enzyme induction and competitive inhibition by alcohol of the meprobamate-oxidizing enzyme system. This hypothesis explains the greater effectiveness of chronic administration of high doses (1600 mg) of meprobamate (cumulative increase in serum drug levels) (3–5) in contrast to single low dose (400 mg) medication in persons under the influence of alcohol (6).

Evaluation of Clinical Data—In one controlled experiment with 22 subjects (3), small amounts of alcohol (blood alcohol level, 50 mg/100 ml, approximately 1–2 drinks) with meprobamate (400 mg four times daily, started 1 week before testing) produced a significantly greater impairment of performance and judgment than either agent given individually.

The behavioral and physiological effects of meprobamate (800 mg) and alcohol (0.33–0.66 g/kg or 0.9–1.8 ml of whiskey/kg) were measured in a double-blind controlled study of eight patients (7). Meprobamate increased the subjective symptoms and the objective signs (during the first 3–4 hr after intake) of alcohol-induced CNS depression.

The effects of alcohol and meprobamate (800 mg) (blood alcohol level, 80 mg/100 ml) on driving ability were evaluated in 20 healthy subjects under double-blind conditions (8). Meprobamate alone slightly decreased the driving performance, but the addition of alcohol caused a statistically significant decrease in the driving performance scores.

Only a slight enhancement of CNS depression occurred when alcohol (0.3–0.82 g/kg) was ingested by patients taking meprobamate (800–1600 mg/day po) (4, 5). Low doses of meprobamate (400 mg) did not enhance the effects of alcohol (5) and some studies indicate that the drug interaction may only occur in certain labile patients (9, 10).

■ Based on these clinical studies, it appears that alcohol enhances the CNS depressant effects of meprobamate at certain doses which may differ among patients. These effects are predominantly impairment of mental performance and judgment, reduction of motor skills and coordination, increased drowsiness, and sleepiness (3, 7, 8). If either drug is taken in large doses (16–20 g of meprobamate or 300–400 ml of 100% alcohol), these agents can enhance CNS depression, possibly causing death (11).

Recommendations—Patients taking meprobamate should be informed that the CNS depressant effects of alcohol may be increased by meprobamate and that concurrent use of alcohol may produce greater impairment of their ability to drive an automobile and that it could endanger their safety in operating hazardous machinery.

Other CNS depressant drugs such as the barbiturates (see *Phenobarbital–Alcohol*, p. 180), the benzodiazepines (see *Diazepam–Alcohol*, p. 47), chloral hydrate (see *Chloral Hydrate–Alcohol*, p. 20), ethchlorvynol (12), glutethimide (13), and possibly methaqualone (14) interact with alcohol in a manner similar to meprobamate.

References

(1) P. S. Misra *et al.*, "Increase of Ethanol, Meprobamate and Pentobarbital Metabolism after Chronic Ethanol Administration in Man and in Rats," *Amer. J. Med., 51,* 346 (1971).

(2) E. Rubin *et al.*, "Inhibition of Drug Metabolism by Acute Ethanol Intoxication," *Amer. J. Med., 49,* 801 (1970).

(3) G. A. Zirkle *et al.*, "Meprobamate and Small Amounts of Alcohol. Effects on Human Ability, Coordination, and Judgment," *J. Amer. Med. Ass., 173,* 1823 (1960).

(4) R. B. Forney and F. W. Hughes, "Meprobamate, Ethanol or Meprobamate–Ethanol Combinations on Performance of Human Subjects under Delayed Audiofeedback (DAF)," *J. Psychol., 57,* 431 (1964).

(5) N. Reisby and A. Theilgaard, "The Interaction of Alcohol and Meprobamate in Man," *Acta Psychiat. Scand., 208,* suppl., 5 (1969).

(6) P. Kielholz *et al.*, "Road Traffic, Tranquilizers, and Alcohol," *Deut. Med. Wochenschr., 92,* 1525 (1967).

(7) L. Goldberg, "Behavioral and Physiological Effects of Alcohol on Man," *Psychosom. Med., 28,* 570 (1966).

(8) P. Kielholz *et al.*, "Tests of Driving Ability for Estimating the Effects of Alcohol, Tranquilizers, and Hypnotics," *Deut. Med. Wochenschr., 94,* 301 (1969).

(9) W. J. Eicke, "Incidents during Treatment with Meprobamate and Simultaneous Consumption of Alcohol," *Int. Pharmacopsychiat., 3,* 203 (1969).

(10) P. Munkelt and G. A. Lienert, "Blood Alcohol Level and Psychophysical Constitution," *Arzneim.-Forsch., 14,* 573 (1964).

(11) S. Felby, "Concentrations of Meprobamate in the Blood and Liver following Fatal Meprobamate Poisoning," *Acta Pharmacol. Toxicol., 28,* 334 (1970).

(12) A. Flemenbaum and B. Gunby, "Ethchlorvynol (Placidyl) Abuse and Withdrawal (Review of Clinical Picture and Report of Two Cases)," *Dis. Nerv. Syst., 32,* 188 (1971).

(13) G. P. Mould *et al.*, "Interaction of Glutethimide and Phenobarbitone with Ethanol in Man," *J. Pharm. Pharmacol., 24,* 894 (1972).

(14) D. S. Inaba *et al.*, "Methaqualone Abuse. 'Luding Out'," *J. Amer. Med. Ass., 224,* 1505 (1973).

[For additional information, see *Sedative–Hypnotic Therapy*, p. 442.]

Nonproprietary and Trade Names of Drugs

Alcohol—*Various products and beverages*
Carisoprodol—*Rela, Soma*
Chlormezanone—*Trancopal*
Chlorphenesin carbamate—*Maolate*
Ethchlorvynol—*Placidyl*
Glutethimide—*Doriden*

Meprobamate—*Equanil, Meprospan, Miltown, and various combination products*
Methaqualone—*Quaalude, Sopor*
Methocarbamol—*Robaxin*
Tybamate—*Solacen, Tybatran*

Prepared and evaluated by the Scientific Review Subpanel on Psychotropic Agents and reviewed by Practitioner Panel I.

Meprobamate—Imipramine

Summary—Imipramine enhances the central nervous system (CNS) effect of meprobamate in animals, but the clinical significance of this effect has not been established in humans. Until more clinical data are available, patients receiving meprobamate and imipramine concurrently should be warned about possible enhanced CNS depression.

Related Drugs—Agents structurally related to meprobamate include **carisoprodol,** **chlormezanone, chlorphenesin, methocarbamol,** and **tybamate.** Related tricyclic antidepressants include **amitriptyline, desipramine, doxepin, nortriptyline,** and **protriptyline.** Meprobamate also is available in combination products.

Pharmacological Effect and Mechanism—Meprobamate is metabolized by hepatic microsomal enzymes and is capable of accelerating the metabolism of a large number of drugs and of stimulating its own metabolism upon prolonged administration in humans (1).

Nortriptyline is metabolized by hepatic microsomal enzymes to demethylated and hydroxylated derivatives in rats (2). Other tricyclic antidepressants are presumably metabolized by the same mechanism.

Imipramine enhanced the sedative effects of meprobamate and carisoprodol in rats and inhibited the *in vitro* metabolism of these drugs in rat liver microsomal enzyme preparations (3). This evidence suggests that the mechanism of imipramine-enhanced sedative effects of meprobamate and carisoprodol in rats is hepatic microsomal enzyme inhibition rather than additive central depression.

Evaluation of Clinical Data—In a double-blind study (4) in depressed neurotic outpatients, meprobamate administered concurrently with protriptyline was compared with meprobamate alone in improving the clinical state of depression and anxiety. Patients received meprobamate (1600 mg/day po) alone or with protriptyline (40 mg/day po) for 4 weeks. Evaluation of side effects at 2 and 4 weeks revealed that 33% of all patients taking both drugs reported side effects consisting of drowsiness and dizziness. This percentage remained unchanged for the entire study. In contrast, 29% of the patients receiving meprobamate alone complained of drowsiness at the 2-week period, but this figure dropped to 8% at 4 weeks. It was emphasized by the investigators that the conclusions were limited because of the short study period involved.

Both meprobamate (5) and the tricyclic antidepressants (6) may cause drowsiness when used alone.

■ Based on available animal and clinical data, it appears that the interaction between meprobamate and imipramine is of minor clinical significance; enhanced sedation would be the predominant effect.

Recommendations—A few patients may experience enhanced drowsiness and dizziness when imipramine is given concurrently with meprobamate. Patients receiving these drugs concurrently should be advised that these effects may occur.

References

(1) A. H. Conney, "Pharmacological Implications of Microsomal Enzyme Induction," *Pharmacol. Rev., 19,* 317 (1967).
(2) R. E. McMahon *et al.,* "The Metabo-

lism of Nortriptyline-N-Methyl-¹⁴C in Rats," *Biochem. Pharmacol., 12,* 1207 (1963).

(3) R. Kato *et al.*, "Mechanism of Potentiation of Barbiturates and Meprobamate Actions by Imipramine," *Biochem. Pharmacol., 12*, 357 (1963).

(4) K. Rickels *et al.*, "Drug Treatment in Depression. Antidepressant or Tranquilizer?" *J. Amer. Med. Ass., 201*, 105 (1967).

(5) "The Pharmacological Basis of Therapeutics," 5th ed., L. S. Goodman and A. Gilman, Eds., Macmillan, New York, NY 10022, 1975, p. 189.

(6) D. J. Greenblatt and R. I. Shader, "Rational Use of Psychotropic Drugs," *Amer. J. Hosp. Pharm., 32*, 59 (1975).

[For additional information, see *Antidepressant Therapy*, p. 373.]

Nonproprietary and Trade Names of Drugs

Amitriptyline hydrochloride—*Elavil Hydrochloride and various combination products*

Carisoprodol—*Rela, Soma*

Chlormezanone—*Trancopal*

Chlorphenesin carbamate—*Maolate*

Desipramine hydrochloride—*Norpramin, Pertofrane*

Doxepin hydrochloride—*Adapin, Sinequan*

Imipramine hydrochloride—*Presamine, Tofranil, Tofranil PM*

Meprobamate—*Equanil, Meprospan, Miltown, and various combination products*

Methocarbamol—*Robaxin*

Nortriptyline hydrochloride—*Aventyl Hydrochloride*

Protriptyline hydrochloride—*Vivactil Hydrochloride*

Tybamate—*Solacen, Tybatran*

Prepared and evaluated by the Scientific Review Subpanel on Psychotropic Agents and reviewed by Practitioner Panel II.

Mercaptopurine—Allopurinol

Summary—The administration of allopurinol inhibits the enzymatic oxidation of mercaptopurine within 24 hr when administered concurrently in therapeutic doses. This interaction is clinically significant and requires an immediate reduction in the mercaptopurine dose.

Related Drugs—**Azathioprine** is chemically and pharmacologically related to mercaptopurine and follows the same catabolic pathways to 6-thiouric acid (approximately 10% of the drug is excreted unchanged). Although not documented, it may be expected to interact with allopurinol in a similar manner. **Thioguanine** is also related to mercaptopurine but is metabolized differently (1) and should not interact with allopurinol.

Pharmacological Effect and Mechanism—Mercaptopurine (active) is normally metabolized to 6-thiouric acid (inactive) by enzymatic oxidation which is catalyzed by the enzyme xanthine oxidase (2, 3). Allopurinol inhibits the action of xanthine oxidase, thereby reducing the rate at which mercaptopurine is inactivated (4). Allopurinol is often given concurrently with mercaptopurine to decrease urate production and to prevent uric acid nephropathy (5). Concurrent administration of allopurinol has increased the cytotoxic effects of mercaptopurine approximately fourfold (5).

Evaluation of Clinical Data—Controlled clinical studies demonstrated that allopurinol administered concurrently with oral mercaptopurine inhibits the conversion of mercaptopurine to 6-thiouric acid. This inhibition has been observed in three patients who received concurrent mercaptopurine–allopurinol therapy (6). In one patient, increasing the dose of allopurinol to 800 mg po caused the amount of free mercaptopurine (dose of 100 mg po) in the urine to rise from 3.1 to 27.8% while 6-thiouric acid fell from 24 to 2.4%.

This drug interaction was studied in two patients with chronic granulocytic leukemia (5). One patient showed an increase from 7.2 to 29% of free mercaptopurine in the urine and a decrease in 6-thiouric acid from 25.5 to 3.4% when mercaptopurine (150 mg po) and allopurinol (75 mg po) were administered concurrently. The second patient showed comparable results. A later study (7) involving six patients verified the previous data (5) by reporting an increase of free mercaptopurine in the urine from less than 3% to as much as 27%.

This drug interaction has been used in an attempt to increase the effectiveness of mercaptopurine in the treatment of acute leukemia in children but did not improve the initial incidence of remission (8).

■ Although the clinical effects of the drug interaction have not been identified, some studies, involving a small number of subjects, show a significant increase in the quantity of free mercaptopurine in the urine when allopurinol was administered concurrently with mercaptopurine (5–7). Some evidence indicates that intravenously administered mercaptopurine does not require a reduction in dosage as does the orally administered mercaptopurine with allopurinol (9). However, until the pharmacokinetics and the clinical outcome of the mercaptopurine–allopurinol interaction are elucidated fully, the current practice of reducing the mercaptopurine dosage should continue when allopurinol is administered concurrently.

Recommendations—The initial dose of mercaptopurine should be reduced to one-third or one-fourth of the presently recommended dosage level when allopurinol (200–300 mg po) is administered concurrently (5). Subsequent adjustments of mercaptopurine dosages should be made on the basis of clinical response and/or toxicity.

References

(1) "The Pharmacological Basis of Therapeutics," 5th ed., L. S. Goodman and A. Gilman, Eds., Macmillan, New York, NY 10022, 1975, p. 1283.

(2) G. B. Elion et al., "The Fate of 6-Mercaptopurine in Mice," Ann. N.Y. Acad. Sci., 60, 297 (1954).

(3) L. Hamilton and G. B. Elion, "The Fate of 6-Mercaptopurine in Man," Ann. N.Y. Acad. Sci., 60, 304 (1954).

(4) G. B. Elion et al., "Relationship between Metabolic Fates and Antitumor Activities of Thiopurines," Cancer Res., 23, 1207 (1963).

(5) R. W. Rundles et al., "Effects of a Xanthine Oxidase Inhibitor on Thiopurine Metabolism, Hyperuricemia and Gout," Trans. Ass. Amer. Physician, 76, 126 (1963).

(6) G. H. Hitchings, "Summary of Informal Discussion on the Role of Purine Antagonists," Cancer Res., 23, 1218 (1963).

(7) W. R. Vogler et al., "Metabolic and Therapeutic Effects of Allopurinol in Patients with Leukemia and Gout," Amer. J. Med., 40, 548 (1966).

(8) A. S. Levine et al., "Combination Therapy with 6-Mercaptopurine (NSC-755) and Allopurinol (NSC-1390) during Induction and Maintenance of Remission of Acute Leukemia in Children," Cancer Chemother. Rep., 53, 53 (1969).

(9) J. J. Coffey et al., "Effect of Allopurinol on the Pharmacokinetics of 6-Mercaptopurine (NSC 755) in Cancer Patients," Cancer Res., 32, 1283 (1972).

[For additional information, see Antineoplastic Therapy, p. 395.]

Nonproprietary and Trade Names of Drugs

Allopurinol—*Zyloprim*
Azathioprine—*Imuran*
Mercaptopurine—*Purinethol*

Thioguanine—*Available under nonproprietary name*

Prepared and evaluated by the Scientific Review Subpanel on Antineoplastic Agents and reviewed by Practitioner Panel VI.

Methotrexate—Aspirin

Summary—Limited clinical data suggest that the concurrent administration of methotrexate and aspirin may result in elevated and/or prolonged serum levels of free methotrexate which may increase the potential for methotrexate toxicity. Administration of aspirin should be avoided in patients receiving methotrexate when an acceptable alternative drug is available.

Related Drugs—All **salicylates** and **salicylamide** and **their combination products** should be expected to interact with methotrexate.

Pharmacological Effect and Mechanism—The interaction between methotrexate and aspirin may occur by two different mechanisms acting simultaneously. Methotrexate and aspirin are bound to plasma proteins by approximately the same amount (70%) (1, 2). Aspirin and other protein-bound drugs, in concentrations 50–500 times that of methotrexate, are capable of displacing methotrexate from plasma proteins *in vitro* (3). Methotrexate and aspirin (or its metabolites) are excreted primarily by the kidney *via* a combination of glomerular filtration and active tubular secretion (2, 4). Because of this common elimination pathway, aspirin competes with and inhibits the renal secretion of methotrexate, resulting in an increase in the serum methotrexate level and half-life (2).

Since methotrexate has a narrow therapeutic index and causes serious adverse reactions [*e.g.*, leukopenia, gastrointestinal (GI) bleeding, oral lesions, renal impairment, and skin eruptions] (5, 6), the increase, however small, in the serum levels and the half-life of methotrexate caused by aspirin may precipitate these toxic effects. Several reports suggest that the duration of exposure may influence methotrexate toxicity more than concentration because continuous low-dose therapy is more toxic than intermittent therapy at higher doses (4, 7, 8).

Evaluation of Clinical Data—The effects of sodium salicylate on plasma protein binding and renal excretion were measured in a controlled trial of 15 patients with disseminated malignancies who were treated with methotrexate (5–15 mg/day iv) (2). Methotrexate clearance was reduced 35% (mean) when an intravenous infusion of sodium salicylate was added to the regimen. Interpretation of these results is difficult because the influence of other drugs in the regimen was not evaluated. Also, the results were not analyzed statistically.

Aspirin was suggested as contributing to methotrexate toxicity in two patients described in another report (9). However, the conditions were not well controlled and a causal relationship between methotrexate and aspirin toxicity was not definitely established.

■ Although the clinical evidence is limited, there are sufficient data to suggest that concurrent administration of aspirin may increase the serum level and the half-life of methotrexate and may precipitate toxic reactions to the antineoplastic drug. There is no clinical evidence to indicate that a change in the administration schedule of methotrexate lessens the influence of concurrent aspirin administration.

Recommendations—Because methotrexate has a narrow therapeutic index and even a small increase in its serum level and/or half-life may produce serious toxic reactions, it would be prudent to avoid concurrent use of aspirin if alternative drugs are available. If the drugs must be given concurrently, the patients should be observed closely for any symptoms of methotrexate toxicity (2, 6). Particular attention should be given to patients with renal impairment.

Acetaminophen and indomethacin have been used concurrently with methotrexate in psoriatic patients without causing methotrexate toxicity (10). Although acetaminophen may be used instead of aspirin for analgesia and antipyresis, indomethacin has a high incidence of side effects (11) and may not be a desirable alternative to aspirin.

References

(1) "The Pharmacological Basis of Therapeutics," 5th ed., L. S. Goodman and A. Gilman, Eds., Macmillan, New York, NY 10022, 1975, pp. 326–339.

(2) D. G. Liegler *et al.*, "The Effect of Organic Acids on Renal Clearance of Methotrexate in Man," *Clin. Pharmacol. Ther.*, 10, 849 (1969).

(3) R. L. Dixon *et al.*, "Plasma Protein Binding of Methotrexate and Its Displacement by Various Drugs," abstract, *Fed. Proc.*, 24, 454 (1965).

(4) G. Levy, "Pharmacokinetics of Salicylate Elimination in Man," *J. Pharm. Sci.*, 54, 959 (1965).

(5) H. B. Baden and M. M. Pugliese, "Psoriasis," *Disease-a-Month*, September 1973, pp. 30–34.

(6) I. C. D. Douglas and L. A. Price, "Bone-Marrow Toxicity of Methotrexate: A Reassessment," *Brit. J. Haematol.*, 24, 625 (1973).

(7) J. H. Goldie *et al.*, "Methotrexate Toxicity: Correlation with Duration of Administration, Plasma Levels, Dose and Excretion Pattern," *Eur. J. Cancer*, 8, 409 (1972).

(8) D. H. Huffman *et al.*, "Pharmacokinetics of Methotrexate," *Clin. Pharmacol. Ther.*, 14, 572 (1973).

(9) H. Baker, "Intermittent High Dose Oral Methotrexate Therapy in Psoriasis," *Brit. J. Dermatol.*, 82, 65 (1970).

(10) M. G. Dahl *et al.*, "Methotrexate Hepatotoxicity in Psoriasis—Comparison of Different Dosage Regimens," *Brit. Med. J.*, 1, 654 (1972).

(11) G. L. Bach, "Adverse Reactions of Antirheumatic Drugs," *Int. J. Clin. Pharmacol.*, 7, 198 (1973).

[For additional information, see *Antineoplastic Therapy*, p. 395.]

Nonproprietary and Trade Names of Drugs

Acetaminophen—*Datril, Nebs, SK-APAP, Tempra, Tenlap, Tylenol, Valadrol, and various combination products*
Aluminum aspirin—*Available in combination products*
Aspirin—*Available alone or as a fixed combination in many trade name products, especially over-the-counter preparations*
Carbethyl salicylate—*Sal-Ethyl Carbonate*

Choline salicylate—*Actasal, Arthropan*
Indomethacin—*Indocin*
Magnesium salicylate—*Various manufacturers*
Methotrexate—*Available under nonproprietary name*
Potassium salicylate—*Various manufacturers*
Salicylamide—*Various manufacturers*
Sodium salicylate—*Various manufacturers*

Prepared and evaluated by the Scientific Review Subpanel on Antineoplastic Agents and reviewed by Practitioner Panel I.

Methotrexate—Cytarabine

Summary—Cytarabine enhances the cell-kill effects of methotrexate when administered 48 hr before initiation of methotrexate therapy. Conversely, methotrexate enhances the cell-kill effects of cytarabine when administered at least 10 min before initiation of cytarabine therapy. Methotrexate also has antagonized the effects of cytarabine *in vitro* and in animals but not in humans. However, the data to support the synergistic or antagonistic effects of concurrent use of these drugs are inconclusive. The routine parameters used to evaluate antineoplastic therapy (*e.g.*, percent of immature and abnormal cell forms in the bone marrow) would be the best method to determine the unpredictable clinical outcome of concurrent use of these drugs.

Related Drugs—There are no drugs related to cytarabine or methotrexate commercially available in the United States.

Pharmacological Effect and Mechanism—The mechanism of interaction is dependent upon which drug is administered first, the time interval between the administration of the two drugs, and the complexities of the enzymes and substrates in each patient. Because of the latter, the interaction may vary from patient to patient.

Methotrexate, through its inhibitory action on dihydrofolate reductase, prevents the conversion of deoxyuridylate (dUMP) to deoxythymidylate (dTMP) (1). This inhibition results in accumulation of deoxycytidine triphosphate (dCTP), a substrate for DNA polymerase. Cytarabine, following metabolism to the 5-triphosphate derivative, acts by inhibiting DNA polymerase (1, 2) and is antagonized by the excess substrate (dCTP) produced by methotrexate (1).

Results in L-5178Y lymphoma cells showed strong antagonism when the two drugs were administered at the same time and when methotrexate preceded cytarabine by 6 hr (1). Only slight antagonism occurred when cytarabine was added to the cell culture first and methotrexate was added 6 hr later. A similar result was reported in mice with TLX/5 lymphoma (3).

After the administration of cytarabine *in vivo,* the subsequent administration of methotrexate 48 hr later resulted in significant cell kill (4, 5). This result suggested that cytarabine increases the susceptibility of leukemic cells to subsequent cycle-active (*e.g.,* methotrexate) drugs by increasing the relative growth fraction (6).

Other reports (7, 8) showed that cytarabine killed a larger fraction of cells pretreated with methotrexate. It is postulated that pretreatment with methotrexate sensitizes cells to the action of cytarabine, resulting in a synergistic effect on cell death (8). Methotrexate pretreatment affects the distribution of cytarabine by increasing its phosphorylation. The higher levels of cytarabine nucleosides may increase the incorporation of cytarabine into the DNA fraction and increase the inhibition of DNA polymerase, thereby resulting in enhanced cell death.

Evaluation of Clinical Data—Cytarabine (5 mg/kg/week iv) and methotrexate (1 mg/kg/week iv) were studied in two patients with acute lymphoblastic leukemia, one patient with acute myeloblastic leukemia, and one patient with leukemic transformation of lymphosarcoma (5). Methotrexate was administered 48 hr after cytarabine. These cycles of cytarabine and methotrexate were repeated at weekly intervals; the dose of methotrexate was increased by 1 mg/kg/week.

After three cycles of therapy, one patient with acute lymphoblastic leukemia had a complete remission and remained in remission upon evaluation 18 months later. No remission after similar treatment was seen in the other patient with acute lymphoblastic leukemia and patients with acute myeloblastic leukemia or lymphosarcoma.

In 12 patients with acute leukemia (6), cytarabine (100 mg/m^2 iv) was administered rapidly followed in 48 hr by methotrexate (50 mg/m^2 po every 6 hr for four doses) and then vincristine (1 mg/m^2 iv). Prednisone (100 mg/m^2 po every day for 1 week) also was administered to patients with acute lymphoblastic leukemia. All patients were evaluated for response by marrow labeling index determinations. Four patients (three with acute myeloblastic leukemia and one with acute lymphoblastic leukemia) had no clinical response. Three patients (one with acute lymphoblastic leukemia and two with acute myeloblastic leukemia) responded with a complete remission; three patients (one with acute lymphoblastic leukemia and two with acute myeloblastic leukemia) responded with partial remission; and two patients with acute myeloblastic leukemia had marked improvement but succumbed to infection.

Twenty-two adult patients with acute myeloblastic leukemia or with acute lymphoblastic leukemia were treated with cyclophosphamide, cytarabine, and methotrexate or cyclophosphamide, cytarabine, methotrexate, and leucovorin, respectively (9). Methotrexate (80 mg/m²) was initially administered as a 24-hr iv infusion. During the first 0.5 hr, cyclophosphamide (1 g/m²) was infused; during the second 0.5 hr, cytarabine (300 mg/m²) was infused concurrently with methotrexate. Leucovorin (25 mg/m² as a 6-hr iv infusion) was administered at the end of the 24-hr methotrexate therapy. Once-weekly cycles were administered until the bone marrow became hypoplastic or until a marrow remission was evident. Then maintenance doses of cyclophosphamide, cytarabine, and methotrexate were administered every 3–4 weeks to both groups. For the patients with acute lymphoblastic leukemia, leucovorin also was administered; in patients with acute myeloblastic leukemia, the doses and routes of the antineoplastic drugs were changed. In either therapeutic regimen, each methotrexate dosage preceded the cytarabine dosage by 10 min. Five of eight patients with acute lymphoblastic leukemia responded with a complete remission lasting 2–14 months. Seven of 14 patients with acute myeloblastic leukemia responded with a complete remission lasting 1–20 months.

Cytarabine (300 mg/m² iv) was given as a rapid injection 16 hr after initiating treatment with methotrexate and leucovorin in 15 patients with advanced reticulum cell sarcoma (10). Allopurinol (100 mg three times daily), cyclophosphamide (1.5 g/m² iv), and vincristine (1.4 mg/m² iv) were administered at different time intervals. Three such cycles were used with 1–2-week intervals between cycles. Nine patients had a complete remission and six had a partial remission after treatment with these drugs. The median survival was 18+ months after chemotherapy was initiated (22 months from diagnosis).

■ Cytarabine enhances the cell-kill effects of methotrexate when administered 48 hr before the initiation of methotrexate therapy (5, 6). Methotrexate enhances the cell-kill effects of cytarabine when administered at least 10 min before initiation of cytarabine therapy (9, 10). However, the clinical data to support these observations are inconclusive. The patient populations tested often were heterogeneous, other antineoplastic drugs were used concurrently, dose and administration time varied, or the results were not statistically analyzed. Methotrexate also has antagonized the effects of cytarabine in animals (3) and *in vitro* (1) but not in humans (9). Until more reliable data are available, the clinical outcome of concurrent use of these drugs cannot be predicted.

Recommendations—Until adequate data are available to evaluate this drug interaction, the following recommendations should be considered when these drugs are used for the treatment of leukemia. If a synergistic effect is desired, cytarabine should be administered 48 hr prior or at least 10 min after the initiation of methotrexate therapy (5, 6, 9, 10).

However, synergism does not occur in all patients (6) and antagonism (1, 3) is also possible. Routine monitoring of antineoplastic therapy (*e.g.*, determining the percent of immature and abnormal cell forms in the bone marrow) would be the best method to determine the unpredictable clinical outcome of concurrent use of these drugs.

References

(1) M. H. N. Tattersall and K. R. Harrap, "Combination Chemotherapy: The Antagonism of Methotrexate and Cytosine Arabinoside," *Eur. J. Cancer, 9,* 229 (1973).

(2) J. J. Furth and S. S. Cohen, "Inhibition of Mammalian DNA Polymerase by the 5′-Triphosphate of 1-β-D-Arabinofuranosylcytosine and the 5′-Triphosphate of 9-β-D-Arabinofuranosyladenine," *Cancer Res., 28,* 2061 (1968).

(3) M. H. N. Tattersall *et al.*, "Interaction of Methotrexate and Cytosine Arabinoside," *Lancet, ii*, 1378 (1972).

(4) A. M. Mauer *et al.*, "Effects of Chemotherapeutic Agents on Cell Cycle and Cellular Proliferation: Basic and Clinical Considerations," *Transplant. Proc., 5*, 1181 (1973).

(5) B. C. Lampkin *et al.*, "Synchronization and Recruitment in Acute Leukemia," *J. Clin. Invest., 50*, 2204 (1971).

(6) L. E. Cooper *et al.*, "The Effect of Drug-Induced Alteration of the Growth Fraction on the Clinical Response in Adult Acute Leukemia," abstract, *Clin. Res., 19*, 38 (1971).

(7) M.-Y. Chu and G. A. Fischer, "Effects of Cytosine Arabinoside on the Cell Viability and Uptake of Deoxypyrimidine Nucleosides in L5178Y Cells," *Biochem. Pharmacol., 17*, 741 (1968).

(8) M. L. Hoovis and M.-Y. Chu, "Enhancement of the Antiproliferative Action of 1-β-D-Arabinofuranosylcytosine by Methotrexate in Murine Leukemic Cells (L5178Y)," *Cancer Res., 33*, 521 (1973).

(9) R. T. Skeel *et al.*, "Development of a Combination Chemotherapy Program for Adult Acute Leukemia: CAM and CAM-L," *Cancer, 32*, 76 (1973).

(10) M. Levitt *et al.*, "Combination Sequential Chemotherapy in Advanced Reticulum Cell Sarcoma," *Cancer, 29*, 630 (1972).

[For additional information, see *Antineoplastic Therapy*, p. 395.]

Nonproprietary and Trade Names of Drugs

Cytarabine—*Cytosar*

Methotrexate—*Available under nonproprietary name*

Prepared and evaluated by the Scientific Review Subpanel on Antineoplastic Agents and reviewed by Practitioner Panel II.

Methotrexate—Leucovorin

Summary—Animal and human studies indicate that the toxicity of methotrexate and other folic acid antagonists may be reduced, without an equivalent reduction in therapeutic response, by the consecutive (within 6 hr) administration of leucovorin (leucovorin rescue). However, simultaneous administration of these two drugs may offset this benefit.

Related Drugs—Any folic acid antagonist that inhibits the action of dihydrofolate reductase probably will act in a manner similar to methotrexate.

Pharmacological Effect and Mechanism—Methotrexate is a folic acid antagonist that combines with dihydrofolate reductase, thereby blocking folate metabolism. The synthesis of thymidylic acid from deoxyuridylic acid, which requires tetrahydrofolate ordinarily supplied by the metabolism of folic acid, is thus blocked, causing an inhibition of nucleic acid synthesis necessary for cell replication. Rapidly proliferating cells characteristically present in diseases such as cancer, pemphigus vulgaris, and psoriasis are more adversely affected than normally proliferating cells. Normal cellular reproduction is also affected and accounts for many of the typical side effects of these drugs such as bone marrow depression, gastrointestinal (GI) disturbances, and stomatitis (1, 2).

Leucovorin (*N*-5-formyltetrahydrofolic acid) is an active metabolite of folic acid. Leucovorin supplies tetrahydrofolate, which bypasses the dihydrofolate reductase enzymatic step, and negates the effect of methotrexate. This action allows nucleic acid synthesis and other biochemical processes to resume (3). The consecutive administration of leucovorin 6 hr or less after methotrexate limits the duration of action of methotrexate and "rescues" normal cells that are not yet irreversibly damaged.

Several animal studies (4–7) appear to confirm this mechanism. These reports also indicate that the simultaneous administration of methotrexate and leucovorin may reduce the therapeutic response of methotrexate as well as the toxicity.

Evaluation of Clinical Data—Methotrexate therapy combined with leucovorin rescue is effective in several clinical disorders including cancer of the head and neck (8), acute leukemia (9, 10), and osteogenic sarcoma (11). Three studies (3, 9, 10) reported only mild and infrequent toxic side effects with intermittent infusions of methotrexate followed immediately by leucovorin in the treatment of acute leukemia.

Methotrexate (up to 3 mg/kg), administered as a 24-hr infusion for the treatment of head and neck cancers, followed immediately by the administration of leucovorin resulted in reduced toxicity of methotrexate (12). Another study (13) of head and neck epidermoid cancers reported improvement in the therapeutic index of high-dose methotrexate using leucovorin rescue. Leucovorin was initiated immediately after completion of a 36–42-hr infusion of methotrexate.

A study (14) of oral methotrexate for the treatment of psoriasis reported a high incidence of mouth ulcerations. This problem usually could be overcome by administering methotrexate intramuscularly followed 2 hr later by leucovorin intramuscularly. Leucovorin did not appear to interfere with the beneficial effects of methotrexate on psoriatic epidermis. The psoriatic skin lesions continued to clear despite the addition of leucovorin, and mouth ulcerations were eliminated.

An attempt to use leucovorin rescue in 10 patients with severe psoriasis, who had been successfully treated with methotrexate, resulted in increased psoriatic activity (15). Administration of leucovorin at intervals of 24–72 hr after the administration of methotrexate produced exacerbation of the psoriasis. Unlike the other studies, leucovorin was administered orally and the interval between drug administrations was much greater.

By administering leucovorin 0.5–3 hr after injection of methotrexate, the immunosuppressive action of methotrexate in the treatment of pemphigus vulgaris was maintained in a majority of patients with a reduction in mouth lesions and GI symptoms (16).

■ The clinical evidence strongly suggests that leucovorin reverses methotrexate-induced inhibition of folic acid antagonism. Beneficial results in some diseases, in the form of reduced toxicity and an improved therapeutic index of methotrexate, may be obtained by intramuscular or intravenous administration of methotrexate followed by intramuscular leucovorin (3, 8–11, 17). Results of oral administration are not so conclusive (14, 15). The optimal interval between the administration of the two drugs has not been determined, although best results were obtained with an interval of 6 hr or less (18). Effective doses of leucovorin have not been firmly established, but they appear to be in the 4–12-mg range. Methotrexate may be used successfully in a higher dose range (up to 600 mg/kg) when consecutive leucovorin administration is used (18). However, the usual methotrexate dose when given with leucovorin is 50–300 mg/kg (18). The simultaneous administration of methotrexate and leucovorin results in decreased toxicity of methotrexate (14, 17), but evidence obtained from animal studies indicates that this may be accompanied by a decrease in the therapeutic activity of the antineoplastic drug (4–7).

Recommendations—Methotrexate and leucovorin therapy should be used in consecutive (6 hr or less) fashion rather than simultaneously. The usual monitoring of methotrexate therapy must be continued.

References

(1) "The Pharmacological Basis of Therapeutics," 5th ed., L. S. Goodman and A. Gilman, Eds., Macmillan, New York, NY 10022, 1975, pp. 1269–1270.

(2) J. R. Bertino, "The Mechanism of Action of the Folate Antagonists in Man," *Cancer Res.*, *23*, 1286 (1963).

(3) M. S. Mitchell *et al.*, "Effectiveness of High-Dose Infusions of Methotrexate followed by Leucovorin in Carcinoma of the Head and Neck," *Cancer Res., 28*, 1088 (1968).

(4) J. S. Sandberg and A. Goldin, "The Use of Leucovorin Orally in Normal and Leukemic L1210 Mice to Prevent the Toxicity and Gastrointestinal Lesions Caused by High Doses of Methotrexate," *Cancer Res., 30*, 1276 (1970).

(5) A. Goldin *et al.*, "Eradication of Leukaemic Cells (L1210) by Methotrexate and Methotrexate plus Citrovorum Factor," *Nature, 212*, 1548 (1966).

(6) G. P. Canellos *et al.*, "The Effect of Treatment with Cytotoxic Agents on Mouse Spleen Dihydrofolate Reductase Activity," *Cancer Res., 27*, 784 (1967).

(7) W. M. Abbott *et al.*, "The Effect of Supralethal Amethopterin and Folinic Acid Rescue on Mouse Skin Allograft Survival," *Proc. Soc. Exp. Biol. Med., 136*, 510 (1971).

(8) R. L. Capizzi *et al.*, "Methotrexate Therapy of Head and Neck Cancer: Improvement in Therapeutic Index by the Use of Leucovorin 'Rescue'," *Cancer Res., 30*, 1782 (1970).

(9) I. Djerassi *et al.*, "Long-Term Remissions in Childhood Acute Leukemia: Use of Infrequent Infusions of Methotrexate; Supportive Roles of Platelet Transfusions and Citrovorum Factor," *Clin. Pediat., 5*, 502 (1966).

(10) W. M. Hryniuk and J. R. Bertino, "Treatment of Leukemia with Large Doses of Methotrexate and Folinic Acid: Clinical-Biochemical Correlates," *J. Clin. Invest., 48*, 2140 (1969).

(11) N. Jaffe, "Progress Report on High-Dose Methotrexate (NSC-740) with Citrovorum Rescue in the Treatment of Metastatic Bone Tumors," *Cancer Chemother. Rep., 58*, 275 (1974).

(12) E. Lefkowitz *et al.*, "Head and Neck Cancer III. Toxicity of 24-Hour Infusions of Methotrexate (NSC-740) and Protection by Leucovorin (NSC-3590) in Patients with Epidermoid Carcinomas," *Cancer Chemother. Rep., 51*, 305 (1967).

(13) M. Levitt *et al.*, "Improved Therapeutic Index of Methotrexate with 'Leucovorin Rescue'," *Cancer Res., 33*, 1729 (1973).

(14) H. H. Roenigk, Jr., *et al.*, "Methotrexate for Psoriasis in Weekly Oral Doses," *Arch. Dermatol., 99*, 86 (1969).

(15) A. P. Cipriano *et al.*, "Failure of Leucovorin 'Rescue' in Methotrexate Treatment of Psoriasis," *Arch. Dermatol., 101*, 651 (1970).

(16) S. M. Peck *et al.*, "Studies in Bullous Diseases. Treatment of Pemphigus Vulgaris with Immunosuppressives (Steroids and Methotrexate) and Leucovorin Calcium," *Arch. Dermatol., 103*, 141 (1971).

(17) F. A. Ive and C. F. W. De Saram, "Methotrexate and the Citrovorum Factor in the Treatment of Psoriasis," *Trans. St. Johns Hosp. Dermatol. Soc., 56*, 45 (1970).

(18) J. S. Penta, "Overview of Protocols on Clinical Studies of High-Dose Methotrexate (NSC-740) with Citrovorum Factor (NSC-3590) Rescue," *Cancer Chemother. Rep., part 3, 6*, 7 (1975).

[For additional information, see *Antineoplastic Therapy*, p. 395.]

Nonproprietary and Trade Names of Drugs

Leucovorin—*Available under nonproprietary name*

Methotrexate—*Available under nonproprietary name*

Prepared and evaluated by the Scientific Review Subpanel on Antineoplastic Agents and reviewed by Practitioner Panel IV.

Methotrexate—Sulfisoxazole

Summary—Methotrexate plasma protein binding is decreased by the administration of sulfisoxazole and other oral sulfonamides; this decreased binding may result in methotrexate toxicity from increased serum levels of free methotrexate. Although the clinical effects of this drug interaction have not been determined, the patient should be observed closely for unexpected symptoms of methotrexate toxicity.

Related Drugs—Because of the similarities in protein binding, all **oral sulfonamides** alone or in combination products may enhance the serum levels of unbound methotrexate to varying degrees.

Pharmacological Effect and Mechanism—Methotrexate is approximately 50% bound to plasma proteins (1). Therefore, displacement from its binding sites can be clinically important, particularly since the therapeutic dosage levels are very close to the toxic levels. *In vitro* studies (2, 3) showed that several types of drugs (aminobenzoic acid, salicylates, and sulfonamides) compete for plasma protein binding sites with methotrexate, leading to a decrease in bound methotrexate. Theoretically, the decrease in bound methotrexate and the subsequent increase in serum methotrexate levels should increase biological effects.

Evaluation of Clinical Data—There are no published reports of methotrexate toxicity due to its displacement from binding sites by sulfonamides. The only human study (4) involved six patients and showed that intravenous sulfisoxazole infusions (2–4 g initially, then 33–66 mg/min) decreased plasma-bound methotrexate in four patients by an average of 28% (22, 22, 42, and 26%) and had negligible effects on the remaining two patients. However, the clinical effects of the drug interaction were not studied. A minor inhibitory effect on the renal tubular secretion of methotrexate also was shown. No statements on toxicity were made in the study. There are no studies concerning the effects of orally administered sulfonamides on methotrexate plasma protein binding.

■ No reports of toxicity directly attributable to concurrent use of methotrexate and sulfisoxazole (or any other sulfonamide) have been published. However, from a theoretical standpoint, enhanced methotrexate toxicity due to increased free drug in the plasma could occur.

Recommendations—Concurrent administration of methotrexate and sulfisoxazole (or any other sulfonamide) should be approached with an awareness that enhanced methotrexate toxicity might occur.

References

(1) "The Pharmacological Basis of Therapeutics," 5th ed., L. S. Goodman and A. Gilman, Eds., Macmillan, New York, NY 10022, 1975, p. 1271.
(2) R. L. Dixon *et al.*, "Plasma Protein Binding of Methotrexate and Its Displacement by Various Drugs," *Fed. Proc.*, *24*, 454 (1965).
(3) B. B. Brodie, "Displacement of One Drug by Another from Carrier or Receptor Sites," *Proc. Roy. Soc. Med.*, *58*, 946 (1965).
(4) D. G. Liegler *et al.*, "The Effect of Organic Acids on Renal Clearance of Methotrexate in Man," *Clin. Pharmacol. Ther.*, *10*, 849 (1969).

[For additional information, see *Antineoplastic Therapy*, p. 395, and *Methotrexate–Aspirin*, p. 150.]

Nonproprietary and Trade Names of Drugs

Methotrexate—*Available under nonproprietary name*
Sulfadiazine—*Various manufacturers*
Sulfameter—*Sulla*
Sulfamethazine—*Various combination products*

Sulfamethizole—*Thiosulfil*
Sulfamethoxazole—*Bactrim, Gantanol, Septra*
Sulfamethoxypyridazine—*Midicel*
Sulfaphenazole—*Orisul, Sulfabid*
Sulfisoxazole—*Gantrisin, SK-Soxazole*

Prepared and evaluated by the Scientific Review Subpanel on Antineoplastic Agents and reviewed by Practitioner Panel V.

Metronidazole—Alcohol

Summary—Because well-controlled studies have not substantiated a reported mild "disulfiram-like" effect (*e.g.,* facial flushing, headache, nausea, and sweating) with metronidazole following alcohol ingestion, the likelihood of this drug interaction occurring is remote. However, the patient should be advised of the possible effects of this drug interaction when alcohol is ingested during metronidazole therapy.

Related Drugs—There are no drugs commercially available that are chemically and pharmacologically related to metronidazole.

Pharmacological Effect and Mechanism—Metronidazole is a trichomonicide that may be useful in the treatment of alcoholism by decreasing the individual's desire for alcohol and making alcohol ingestion unpleasant. This effect possibly is associated with a disulfiram-like reaction. If a disulfiram-like reaction occurs, the mechanism may be similar to that of disulfiram itself, *i.e.,* due to inhibition of the enzyme aldehyde dehydrogenase. *In vitro* studies (1–3) showed that metronidazole produces an inhibition of aldehyde dehydrogenase and other alcohol-oxidizing enzymes. However, a study in rats failed to substantiate the results of the *in vitro* studies (4).

Evaluation of Clinical Data—While studying the side effects of metronidazole in the treatment of trichomoniasis, an alteration in the drinking patterns of some patients was noted (5). Later, a study of 52 alcoholics was reported (5) in whom there appeared to be decreased tolerance for alcohol, decreased compulsion to obtain it, and a mild to moderate disulfiram-like reaction to alcohol.

Early clinical reports and studies of metronidazole (400–500 mg/day) have been contradictory. In one study (6), metronidazole produced a decreased tolerance for alcohol and adverse reactions such as nausea, headache, and increased sweating or flushing on challenge drinking trials. However, a double-blind crossover study (7) did not find significant drug effects on blood pressure, pulse rate, or subjective reports of autonomic side effects to a challenge drink. In addition, several other well-controlled studies (8, 9) evaluating metronidazole in the treatment of outpatient alcoholics also failed to find side effects in patients who resume drinking.

A study of the effects of metronidazole on 12 carefully selected alcoholic subjects failed to confirm either a decrease in the desire to drink or a disulfiram-like reaction to alcohol (10). In this study, of two subjects who reported mild disulfiram-like reactions with alcohol, one continued to experience this reaction when switched to placebo treatment.

In another double-blind study of metronidazole in 169 outpatient alcoholics (11), no evidence was found that metronidazole decreased craving for alcohol or produced mild disulfiram-like side effects in patients who resumed drinking.

Two additional controlled studies (12, 13), one investigating metronidazole (500 mg/day po) in the treatment of alcoholism and the other studying the effect of metronidazole (1 g/day) on social drinkers, found no unusual toxicities in most subjects when metronidazole and alcohol were given concurrently. However, some social drinkers reported a bitter taste to alcohol or no desire to drink (12). This difference was not statistically significant.

■ Although earlier reports seem to indicate the possibility of a disulfiram-like reaction in patients ingesting metronidazole and alcohol, more recent double-blind studies have not documented its existence. In the absence of evidence to the contrary, it must be assumed that this interaction is infrequent and not clinically significant.

Recommendations—Adverse effects of concurrent ingestion of metronidazole and alcohol are infrequent. The possibility exists, however, that a mild disulfiram-like effect (*e.g.*, facial flushing, headache, nausea, and sweating) may occur infrequently in some patients. Therefore, the patient should be advised about these effects in the event that alcohol might be ingested during metronidazole therapy.

References

(1) J. A. Edwards and J. Price, "Metronidazole and Atypical Human Alcohol Dehydrogenase," *Biochem. Pharmacol.*, *16*, 2026 (1967).

(2) R. Fried and L. W. Fried, "The Effect of Flagyl on Xanthine Oxidase and Alcohol Dehydrogenase," *Biochem. Pharmacol.*, *15*, 1890 (1966).

(3) E. Paltrinieri, "Inhibitory Action on Alcohol-Dehydrogenase by Hydroxy-2'-ethyl-1-methyl-2-nitro-5-imidazole," *Farmaco, Ed. Sci.*, *22*, 1054 (1967).

(4) H. Kalant et al., "Metabolic and Pharmacologic Interaction of Ethanol and Metronidazole in the Rat," *Can. J. Physiol. Pharmacol.*, *50*, 476 (1972).

(5) J. T. Taylor, "Metronidazole—A New Agent for Combined Somatic and Psychic Therapy of Alcoholism," *Bull. Los Angeles Neurol. Soc.*, *29*, 158 (1964).

(6) H. E. Lehmann et al., "Metronidazole in the Treatment of the Alcoholic," *Psychiat. Neurol.*, *152*, 395 (1966).

(7) M. C. Gelder and G. Edwards, "Metronidazole in the Treatment of Alcohol Addiction. A Controlled Trial," *Brit. J. Psychiat.*, *114*, 473 (1968).

(8) W. P. Egan and R. Goetz, "Effect of Metronidazole on Drinking by Alcoholics," *Quart. J. Stud. Alc.*, *29*, 899 (1968).

(9) D. M. Dallant et al., "A Six-Month Controlled Evaluation of Metronidazole in Chronic Alcoholic Patients," *Curr. Ther. Res.*, *10*, 82 (1968).

(10) D. W. Goodwin, "Metronidazole in the Treatment of Alcoholism: A Negative Report," *Amer. J. Psychiat.*, *123*, 1276 (1967).

(11) A. Platz et al., "Metronidazole and Alcoholism. (An Evaluation of Specific and Nonspecific Factors in Drug Treatment)," *Dis. Nerv. Syst.*, *31*, 631 (1970).

(12) H. D. Strassman et al., "Metronidazole Effect on Social Drinkers," *Quart. J. Stud. Alc.*, *31*, 394 (1970).

(13) I. Lowenstein, "Metronidazole and Placebo in the Treatment of Chronic Alcoholism," *Psychosomatics*, *10*, 43 (1970).

[For additional information, see *Anti-Infective Therapy*, p. 388.]

Nonproprietary and Trade Names of Drugs

Alcohol—*Various products and beverages*   Metronidazole—*Flagyl*

Prepared and evaluated by the Scientific Review Subpanel on Anti-Infectives and reviewed by Practitioner Panel VI.

Nitrofurantoin—Probenecid

Summary—Concurrent administration of probenecid, particularly in high doses, decreases the renal clearance of nitrofurantoin and increases the serum level of the anti-infective drug. The drug interaction may lead to nitrofurantoin-induced toxicity (*e.g.*, polyneuropathies) or decreased nitrofurantoin efficacy as a urinary tract anti-infective agent. Therefore, concurrent administration of these drugs should be avoided whenever possible.

Related Drugs—Uricosuric agents such as **sulfinpyrazone** may have an effect on nitrofurantoin excretion similar to that of probenecid (1).

Pharmacological Effect and Mechanism—The immediate effects of decreased renal clearance of nitrofurantoin would be the systemic accumulation of the drug and a decreased effectiveness in urinary tract infections due to lower urine nitrofurantoin levels.

Renal tubular secretion of nitrofurantoin and its apparent inhibition by probenecid were demonstrated in dogs and chickens (2). In view of clinical reports of high urine levels and extremely low serum levels of nitrofurantoin, tubular secretion of nitrofurantoin was thought to occur in humans. The interference of probenecid with nitrofurantoin excretion was subsequently reported in humans (3), thus confirming the earlier supposition regarding nitrofurantoin excretion.

Evaluation of Clinical Data—Although therapeutic doses of nitrofurantoin result in extremely low serum levels (about 1 μg/ml or less), urine levels are attained well in excess of the minimum inhibitory concentrations required for the eradication of susceptible urinary tract infections (3, 4). The only clinical data (3) involving the concurrent administration of nitrofurantoin and probenecid demonstrated (a) a 33–66% reduction of nitrofurantoin urinary excretion, depending upon the size of the dose of probenecid employed; (b) an inability to achieve effective urine antibacterial levels; and (c) an increase in serum levels to concentrations greater than 2 μg/ml.

■ The effect of probenecid upon the systemic accumulation of nitrofurantoin should be considered in view of the fact that elevated serum levels of nitrofurantoin appear to be associated with the onset of polyneuropathies, including degeneration of sensory and motor nerves (3, 5, 6). Decreased renal clearance produces urine nitrofurantoin levels which fall below the minimum inhibitory concentration required for control of susceptible urinary tract infections (3).

The significance of this interaction is difficult to determine for several reasons. First, other than the one study (3), no other reports of a nitrofurantoin–probenecid interaction in clinical practice have appeared. Second, the lower doses of probenecid frequently used in clinical practice would not exert as great an effect on nitrofurantoin excretion and systemic accumulation as the doses of 500–1000 mg every 2 hr used experimentally (3).

An additional factor for consideration involves renal dysfunction. Systemic accumulation and decreased urinary excretion of nitrofurantoin occurred in patients in whom serum creatinine levels were greater than about 2.5–3 mg% (normal, 0.6–1.2 mg%) (3). Thus, patients with decreased renal efficiency may not be good candidates for nitrofurantoin therapy.

Recommendations—Drugs, such as probenecid, that interfere with the renal clearance of nitrofurantoin may decrease the effectiveness of nitrofurantoin (as a urinary tract anti-infective agent) if given in sufficiently high doses. An increase in nitrofurantoin dosage in an attempt to enhance urine levels would only serve to increase the likelihood of systemic accumulation and the adverse effects associated with increased serum levels. Thus, concurrent administration of these drugs should be avoided whenever possible.

References

(1) J. Schirmeister et al., "Renal Handling of Nitrofurantoin in Man," Antimicrob. Ag. Chemother., 5, 223 (1966).

(2) J. A. Buzard et al., "Renal Tubular Transport of Nitrofurantoin," Amer. J. Physiol., 202, 1136 (1962).

(3) R. Hubmann and G. Bremer, "Die Ausscheidung von Furadantin bei Manifester Niereninsuffizienz," Med. Welt., 19, 1039 (1965).

(4) J. D. Conklin and F. J. Hailey, "Urinary Drug Excretion in Man during Oral Dosage of Different Nitrofurantoin Formulations," Clin. Pharmacol. Ther., 10, 534 (1969).

(5) M. Hoyest and E. Zachara, "A Case of Polyneuritis during Long-Term Treatment with Nitrofurantoin," *Pol. Tyg. Lek.*, *23*, 1978 (1968); through *FDA Clin. Experience Abstr.*, *29*, 469 (1970).

(6) "The Pharmacological Basis of Therapeutics," 5th ed., L. S. Goodman and A. Gilman, Eds., Macmillan, New York, NY 10022, 1975, p. 1008.

[For additional information, see *Anti-Infective Therapy*, p. 388.]

Nonproprietary and Trade Names of Drugs

Nitrofurantoin—*Furachel, Furadantin, Macrodantin, Trantoin*

Probenecid—*Benemid*
Sulfinpyrazone—*Anturane*

Prepared and evaluated by the Scientific Review Subpanel on Anti-Infectives and reviewed by Practitioner Panel II.

Nortriptyline—Phenobarbital

Summary—Some data indicate that phenobarbital and other barbiturates may decrease the serum level of nortriptyline and other tricyclic antidepressants. Although the therapeutic effect caused by the decreased serum level was not measured, phenobarbital or other barbiturates may be a causative factor in barbiturate-treated patients who are unresponsive to tricyclic antidepressants.

Related Drugs—In addition to nortriptyline, this interaction has been reported to occur with **desipramine** (1). **Amobarbital** (2, 3), **pentobarbital** (4), and **secobarbital** (4) have been shown to interact in a similar manner to phenobarbital, but the data are limited and unreliable. Although not documented, it is likely that a similar interaction occurs between all other **barbiturates** and **tricyclic antidepressants.**

Pharmacological Effect and Mechanism—Tricyclic antidepressants enhanced the actions of barbiturates in animals by inhibiting the enzyme system responsible for barbiturate metabolism (5). This effect has not been observed in humans (6). Other reports suggest that barbiturates stimulate the metabolism of tricyclic antidepressants (1–4).

Evaluation of Clinical Data—The clinical reports about this drug interaction primarily concern decreased serum levels of tricyclic antidepressants. In one report (1), a 50% decrease in the steady-state serum level of desipramine was found in a patient receiving phenobarbital (100 mg po) as a night medication for 14 days.

In a study of serum nortriptyline levels (4), one twin in each of five sets of twins (two identical and three fraternal) was treated with a barbiturate (pentobarbital, 50 mg/day po; phenobarbital, 45–130 mg/day po; or secobarbital, 150 mg/day po) and had considerably lower serum nortriptyline levels (approximately 30% lower) than the nonbarbiturate-treated twin (personal communication, F. Sjoqvist, Karolinska Institute, Huddinge, Sweden). Another pair of identical twins both receiving barbiturates achieved lower steady-state levels of nortriptyline (15 and 17 ng/ml) than the steady-state serum concentrations observed in nonbarbiturate-treated subjects (8–78 ng/ml). This difference in serum levels observed in the first groups of twins probably was due to the effect of the barbiturate and is supported by data from the other sets of identical twins who had similar serum nortriptyline levels when given the same doses of the drugs.

The serum level of nortriptyline decreased significantly in one patient (personal communication, G. D. Burrows, University of Melbourne, Melbourne, Australia) when amobarbital (200 mg po) was given concurrently for 5 days at night (3). In a retrospective analysis (7) of a previously published study (6), it was mentioned that barbiturates were used for nighttime sedation and could have caused the relatively low serum levels of nortriptyline in the patients studied.

Another study (2) also demonstrated a lowering of serum nortriptyline levels (by as much as 40%) in three patients who were given amobarbital (120 mg po) at night. The fall in serum nortriptyline levels was statistically significant only after 10 days of concurrent nortriptyline–amobarbital therapy. There was a less significant fall in nortriptyline levels when the amobarbital dose was decreased to 60 mg po at night (personal communication, G. Silverman, St. Bernard's and King Memorial Hospital, London, England).

■ Although the clinical data are limited, they are sufficient to indicate that barbiturates will probably decrease serum tricyclic antidepressant levels in patients receiving these drugs concurrently. Because the therapeutic effect caused by decreased serum drug levels was not measured, the clinical significance of this drug interaction is not known.

Recommendations—Phenobarbital should be considered a possible causative factor for unresponsiveness to antidepressant therapy in phenobarbital-treated patients.

The addition of other agents to tricyclic antidepressant therapy to treat anxiety states that often accompany depression is usually not necessary. Tricyclic antidepressants produce an anxiolytic or sedative effect (8) and "loading doses" are often administered at bedtime to avoid daytime sedation (9). There is no evidence that these sedative or anxiolytic effects of the tricyclic antidepressants are enhanced by the addition of other drugs (10).

If additional drugs must be used, the benzodiazepines do not affect the metabolism of the tricyclic drugs and may be useful in treating anxiety symptoms (see *Amitriptyline–Chlordiazepoxide*, p. 8). Chloral hydrate and the benzodiazepine flurazepam apparently do not affect the metabolism of tricyclic antidepressants and either might be useful if a hypnotic drug is desired.

References

(1) W. Hammer *et al.*, in "Antidepressant Drugs: Proceedings of the First International Symposium," Excerpta Medica International Congress Series No. 122, S. Garattini and M. N. G. Dukes, Eds., 1967, p. 301.

(2) G. Silverman and R. Braithwaite, "Interaction of Benzodiazepines with Tricyclic Antidepressants," *Brit. Med. J.*, *4*, 111 (1972).

(3) G. D. Burrows and B. Davies, "Antidepressants and Barbiturates," *Brit. Med. J.*, *4*, 113 (1971).

(4) B. Alexanderson *et al.*, "Steady-State Plasma Levels of Nortriptyline in Twins: Influence of Genetic Factors and Drug Therapy," *Brit. Med. J.*, *4*, 764 (1969). (Additional information supplied by F. Sjoqvist.)

(5) A. B. Dobkin, "Potentiation of Thiopental Anesthesia by Derivatives and Analogues of Phenothiazines," *Anesthesiology*, *21*, 292 (1960).

(6) M. Asberg *et al.*, "Relationship between Plasma Level and Therapeutic Effect of Nortriptyline," *Brit. Med. J.*, *3*, 331 (1971).

(7) P. Kragh-Sorensen *et al.*, "Plasma-Nortriptyline Levels in Endogenous Depression," *Lancet*, *i*, 113 (1973).

(8) L. E. Hollister, "Clinical Use of Psychotherapeutic Drugs II: Antidepressant and Antianxiety Drugs and Special Problems in the Use of Psychotherapeutic Drugs," *Drugs*, *4*, 361 (1972).

(9) J. Mendels and J. DiGiacomo, "The Treatment of Depression with a Single Daily Dose of Imipramine Pamoate," *Amer. J. Psychiat.*, *130*, 1022 (1973).

(10) "Benzodiazepines in Clinical Practice," D. J. Greenblatt and R. I. Shader, Eds., Raven, New York, N.Y., 1974, p. 61.

[For additional information, see *Antipsychotic Therapy*, p. 397.]

Nonproprietary and Trade Names of Drugs

Allobarbital—*Diadol*
Amitriptyline hydrochloride—*Elavil
Hydrochloride and various combination
products*
Amobarbital—*Amytal and various
combination products*
Aprobarbital—*Alurate*
Barbital—*Neurondia*
Butabarbital sodium—*Butisol Sodium*
Butalbital—*Available in combination
products*
Chloral hydrate—*Kessodrate, Noctec,
Somnos*
Desipramine hydrochloride—*Norpramin,
Pertofrane*
Doxepin hydrochloride—*Adapin, Sinequan*
Hexobarbital—*Sombulex*

Imipramine hydrochloride—*Presamine,
Tofranil, Tofranil PM*
Mephobarbital—*Mebaral, Mebroin*
Metharbital—*Geminol*
Methohexital sodium—*Brevital Sodium*
Nortriptyline hydrochloride—*Aventyl
Hydrochloride*
Pentobarbital—*Nembutal and various
combination products*
Phenobarbital—*Eskabarb, Luminal*
Protriptyline hydrochloride—*Vivactil
Hydrochloride*
Secobarbital—*Seconal and various
combination products*
Talbutal—*Lotusate*
Thiopental sodium—*Pentothal Sodium*

*Prepared and evaluated by the Scientific Review Subpanel on
Psychotropic Agents and reviewed by Practitioner Panel I.*

Orphenadrine—Propoxyphene

Summary—Orphenadrine has been reported to enhance the central nervous system (CNS) effects of propoxyphene when these drugs are used concurrently. However, the clinical data about this drug interaction are unreliable and the reported toxic effects can be caused by either agent alone. Concurrent use of these drugs need not be avoided when indicated.

Related Drugs—Both orphenadrine and propoxyphene are available as single entities and in dosage forms combined with other drugs, particularly aspirin.

Pharmacological Effect and Mechanism—Orphenadrine is a centrally acting anticholinergic agent used in the treatment of parkinsonism (1) and for the treatment of spasm of voluntary muscles (2, 3). The recommended dose is 100 mg twice daily (1, 2). Side effects reported with the drug include restlessness, mental confusion, and occasionally hallucinations (4).

Propoxyphene is a synthetic analgesic structurally related to the narcotic analgesic methadone. The recommended daily dose for analgesia is 65 mg every 4 hr. Side effects related to propoxyphene include paradoxical excitement and occasionally euphoria. Propoxyphene is prescribed frequently as a combination product containing acetaminophen or aspirin or a combination of aspirin, phenacetin, and caffeine. Mental confusion, apprehension, and tremors are side effects attributed to propoxyphene alone or in combination (5).

Tremors, mental confusion, and anxiety are the symptoms reported following concurrent administration of orphenadrine and propoxyphene according to both the manufacturers (6) and one reported case history (7).

If there is an interaction between orphenadrine and propoxyphene (8, 9), it is difficult to distinguish the reported symptoms from those attributed to the individual drugs.

Evaluation of Clinical Data—There have been no controlled studies reported and the clinical data about this drug interaction consist of 13 unpublished individual reports to the manufacturer, one vague unpublished group report to the manufacturer (8) (personal communications, I. F. Bennett, Lilly Research Laboratories, and O. N. Re, Riker Laboratories), and one published clinical impression (7). The individual reports to one manufacturer were mostly anecdotal, were lacking details, and involved no patient hazard (personal communication, I. F. Bennett, Lilly Research Laboratories). In four of the seven individual reports to another manufacturer, the dose of orphenadrine was twice the recommended dose (personal communication, O. N. Re, Riker Laboratories). In all seven cases, the manifestations of the reactions were similar to those previously reported for orphenadrine alone or propoxyphene alone (8).

In the published study (9), no significant adverse effects were noted in four of five patients receiving orphenadrine and propoxyphene concurrently. One patient was reported to be experiencing some "shaking," but the investigators attributed this effect to the patient's condition. Moreover, the patient had been receiving the two drugs concurrently for 2 weeks without experiencing any adverse effects.

■ Although orphenadrine has been reported to enhance the CNS effects of propoxyphene when these drugs are administered concurrently, there are no reliable data to support this observation. The toxic effects attributed to this drug interaction are likely to have been caused by either drug alone.

Recommendations—The concurrent use of orphenadrine and propoxyphene need not be avoided when indicated. If toxic CNS effects occur, they are probably due to either drug alone and require a reduction in the dose or discontinuation of one or both agents.

References

(1) W. J. Nicholson, "Medicine in Old Age. Diseases of the Motor System," *Brit. Med. J., 4,* 664 (1973).

(2) R. J. Popkin, "Orphenadrine Citrate for the Treatment of 'Restless Legs' and Related Syndromes," *J. Amer. Geriat. Soc., 19,* 76 (1971).

(3) V. B. Whittaker, "The Effect of Orphenadrine Citrate by Injection in Skeletal Muscle Spasm Using an Electromyographic Examination Technique," *J. Clin. Pract., 23,* 115 (1969).

(4) "Side Effects of Drugs," vol. 7, Excerpta Medica, Amsterdam, The Netherlands, 1972, pp. 248–249.

(5) "The Pharmacological Basis of Therapeutics," 5th ed., L. S. Goodman and A. Gilman, Eds., Macmillan, New York, NY 10022, 1975, p. 263.

(6) "Physicians' Desk Reference," 29th ed., Medical Economics, Inc., Oradell, NJ 07649, 1975, pp. 920, 1608.

(7) W. Renforth, "Orphenadrine and Propoxyphene," *N. Engl. J. Med., 283,* 998 (1970).

(8) R. E. Pearson and F. J. Salter, "Drug Interaction?—Orphenadrine with Propoxyphene," *N. Engl. J. Med., 282,* 1215 (1970).

(9) W. H. Puckett and J. A. Visconti, "Orphenadrine and Propoxyphene (cont.)," *N. Engl. J. Med., 283,* 544 (1970).

[For additional information, see *Analgesic Therapy (Nonnarcotic),* p. 341.]

Nonproprietary and Trade Names of Drugs

Orphenadrine citrate—*Norflex and various combination products*
Orphenadrine hydrochloride—*Disipal*

Propoxyphene hydrochloride—*Darvon, Dolene, SK-65*
Propoxyphene napsylate—*Darvon-N*

Prepared and evaluated by the Scientific Review Subpanel on Analgesics and reviewed by Practitioner Panel I.

Oxyphenbutazone—Methandrostenolone

Summary—When oxyphenbutazone and methandrostenolone are administered concurrently in humans, serum oxyphenbutazone levels may be elevated. Patients treated with these drugs concurrently should be monitored for signs of oxyphenbutazone-induced adverse effects.

Related Drugs—**Phenylbutazone** is partially metabolized to oxyphenbutazone (1, 2) but apparently is not affected by methandrostenolone (3). **Aminopyrine, antipyrine,** and **sulfinpyrazone** are structurally related to oxyphenbutazone and might be expected to interact with methandrostenolone, although such interactions have not been reported.

Anabolic steroids related to methandrostenolone (*e.g.*, **methyltestosterone, nandrolone, norethandrolone, oxymetholone, stanozolol,** and **testosterone**) may also increase serum oxyphenbutazone levels.

Pharmacological Effect and Mechanism—There are insufficient data to determine the mechanism by which methandrostenolone affects oxyphenbutazone. However, two mechanisms have been proposed: inhibition of oxyphenbutazone metabolism (3), and displacement of oxyphenbutazone from its binding site on serum albumin (4, 5).

Phenylbutazone is unaffected by concurrent administration of methandrostenolone. Although the mechanism of action is unclear, phenylbutazone binds more strongly to albumin than oxyphenbutazone and apparently is not displaced by methandrostenolone. The metabolism of phenylbutazone is also unaffected by methandrostenolone (3).

Evaluation of Clinical Data—Clinical data concerning the interaction of these two agents are limited but indicate that methandrostenolone may cause at least a 25–75% increase in serum oxyphenbutazone levels (3, 4, 6, 7). Evaluation of the data is difficult primarily because of the small number of subjects in whom the interaction has been studied. One study (4) utilized six subjects, and another study (3) utilized only two subjects; both groups showed increased serum oxyphenbutazone levels when methandrostenolone was added to the therapy. The validity of these conclusions can be determined only after further study.

Clinical data relating to a mechanism for a methandrostenolone-induced increase in serum oxyphenbutazone levels are insufficient and conflicting. Only one patient was studied to demonstrate that methandrostenolone did not affect the serum half-life of oxyphenbutazone (4), and one subject was evaluated to determine that the urinary excretion of oxyphenbutazone glucuronide was also unaffected (8).

Although methandrostenolone administration increased the serum half-life of oxyphenbutazone in another study (3), only one subject was evaluated. This patient was an alcoholic and, while it has been reported that the metabolism of phenylbutazone is not different in cirrhotic patients (9), the possibility remains that liver disease resulted in abnormal metabolism of oxyphenbutazone.

Although it has been stated that methandrostenolone interferes with the metabolism of oxyphenbutazone (10), it is not possible to conclude from the data that such interference occurs.

■ Although a greater incidence of untoward effects due to increased serum oxyphenbutazone levels may be expected in the presence of methandrostenolone, no adverse effects have been reported. Additionally, there are no studies showing that a clinical response to lower doses of oxyphenbutazone is attained when methandrostenolone is administered concurrently.

Recommendations—When oxyphenbutazone is administered concurrently with methandrostenolone, the increased serum oxyphenbutazone levels increase the risk of adverse reactions. Patients receiving both agents should be monitored closely for oxyphenbutazone-induced toxicity.

Phenylbutazone is reportedly unaffected by concurrent administration of methandrostenolone (3). Until more clinical data are available, phenylbutazone may be considered as an alternative drug to oxyphenbutazone when methandrostenolone is used concurrently.

References

(1) J. J. Burns *et al.,* "The Physiological Disposition of Phenylbutazone (Butazolidin) in Man and a Method for Its Estimation in Biological Material," *J. Pharmacol. Exp. Ther., 109,* 346 (1953).

(2) J. J. Burns *et al.,* "Biochemical Pharmacological Considerations of Phenylbutazone and Its Analogues," *Ann. N.Y. Acad. Sci., 86,* 253 (1960).

(3) E. F. Hvidberg *et al.,* "Studies of the Interaction of Phenylbutazone, Oxyphenbutazone, and Methandrostenolone in Man," *Proc. Soc. Exp. Biol. Med., 129,* 438 (1968).

(4) M. Weiner *et al.,* "Effect of Steroids on Disposition of Oxyphenbutazone in Man," *Proc. Soc. Exp. Biol. Med., 124,* 1170 (1967).

(5) B. B. Brodie, "Displacement of One Drug by Another from Carrier or·Receptor Sites," *Proc. Roy. Soc. Med., 58,* 946 (1965).

(6) P. G. Dayton *et al.,* "Interaction of Phenylbutazone, Oxyphenbutazone and Methandrostenolone in Man," *Fed. Proc., 27,* 531 (1968).

(7) M. Weiner *et al.,* "Drug Interactions: The Effect of Combined Administration on the Half-Life of Coumarin and Pyrazolone Drugs in Man," *Fed. Proc., 24,* 153 (1965).

(8) J. M. Perel *et al.,* "A Study of Structure–Activity Relationships in Regard to Species Differences in the Phenylbutazone Series," *Biochem. Pharmacol., 13,* 1305 (1964).

(9) M. Weiner *et al.,* "Observations on the Metabolic Transformation and Effects of Phenylbutazone in Subjects with Hepatic Disease," *Amer. J. Med. Sci., 228,* 36 (1954).

(10) T. M. King and J. K. Burgard, "Drug Interaction," *Amer. J. Obstet. Gynecol., 98,* 128 (1967).

[For additional information, see *Analgesic Therapy (Nonnarcotic),* p. 341.]

Nonproprietary and Trade Names of Drugs

Aminopyrine—*Various manufacturers*
Antipyrine—*Various manufacturers*
Methandrostenolone—*Dianabol*
Methyltestosterone—*Metandren, Oreton Methyl, and various combination products*
Nandrolone phenpropionate—*Durabolin*
Norethandrolone—*Various manufacturers*

Oxymetholone—*Adroyd, Anadrol*
Oxyphenbutazone—*Oxalid, Tandearil*
Phenylbutazone—*Azolid, Butazolidin*
Stanozolol—*Winstrol*
Sulfinpyrazone—*Anturane*
Testosterone—*Oreton*

Prepared and evaluated by the Scientific Review Subpanel on Analgesics and reviewed by Practitioner Panel II.

Penicillin—Aspirin

Summary—Limited clinical data indicate that aspirin, in large doses, increases the serum level and half-life of penicillin when these drugs are given concurrently. Although concurrent use of high doses of aspirin has been suggested to increase the clinical benefits of penicillin, the possible toxicities due to high-dose aspirin administration discourage such therapy.

Related Drugs—Serum binding of **cloxacillin, dicloxacillin, diphenicillin, nafcillin,** and **oxacillin** also is reduced when administered concurrently with aspirin (1). A similar effect could be expected to occur with other **penicillins.**

The effects of other salicylates on the displacement and serum half-life of penicillin have not been evaluated.

Pharmacological Effect and Mechanism—The mechanism for this drug interaction is unclear, but it appears to involve two separate effects. Aspirin may displace penicillin from its plasma protein binding site. The acetyl group of aspirin binds covalently to the ϵ-amino group of lysine residues on albumin (2), resulting in an altered secondary structure of the protein. The altered secondary structure may result in altered protein binding to other drugs. An *in vivo* study (3) indicated that low concentrations of salicylates did not significantly displace penicillin G from its protein binding sites, although high concentrations did. Adjustment of the salicylate or penicillin concentration in this study did not further affect the percentage of free penicillin, indicating that the protein displacement is noncompetitive. Another *in vivo* study (1) indicated that the free unbound serum penicillin level increased approximately twofold after concurrent administration of aspirin, although the total serum penicillin level decreased.

Penicillin and aspirin also may compete for the same renal secretory sites. Aspirin and the other acidic drugs are secreted by the same proximal tubular active transport system as penicillin. The increase in the penicillin half-life that occurs when penicillin and aspirin are administered concurrently may be the result of competition between the two drugs for the same excretory system (4).

Evaluation of Clinical Data—In the only clinical study (4), 11 patients with arteriosclerotic disorders were given penicillin G (600 mg iv) before and after 5–7 days of aspirin (3 g/day po). All patients had normal serum creatinine levels but had a wide variation in the creatinine clearance, indicating differences in age and in renal function. Aspirin administration significantly increased the penicillin half-life from 44.5 to 72.4 min ($p < 0.05$). The clinical effects of this increase were not determined.

■ The limited clinical data prevent an authoritative assessment of the clinical significance of this drug interaction. In the only clinical report, some patients may have had preexisting renal dysfunction which would have influenced the results (4). If a drug interaction does occur, it probably only occurs when large doses of aspirin (~ 3 g) are given for a long period (3).

Recommendations—Although concurrent use of high doses of aspirin has been suggested to increase the clinical benefits of penicillin (3), the possible toxicities of high-dose aspirin administration discourage such therapy.

References

(1) C. M. Kunin, "Clinical Pharmacology of the New Penicillins II. Effect of Drugs which Interfere with Binding to Serum Proteins," *Clin. Pharmacol. Ther., 7,* 180 (1966).

(2) D. Hawkins *et al.,* "Structural Changes in Human Serum Albumin Induced by Ingestion of Acetylsalicylic Acid," *J. Clin. Invest., 48,* 536 (1969).

(3) B. Moskowitz *et al.,* "Salicylate Interaction with Penicillin and Secobarbital Binding Sites on Human Serum Albumin," *Clin. Toxicol., 6,* 247 (1973).

(4) J. Kampmann *et al.,* "Effect of Some Drugs on Penicillin Half-life in Blood," *Clin. Pharmacol. Ther., 13,* 516 (1972).

[For additional information, see *Anti-Infective Therapy,* p. 388.]

Nonproprietary and Trade Names of Drugs

Amoxicillin—*Amoxil*

Ampicillin—*Alpen, Amcill, Omnipen, Penbritin, Polycillin, Principen, Totacillin*

Aspirin—*Available alone or as a fixed combination in many trade name products, especially over-the-counter preparations*

Carbenicillin disodium—*Geopen, Pyopen*

Cloxacillin sodium monohydrate—*Tegopen*

Dicloxacillin sodium monohydrate—*Dynapen, Pathocil, Veracillin*

Diphenicillin sodium—*Ancillin*

Methicillin sodium—*Staphcillin*

Nafcillin sodium—*Unipen*

Oxacillin sodium—*Bactocill, Prostaphlin*

Penicillin G benzathine—*Bicillin, Permapen*

Penicillin G potassium—*Dramcillin, G-Recillin, Hyasorb, Kesso-Pen, Palocillin S-10, Pedacillin, Pentids, Pfizerpen, Sugracillin*

Penicillin G procaine—*Crysticillin AS, Diurnal-Penicillin, Duracillin A.S., Pentids-P, Pfizerpen-AS, Wycillin*

Penicillin V benzathine—*Pen-Vee*

Penicillin V potassium—*Compocillin-VK, Ledercillin VK, Robicillin VK, Uticillin VK, V-Cillin K, Veetids*

Phenethicillin potassium—*Darcil, Maxipen, Syncillin*

Propicillin potassium—*Brocillin, Ultrapen*

Prepared and evaluated by the Scientific Review Subpanel on Anti-Infectives and reviewed by Practitioner Panel III.

Penicillin—Chloramphenicol

Summary—*In vitro* and *in vivo* data indicate that the bacteriostatic action of chloramphenicol may antagonize the bactericidal action of penicillin in the early growth phase of an organism. However, this antagonism has not been unequivocally demonstrated clinically. Therefore, concurrent use of these antibiotics need not be avoided in the limited circumstances where such therapy is indicated.

Related Drugs—There are various antibiotics related to penicillin that are commercially available.

Pharmacological Effect and Mechanism—Chloramphenicol inhibits protein synthesis specifically by inhibiting the function of messenger RNA at the 50 S ribosomal subunit (1, 2). Bacteriostatic action occurs because of immediate cessation of new protein formation within the cell, thus preventing bacterial multiplication. Penicillin exerts a bactericidal effect by inhibition of a specific step in cell wall synthesis and exerts its greatest activity during the early phase of bacterial growth. When the static phase of bacterial growth is reached, the activity of penicillin is considerably reduced (3).

Chloramphenicol, when administered in the early growth phase, may affect the bacterial population in such a way that it resembles a static phase. This effect has been demonstrated with certain organisms both *in vitro* and *in vivo* (4). However, there are no studies that have proven that this antagonism will occur clinically.

Evaluation of Clinical Data—Ampicillin and chloramphenicol alone and concurrently have been evaluated in the treatment of *Salmonella* and nonspecific enteric fevers (5). Concurrent therapy and chloramphenicol alone proved similarly more successful than ampicillin alone, although the patients receiving ampicillin had fewer relapses. Chloramphenicol was administered at 50 mg/kg/day po and ampicillin was used at 100 mg/kg/day po, alone or concurrently. No particular advantage or disadvantage was noted for the concurrent therapy *versus* chloramphenicol alone.

Concurrent treatment with ampicillin (4 g/24 hr im) and chloramphenicol (2 g/24 hr po) was compared with chloramphenicol alone in 100 patients with typhoid fever (6). Concurrent treatment significantly shortened the febrile period compared with the single treatment. However, the dose of chloramphenicol used in the single treatment (2 g/day) was lower than the dose of chloramphenicol normally recommended for treatment of typhoid fever (3–4 g/day) (7, 8).

A study (9) comparing one dose of chloramphenicol (1 g po) alone and with procaine penicillin (600,000 units im) was conducted in 700 patients with gonorrhea. Concurrent treatment again was superior to chloramphenicol alone and the investigators were unable to demonstrate antagonism in limited *in vitro* studies using gonococcal cultures and a diffusion method. No comparison of concurrent therapy was made with penicillin administered alone.

Data were reported for 268 patients (various ages) with acute bacterial meningitis treated with either ampicillin (150 mg/kg/day iv) alone or ampicillin at the same dosage administered with both chloramphenicol (100 mg/kg/day iv, maximum 4 g/day) and streptomycin (40 mg/kg/day im, maximum 2 g/day) (10). Ampicillin and chloramphenicol were given for the total duration of therapy while streptomycin was given only for the initial 2 days of treatment. The administration of chloramphenicol was delayed until 30 min after ampicillin had been administered to avoid antibiotic interference. These results indicated that the case fatality ratio was significantly higher in the group receiving concurrent therapy in comparison with ampicillin alone ($\chi = 5.01$, $p = 0.02$).

■ Although *in vitro* and *in vivo* data indicate that chloramphenicol may antagonize penicillin's bactericidal action, the clinical significance of this interaction has not been evaluated adequately. Most data involve *in vitro* and animal studies (4, 11–14) with only limited human data. The human data indicate that administration of the two drugs simultaneously does not compromise clinical effectiveness in many situations (15, 16). Many variables such as the organisms involved and the doses used can affect the potential interaction. In situations such as meningitis, where early bacterial kill is important in the proliferative phase, the potential antagonism could be detrimental to the clinical status of the patient (10, 15, 16), but this antagonism has not been demonstrated clinically.

Recommendations—There is no unequivocal clinical evidence that chloramphenicol causes any significant antagonism of the bactericidal effect of penicillin. Therefore, concurrent use of these antibiotics need not be avoided in the limited circumstances where such therapy is indicated.

References

(1) C. Coutsogeorgopoulos, "Inhibitors of the Reaction between Puromycin and Polylysyl-RNA in the Presence of Ribosomes," *Biochem. Biophys. Res. Commun.,* 27, 46 (1967).

(2) A. D. Wolfe and F. E. Hahn, "Mode of Action of Chloramphenicol. IX. Effects of Chloramphenicol upon a Ribosomal Amino Acid Polymerization System and Its Binding to Bacterial Ribosome," *Biochim. Biophys. Acta,* 95, 146 (1965).

(3) "Drill's Pharmacology in Medicine," J. R. DiPalma, Ed., McGraw-Hill, New York, N.Y., 1971, pp. 1680, 1683.

(4) J. F. Wallace *et al.,* "Studies on the Pathogenesis of Meningitis. VI. Antagonism between Penicillin and Chloramphenicol in Experimental Pneumococcal Meningitis," *J. Lab. Clin. Med.,* 70, 408 (1967).

(5) R. P. Robertson *et al.,* "Evaluation of Chloramphenicol and Ampicillin in Salmonella Enteric Fever," *N. Engl. J. Med.,* 278, 171 (1968).

(6) F. De Ritis *et al.,* "Chloramphenicol Combined with Ampicillin in Treatment of Typhoid," *Brit. Med. J.,* 4, 17 (1972).

(7) "The Pharmacological Basis of Therapeutics," 5th ed., L. S. Goodman and A. Gilman, Eds., Macmillan, New York, NY 10022, 1975, p. 1198.

(8) "Antibiotics in Clinical Practice," H. Smith, Ed., Williams and Wilkins, Baltimore, Md., 1972, p. 76.

(9) H. C. Gjessing and K. Odegaard, "Oral Chloramphenicol Alone and with Intramuscular Procaine Penicillin in the Treatment of Gonorrhea," *Brit. J. Vener. Dis.*, *43*, 133 (1967).

(10) P. F. Wehrle *et al.*, "Bacterial Meningitis," *Ann. N.Y. Acad. Sci.*, *145*, 488 (1967).

(11) E. Jawetz *et al.*, "The Combined Action of Penicillin with Streptomycin or Chloromycetin on Enterococci *In Vitro*," *Science*, *111*, 254 (1950).

(12) E. Jawetz *et al.*, "Studies on Antibiotic Synergism and Antagonism," *Arch. Intern. Med.*, *87*, 349 (1951).

(13) E. Yourassowsky and R. Monsieur, "Antagonism Limit of Penicillin G and Chloramphenicol against *Neisseria meningtides*," *Arzneim.-Forsch.*, *21*, 1385 (1971).

(14) P. Ardalan, "Zur Frage des Antagonismus von Penicillin und Chloramphicolus Klinischer Sicht," *Praxis Pneumol.*, *23*, 772 (1969). (English abstract)

(15) E. Jawetz, "The Use of Combinations of Antimicrobial Drugs," *Ann. Rev. Pharmacol.*, *8*, 151 (1968).

(16) J. Crofton, "Some Principles in the Chemotherapy of Bacterial Infections," *Brit. Med. J.*, *2*, 137 (1969).

[For additional information, see *Anti-Infective Therapy*, p. 388.]

Nonproprietary and Trade Names of Drugs

Amoxicillin—*Amoxil*
Ampicillin—*Alpen, Amcill, Omnipen, Penbritin, Polycillin, Principen, Totacillin*
Carbenicillin disodium—*Geopen, Pyopen*
Chloramphenicol—*Amphicol, Chloromycetin, Mychel*
Cloxacillin sodium monohydrate—*Tegopen*
Dicloxacillin sodium monohydrate—
Dynapen, Pathocil, Veracillin
Diphenicillin sodium—*Ancillin*
Methicillin sodium—*Staphcillin*
Nafcillin sodium—*Unipen*
Oxacillin sodium—*Bactocill, Prostaphlin*
Penicillin G benzathine—*Bicillin, Permapen*

Penicillin G potassium—*Dramcillin, G-Recillin, Hyasorb, Kesso-Pen, Palocillin S-10, Pedacillin, Pentids, Pfizerpen, Sugracillin*
Penicillin G procaine—*Crysticillin AS, Diurnal-Penicillin, Duracillin A.S., Pentids-P, Pfizerpen-AS, Wycillin*
Penicillin V benzathine—*Pen-Vee*
Penicillin V potassium—*Compocillin-VK, Ledercillin VK, Robicillin VK, Uticillin VK, V-Cillin K, Veetids*
Phenethicillin potassium—*Darcil, Maxipen, Syncillin*
Propicillin potassium—*Brocillin, Ultrapen*

Prepared and evaluated by the Scientific Review Subpanel on Anti-Infectives and reviewed by Practitioner Panel V.

Penicillin—Chlortetracycline

Summary—Tetracycline may antagonize the bactericidal effect of penicillin, but a clinically significant interaction occurs only in situations where a rapid bactericidal effect is necessary (*e.g.*, pneumococcal meningitis). Concurrent use of these agents should be avoided because of potential antagonism or a lack of enhanced therapeutic effect.

Related Drugs—Penicillin G is the only penicillin for which there is documented antagonism by a tetracycline preparation (1, 2). Antagonism of the action of all other **penicillins** might be expected due to their common mechanism of action. The evidence primarily involves the antagonism of the action of penicillin by chlortetracycline, but there are also data to suggest a similar effect by **oxytetracycline** and **tetracycline** (3). All **tetracyclines** may be expected to interact in a similar manner with penicillin.

Pharmacological Effect and Mechanism—Penicillin exerts its bactericidal effect by blocking synthesis of cell wall mucopeptides and exhibits its maximal effect during the early, more rapid phase of bacterial growth. Tetracycline, a bacteriostatic antibiotic, primarily inhibits protein synthesis within the microorganism. Since active protein synthesis within the cell wall may be necessary for mucopeptide synthesis to proceed, agents that inhibit protein synthesis may antagonize inhibitors of cell wall synthesis (4).

Spheroplast formation has been observed as a step preceding lysis of the bacteria exposed to penicillin. Tetracycline, when used with penicillin *in vitro*, inhibits the formation of spheroplasts, suggesting suppression of the bactericidal activity of penicillin G (5).

Other *in vitro* and *in vivo* animal studies failed to elucidate the mechanism of the interaction, but they indicate that the interaction may be dependent upon factors which determine the bactericidal or bacteriostatic effects of the antibiotics used, *i.e.*, the organism involved (6), the relative doses of the drugs (7, 8), and the relative times of drug administration (8).

Evaluation of Clinical Data—The effectiveness of penicillin therapy (1,000,000 units im every 2 hr) in 14 patients with pneumococcal meningitis was compared to the effectiveness of concurrent therapy with penicillin (same dose) and chlortetracycline (0.5 g iv every 6 hr for 2–4 days, then every 3 hr during recovery) in another group of 14 patients (1). The mortality rate in patients receiving penicillin alone was 30% compared to 79% for the group receiving both drugs. There was no major difference in patient characteristics between the two groups except that the penicillin only group had a larger percentage of patients who were comatose or in whom treatment was started relatively late.

In another study (2), 315 patients with uncomplicated Scarlatina (scarlet fever) were divided into three groups each with 105 patients of various ages. One group received penicillin alone (150,000–750,000 units/day po), one group received chlor-tetracycline alone (100–1000 mg/day po), and the third group received both drugs. All antibiotic regimens lasted 14 days. There was no statistically significant difference in the response of the three groups during the acute phase. A statistically significant difference was noted in the incidence of spontaneous reinfection in these patients after therapy was discontinued. In patients treated with chlortetracycline alone or with chlortetracycline and penicillin, the streptococcal infection returned 3 weeks after discharge in numbers far greater than in those treated with penicillin alone. It was concluded that the use of chlortetracycline and penicillin concurrently was unsuited for the treatment of this infection (2).

A later investigation of the treatment of pneumococcal meningitis (3) noted results similar to those of the initial study (1). By employing essentially the same dosage regimen (some patients received oxytetracycline or tetracycline instead of chlortetracycline), an 85% mortality rate (six of seven patients) was noted in the group receiving both drugs compared to a 54–59% rate in the patients receiving only penicillin (20 patients). These results support the previous observations, but the small number of patients involved prevents a definite correlation.

The effects of concurrent chlortetracycline (1 g/day po) and penicillin (600,000 units im upon admission and 300,000 units im every 12 hr) therapy were compared with penicillin alone (same dose) in 50 patients with pneumococcal pneumonia (9). Each therapeutic regimen lasted 5–7 days. The response in both groups was essentially the same. It was suggested that the antagonism was not seen because rapid kill of bacteria was not essential in this situation.

■ Tetracycline may cause a clinically significant antagonism of penicillin in situations where rapid bactericidal activity is necessary (*e.g.*, pneumococcal meningitis). With infections where rapid bacterial kill is not critical, there is no clinical evidence supporting a penicillin–tetracycline interaction. Even in those cases where no antagonism occurs, there is no justification for concurrent use of penicillin and tetracycline.

Recommendations—Penicillin and tetracycline should not be administered concurrently in situations where rapid bactericidal activity is necessary (*e.g.*, pneumococcal meningitis). No antagonism has been demonstrated in less critical infections but the therapeutic benefit is not increased by using penicillin and tetracycline concurrently compared to penicillin alone.

References

(1) M. H. Lepper and H. F. Dowling, "Treatment of Pneumococcic Meningitis with Penicillin Compared with Penicillin plus Aureomycin," *Arch. Intern. Med.*, *88*, 489 (1951).

(2) J. Strom, "The Question of Antagonism between Penicillin and Chlortetracycline, Illustrated by Therapeutical Experiments in Scarlatina," *Antibiot. Med.*, *1*, 6 (1955).

(3) R. A. Olsson *et al.*, "Pneumococcal Meningitis in the Adult. Clinical, Therapeutic, and Prognostic Aspects in Forty-three Patients," *Ann. Intern. Med.*, *55*, 545 (1961).

(4) E. Jawetz, "The Use of Combinations of Antimicrobial Drugs," *Ann. Rev. Pharmacol.*, *8*, 151 (1968).

(5) T. W. Chang and L. Weinstein, "Inhibitory Effects of Other Antibiotics on Bacterial Morphologic Changes Induced by Penicillin G," *Nature*, *211*, 763 (1966).

(6) L. P. Garrod and P. M. Waterworth, "Methods of Testing Combined Antibiotic Bactericidal Action and the Significance of the Results," *J. Clin. Pathol.*, *15*, 328 (1962).

(7) A. Manten and J. I. Terra, "The Antagonism between Penicillin and Other Antibiotics in Relation to Drug Concentration," *Chemotherapy*, *8*, 21 (1964).

(8) R. S. Speck *et al.*, "Studies on Antibiotic Synergism and Antagonism," *Arch. Intern. Med.*, *88*, 168 (1951)

(9) J. J. Ahern and W. M. M. Kirby, "Lack of Interference of Aureomycin with Penicillin in Treatment of Pneumococcic Pneumonia," *Arch. Intern. Med.*, *91*, 197 (1953).

[For additional information, see *Anti-Infective Therapy*, p. 388.]

Nonproprietary and Trade Names of Drugs

Amoxicillin—*Amoxil*
Ampicillin—*Alpen, Amcill, Omnipen, Penbritin, Polycillin, Principen, Totacillin*
Carbenicillin disodium—*Geopen, Pyopen*
Chlortetracycline hydrochloride—*Aureomycin*
Cloxacillin sodium monohydrate—*Tegopen*
Demeclocycline—*Declomycin*
Dicloxacillin sodium monohydrate—*Dynapen, Pathocil, Veracillin*
Diphenicillin sodium—*Ancillin*
Doxycycline monohydrate—*Doxy-II Monohydrate, Doxychel, Vibramycin Monohydrate*
Methacycline hydrochloride—*Rondomycin*
Methicillin sodium—*Staphcillin*
Minocycline hydrochloride—*Minocin, Vectrin*
Nafcillin sodium—*Unipen*
Oxacillin sodium—*Bactocill, Prostaphlin*
Oxytetracycline—*Dalimycin, Terramycin*
Oxytetracycline hydrochloride—*Oxy-Kesso-Tetra, Oxy-Tetrachel, Terramycin Hydrochloride*

Penicillin G benzathine—*Bicillin, Permapen*
Penicillin G potassium—*Dramcillin, G-Recillin, Hyasorb, Kesso-Pen, Palocillin S-10, Pedacillin, Pentids, Pfizerpen, Sugracillin*
Penicillin G procaine—*Crysticillin AS, Diurnal-Penicillin, Duracillin A.S., Pentids-P, Pfizerpen-AS, Wycillin*
Penicillin V benzathine—*Pen-Vee*
Penicillin V potassium—*Compocillin-VK, Ledercillin VK, Robicillin VK, Uticillin VK, V-Cillin K, Veetids*
Phenethicillin potassium—*Darcil, Maxipen, Syncillin*
Propicillin potassium—*Brocillin, Ultrapen*
Rolitetracycline—*Syntetrin*
Tetracycline—*Achromycin, Panmycin, Panmycin KM, Sumycin, Tetracyn, Tetrex-S*
Tetracycline hydrochloride—*Achromycin, Bristacycline, Cyclopar, Panmycin, Robitet, Steclin, Sumycin, Tetracyn*
Tetracycline phosphate complex—*Tetrex*

Prepared and evaluated by the Scientific Review Subpanel on Anti-Infectives and reviewed by Practitioner Panel I.

Penicillin—Erythromycin

Summary—Although the clinical data are limited and unreliable, concurrent administration of penicillin and erythromycin may result in synergism of the anti-bacterial activity. This action is dependent on the microorganism involved and its susceptibility to these antibiotics. However, these drugs should not be used concurrently in place of equally effective individual agents.

Related Drugs—Of the penicillin analogs, **diphenicillin** (1), **methicillin** (1, 2), **penicillin G** (1, 3–5), **penicillin V** (1, 6), **phenethicillin** (1), and **propicillin** (7) are documented to interact *in vivo* and *in vitro* with erythromycin as erythromycin estolate (7) and crystalline erythromycin (8). Although there is no published documentation, all other **penicillins** and **erythromycins** may theoretically be expected to behave in a similar manner.

Pharmacological Effect and Mechanism—*In vitro* studies with penicillin and erythromycin indicated that this drug interaction may result in either antagonism or synergism of the antibacterial activity. There are no absolute rules in predicting results when a bactericidal and a bacteriostatic antibiotic are used together. Erythromycin, in low concentrations, is bacteriostatic and may antagonize the action of penicillin. In higher concentrations, it may be bactericidal and the use of both drugs may result in synergism (2, 4, 9). Another important factor is the concentration attained by either antibiotic at the infected site (9).

Penicillin exerts its bactericidal activity by inhibition of bacterial cell wall synthesis, leaving the formation of cytoplasm unaffected. If cell growth occurs, rupture of the membrane with lysis results in cell death (4). Erythromycin affects cytoplasm formation by selectively inhibiting the synthesis of essential protein and enzymes with resultant bacteriostasis (4). Erythromycin's bacteriostatic action results in decreased bacterial cytoplasmic growth and less susceptibility to penicillin-induced cell lysis. The bacteriostatic action of erythromycin remains unimpaired. This antagonism is frequent if one or both agents are present at levels below the minimum inhibitory concentrations (2, 10).

Concurrent use of penicillin G and erythromycin suppressed the development of resistant staphylococcal mutants (1) and has been effective against penicillinase-producing staphylococci that show limited resistance to erythromycin (1). The synergism between these antibiotics appears to be limited. The phenomenon does not occur with highly active penicillinase-producing strains. Erythromycin may also protect penicillin from penicillinase inactivation when tested on staphylococci producing this enzyme (1, 4).

Evaluation of Clinical Data—Penicillin–erythromycin synergism was demonstrated in an uncontrolled study of six patients who received equal amounts of propicillin (1 g/day po) and erythromycin estolate (1 g/day po) concurrently for 7–28 days (7). Excellent clinical results were reported. In three cases, concurrent administration was useful for severe staphylococcal infections caused by organisms resistant to either agent alone.

The antibacterial activity of penicillin was unaffected by erythromycin in 315 hospitalized patients (children and adults) who had Scarlatina (scarlet fever) (6). The patients were divided into three groups of 105 patients. One group received penicillin alone, another group received erythromycin alone, and the third group received both drugs. The drugs were given orally and the dosage varied with the age of the patient. The dose ranges for penicillin and erythromycin were 300,000–750,000 units/day and 300–1150 mg/day, respectively. The duration of fever was longer in those patients receiving both drugs concurrently than in the group receiving penicillin alone. Although this difference was statistically significant ($p<0.01$), the possibility that the fever was induced by penicillin or erythromycin was not investigated. The disappearance of streptococci was fastest in the penicillin group and was slowest with the erythromycin group. The rate also was slower in the group receiving both drugs than in the group receiving penicillin alone, but none of the differences was statistically significant. About the same degree of difference was observed in the percentage of patients showing a return of hemolytic streptococcal infection after 3 weeks of treatment. These results seem to indicate that penicillin alone was as effective in the treatment of hemolytic streptococci as erythromycin alone or both drugs administered concurrently.

■ Based on these reports, it appears that the concurrent administration of penicillin and erythromycin may result in either indifference (6) or synergism (7) depending on the microorganism involved and its susceptibility to these antibiotics. Since the study demonstrating synergism involved a relatively small number of patients, concurrent therapy does not seem to offer any advantage over individual drug therapy.

Recommendations—The penicillins should not be routinely administered with erythromycin. Although concurrent therapy has been used in resistant staphylococcal infections not responding to penicillins alone (11), other primary drugs of choice [such as cloxacillin or methicillin (12)] would be preferable to concurrent administration of penicillin and erythromycin. These drugs should not be used concurrently to treat streptococcal infections.

References

(1) J. A. Gronroos, "Changes in the Sensitivity of Staphylococci during Passages in Combinations of Erythromycin and Various Penicillin Derivatives and Cephaloridine," *Curr. Ther. Res., 8*, 61 (1966).

(2) L. P. Garrod and P. M. Waterworth, "Methods of Testing Combined Antibiotic Bactericidal Action and the Significance of the Results," *J. Clin. Pathol., 15*, 328 (1962).

(3) T. W. Chang and L. Weinstein, "Inhibitory Effects of Other Antibiotics on Bacterial Morphologic Changes Induced by Penicillin G," *Nature, 211*, 763 (1966).

(4) A. Manten and J. I. Terra, "The Antagonism between Penicillin and Other Antibiotics in Relation to Drug Concentration," *Chemotherapia, 8*, 21 (1964).

(5) C. Simon and E. Latz, "Contributions to the Antibiotic Therapy of Staphylococci Infections. On the Influence of Chloramphenicol and Erythromycin on the Bactericidal Actions of Penicillin G and Methicillin In Vitro," *Med. Welt., 4*, 277 (1968).

(6) J. Strom, "Penicillin and Erythromycin Singly and in Combination in Scarlatina Therapy and the Interference between Them," *Antibiot. Chemother., 11*, 694 (1961).

(7) W. E. Herrell *et al.*, "Alpha-Phenoxypropyl Penicillin and Propinyl Erythromycin Against Resistant Staphylococci," *Antimicrob. Ag. Chemother., 1961*, 727–733.

(8) A. Manten, "Synergism and Antagonism between Antibiotic Mixtures Containing Erythromycin," *Antibiot. Chemother., 4*, 1228 (1954).

(9) M. Barber, "Drug Combinations in Antibacterial Chemotherapy," *Proc. Roy. Soc. Med., 58*, 990 (1965).

(10) "Chemotherapy with Antibiotics and Allied Drugs," 3rd ed., J. C. Tolhurst *et al.*, Eds., Australian Government Printing Service, 1972, p. 135.

(11) "The Use of Antibiotics," 2nd ed., A. Kucers and N. McK. Bennett, Eds., Lippincott, Philadelphia, Pa., 1975, p. 314.

(12) "Antimicrobial Agents in Medicine," B. M. Barker and F. Prescott, Eds., Blackwell Scientific Publications, Oxford, England, 1973, p. 147.

[For additional information, see *Anti-Infective Therapy*, p. 388.]

Nonproprietary and Trade Names of Drugs

Amoxicillin—*Amoxil*
Ampicillin—*Alpen, Amcill, Omnipen, Penbritin, Polycillin, Principen, Totacillin*
Carbenicillin disodium—*Geopen, Pyopen*
Cloxacillin sodium monohydrate—*Tegopen*

Dicloxacillin sodium monohydrate—*Dynapen, Pathocil, Veracillin*
Diphenicillin sodium—*Ancillin*
Erythromycin—*E-Mycin, Erythrocin, Ilotycin*
Erythromycin estolate—*Ilosone*

Erythromycin ethylsuccinate—*Erythrocin*
  Ethyl Succinate, Pediamycin
Erythromycin gluceptate—*Ilotycin*
  Gluceptate
Erythromycin stearate—*Bristamycin,*
  Erythrocin Stearate, Ethril
Methicillin sodium—*Staphcillin*
Nafcillin sodium—*Unipen*
Oxacillin sodium—*Bactocill, Prostaphlin*
Penicillin G benzathine—*Bicillin,*
  Permapen
Penicillin G potassium—*Dramcillin,*
  G-Recillin, Hyasorb, Kesso-Pen,

Palocillin S-10, Pedacillin, Pentids,
  Pfizerpen, Sugracillin
Penicillin G procaine—*Crysticillin AS,*
  Diurnal-Penicillin, Duracillin A.S.,
  Pentids-P, Pfizerpen-AS, Wycillin
Penicillin V benzathine—*Pen-Vee*
Penicillin V potassium—*Compocillin-VK,*
  Ledercillin VK, Robicillin VK, Uticillin
  VK, V-Cillin K, Veetids
Phenethicillin potassium—*Darcil, Maxipen,*
  Syncillin
Propicillin potassium—*Brocillin, Ultrapen*

*Prepared and evaluated by the Scientific Review Subpanel
on Anti-Infectives and reviewed by Practitioner Panel VI.*

Penicillin—Probenecid

Summary—Concurrent administration of penicillin and probenecid results in higher and more sustained serum antibiotic levels. Concurrent therapy, however, should be limited to certain infections where high single-dose levels of penicillin are desirable (*e.g.*, venereal disease).

Related Drugs—Other penicillin analogs shown to interact with probenecid are **amoxicillin** (1), **ampicillin** (2), **carbenicillin** (3), **cloxacillin** (4), **methicillin** (5), and **oxacillin** (5). All other **penicillins** also should be expected to interact in a similar manner.

Pharmacological Effect and Mechanism—Two mechanisms have been proposed to explain the well-documented enhancement of serum penicillin levels. One possibility is that probenecid actively competes with other weak organic acids for the renal transport process and thus diminishes tubular secretion of such compounds (*e.g.*, penicillins) (6). A second possibility is that probenecid decreases the apparent volume of distribution of the penicillins, resulting in a larger penicillin fraction in the central (plasma and extracellular water) compartment (7). The pharmacokinetic interpretation (8) of literature data indicates that the limitation of penicillin distribution has a greater effect on enhancement and prolongation of serum penicillin levels than the decreased renal transport of the antibiotic.

Evaluation of Clinical Data—Several studies indicate that probenecid increases and prolongs the serum levels achieved with a specific penicillin dose. The probenecid dosages usually employed as an adjuvant in penicillin therapy range from 1 to 4 g/day for adults. Single doses of penicillins in conjunction with a probenecid regimen resulted in serum level–time curves approximately twofold greater in area than without probenecid (3, 7, 9).

In another study (10), ampicillin (2 g/day im) was administered along with probenecid (2 g/day po) to persistent excreters of typhoid bacteria. After 18 days of treatment, one patient had a serum ampicillin level of 2000 μg/ml (well in excess of the 10–20 μg/ml normally encountered after a single 2-g im ampicillin dose) and became febrile, necessitating discontinuation of the drug.

The high levels of penicillin achieved by the concurrent administration of probenecid are seldom a problem in terms of adverse effects because of the low toxicity of penicillins in general. However, hypersensitivity reactions (particularly skin reactions) occur with probenecid as well as with penicillin, making diagnosis of hypersensitivity to the antibiotic more difficult (11). As noted previously, probenecid also can have an effect on other drugs.

■ The use of probenecid to increase and prolong serum penicillin levels was promoted at a time when the penicillins were relatively expensive and in short supply. Severe systemic *Pseudomonas* infections may necessitate the use of large doses of carbenicillin —a relatively expensive semisynthetic penicillin. Because probenecid enhances serum carbenicillin levels by about 50% (3), it may prove beneficial, both therapeutically and economically, to use probenecid as an adjuvant to carbenicillin. Ordinarily, however, there is seldom need to resort to penicillin–probenecid therapy since adequately high penicillin levels can be achieved by the use of larger penicillin doses. The recent resurgence of venereal disease presents another potential indication for penicillin–probenecid therapy since the attainment of relatively high penicillin levels after a single dose, for a prolonged period, may be necessary if maximal control is to be achieved (9, 12, 13). Ampicillin (3.5 g po) and penicillin G procaine (4.8 million units as a single intramuscular dose) both have been recommended for the treatment of venereal disease in conjunction with probenecid (1 g po) (14).

Recommendations—Unless the expense of the penicillin or the necessity for single-dose treatment is a factor (such as in the treatment of venereal disease), there is seldom need to resort to probenecid as an adjuvant to penicillin therapy.

Complications during concurrent administration of these drugs are due to increased antibiotic levels and are encountered most frequently during chronic treatment. Elimination of the penicillin-induced adverse reactions (with the exception of penicillin anaphylaxis) can usually be achieved by reduction in antibiotic dosage.

References

(1) R. Sutherland *et al.*, "Amoxycillin: A New Semi-Synthetic Penicillin," *Brit. Med. J.*, *3*, 13 (1972).

(2) "Treatment and Prevention of Syphilis and Gonorrhea," *Med. Lett.*, *13*, 85 (1971).

(3) H. C. Standiford *et al.*, "Clinical Pharmacology of Carbenicillin Compared with Other Penicillins," *J. Infec. Dis.*, *122*, suppl., S9 (1970).

(4) E. H. Nauta *et al.*, "Effect of Probenecid on the Apparent Volume of Distribution and Elimination of Cloxacillin," *Antimicrob. Ag. Chemother.*, *6*, 300 (1974).

(5) H. J. Simon and L. A. Rantz, "The Newer Penicillins I. Bacteriological and Clinical Pharmacological Investigations with Methicillin and Oxacillin," *Ann. Intern. Med.*, *57*, 335 (1962).

(6) I. M. Weiner *et al.*, "On the Mechanism of Action of Probenecid on Renal Tubular Secretion," *Bull. Johns Hopkins Hosp.*, *106*, 333 (1960).

(7) M. Gibaldi and M. A. Schwartz, "Apparent Effect of Probenecid on the Distribution of Penicillins in Man," *Clin. Pharmacol. Ther.*, *9*, 345 (1968).

(8) K. H. Beyer *et al.*, "Benemid, *p*-(Di-*n*-Propylsulfamyl)-Benzoic Acid: Its Renal Affinity and Its Elimination," *Amer. J. Physiol.*, *166*, 625 (1951).

(9) D. W. Johnson *et al.*, "Single-Dose Antibiotic Treatment of Asymptomatic Gonorrhea in Hospitalized Women," *N. Engl. J. Med.*, *283*, 1 (1970).

(10) D. Munnich *et al.*, "Langfristige, Parenterale (i.m.) Ampicillin- und Orale Probenecid-Behandlung der Typhus-Bakterien-Dauerausscheider," *Chemotherapia*, *10*, 253 (1965–1966).

(11) "Probenecid as an Aid to Penicillin Therapy," *Med. Lett.*, *8*, 11 (1966).

(12) K. K. Holmes *et al.*, "Studies of Venereal Disease. I. Probenecid-Procaine Penicillin G Combination and Tetracycline Hydrochloride in the Treatment of 'Penicillin-Resistant' Gonorrhea in Men," *J. Amer. Med. Ass.*, *202*, 461 (1967).

(13) K. K. Holmes *et al.*, "Single-Dose Aqueous Procaine Penicillin G Therapy for Gonorrhea: Use of Probenecid and Cause of Treatment Failure," *J. Infec. Dis.*, *127*, 455 (1973).

(14) "Handbook of Antimicrobial Therapy," The Medical Letter, New Rochelle, NY 10801, 1974, p. 48.

[For additional information, see *Anti-Infective Therapy*, p. 388.]

Nonproprietary and Trade Names of Drugs

Amoxicillin—*Amoxil*

Ampicillin—*Alpen, Amcill, Omnipen, Penbritin, Polycillin, Principen, Totacillin*

Carbenicillin disodium—*Geopen, Pyopen*

Cloxacillin sodium monohydrate—*Tegopen*

Dicloxacillin sodium monohydrate— *Dynapen, Pathocil, Veracillin*

Diphenicillin sodium—*Ancillin*

Methicillin sodium—*Staphcillin*

Nafcillin sodium—*Unipen*

Oxacillin sodium—*Bactocill, Prostaphlin*

Penicillin G benzathine—*Bicillin, Permapen*

Penicillin G potassium—*Dramcillin,*

G-Recillin, Hyasorb, Kesso-Pen, Palocillin S-10, Pedacillin, Pentids, Pfizerpen, Sugracillin

Penicillin G procaine—*Crysticillin AS, Diurnal-Penicillin, Duracillin A.S., Pentids-P, Pfizerpen-AS, Wycillin*

Penicillin V benzathine—*Pen-Vee*

Penicillin V potassium—*Compocillin-VK, Ledercillin VK, Robicillin VK, Uticillin VK, V-Cillin K, Veetids*

Phenethicillin potassium—*Darcil, Maxipen, Syncillin*

Probenecid—*Benemid*

Propicillin potassium—*Brocillin, Ultrapen*

Prepared and evaluated by the Scientific Review Subpanel on Anti-Infectives and reviewed by Practitioner Panel IV.

Phenformin—Alcohol

Summary—Diabetic patients treated with phenformin should avoid ingestion of alcoholic beverages because concurrent use may cause hypoglycemic reactions or lead to life-threatening lactic acidosis with shock. Some patients receiving phenformin also experience a pronounced anorexia and intolerance to alcohol. Since abstinence from alcohol is not always feasible, phenformin-treated patients should be warned to drink only small amounts of alcohol and should be cautioned about the severe effects caused by concurrent ingestion of these agents.

Related Drugs—Phenformin is the only biguanide derivative presently used in the United States for the treatment of diabetes mellitus.

Pharmacological Effect and Mechanism—Alcohol [in amounts as small as 35 ml of 100% alcohol (equivalent to 70 ml of 100-proof whiskey) (1)] lowers serum glucose levels by two mechanisms: one is related to suppression of hepatic gluconeogenesis (2), and the other is a less well-defined effect which modifies pancreatic β-cell function as indicated by increased plasma insulin responses to glucose loading (3). The effect on gluconeogenesis has been attributed to the shift in the NAD:NADH (oxidized and reduced forms of diphosphopyridine nucleotide, respectively) ratio and inhibition of the tricarboxylic acid cycle which take place during the oxidation of alcohol. These changes impair the utilization and conversion of lactic acid, amino acids, and glycerol to glucose (4). Alcoholic beverages, particularly beer, also may increase serum glucose levels because of their high carbohydrate content (5).

Both phenformin (6, 7) and alcohol (8, 9) increase serum lactic acid levels. The mechanism of action of phenformin is poorly understood. Facilitation of glucose utilization, activation of anaerobic glycolysis, and reduced oxidative metabolism have been proposed (10). Phenformin also appears to interfere with the utilization of endogenous and exogenous lactic acid (7, 11) which could be related to an inhibition of the citric acid cycle and oxidative phosphorylation (12). It is unclear which specific factors are responsible for the development of severe and life-threatening lactic acidosis observed in some phenformin-treated patients.

The serum lactic acid level increase caused by alcohol is variable. It has been associated with the decrease of the NAD:NADH ratio which favors the conversion of pyruvate to lactate (13), but tissue hypoxia due to central nervous system depression, especially with severe levels of intoxication, can be expected to contribute to it considerably.

The mechanism of the alcohol anorexia (14) remains to be elucidated. While it has the characteristics of an aversion reaction, it differs significantly from those elicited by disulfiram, the oral sulfonylureas, and metronidazole. Blood acetaldehyde levels have not yet been studied in this syndrome.

Studies on 20 volunteers (15), two of whom had abnormally high serum glucose levels, indicated that: (*a*) the hyperlacticacidemia produced by phenformin and alcohol is a result of both increased lactate production and decreased lactate utilization; (*b*) phenformin and alcohol exert an enhanced effect on blood lactate levels; and (*c*) the inhibitory effects of alcohol on gluconeogenesis from lactate are partially blocked by phenformin.

Evaluation of Clinical Data—Alcoholic hypoglycemia is a clinical entity usually observed in chronic malnourished alcoholic subjects who have glycogen-depleted livers (4). However, it also occurs after prolonged drinking sprees, in the occasional drinker [hypoglycemia has occurred in adults who have ingested 35–50 ml of 100% alcohol (equivalent to 70–100 ml of 100-proof whiskey) after a 2-day fast (1)], and in infants and children who have accidentally ingested alcohol. In the latter group, ingestion of 1 ml/kg of absolute alcohol resulted in blood alcohol levels of 100 mg/100 ml 2 hr after ingestion. This level is associated with development of hypoglycemia and coma (16). Alcohol enhances the hypoglycemic activity of the oral hypoglycemic agents and insulin (17), which could result in nervousness, anxiety, diaphoresis, tachycardia, convulsion, coma, and, in some cases, eventual death.

Numerous publications discuss phenformin and lactic acidosis (7, 11, 18–21). The fact that lactic acidosis occurs in diabetic subjects not treated with phenformin has made it difficult to assess the role that the drug plays in the elicitation of the syndrome.

Since alcohol alone can increase lactic acid levels, it is not surprising to find that alcohol ingestion preceded the onset of clinical illness in several cases (7, 19, 22, 23). The patient's condition rapidly deteriorates as acidosis develops. Severe abdominal pain, acute pulmonary hypertension, hypothermia, hypotension, and coma have been described. Serum glucose values need not be grossly abnormal, urinary ketone bodies are negative or only moderately increased, and blood lactic acid values may range from 80 to 130 mg/100 ml. Lethal outcome may be prevented by intensive use of sodium bicarbonate to correct the acidosis, although deterioration and death have occurred despite sodium bicarbonate therapy (24, 25).

The alcohol anorexia manifests itself with a bad metallic taste as well as nausea and vomiting (14, 20). However, it should not be overlooked that similar symptoms are occasionally caused by phenformin alone (26).

■ The enhancement of the hypoglycemic effects of phenformin and the elicitation of lactic acidosis in diabetic patients are dangerous and potentially life-threatening interactions of the drug with alcohol. Even if statistical data concerning the frequency of these interactions are not available, the practitioner must anticipate this interaction and recognize its pathogenesis. Alcohol anorexia affects approximately 30% of those patients who regularly consume alcohol (14), although these symptoms also may be caused by phenformin alone (26).

Recommendations—Patients receiving phenformin should avoid concurrent ingestion of alcohol. In those rare cases where abstinence is not feasible, ingestion of small amounts of low alcoholic wines is suggested. The patient also should be warned about the harmful effects (*e.g.*, symptoms of severe hypoglycemia and lactic acidosis) that may occur when these drugs are used concurrently.

Switching to other hypoglycemic drugs will not avoid a drug interaction with alcohol, although it may result in a decreased potential for precipitating lactic acidosis (see *Tolbutamide–Alcohol*, p. 240).

References

(1) J. B. Field *et al.*, "Studies on the Mechanism of Ethanol-Induced Hypoglycemia," *J. Clin. Invest.*, *42*, 497 (1963).

(2) L. Madison *et al.*, "Ethanol-Induced Hypoglycemia: II. Mechanism of Suppression of Hepatic Gluconeogenesis," *Diabetes*, *16*, 252 (1967).

(3) R. Metz *et al.*, "Potentiation of the Plasma Insulin Response to Glucose by Prior Administration of Alcohol, an Apparent Islet-Priming Effect," *Diabetes*, *18*, 517 (1969).

(4) L. L. Madison, "Ethanol-Induced Hypoglycemia," *Advan. Metab. Disord.*, *3*, 85 (1968).

(5) C. H. Walsh and D. J. O'Sullivan, "Effect of Moderate Alcohol Intake on Control of Diabetes," *Diabetes*, *23*, 440 (1974).

(6) G. M. Bernier *et al.*, "Lactic Acidosis and Phenformin Hydrochloride," *J. Amer. Med. Ass.*, *184*, 43 (1963).

(7) J. Lacher and L. Lasagna, "Phenformin and Lactic Acidosis," *Clin. Pharmacol. Ther.*, *7*, 477 (1966).

(8) H. E. Himwich *et al.*, "The Metabolism of Alcohol," *J. Amer. Med. Ass.*, *100*, 651 (1933).

(9) W. M. Nicholson and H. M. Taylor, "The Effect of Alcohol on the Water and Electrolyte Balance in Man," *J. Clin. Invest.*, *17*, 279 (1938).

(10) "Textbook of Endocrinology," 4th ed., R. Williams, Ed., Saunders, Philadelphia, Pa., 1968, pp. 803–846.

(11) H. K. Johnson and C. Waterhouse, "Relationship of Alcohol and Hyperlactatemia in Diabetic Subjects Treated with Phenformin," *Amer. J. Med.*, *45*, 98 (1968).

(12) G. Ungar *et al.*, "Action of Phenethylbiguanide, a Hypoglycemic Agent, on Tricarboxylic Acid Cycle," *Metabolism*, *9*, 36 (1960).

(13) O. A. Forsander, "Influence of Ethanol on the Redox State of the Liver," *Quart. J. Stud. Alc.*, *31*, 550 (1970).

(14) P. E. Lisboa *et al.*, "Anorexia for Alcohol: A Side-Effect of Phenethylbiguanide," letter to the editor, *Lancet, i*, 678 (1961).

(15) R. A. Kreisberg *et al.*, "Hyperlacticacidemia in Man: Ethanol-Phenformin Synergism," *J. Clin. Endocrinol. Metab.*, *34*, 29 (1972).

(16) M. H. Moss, "Alcohol Induced Hypoglycemia Caused by Alcohol Sponging," *Pediatrics*, *46*, 445 (1955).

(17) R. A. Arky *et al.*, "Irreversible Hypoglycemia: A Complication of Alcohol and Insulin," *J. Amer. Med. Ass.*, *206*, 575 (1968).

(18) G. A. Ewy *et al.*, "Lactate Acidosis Associated with Phenformin Therapy and Localized Tissue Hypoxia: Report of a Case Treated by Hemodialysis," *Ann. Intern. Med.*, *59*, 878 (1963).

(19) B. J. Sproule *et al.*, "Acute Pulmonary Hypertension in Idiopathic Lactic Acidosis," *Can. Med. Ass. J.*, *94*, 141 (1966).

(20) A. Gottlieb *et al.*, "Phenformin Acidosis," *N. Engl. J. Med.*, *267*, 806 (1962).

(21) P. Isaacs, "Alcohol and Phenformin in Diabetes," letter to the editor, *Brit. Med. J.*, *3*, 773 (1970).

(22) M. B. Davidson *et al.*, "Phenformin, Hypoglycemia and Lactic Acidosis, Report of Attempted Suicide," *N. Engl. J. Med.*, *275*, 886 (1966).

(23) G. G. Shirriffs and P. D. Bewsher, "Hypothermia, Abdominal Pain, and Lactic Acidosis in Phenformin-Treated Diabetic," *Brit. Med. J.*, *3*, 506 (1970).

(24) R. Assan *et al.*, "Phenformin-Induced Lactic Acidosis in Diabetic Patients," *Diabetes*, *24*, 791 (1975).

(25) O. Kristensen *et al.*, "Glucose-Insulin Treatment of Lactic Acidosis in Phenformin-Treated Diabetics," *Acta Med. Scand.*, *197*, 463 (1975).

(26) "Drill's Pharmacology in Medicine," 4th ed., J. R. DiPalma, Ed., McGraw-Hill, New York, N.Y., 1971, p. 1520.

[For additional information, see *Hypoglycemic Therapy*, p. 422.]

Nonproprietary and Trade Names of Drugs

Alcohol—*Various products and beverages*   Phenformin hydrochloride—*DBI, Meltrol*

Prepared and evaluated by the Scientific Review Subpanels on Hypoglycemic Agents and Sedative–Hypnotics and reviewed by Practitioner Panel VI.

Phenobarbital—Alcohol

Summary—Concurrent ingestion of phenobarbital and alcohol leads to intensification of their central nervous system (CNS) depressant effects. Patients should be advised that relatively moderate amounts of alcohol (90–120 ml of 100-proof whiskey) will impair their ability to drive an automobile or operate hazardous machinery and that this danger is increased when barbiturates are given concurrently.

Related Drugs—There are numerous reports of similar interactions involving long-, intermediate-, short-, and ultrashort-acting **barbiturates** (1, 2), and it can be assumed that all barbiturates intensify the depressant effects of alcohol.

Pharmacological Effect and Mechanism—The combined actions of barbiturates and alcohol have been described as antagonistic (3), additive (4), potentiating (5), and synergistic (6). The studies cannot be compared easily since they utilized different animal species, employed varying dose levels, and used diverse experimental designs. For example, one study (7) showed an additive effect with moderate dosages in mice tested for their ability to stay on a 60-degree inclined screen but a supraadditive effect with higher dosages using loss of righting reflex as the criterion of response.

While the mechanism of the intensification of effect at the CNS level is not well understood, several theories have been proposed. One theory concerns a hepatic microsomal enzyme system that not only is involved in metabolic transformations of numerous drugs but also acts as an ethanol-oxidizing system and is responsible for adaptive increases of the rate of alcohol metabolism in alcoholics. When it is induced by phenobarbital, alcohol metabolism accelerates, and there is a greater tolerance to alcohol. When it is induced by chronic consumption of alcohol, phenobarbital is metabolized more quickly and the person becomes more tolerant to barbiturates. When barbiturates and alcohol are ingested concurrently, competition for the system leads to inhibition of oxidation and enhancement of CNS depressant effects (8, 9). However, this theory has been disputed (10, 11), because the physiological significance of the microsomal ethanol-oxidizing system has been questioned (12, 13). Another theory is that alcohol facilitates the passage of barbiturates into the brain (14), but the evidence that supports this theory is inconclusive.

The clinical results of this drug interaction are similar to the effects of either agent given alone, except more intense. The major system affected is the CNS; motor impairment and drowsiness are the most common symptoms (2, 15–18). Respiratory depression is mild at low doses of either drug (17, 19) but can become serious at higher doses and may result in death (2, 17).

Evaluation of Clinical Data—Clinical data about the effects of the barbiturate–alcohol interaction were derived from tests of reaction times, skills related to driving an automobile, and behavior analysis. In most investigations, concurrent administration was preceded by separate tests of individual effects.

A study performed on 200 healthy volunteers involved actual driving of an automobile combined with tests of reaction times and self-evaluation (15). Alcohol intake was adjusted to produce average peak blood levels of 87 mg/100 ml (equivalent to 90–120 ml of 100-proof whiskey); the phenobarbital dose was 200 mg. Each agent taken alone caused an increase of the error score. Concurrent administration led to a significant ($p < 0.001$) increase in errors indicating an intensification of each agent's effect.

Amobarbital sodium (150 mg po during a 36-hr period) was given alone and concurrently with alcohol (0.5 g/kg) to 20 healthy subjects (20). The study was double blind with a control group and the average blood alcohol level in these subjects was 50 mg/100 ml. The subject's ability to control a vehicle was determined and an objective assessment scale of the emotional, behavioral, and neurological characteristics of each person was utilized. The results showed that amobarbital alone impaired the subject's ability to perform the various experimental tests correctly. There was no significant change in the subject's performance when alcohol was ingested concurrently. The investigators suggested that the lack of enhanced effect with alcohol was probably due to the relatively low dose used (<90 ml of 100-proof whiskey).

Information about the toxic blood levels of barbiturates and alcohol is generally restricted to data obtained through postmortem analysis. Fatalities in humans have occurred with blood alcohol levels as low as 100 mg/100 ml or serum phenobarbital levels as low as 0.5 mg/ml when these drugs were used concurrently (21). Since the fatal blood levels of alcohol alone are usually between 400 and 500 mg/100 ml (22, 23) and of phenobarbital alone is 10 mg/ml (17), it can be concluded that concurrent use of phenobarbital and alcohol in normally nonfatal quantities can cause death.

■ Clinical evidence indicates that alcohol (in doses of at least 90–120 ml of 100-proof whiskey) enhances the CNS depressant effects of phenobarbital when these drugs are ingested concurrently. The effects of this drug interaction are dose related. With relatively moderate amounts of alcohol (90–120 ml of 100-proof whiskey), impairment of motor performance and physical alertness sometimes, but not always, occurs (20); with higher amounts (150–200 ml of 100-proof whiskey), significant respiratory depression and possibly death may result (21). Initial CNS depression occurs approximately 30 min after concurrent ingestion (16, 18).

Recommendations—Patients should be informed that relatively moderate amounts of alcohol (90–120 ml of 100-proof whiskey ingested during a 1-hr period) may impair their ability to drive an automobile or operate hazardous machinery and that this danger is increased when barbiturates are taken concurrently. Moreover, patients receiving barbiturates should be warned that ingestion of large amounts of alcohol (150–200 ml of 100-proof whiskey) should be avoided.

Although the benzodiazepines also interact with alcohol (see *Diazepam–Alcohol*, p. 47), some investigators prefer benzodiazepines to barbiturates for the treatment of alcohol withdrawal because they do not significantly depress respiration or disturb sleep patterns (24, 25).

Other CNS depressant drugs such as chloral hydrate (see *Chloral Hydrate–Alcohol*, p. 20), ethchlorvynol (26), glutethimide (27), and possibly methaqualone (28) interact with alcohol in a manner similar to phenobarbital.

References

(1) "Interaction of Alcohol and Other Drugs," E. Polacsek *et al.*, Eds., Addiction Research Foundation, Toronto, Canada, 1972.

(2) "Combined Effects of Alcohol and Other Drugs," R. F. Forney and F. Hughes, Eds., Charles C. Thomas, Springfield, Ill., 1968, p. 48.

(3) G. Carriere *et al.*, "Etude Experimental des Injections Intraveineuses d'Alcool au Cours d' Intoxications par le Gardenal," *C. R. Soc. Biol.*, *116*, 188 (1934).

(4) C. M. Gruber, Jr., "A Theoretical Consideration of Additive and Potentiated Effects between Drugs with a Practical Example Using Alcohol and Barbiturates," *Arch. Int. Pharmacodyn. Ther.*, *102*, 17 (1955).

(5) P. L. Morselli *et al.*, "Further Ob-

servations on the Interaction between Ethanol and Psychotrophic Drugs," *Arzneim.-Forsch.*, *21*, 20 (1971).

(6) W. W. Jetter and R. McLean, "Poisoning by the Synergistic Effect of Phenobarbital and Ethyl Alcohol. An Experimental Study," *Arch. Pathol.*, *36*, 112 (1943).

(7) G. F. Gebhart *et al.*, "The Effects of Ethanol Alone and in Combination with Phenobarbital, Chlorpromazine or Chlordiazepoxide," *Toxicol. Appl. Pharmacol.*, 15, 405 (1969).

(8) C. S. Lieber and L. M. DeCarli, "Effect of Drug Administration on the Activity of the Hepatic Microsomal Ethanol Oxidizing System," *Life Sci.*, *9*, 267 (1970).

(9) C. S. Lieber and L. M. DeCarli, "The Role of the Hepatic Microsomal Ethanol Oxidizing System (MEOS) for Ethanol Metabolism *In Vivo*," *J. Pharmacol. Exp. Ther.*, *181*, 279 (1972).

(10) J. M. Khanna *et al.*, "Significance *In Vivo* of the Increase in Microsomal Ethanol-Oxidizing System after Chronic Administration of Ethanol, Phenobarbital and Chlorcyclizine," *Biochem. Pharmacol.*, *21*, 2215 (1972).

(11) M. K. Roach *et al.*, "Ethanol Metabolism In Vivo and the Role of Hepatic Microsomal Ethanol Oxidation," *Quart. J. Stud. Alc.*, *33*, 751 (1972).

(12) J. M. Khanna and H. Kalant, "Effect of Inhibitors and Inducers of Drug Metabolism on Ethanol Metabolism *In Vivo*," *Biochem. Pharmacol.*, *19*, 2033 (1970).

(13) E. A. Carter and K. J. Isselbacher, "Hepatic Microsomal Ethanol Oxidation. Mechanism and Physiologic Significance," *Lab. Invest.*, *27*, 283 (1972).

(14) B. B. Coldwell *et al.*, "Some Effects of Ethanol on the Toxicity and Distribution of Barbiturates in Rats," *Can. J. Physiol. Pharmacol.*, *48*, 254 (1970).

(15) P. Kielholz *et al.*, "Fahrversuche zur Frage der Beeintrachtigung der Verkehrstuchtigkeit durch Alkohol, Tranquilizer und Hypnotika," *Deut. Med. Wochenschr.*, *94*, 301 (1969).

(16) C. R. B. Joyce *et al.*, "Potentiation by Phenobarbitone of Effects of Ethyl Alcohol on Human Behaviour," *J. Ment. Dis.*, *105*, 51 (1959).

(17) "Acute Barbiturate Poisoning," H. Mathew, Ed., Excerpta Medica Foundation, Amsterdam, The Netherlands, 1971, p. 87.

(18) M. A. Evans *et al.*, "Quantitative Relationship between Blood Alcohol Concentration and Psychomotor Performance," *Clin. Pharmacol. Ther.*, *15*, 253 (1974).

(19) R. E. Johnstone and C. E. Reier, "Acute Respiratory Effects of Ethanol in Man," *Clin. Pharmacol. Ther.*, *14*, 501 (1973).

(20) T. A. Betts *et al.*, "Effects of Four Commonly-Used Tranquillizers on Low-Speed Driving Performance Tests," *Brit. Med. J.*, *4*, 580 (1972).

(21) R. C. Gupta and J. Kofoed, "Toxicological Statistics for Barbiturates, Other Sedatives and Tranquilizers in Ontario: A 10-year Survey," *Can. Med. Ass. J.*, *94*, 863 (1966).

(22) D. C. MacGregor *et al.*, "Acute Toxicity Studies on Ethanol, Propranolol, and Butanol," *Can. J. Physiol. Pharmacol.*, *42*, 689 (1964).

(23) "The Pharmacological Basis of Therapeutics," 5th ed., L. S. Goodman and A. Gilman, Eds., Macmillan, New York, NY 10022, 1975, p. 143.

(24) D. J. Greenblatt and M. Greenblatt, "Which Drug for Alcohol Withdrawal?" *J. Clin. Pharmacol.*, *12*, 429 (1972).

(25) E. Rothstein, "Prevention of Alcohol Withdrawal Seizures: The Roles of Diphenylhydantoin and Chlordiazepoxide," *Amer. J. Psychol.*, *130*, 1381 (1973).

(26) A. Flemenbaum and B. Gunby, "Ethchlorvynol (Placidyl) Abuse and Withdrawal (Review of Clinical Picture and Report of Two Cases)," *Dis. Nerv. Syst.*, *32*, 188 (1971).

(27) G. P. Mould *et al.*, "Interaction of Glutethimide and Phenobarbitone with Ethanol in Man," *J. Pharm. Pharmacol.*, *24*, 894 (1972).

(28) D. S. Inaba *et al.*, "Methaqualone Abuse. 'Luding Out'," *J. Amer. Med. Ass.*, *224*, 1505 (1973).

[For additional information, see *Sedative–Hypnotic Therapy*, p. 442; *Chloral Hydrate–Alcohol*, p. 20; *Diazepam–Alcohol*, p. 47; and *Meprobamate–Alcohol*, p. 145.]

Nonproprietary and Trade Names of Drugs

Alcohol—*Various products and beverages*
Allobarbital—*Diadol*
Amobarbital—*Amytal and various combination products*
Aprobarbital—*Alurate*
Barbital—*Neurondia*
Butabarbital sodium—*Butisol Sodium*
Butalbital—*Available in combination products*
Ethchlorvynol—*Placidyl*
Glutethimide—*Doriden*
Hexobarbital—*Sombulex*

Mephobarbital—*Mebaral, Mebroin*
Methaqualone—*Quaalude, Sopor*
Metharbital—*Gemonil*
Methohexital sodium—*Brevital Sodium*
Pentobarbital—*Nembutal and various combination products*
Phenobarbital—*Eskabarb, Luminal*
Secobarbital—*Seconal and various combination products*
Talbutal—*Lotusate*
Thiopental sodium—*Pentothal Sodium*

Prepared and evaluated by the Scientific Review Subpanel on Sedative–Hypnotics and reviewed by Practitioner Panel I.

Phenobarbital—Chlorpromazine

Summary—When administered parenterally as a preanesthetic medication, chlorpromazine enhances the central nervous system (CNS) depressant effect of barbiturates, resulting in prolonged sleeping times and hypotension. The barbiturate dose should be decreased to avoid this effect. Prolonged phenobarbital administration may decrease serum chlorpromazine levels and increase the urinary excretion of chlorpromazine metabolites possibly through alterations in microsomal enzyme activity. The clinical effects of this interaction have not been evaluated; patients receiving these drugs concurrently should be monitored for a possible decrease in the effect of chlorpromazine.

Related Drugs—**Thiamylal** (1, 2) and **thiopental** (2, 3) are short-acting barbiturates commonly used intravenously in anesthesia and have been reported to interact with chlorpromazine in animals. Thiopental interacts with chlorpromazine in humans (4). Other barbiturates shown to interact in a similar manner are **pentobarbital** (5) and **secobarbital** (1, 5), although all **barbiturates** should also be expected to interact.

The only other phenothiazine reported to interact with the barbiturates is **promazine** (3).

Pharmacological Effect and Mechanism—Chlorpromazine enhances the intensity and duration of activity of CNS depressants including hypnotics (6). Chlorpromazine depresses the CNS in many areas, but perhaps certain segments more than others (6). The sedative action of barbiturates is due primarily to depression of the ascending reticular arousal system (7). It is probable that some of the effects of barbiturates and chlorpromazine are due to action on the same CNS sites.

The chief metabolic pathway of chlorpromazine is hydroxylation and subsequent conjugation with glucuronic acid (6). Phenobarbital increased the rate of urinary chlorpromazine excretion, primarily in the conjugated fraction, in psychotic patients receiving large doses of both agents (8) and also decreased the serum chlorpromazine level in one patient (9). Both agents are inducers of microsomal drug-metabolizing enzymes (10–12).

Evaluation of Clinical Data—Chlorpromazine (25–50 mg po) enhanced the hypnotic effect of pentobarbital, phenobarbital, secobarbital, and a combination of amobarbital and secobarbital in 17 patients (5). Practically no failures (number not given) were reported when these drug regimens were used to induce sleep. In 13 patients, chlorpromazine (25 mg three times daily) was effective in treatment of anxiety states when used with phenobarbital. In some patients, previously ineffective doses of barbiturate became effective when administered concurrently with chlorpromazine. There was no evidence for development of tolerance to either drug, although both agents are known to induce microsomal drug-metabolizing enzymes (10–12).

In another report, the value of chlorpromazine as a preanesthetic medication was evaluated in 292 patients (4). The average dose of thiopental required for anesthesia was reduced from 580 mg in controls to 240 mg in patients pretreated with chlorpromazine. There was also a trend toward more prolonged postoperative CNS depression (*e.g.,* prolonged sleeping time and hypotension) in the chlorpromazine-treated patients. It was suggested (4) that the ability of chlorpromazine to cause hypotension and tachycardia was a serious drawback to its preoperative use.

In another study (8), phenobarbital (180–300 mg/day po) was administered for 2–7 days to 10 male patients who had been receiving chlorpromazine (400–1200 mg/day po) for periods ranging from 3 months to several years. The rate of urinary chlorpromazine metabolite excretion increased by 10–18%. The report did not indicate whether the therapeutic action of chlorpromazine was altered by concurrent administration of phenobarbital.

■ The therapeutic significance of the enhanced metabolism of chlorpromazine by phenobarbital has not been determined. Chlorpromazine, administered as an adjunct to anesthesia or in preanesthetic medication, enhances the action of ultrashort-acting or short-acting barbiturates (4, 13). The amount of sedatives given postoperatively to chlorpromazine-treated patients must be adjusted to compensate for possible enhanced CNS depression (*e.g.*, prolonged sleeping time and hypotension) (13).

Recommendations—Because of the complexity of potential pharmacological interactions between barbiturates and chlorpromazine, these drugs should not be used together without close patient monitoring. Chronic administration of barbiturates might decrease the effectiveness of chlorpromazine. Conversely, the toxicity to chlorpromazine may increase once a barbiturate is discontinued from the drug regimen.

Preanesthetic sedation with barbiturates does not preclude use of chlorpromazine during or after surgery. However, the barbiturate dose should be decreased and the patient should be observed closely to avoid hypotension and prolonged CNS depression.

Although there is no documentation, other phenothiazine-related compounds such as the butyrophenones (*e.g.*, haloperidol) and thioxanthenes (*e.g.*, thiothixene) could be expected to interact similarly.

References

(1) M. S. Sadove *et al.*, "The Potentiating Action of Chlorpromazine," *Curr. Res. Anesth. Analg.*, *35*, 165 (1956).

(2) J. W. Dundee and W. E. B. Scott, "The Effect of Phenothiazine Derivates on Thiobarbiturate Narcosis," *Anesth. Analg.*, *37*, 12 (1958).

(3) E. Tonuma, "Some Ataractic Drugs as Adjuvants to Thiopental Sodium Anesthesia in Small Animals," *Can. Vet. J.*, *7*, 128 (1966).

(4) R. D. Dripps *et al.*, "The Use of Chlorpromazine in Anesthesia and Surgery," *Ann. Surg.*, *142*, 774 (1955).

(5) R. Wallis, "Potentiation of Hypnotics and Analgesics—Clinical Experience with Chlorpromazine," *N.Y. State J. Med.*, *55*, 243 (1955).

(6) "The Pharmacological Basis of Therapeutics," 5th ed., L. S. Goodman and A. Gilman, Eds., Macmillan, New York, NY 10022, 1975, pp. 158–165.

(7) H. W. Magoun, "Symposium on Sedative and Hypnotic Drugs," Williams and Wilkins, Baltimore, Md., 1954.

(8) F. M. Forrest *et al.*, "Modification of Chlorpromazine Metabolism by Some Other Drugs Frequently Administered to Psychiatric Patients," *Biol. Psychiat.*, *2*, 53 (1970).

(9) S. H. Curry *et al.*, "Factors Affecting Chlorpromazine Plasma Levels in Psychiatric Patients," *Arch. Gen. Psychiat.*, *22*, 209 (1970).

(10) L. W. Wattenberg and J. L. Leong, "Inhibition of 9,10-Dimethylbenzanthracene (DMBA) Induced Mammary Tumorigenesis by Phenothiazines," *Fed. Proc.*, *26* (2), abstract 2435, 1967, p. 692.

(11) A. H. Conney, "Pharmacological Implications of Microsomal Enzyme Induction," *Pharmacol. Rev.*, *19*, 317 (1967).

(12) J. J. Burns *et al.*, "Stimulatory Effect of Chronic Drug Administration on Drug-Metabolizing Enzymes in Liver Microsomes," *Ann. N.Y. Acad. Sci.*, *104*, 881 (1963).

(13) E. G. Cutright, "The Effects of Chlorpromazine Premedication on Anesthesia and Postanesthetic Symptoms," *J. Amer. Med. Women's Ass.*, *11*, 45 (1956).

[For additional information, see *Sedative–Hypnotic Therapy*, p. 442.]

Nonproprietary and Trade Names of Drugs

Acetophenazine maleate—*Tindal*
Allobarbital—*Diadol*
Amobarbital—*Amytal and various combination products*
Aprobarbital—*Alurate*

Barbital—*Neurondia*
Butabarbital sodium—*Butisol Sodium*
Butalbital—*Available in combination products*
Butaperazine maleate—*Repoise Maleate*

Carphenazine maleate—*Proketazine*
Chlorpromazine—*Chlor-PZ, Promapar, Thorazine*
Chlorprothixene—*Taractan*
Fluphenazine enanthate—*Prolixin Enanthate*
Fluphenazine hydrochloride—*Permitil, Prolixin*
Haloperidol—*Haldol*
Hexobarbital—*Sombulex*
Mephobarbital—*Mebaral, Mebroin*
Mesoridazine—*Serentil*
Metharbital—*Gemonil*
Methohexital sodium—*Brevital Sodium*
Pentobarbital—*Nembutal and various combination products*
Perphenazine—*Trilafon and various combination products*

Phenobarbital—*Eskabarb, Luminal*
Piperacetazine—*Quide*
Prochlorperazine—*Compazine and various combination products*
Promazine hydrochloride—*Sparine*
Secobarbital—*Seconal and various combination products*
Talbutal—*Lotusate*
Thiamylal sodium—*Surital Sodium*
Thiopental sodium—*Pentothal Sodium*
Thiopropazate hydrochloride—*Dartal*
Thioridazine hydrochloride—*Mellaril*
Thiothixene—*Navane*
Trifluoperazine hydrochloride—*Stelazine*
Triflupromazine hydrochloride—*Vesprin*

Prepared and evaluated by the Scientific Review Subpanel on Sedative–Hypnotics and reviewed by Practitioner Panel III.

Phenylbutazone—Cholestyramine

Summary—The significance of the interaction between phenylbutazone and cholestyramine resin has yet to be determined in humans. However, since cholestyramine delays the absorption of phenylbutazone in animals, it may be prudent to avoid simultaneous administration in humans.

Related Drugs—**Oxyphenbutazone** is chemically and pharmacologically related to phenylbutazone and might be expected to interact in a similar manner with cholestyramine resin.

Polyamine-methylene resin is an anion-exchange resin similar to cholestyramine that might also bind organic acids such as phenylbutazone if administered concurrently.

Pharmacological Effect and Mechanism—Cholestyramine is a nonabsorbable anion-exchange resin that binds to bile acids by exchanging chloride ions for cholates in the lumen of the intestine (1). Phenylbutazone is an acidic drug and may bind to cholestyramine in a manner similar to the bile acids, resulting in a delay in phenyl-butazone absorption (2). *In vitro* results indicated that phenylbutazone was 98% bound by cholestyramine (2).

In *in vivo* studies by the same investigators (2), fasted rats received cholestryramine (71.5 or 357.5 mg/kg) and a concurrent single dose of phenylbutazone (dose not reported). When compared to control values after 1 hr, serum phenylbutazone levels were reduced 32% by the low dose of cholestyramine and 49% by the higher dose. After 2 hr, reductions in serum phenylbutazone levels of 22 and 47% were attributed to the low and high dose of cholestyramine, respectively. However, after 4 hr, rats receiving the lower dose of cholestyramine had serum phenylbutazone levels 29% higher than rats serving as controls. All results (2) were statistically significant, and the investigators suggested that the resin delayed phenylbutazone absorption.

Evaluation of Clinical Data—There are no studies in humans supporting this interaction.

■ Until clinical data are published, the clinical significance of this interaction cannot be assessed.

Recommendations—Although there are no published studies indicating that this drug interaction occurs in humans, data obtained from rat studies (2) indicate that it may be prudent to avoid simultaneous use of phenylbutazone and cholestyramine. The lack of clinical data makes selection of an appropriate time interval between administration of phenylbutazone and cholestyramine difficult, but it appears that a safe time to administer phenylbutazone would be 1 hr prior to or 4–6 hr after cholestyramine administration (2, 3).

References

(1) "The Pharmacological Basis of Therapeutics," 5th ed., L. S. Goodman and A. Gilman, Eds., Macmillan, New York, NY 10022, 1975, p. 748.
(2) D. G. Gallo *et al.*, "The Interaction between Cholestyramine and Drugs," *Proc. Soc. Exp. Biol. Med.*, *120*, 60 (1965).
(3) Package insert, Questran, Mead Johnson, Evansville, Ind., 1974.

[For additional information, see *Analgesic Therapy (Nonnarcotic)*, p. 341.]

Nonproprietary and Trade Names of Drugs

Cholestyramine resin—*Cuemid, Questran*
Oxyphenbutazone—*Oxalid, Tandearil*

Phenylbutazone—*Azolid, Butazolidin*
Polyamine-methylene resin—*Resinat*

Prepared and evaluated by the Scientific Review Subpanel on Analgesics and reviewed by Practitioner Panel III.

Phenylephrine—Guanethidine

Summary—Topically administered guanethidine enhances the response of the eye to topically administered phenylephrine, resulting in increased mydriasis. The drug interaction also may occur when the drugs are administered systemically, resulting in an enhanced blood pressure response to phenylephrine. However, data about the systemic effects of the drug interaction are limited and unreliable. Nevertheless, concurrent administration of these drugs should be avoided. Reversal of the interaction is achieved by administering an a-adrenergic receptor blocking drug such as phentolamine.

Related Drugs—The direct-acting a-adrenergic sympathomimetic amine **methoxamine** has been reported to interact with guanethidine in the eye (1, 2). Other predominantly direct-acting amines such as **dopamine, epinephrine,** and **levarterenol** also may be expected to interact with guanethidine. **Metaraminol** has both direct and indirect effects on the adrenergic receptor (3) and an enhanced pressor response to metaraminol has occurred in a patient stabilized on guanethidine (4).

Debrisoquin is pharmacologically and chemically related to guanethidine and has enhanced the pressor response to phenylephrine in one patient (4). **Bethanidine** also is related to guanethidine and would be expected to interact with sympathomimetics.

Pharmacological Effect and Mechanism—The main site of action of guanethidine is at the sympathetic adrenergic nerve terminal where it initially inhibits the release of norepinephrine. Continued administration of guanethidine also causes a depletion of tissue norepinephrine (5).

The responses to exogenously administered norepinephrine and other direct-acting sympathomimetics often are enhanced after guanethidine-induced adrenergic neuron blockade (1, 2, 4–7). This enhanced response to the sympathomimetic amines closely resembles the supersensitivity often caused by surgical sympathetic postganglionic denervation (6, 8, 9). Prolonged interference with the transmission of nerve impulses caused by the adrenergic neuron blockers (such as guanethidine) increases the re-activity of the effector cells to direct stimulation which may produce an acute increase in the response to certain direct-acting sympathomimetic amines. This type of super-sensitivity may be related to the ability of guanethidine to indirectly interfere with the adrenergic neuron amine uptake mechanism (10–12) and/or to a direct "sensitizing" action of the drug on the adrenergic receptor (13, 14).

Evaluation of Clinical Data—By using the iris as a convenient model for investigating drug interactions, the mydriatic action of locally administered phenylephrine (5%), methoxamine (2%), and epinephrine (1%) was markedly enhanced in patients undergoing treatment with guanethidine eye drops for thyrotoxic lid retraction (1, 2). Increased sensitivity of the iris to phenylephrine became quite apparent 6 hr after the administration of 1 drop of guanethidine (10%) and was clearly established after 24 hr. In another preliminary observation, the duration of the mydriasis caused by phenylephrine (10%) eye drops was also prolonged (up to 10 hr) in one patient receiving oral guanethidine (dose not specified) for the treatment of hypertension (15).

Two anecdotal reports with limited documentation described the effects of an interaction between adrenergic neuron blocking drugs and noncatechol sympathomimetic amines on the cardiovascular system in humans. In one instance, a hypertensive female patient with mild hypertension previously controlled with guanethidine (20 mg/day po) was given metaraminol (10 mg im) during therapy for myocardial infarction. Within a few minutes after injection of the pressor amine, blood pressure increased dramatically from 75 mm Hg systolic to 220/130 mm Hg (7). In another case, a hypertensive male patient treated with debrisoquin (20 mg po three times daily) consented to taking phenylephrine (50 mg po) to examine a possible interaction between the two drugs. Twenty minutes after taking phenylephrine, blood pressure was increased to 180 mm Hg diastolic. This type of response was never observed with patients who were not receiving debrisoquin (4). In a more detailed account of the drug interaction, the magnitude and duration of the circulatory effects of phenylephrine (0.5–0.75 mg/kg po) were enhanced significantly after debrisoquin (30–60 mg/kg po) (16).

■ There is conclusive evidence that guanethidine administered topically to the eye causes increased mydriatic response to phenylephrine administered by the same route. The data about the systemic effects of concurrent use of these drugs are not reliable, but guanethidine may increase the hypertensive response to phenylephrine, resulting in a rapid rise in blood pressure.

Recommendations—The practitioner should be alert to the possibility of an enhanced pharmacological response to phenylephrine and the other predominantly direct-acting a-adrenergic sympathomimetic amines (*e.g.*, dopamine, levarterenol, and methoxamine) in patients who are receiving or have recently received guanethidine. Reversal of the interaction can be achieved by administering an adrenergic receptor blocking drug such as phentolamine (4).

References

(1) J. M. Sneddon and P. Turner, "Structure–Activity Relationship of Some Sympathomimetic Amines in the Guanethidine-Treated Human Eye," *J. Physiol., 192*, 23P (1967).

(2) J. M. Sneddon and P. Turner, "The Interactions of Local Guanethidine and Sympathomimetic Amines in the Human Eye," *Arch. Ophthalmol., 81*, 622 (1969).

(3) J. Axelrod and R. Weinshilboum, "Catecholamines," *N. Engl. J. Med.*, *287*, 237 (1972).

(4) J. Aminu *et al.*, "Interaction between Debrisoquin and Phenylephrine," *Lancet*, *ii*, 935 (1970).

(5) A. L. A. Boura and A. F. Green, "Adrenergic Neurone Blocking Agents," *Ann. Rev. Pharmacol.*, *5*, 183 (1965).

(6) N. Emmelin, "Supersensitivity following 'Pharmacological Denervation'," *Pharmacol. Rev.*, *13*, 17 (1961).

(7) F. R. T. Stevens, "A Danger of Sympathomimetic Drugs," letter to the editor, *Med. J. Aust.*, *2*, 576 (1966).

(8) A. L. A. Boura and A. F. Green, "Comparison of Bretylium and Guanethidine: Tolerance, and Effects on Adrenergic Nerve Function and Responses to Sympathomimetic Amines," *Brit. J. Pharmacol.*, *19*, 13 (1962).

(9) N. Emmelin and J. Engstrom, "Supersensitivity of Salivary Glands following Treatment with Bretylium or Guanethidine," *Brit. J. Pharmacol.*, *16*, 315 (1961).

(10) G. Hertting *et al.*, "Effect of Drugs on the Uptake and Metabolism of H^3-Norepinephrine," *J. Pharmacol. Exp. Ther.*, *134*, 146 (1961).

(11) L. L. Iverson, "Catecholamine Uptake Processes," *Brit. Med. Bull.*, *29*, 130 (1973).

(12) U. Trendelenburg, "Classification of Sympathomimetic Amines," *Handb. Exp. Pharmakol.*, *33*, 336 (1972).

(13) R. A. Maxwell, "Concerning the Mode of Action of Guanethidine and Some Derivatives in Augmenting Vasomotor Action of Adrenergic Amines in Vascular Tissues of the Rabbit," *J. Pharmacol. Exp. Ther.*, *148*, 320 (1965).

(14) F. M. Abboud *et al.*, "Early Potentiation of the Vasoconstrictor Action of Norepinephrine by Guanethidine," *Proc. Soc. Exp. Biol. Med.*, *110*, 489 (1962).

(15) B. Cooper, " 'Neo-Synephrine' (10%) Eye Drops," letter to the editor, *Med. J. Aust.*, *2*, 420 (1968).

(16) W. Allum *et al.*, "Interaction between Debrisoquine and Phenylephrine in Man," *Brit. J. Clin. Pharmacol.*, *1*, 51 (1974).

[For additional information, see *Adrenergic Therapy*, p. 332.]

Nonproprietary and Trade Names of Drugs

Bethanidine sulfate*—*Esbatal*
Debrisoquin sulfate—*Declinax*
Dopamine hydrochloride—*Intropin*
Epinephrine hydrochloride—*Adrenalin Chloride*
Guanethidine sulfate—*Ismelin Sulfate*
Levarterenol bitartrate—*Levophed Bitartrate*

Metaraminol bitartrate—*Aramine*
Methoxamine hydrochloride—*Vasoxyl*
Phentolamine—*Regitine*
Phenylephrine hydrochloride—*Neo-Synephrine Hydrochloride and various combination products*

* Not yet commercially available in the United States.

Prepared and evaluated by the Scientific Review Subpanel on Autonomic Agents and reviewed by Practitioner Panel IV.

Phenylpropanolamine—Tranylcypromine

Summary—Phenylpropanolamine and other indirect-acting sympathomimetic amines (*e.g.*, tyramine) produce a hypertensive crisis and related symptoms in some individuals currently receiving or previously being treated with tranylcypromine or other monoamine oxidase inhibitors. The incidence of this interaction is not frequent, but when it occurs it is usually severe and may be fatal. Sympathomimetics and tyramine-containing foods should be avoided in patients receiving monoamine oxidase inhibitors. The hypertensive crisis may be reversed by administering phentolamine (5 mg im or iv).

Related Drugs—Other drugs with monoamine oxidase inhibitory activity reported to interact with sympathomimetic drugs are **isocarboxazid** (1), **pargyline** (2), and **phenelzine** (3).

Sympathomimetic amines having an indirect effect and reported to interact with monoamine oxidase inhibitors include **amphetamines** (1, 4–7), **ephedrine** (8, 9), **methylphenidate** (10), and **tyramine** (11).

Certain foods in which aging or fermentation is used to enhance flavor (*e.g.*, aged cheese, chianti wine, pickled herring, and chicken livers) have a high tyramine content and interact with monoamine oxidase inhibitors causing hypertensive episodes (11–14). Although there is no documentation, all other indirect-acting sympathomimetic agents such as **cyclopentamine** and **pseudoephedrine** could also be expected to interact with monoamine oxidase inhibitors.

The direct-acting sympathomimetic amines that also have indirect effects and that have been shown to interact with monoamine oxidase inhibitors are **metaraminol** (2) and **phenylephrine** (9). Other direct-acting amines, **epinephrine, isoproterenol, levarterenol (norepinephrine),** and **methoxamine,** have been reported not to interact with monoamine oxidase inhibitors (9, 15–17).

Dopamine, a direct-acting sympathomimetic amine, is metabolized by monoamine oxidase, and its pressor effect is enhanced by monoamine oxidase inhibitors (9, 18) (see *Levodopa–Phenelzine,* p. 128).

Pharmacological Effect and Mechanism—The use of monoamine oxidase inhibitors in animals and humans significantly enhances the peripheral adrenergic stimulation produced by the indirect sympathomimetic amines (9, 19–21). A similar enhancement of some of the direct-acting adrenergic mediators does not occur because they are primarily inactivated by catechol-*O*-methyltransferase, not by monoamine oxidase (9, 16, 17, 22). Metaraminol and phenylephrine exhibit both direct and indirect adrenergic effects (9, 22). The indirect effects are probably enhanced by monoamine oxidase inhibitors (2, 9). Dopamine exerts a direct action on the adrenergic receptors, but it is metabolized by monoamine oxidase (23) and its pressor effects are reported to be enhanced by monoamine oxidase inhibitors (15, 18) (see *Levodopa–Phenelzine,* p. 128).

The apparent selectivity of the monoamine oxidase inhibitor enhancement of sympathomimetic amines having a norepinephrine-releasing function indicates that monoamine oxidase plays a role either in the regulation of viable stores of active mediator or in the amount released (24, 25). It has been shown (25–27) that monoamine oxidase inhibition is accompanied by an increase in norepinephrine stores in various tissues including adrenergic neurons. The increase in neuronal norepinephrine or other amine mediators probably results from a failure (by inhibition) of the intraneuronal monoamine oxidase to regulate properly the amount of active mediator accumulated by the neurons to be stored in synaptic vesicles (25–27). Therefore, the enhancement of adrenergic function induced by the indirect-acting agents could be due to a marked increase in the amount of active mediator released (9, 24–26).

This mechanism of indirect sympathomimetic amine enhancement by monoamine oxidase inhibition has been challenged (20) by a suggestion that the enhancement is due to an inhibition of those hepatic microsomal enzymes that catabolize α-methylated amines resistant to monoamine oxidase degradation rather than an inhibition of monoamine oxidase itself. Regardless of the specific mechanism of action, there is considerable evidence showing that the peripheral actions of the indirect or norepinephrine-releasing amines are enhanced more than the direct-acting amines by effective inhibition of monoamine oxidase and that this interaction occurs in humans with tyramine-containing foods and beverages (11, 14) and all indirect-acting amines (9, 16).

The specific interaction problems involving tranylcypromine also may be complicated by the amphetamine-like actions of tranylcypromine in addition to its monoamine oxidase inhibition (12). Tranylcypromine causes norepinephrine accumulation in adrenergic neurons by virtue of its monoamine oxidase inhibitory activity, and it also induces an enhanced indirect adrenergic stimulation *via* a mediator-releasing function (28). This stimulation would explain paradoxical hypertensive problems observed in some patients given only this drug (29). However, this theory has not been substantiated in animals (30) and has not been examined in humans.

The monoamine oxidase inhibitors exhibited the following potency (on a dose basis) in rats with regard to the enhancement of the action of indirect-acting amines (amphetamine): isocarboxazid = tranylcypromine > phenelzine > nialamide > pargyline (30).

Evaluation of Clinical Data—Adverse effects in humans following the use of monoamine oxidase inhibitors have been reported and reviewed (11–13, 24, 31). Specific problems with tranylcypromine alone and with tyramine-containing foods or beverages have also been reviewed (11, 12, 14, 32, 33). The evidence indicates that tranylcypromine is capable of producing an adrenergic crisis with severe hypertension in some patients when given alone or with indirect sympathomimetic amines. In either case, the syndrome is similar to the hypertensive crisis encountered in pheochromocytoma (12).

The symptoms, which occur rapidly, may include a significant increase in blood pressure with a pounding heart, an intense occipital headache, and, in severe cases, nausea, vomiting, neck stiffness, intracranial hemorrhage, and death (11, 13, 14, 29, 31). Hyperpyrexia has been associated with concurrent administration of monoamine oxidase inhibitors and amphetamines (5, 7). The random occurrence of paradoxical hypertension caused by tranylcypromine suggests an interaction rather than an idiosyncratic response. In one report (34) of 10 patients who were thought to have experienced a paradoxical tranylcypromine hypertensive crisis, eight had consumed tyramine-containing cheeses (*i.e.*, cheddar cheese) within 2 hr after tranylcypromine administration (10 mg two or three times daily).

Specific clinical evidence of hypertensive episodes induced by the concurrent use of tranylcypromine and an indirect sympathomimetic amine is available (1–8), but interactions occurring with tyramine-containing foods or beverages have been reported more frequently (11–14).

Four healthy subjects (9) were pretreated with phenelzine (45 mg/day po) or tranylcypromine (30 mg/day po) and were given either ephedrine (3–12 mg iv or 30 mg/day po), phenylephrine (1–2 mg iv or 3–45 mg/day po), or levarterenol (12–48 μg iv). The pressor response elicited by the intravenous and the oral doses of ephedrine and phenylephrine, but not by levarterenol, was enhanced after monoamine oxidase inhibition. In two experiments with phenylephrine (45 mg po), phentolamine administration (5 mg iv) was necessary to prevent the blood pressure from reaching a harmful level. Phenylephrine at a lower dose (3 mg po) and in a combination product for colds (10 mg) also increased the blood pressure, but not as much as the higher phenylephrine dose.

Four volunteers in another study (16) received intravenous infusions of phenylephrine (average dose, 225 μg/min) after pretreatment with phenelzine (45 mg/day po) or tranylcypromine (30 mg/day po). In each case, the pressor effect of phenylephrine was increased at least twofold.

In another study (35), three healthy males pretreated with tranylcypromine (30 mg/day po for 20–30 days) received nonprescription combination products containing phenylpropanolamine. These products contained 50 mg of phenylpropanolamine in a capsule or 25 mg in a liquid form. Pretreatment administration of these products (100 mg of phenylpropanolamine) caused a modest rise in the systolic blood pressure, but when the same dose was given after 20–30 days of treatment with the monoamine oxidase inhibitor, there was a rapid and significant increase in blood pressure accompanied by an intense, throbbing headache. Administration of a lower dose of phenylpropanolamine (50 mg) caused similar results, but a sustained-release preparation containing 50 mg of phenylpropanolamine caused only a gradual rise in blood pressure.

There have also been numerous case reports of hyperpyrexia, severe hypertensive episodes, or death caused by concurrent administration of sympathomimetics and monoamine oxidase inhibitors (1–8, 36–39).

■ Tranylcypromine and other monoamine oxidase inhibitors are capable of producing a serious adrenergic crisis in certain individuals receiving indirect-acting sympathomimetics concurrently. The symptoms associated with this adrenergic crisis may include a significant increase in blood pressure accompanied by a pounding heart, an intense occipital headache, and in severe cases, nausea, vomiting, neck stiffness, intracranial hemorrhage, and death (11, 13, 14, 29, 31). Comparative studies in humans showed little difference between tranylcypromine and other monoamine oxidase inhibitors (9, 16).

In 1964 (32), it was estimated that, of 3.5 million patients who had received treatment with tranylcypromine, only 50 patients experienced a hypertensive crisis. Of these, 15 died from intracranial hemorrhage. Although this number is not large, the untreated consequences of this drug interaction are serious. This report did not indicate how many of these adverse reactions were paradoxical or were associated with tyramine-containing foods or beverages, with indirect-acting sympathomimetics, or with other drug classes such as the tricyclic antidepressants which also interact with the monoamine oxidase inhibitors to produce a somewhat similar adrenergic crisis (39) (see *Imipramine–Tranylcypromine*, p. 103).

Although the majority of hypertensive episodes reported with the use of monoamine oxidase inhibitors has involved an interaction with tyramine-containing foods or beverages (11, 12, 14, 32), tranylcypromine and other monoamine oxidase inhibitors are capable of causing a similar hypertensive response in patients also receiving phenylpropanolamine or other indirect-acting sympathomimetic amines (1–9, 37–39).

Recommendations—A low tyramine diet should be maintained by patients receiving tranylcypromine. Foods in which aging or protein breakdown is used to enhance flavor (*e.g.,* aged cheese, chianti wine, pickled herring, and chicken livers) should be avoided (11, 30, 40). The patient also should be warned to consult with a pharmacist or physician before taking any nonprescription medications. This drug interaction can occur as early as 3 days after initiation of monoamine oxidase inhibitor therapy (11) or as long as 2 weeks after discontinuation of the monoamine oxidase inhibitor (13).

While the direct-acting sympathomimetics (*e.g.,* epinephrine, isoproterenol, levarterenol, and methoxamine) apparently are not significantly affected by concurrent administration of monoamine oxidase inhibitors (9, 15–17), these drugs should be administered carefully to patients with cardiovascular disease particularly if they are also receiving a monoamine oxidase inhibitor (16).

Since the critical clinical problem of this interaction is the result of excessive adrenergic activation with peripheral vasoconstriction due to a-adrenergic receptor activation, the hypertensive crisis, when encountered, can safely and preferably be aborted by using phentolamine (5 mg im or iv) (9, 13, 30).

References

(1) A. Mason, "Fatal Reaction Associated with Tranylcypromine and Methylamphetamine," letter to the editor, *Lancet, i,* 1073 (1962).

(2) A. R. Horler and N. A. Wynne, "Hypertensive Crisis Due to Pargyline and Metaraminol," *Brit. Med. J., 2,* 460 (1965).

(3) P. M. Humberstone, "Hypertension from Cold Remedies," letter to the editor, *Brit. Med. J., 1,* 846 (1969).

(4) P. Zeck, "The Dangers of Some Antidepressant Drugs," letter to the editor, *Med. J. Aust., 2,* 607 (1961).

(5) E. Lewis, "Hyperpyrexia with Antidepressant Drugs," letter to the editor, *Brit. Med. J.*, *2*, 1671 (1965).

(6) C. M. Tonks and D. Livingston, "Monoamineoxidase Inhibitors," letter to the editor, *Lancet*, *i*, 1323 (1963).

(7) I. Krisko *et al.*, "Severe Hyperpyrexia Due to Tranylcypromine-Amphetamine Toxicity," *Ann. Intern. Med.*, *70*, 559 (1969).

(8) M. S. Hirsch *et al.*, "Subarachnoid Hemorrhage following Ephedrine and MAO Inhibitor," letter to the editor, *J. Amer. Med. Ass.*, *194*, 1259 (1965).

(9) J. Elis *et al.*, "Modification by Monoamine Oxidase Inhibitors of the Effect of Some Sympathomimetics on Blood Pressure," *Brit. Med. J.*, *2*, 75 (1967).

(10) M. Sherman *et al.*, "Toxic Reactions to Tranylcypromine," *Amer. J. Psychiat.*, *120*, 1019 (1964).

(11) B. Blackwell *et al.*, "Hypertensive Interactions between Monoamine Oxidase Inhibitors and Foodstuffs," *Brit. J. Psychiat.*, *113*, 349 (1967).

(12) F. Sjoqvist, "Psychotropic Drugs (2): Interaction between Monoamine Oxidase (MAO) Inhibitors and Other Substances," *Proc. Roy. Soc. Med.*, *58*, 967 (1965).

(13) H. C. Bethune *et al.*, "Vascular Crisis Associated with Monoamine-Oxidase Inhibitors," *Amer. J. Psychiat.*, *121*, 245 (1964).

(14) D. Horwitz *et al.*, "Monoamine Oxidase Inhibitors, Tyramine, and Cheese," *J. Amer. Med. Ass.*, *188*, 1108 (1964).

(15) D. Horwitz *et al.*, "Increased Blood Pressure Responses to Dopamine and Norepinephrine Produced by Monoamine Oxidase Inhibitors in Man," *J. Lab. Clin. Med.*, *56*, 747 (1960).

(16) A. J. Boakes *et al.*, "Interactions between Sympathomimetic Amines and Antidepressant Agents in Man," *Brit. Med. J.*, *1*, 311 (1973).

(17) M. F. Cuthbert and D. W. Vere, "Potentiation of the Cardiovascular Effects of Some Catecholamines by a Monoamine Oxidase Inhibitor," *Brit. J. Pharmacol.*, *43*, 471P (1971).

(18) O. Hornykiewicz, "Dopamine (3-Hydroxytyramine) and Brain Function," *Pharmacol. Rev.*, *18*, 925 (1966).

(19) L. I. Goldberg and A. Sjoerdsma, "Effects of Several Monoamine Oxidase Inhibitors on the Cardiovascular Actions of Naturally Occurring Amines in the Dog," *J. Pharmacol. Exp. Ther.*, *127*, 212 (1959).

(20) M. J. Rand and F. R. Trinker, "The Mechanism of the Augmentation of Responses to Indirectly Acting Sympathomimetic Amines by Monoamine Oxidase Inhibitors," *Brit. J. Pharmacol. Chemother.*, *33*, 287 (1968).

(21) A. M. Asatoor *et al.*, "Tranylcypromine and Cheese," letter to the editor, *Lancet*, *ii*, 733 (1963).

(22) J. Axelrod and R. Weinshilboum, "Catecholamines," *N. Engl. J. Med.*, *287*, 237 (1972).

(23) D. B. Calne and J. L. Reid, "Antiparkinsonian Drugs: Pharmacological and Therapeutic Aspects," *Drugs, 4*, 49 (1972).

(24) L. I. Goldberg, "Monoamine Oxidase Inhibitors: Adverse Reactions and Possible Mechanisms," *J. Amer. Med. Ass.*, *190*, 456 (1964).

(25) I. J. Kopin, "Biochemical Aspects of Release of Norepinephrine and Other Amines from Sympathetic Nerve Endings," *Pharmacol. Rev.*, *18*, 513 (1966).

(26) H. G. Schoepke and R. G. Wiegand, "Relation between Norepinephrine Accumulation or Depletion and Blood Pressure Responses in the Cat and Rat following Pargyline Administration," *Ann. N.Y. Acad. Sci.*, *107*, 924 (1963).

(27) W. A. Pettinger and J. A. Oates, "Supersensitivity to Tyramine during Monoamine Oxidase Inhibition in Man: Mechanism at the Level of the Adrenergic Neuron," *Clin. Pharmacol. Ther.*, *9*, 341 (1968).

(28) D. B. Frewin *et al.*, "Modification of the Vasoconstrictor Action of Sympathomimetic Agents by Bretylium Tosylate and Tranylcypromine in Man," *Brit. J. Pharmacol.*, *36*, 602 (1969).

(29) "Paradoxical Hypertension from Tranylcypromine Sulfate, Report of the Council on Drugs," *J. Amer. Med. Ass.*, *186*, 854 (1963).

(30) K. O'Dea and M. J. Rand, "Interaction between Amphetamine and Monoamine Oxidase Inhibitors," *Eur. J. Pharmacol.*, *6*, 115 (1969).

(31) A. Raskin, "Adverse Reactions to Phenelzine: Results of a Nine-Hospital Depression Study," *J. Clin. Pharmacol.*, *12*, 22 (1972).

(32) S. H. Kraines, "The Public Interest and Drug Recall," letter to the editor, *J. Amer. Med. Ass.*, *188*, 612 (1964).

(33) B. Blackwell and E. Marley, "Interactions of Yeast Extracts and Their Constituents with Monoamine Oxidase Inhibitors," *Brit. J. Pharmacol.*, *26*, 142 (1966).

(34) B. Blackwell, "Hypertensive Crisis Due to Monoamine-Oxidase Inhibitors," *Lancet*, *ii*, 849 (1963).

(35) M. F. Cuthbert *et al.*, "Cough and Cold Remedies: A Potential Danger to Patients on Monoamine Oxidase

Inhibitors," *Brit. Med. J.*, *1*, 404
(1969).

(36) C. M. Tonks and A. T. Lloyd,
"Hazards with Monoamine-Oxidase
Inhibitors," letter to the editor, *Brit.
Med. J.*, *1*, 589 (1963).

(37) J. T. A. Lloyd and D. R. H. Walker,
"Death after Combined Dexamphetamine and Phenelzine," letter to the
editor, *Brit. Med. J.*, *2*, 168 (1965).

(38) A. M. S. Mason and R. M. Buckle,
"'Cold' Cures and Monoamine-

Oxidase Inhibitors," letter to the editor, *Brit. Med. J.*, *1*, 845 (1969).

(39) L. E. Hollister, "Clinical Use of
Psychotherapeutic Drugs II: Antidepressant and Antianxiety Drugs
and Special Problems in the Use of
Psychotherapeutic Drugs," *Drugs*, *4*,
361 (1972).

(40) W. Sargant, "Interactions with Monoamine Oxidase Inhibitors," letter to
the editor, *Brit. Med. J.*, *4*, 101 (1975).

[For additional information, see *Adrenergic Therapy*, p. 332; *Antidepressant Therapy*, p. 373; *Imipramine–Tranylcypromine*, p. 103; *Levodopa–Phenelzine*, p. 128; and *Meperidine–Phenel-zine*, p. 142.]

Nonproprietary and Trade Names of Drugs

Amphetamine complex—*Biphetamine*
Amphetamine sulfate—*Benzedrine*
Cyclopentamine hydrochloride—*Clopane Hydrochloride*
Dextroamphetamine sulfate—*Dexedrine and various combination products*
Dopamine hydrochloride—*Intropin*
Ephedrine hydrochloride and sulfate—*Various manufacturers*
Epinephrine hydrochloride—*Adrenalin Chloride*
Isocarboxazid—*Marplan*
Isoproterenol hydrochloride—*Isuprel Hydrochloride*
Levarterenol bitartrate—*Levophed Bitartrate*
Metaraminol bitartrate—*Aramine*

Methamphetamine hydrochloride—*Desoxyn, Norodin Hydrochloride, Syndrox*
Methoxamine hydrochloride—*Vasoxyl*
Methylphenidate hydrochloride—*Ritalin Hydrochloride*
Pargyline hydrochloride—*Eutonyl and various combination products*
Phenelzine sulfate—*Nardil*
Phentolamine—*Regitine*
Phenylephrine hydrochloride—*Neo-Synephrine Hydrochloride and various combination products*
Phenylpropanolamine hydrochloride—*Various combination products*
Pseudoephedrine hydrochloride—*Sudafed*
Tranylcypromine—*Parnate*
Tyramine—*Various foods and beverages*

Prepared and evaluated by the Scientific Review Subpanels on Autonomic Agents and Psychotropic Agents and reviewed by Practitioner Panel V.

Phenytoin*—Dicumarol

Summary—Dicumarol may increase the serum levels and half-life of phenytoin. In addition, the concurrent administration of phenytoin and dicumarol decreases the serum levels and anticoagulant effect of dicumarol. Patients receiving these drugs concurrently should be monitored closely for signs of toxicity from pheny-toin or for a decrease in the anticoagulant effect of dicumarol.

Related Drugs—In addition to dicumarol, **warfarin** has been reported to cause phenytoin toxicity (1). However, phenytoin's effects on warfarin have not been studied. **Phenindione** has no effect on phenytoin metabolism (2). Other anticoagulants include **acenocoumarol, anisindione, diphenadione,** and **phenprocoumon.**

Although there is no documentation, other hydantoin anticonvulsants (*e.g.*, **ethotoin** and **mephenytoin** and their combination products) and other chemically related anticonvulsants (*e.g.*, **primidone**) may interact with dicumarol in a similar manner.

---

*Phenytoin is the new official name for diphenylhydantoin.

Pharmacological Effect and Mechanism—Dicumarol may inhibit *para*-hydroxylation of phenytoin in the liver causing an increase in the phenytoin half-life.

The rapid change in phenytoin metabolism after an intravenous dose of dicumarol suggests that dicumarol is an inhibitor of the aromatic ring hydroxylating enzyme system rather than an inhibitor of the synthesis of the enzyme protein system. The inhibition of phenytoin metabolism resulted in an increase of 126% in serum phenytoin levels in patients receiving dicumarol and phenytoin concurrently compared to those receiving phenytoin alone (2).

Phenytoin increased the metabolism of other agents through induction of hepatic enzyme systems (3, 4) and decreased serum dicumarol levels in normal subjects (5). Since serum dicumarol levels were depressed for 2–3 weeks after discontinuation of phenytoin in these subjects, it was suggested that phenytoin increased dicumarol metabolism (5).

Evaluation of Clinical Data—The documentation for this drug interaction consists of two studies and one case report (1, 2, 5). The case report (1) discusses phenytoin intoxication related to concurrent warfarin administration. In the first study (2), six healthy volunteers were given phenytoin (300 mg/day po). After 1 week, the serum phenytoin levels were stabilized and each patient was given dicumarol (dosage was adjusted to give a prothrombin level of 30%). The serum phenytoin level was measured during dicumarol administration and 1 week after it was discontinued. An increase in the serum phenytoin level (range, 5–14 μg/ml; mean, 9.7 μg/ml) was observed in the six subjects during dicumarol therapy. Two other volunteers received radiolabeled phenytoin intravenously (100 mg) and the drug's half-life was measured before and after 1 week of dicumarol therapy. The phenytoin half-life increased from 9 to 36 hr and from 9.75 to 44 hr after the two volunteers had received dicumarol.

In another study (5), six volunteers were treated with a constant dose of dicumarol (40–160 mg/day po) during and after treatment with phenytoin (300 mg/day po). Three days after discontinuing phenytoin, the plasma prothrombin–proconvertin concentration (PP%) started to increase from 20 to 50% (mean values) during a 5-day period, indicating a decrease in anticoagulant effect. The mean serum dicumarol level gradually decreased from 29 μg/ml on the fifth day of phenytoin treatment to a low of 21 μg/ml 5 days after phenytoin was withdrawn.

In the same study, using a longer time interval, the return of dicumarol and plasma prothrombin–proconvertin concentrations to pretreatment levels was slow after the withdrawal of phenytoin (3.5 weeks for serum dicumarol levels and 5.5 weeks for plasma prothrombin–proconvertin concentrations). The dicumarol half-life also was measured before and after phenytoin treatment. Four of five subjects showed an increase and the other subject showed a decrease in the dicumarol half-life during and after phenytoin treatment. Since the serum dicumarol half-life would be expected to decrease in all patients, the investigators suggested that the inconsistent results may be attributed to the fact that dicumarol was administered before and after, but not during, phenytoin administration. The separate administration schedules may have prevented phenytoin from inducing the hepatic microsomal system responsible for dicumarol metabolism.

■ Dicumarol may increase serum phenytoin levels and cause phenytoin toxicity when these drugs are given concurrently (2). Phenytoin may decrease serum dicumarol levels and decrease its anticoagulant effect (5). Either effect appears to occur when one drug was added to the drug regimen after a subject was stabilized on the other drug. Although the data indicate that a clinically significant drug interaction may occur if these drugs are used together, the data were obtained from studies in normal subjects. Additional studies in the appropriate patient population are needed before the clinical significance of the drug interaction can be assessed.

Recommendations—Patients receiving phenytoin and dicumarol (or warfarin) concurrently should be monitored closely for the early signs of phenytoin toxicity (*e.g.*, nystagmus, blurring of vision, lethargy, and poor muscular tone), particularly when the anticoagulant is added to the drug regimen of a patient previously stabilized on phenytoin. Similarly, prothrombin times should be monitored closely. Caution should be exercised when reestablishing anticoagulant doses following discontinuation of phenytoin because of the possibility of a subsequent increase in anticoagulant effect. The increased anticoagulant effect takes approximately 3 weeks to develop (5).

References

(1) N. O. Rothermich, "Diphenylhydantoin Intoxication," letter to the editor, *Lancet*, ii, 640 (1966).

(2) J. M. Hansen *et al.*, "Dicumarol-Induced Diphenylhydantoin Intoxication," *Lancet*, ii, 265 (1966).

(3) A. H. Conney, "Pharmacological Implications of Microsomal Enzyme In-duction," *Pharmacol. Rev.*, *19*, 317 (1967).

(4) R. Kuntzman, "Drugs and Enzyme In-duction," *Ann. Rev. Pharmacol.*, *9*, 21 (1969).

(5) J. M. Hansen *et al.*, "Effect of Di-phenylhydantoin on the Metabolism of Dicumarol in Man," *Acta Med. Scand.*, *189*, 15 (1971).

[For additional information, see *Anticoagulant Therapy*, p. 358, and *Anticonvulsant Therapy*, p. 369.]

Nonproprietary and Trade Names of Drugs

Acenocoumarol—*Sintrom*
Anisindione—*Miradon*
Dicumarol—*Various manufacturers*
Diphenadione—*Dipaxin*
Ethotoin—*Peganone*
Mephenytoin—*Mesantoin*
Phenindione—*Hedulin*

Phenprocoumon—*Liquamar*
Phenytoin—*Dilantin*
Primidone—*Mysoline*
Warfarin potassium—*Athrombin-K*
Warfarin sodium—*Coumadin Sodium, Panwarfin*

Prepared and evaluated by the Scientific Subpanels on Anticon-vulsants and Anticoagulants and reviewed by Practitioner Panel V.

Phenytoin*—Disulfiram

Summary—Disulfiram increases serum phenytoin levels in patients previously stabilized on phenytoin. Adjustment of the phenytoin dose during concurrent therapy may be sufficient to avoid phenytoin toxicity in some patients, but dis-continuation of disulfiram also may be necessary. Determinations of the pheny-toin effect by clinical assessment and serum levels are necessary when these drugs are administered concurrently.

Related Drugs—Disulfiram apparently also interacts with the anticonvulsant **primi-done** (1). Although there is no documentation, other hydantoin anticonvulsants such as **ethotoin** and **mephenytoin** may be expected to interact with disulfiram in a similar manner.

Pharmacological Effect and Mechanism—Disulfiram may exert a biphasic effect in animals, *i.e.*, an acute metabolic inhibitory action followed by induction of drug

---
* Phenytoin is the new official name for diphenylhydantoin.

metabolism (2). In humans, disulfiram caused an elevation of plateau serum levels of several chronically administered drugs including phenytoin (3). The elevated serum phenytoin levels occurring after concurrent administration of disulfiram have been attributed to disulfiram inhibition of phenytoin metabolism. Whether or not disulfiram causes a significant inductive effect on liver enzymes in humans has not been reported.

Evaluation of Clinical Data—In a study of three alcoholic patients receiving phenytoin (4), symptoms of phenytoin intoxication were observed 1–3 weeks after initiation of disulfiram (400–800 mg/day po). Exact timing of the onset of symptoms relative to dose was not possible due to a suspected lack of patient compliance. In this study (4), lowering the doses of phenytoin and disulfiram did not completely eliminate symptoms of phenytoin toxicity (particularly dizziness) in one patient. Complete resolution of symptoms came only after disulfiram was discontinued. Since the patient was an alcoholic, the symptoms may have been due to a disulfiram–alcohol interaction.

In a study of four epileptic patients given disulfiram (400 mg/day po), serum phenytoin levels were higher than controls 4 hr after the first dose of disulfiram (1). Phenytoin levels continued to rise throughout the 9 days of disulfiram administration. In one subject (whose phenytoin level had been the highest of the four subjects), the serum level rose to 35 μg/ml (normal level, 7–20 μg/ml). Serum phenytoin levels continued to rise for 1–3 days after cessation of disulfiram therapy and then declined. Another patient in this group received phenobarbital and phenytoin concurrently. After subsequent treatment with disulfiram, there was no change in serum phenobarbital levels at a time when the serum phenytoin level was rising and the excretion rate of the phenytoin metabolite was falling. Three of the patients also received primidone. In these patients, serum phenobarbital (a metabolite of primidone) levels rose after disulfiram administration, indicating that a more rapid conversion of primidone to phenobarbital may have occurred.

■ Although this drug interaction has occurred only in a small number of patients, it seems likely that therapeutic doses of disulfiram increase serum phenytoin levels, possibly leading to toxic symptoms. The low number of reports may be due to the infrequent use of these drugs concurrently, not to a low incidence rate.

Recommendations—Whenever possible, disulfiram should not be given concurrently with phenytoin. If the drugs are administered concurrently, serum phenytoin levels should be determined before disulfiram is added to the drug regimen. In the 2–4 days after initiation of concurrent therapy, serum phenytoin levels should be checked and the clinical response must be monitored closely. Although considerable individual variation exists, nystagmus generally appears when the serum phenytoin level reaches 20 μg/ml or higher. Gait ataxia is observed at levels around 30 μg/ml with constant lethargy seen at levels approaching 40 μg/ml (5). If increased serum phenytoin levels occur, a decrease in the dose of the anticonvulsant is appropriate to avoid toxicity. An increase in the phenytoin dose may be necessary to avoid loss of seizure control when disulfiram is withdrawn from the drug regimen.

The interaction between disulfiram and phenytoin is particularly important in alcoholic patients when concurrent phenytoin–disulfiram therapy is used for treatment of alcohol withdrawal (6).

References

(1) O. V. Olesen, "Disulfiramum (Antabuse) as Inhibitor of Phenytoin Metabolism," *Arch. Pharmacol. Toxicol.*, *24*, 317 (1966).

(2) W. R. F. Notten and P. T. Henderson, "Effect of Disulfiram on the Urinary D-Glucuric Acid Excretion and Activity of Some Enzymes Involved in Drug Metabolism in Guinea-Pig," *Arch. Int. Pharmacodyn. Ther.*, *205*, 199 (1973).

(3) O. V. Olesen, "The Influence of Disulfiram and Calcium Carbimide on the Serum Diphenylhydantoin. Excretion of HPPH in the Urine," *Arch. Neurol.*, *16*, 642 (1967).

(4) E. Kiorboe, "Phenytoin Intoxication during Treatment with Antabuse (Disulfiram)," *Epilepsia*, *7*, 246 (1966).

(5) H. Kutt and F. McDowell, "Manage-

ment of Epilepsy with Diphenylhydantoin Sodium. Dosage Regulation for Problem Patients," *J. Amer. Med. Ass.*, *203*, 969 (1968).

(6) R. Sampliner and F. L. Iber, "Diphenylhydantoin Control of Alcohol Withdrawal Seizures. Results of a Controlled Study," *J. Amer. Med. Ass.*, *230*, 1430 (1974).

[For additional information, see *Anticonvulsant Therapy*, p. 369.]

Nonproprietary and Trade Names of Drugs

Disulfiram—*Antabuse*
Ethotoin—*Peganone*
Mephenytoin—*Mesantoin*

Phenytoin—*Dilantin*
Primidone—*Mysoline*

Prepared and evaluated by the Scientific Review Subpanel on Anticonvulsants and reviewed by Practitioner Panel VI.

Phenytoin*—Folic Acid

Summary—Long-term administration of phenytoin may cause low serum folate levels in some patients and may precipitate symptoms of folic acid deficiency (*e.g.*, mental dysfunction, neuropathy, psychiatric disorders, and, rarely, megaloblastic anemia). Patients receiving phenytoin should be observed for symptoms of folic acid deficiency and, where indicated, serum folate levels should be determined. If desirable, folic acid (0.1–1 mg/day po) may be added as supplemental therapy. Daily administration of 5 mg or more of folic acid is not more effective than smaller doses in correcting folate deficiency and has been associated with an increased seizure frequency in some patients.

Related Drugs—The anticonvulsant **primidone** also has been associated with decreased serum folate levels (1, 2). The hydantoin derivatives, *e.g.*, **ethotoin** and **mephenytoin,** also may decrease serum folate levels in a manner similar to phenytoin, but this decrease has not been documented.

There are no compounds chemically or pharmacologically related to folic acid that might be expected to interact similarly.

Pharmacological Effect and Mechanism—The mechanism of action of the phenytoin-induced folate deficiency in epileptic patients is unclear. An early theory, since disputed (3), was that phenytoin inhibited the intestinal absorption of folic acid (4, 5). A second hypothesis is that the phenytoin-induced increase in drug-metabolizing enzymes causes an increased demand for folate as a coenzyme for drug metabolism (6). A more recent postulation states that folate deficiency in the cerebrospinal fluid caused by phenytoin is due to an interference by phenytoin of the conversion of folate to a form which is transported into the brain and cerebrospinal fluid. This interference results in higher serum folate levels and less folate in the cerebrospinal fluid (7).

Folic acid, when administered in doses of 5 mg or more, enhances the *para*-hydroxylation of phenytoin (8), perhaps altering it to an unknown pathway (9, 10). This observation has been challenged by others (11) who could not find a change in the phenytoin half-life after folic acid administration. Folic acid alone has caused

---

*Phenytoin is the new official name for diphenylhydantoin.

seizures in animals (12) and the anticonvulsant properties of phenytoin may be a result of its antifolate action (1).

Evaluation of Clinical Data—Studies have shown that 27–91% of epileptic patients treated with phenytoin have low serum folate levels (between 2 and 5 ng/ml) (1). Other studies reported correspondingly low folic acid levels in the cerebrospinal fluid and red blood cells of patients after long-term treatment with phenytoin (7, 13).

The clinical manifestations of this deficiency are megaloblastic anemia (in <1% of the cases treated) (1, 14), mental dysfunction, psychiatric disorders, and neuropathy (14). Phenytoin-induced folate deficiency may be responsible for congenital malformations, but a causal relationship has not been established (2, 15, 16).

Folic acid administration (in doses of 5 mg or more) may increase the seizure frequency in patients stabilized on phenytoin (8, 17, 18), possibly resulting in death (13). Most of these reports consisted of individual cases (8, 13, 18). Other studies demonstrated a significant decrease (as much as 50% in some cases) in serum phenytoin levels when folic acid was administered (6, 8, 18, 19). In one study (17), folic acid (15 mg/day po for 1–3 years) resulted in increased seizure frequency in 13 of 26 patients studied. The longer the patient was taking folic acid and phenytoin concurrently, the more apparent was the loss of seizure control. In nine patients, it became necessary to stop folic acid therapy, and in six patients, the loss of seizure control did not occur until after at least 5 months of therapy.

Other studies (10, 20–22) did not corroborate these results. Most of these studies were done over 3 months or less, which may be insufficient time for an accumulation of folate to occur in the tissues and the cerebrospinal fluid and for deterioration of seizure control (1). The only study done for a longer period (22) was double blind with 51 patients receiving 15 mg/day po of folic acid. Each patient had a serum folate level below 3.6 ng/ml (normal, 5–25 ng/ml), and subsequent treatment was for a minimum of 6 months; in 41 patients, it continued for more than 1 year. No significant changes in seizure frequency were observed. These conclusions were later debated (23, 24).

■ The results from these studies and observations offer no conclusive information about the probability of folic acid administration decreasing the seizure control of phenytoin in epileptic patients. Some investigators commented that in many of the controlled studies (10, 17, 20–22) trial design was poor (23), measurement of seizure frequency was vague and subjective (19, 23, 25), and the selected patient population may not have been indicative of the general epileptic population (23).

Additionally, many studies used serum folate levels to identify the folic acid-deficient patient. The limitations of this test for such purposes have been widely acknowledged (22, 23, 26). Finally, in most studies, the patients were receiving other anticonvulsants in addition to phenytoin (usually primidone and/or phenobarbital) which also have been implicated in folate depletion (1, 2, 17, 27). Therefore, no definite causal relationship can be established between loss of seizure control and folic acid administration (6, 8, 28).

Recommendations—Patients receiving phenytoin should be observed closely for symptoms of folic acid deficiency (*e.g.*, mental dysfunction, neuropathy, psychiatric disorders, and, rarely, megaloblastic anemia). If these symptoms are observed, serum folate levels should be obtained to determine if the patient is folate deficient. If desirable, folic acid (0.1–1 mg/day po) may be added as supplemental therapy (29), although its value in correcting the neurological symptoms has not been established. Larger doses of folic acid should not be used since they are not more effective in correcting folate deficiency (29) and may increase the seizure frequency in patients stabilized on phenytoin (8, 17, 18).

In pregnant patients receiving phenytoin who have folate requirements greater than normal, it has been suggested that folic acid should be added to the drug regimen as a prophylactic measure (2). Others, however, feel that the potential harm resulting from the possibility of more seizures caused by folic acid outweighs any benefit gained by folic acid replacement therapy and advise against this approach (16, 18).

Phenobarbital has also been associated with folate deficiency and may interact with folic acid in a manner similar to phenytoin (1, 2, 17, 27).

References

(1) E. H. Reynolds, "Anticonvulsants, Folic Acid, and Epilepsy," *Lancet, i*, 1376 (1973).

(2) B. D. Speidel and S. R. Meadow, "Epilepsy, Anticonvulsants and Congenital Malformations," *Drugs, 8*, 354 (1974).

(3) C. M. Houlihan *et al.*, "The Effect of Phenytoin on the Absorption of Synthetic Folic Acid Polyglutamate," *Gut, 13*, 189 (1972).

(4) A. V. Hoffbrand and T. F. Necheles, "Mechanism of Folate Deficiency in Patients Receiving Phenytoin," *Lancet, ii*, 528 (1968).

(5) R. E. Davis and H. J. Woodliff, "Folic Acid Deficiency in Patients Receiving Anticonvulsant Drugs," *Med. J. Aust., 2*, 1070 (1971).

(6) J. D. Maxwell *et al.*, "Folate Deficiency after Anticonvulsant Drugs: An Effect of Hepatic Enzyme Induction?" *Brit. Med. J., 1*, 297 (1972).

(7) R. H. Mattson *et al.*, "Folate Therapy in Epilepsy: A Controlled Study," *Arch. Neurol., 29*, 78 (1973).

(8) E. M. Baylis *et al.*, "Influence of Folic Acid on Blood-Phenytoin Levels," *Lancet, i*, 62 (1971).

(9) O. V. Olesen and O. N. Jensen, "The Influence of Folic Acid on Phenytoin (DPH) Metabolism and the 24-Hours Fluctuation in Urinary Output of 5-(*p*-Hydroxyphenyl)-5-phenyl-hydantoin (HPPH)," *Acta Pharmacol. Toxicol., 28*, 265 (1970).

(10) A. J. Glazko, "Diphenylhydantoin Metabolism. A Prospective Review," *Drug Metab. Dispos., i*, 711 (1973).

(11) P. B. Andreasen *et al.*, "Folic Acid and Phenytoin Metabolism," *Lancet, i*, 645 (1971).

(12) O. R. Hommes and E. A. M. T. Obbens, "The Epileptogenic Action of Na-folate in the Rat," *J. Neurol. Sci., 16*, 271 (1972).

(13) D. G. Wells, "Folic Acid and Neuropathy in Epilepsy," *Lancet, i*, 146 (1968).

(14) J. W. Norris and R. F. Pratt, "Folic Acid Deficiency and Epilepsy," *Drugs, 8*, 366 (1974).

(15) Y. Baile *et al.*, "Congenital Malformations Due to Anticonvulsant Drugs," *Obstet. Gynecol., 45*, 439 (1975).

(16) D. Janz, "The Teratogenic Risk of Antiepileptic Drugs," *Epilepsia, 16*, 159 (1975).

(17) E. H. Reynolds, "Effects of Folic Acid on the Mental State and Fit-Frequency of Drug-Treated Epileptic Patients," *Lancet, i*, 1086 (1967).

(18) R. G. Strauss and R. Bernstein, "Folic Acid and Dilantin Antagonism in Pregnancy," *Obstet. Gynecol., 44*, 345 (1974).

(19) J. W. Norris and R. F. Pratt, "A Controlled Study of Folic Acid in Epilepsy," *Neurology, 21*, 659 (1971).

(20) O. N. Jensen and O. V. Olesen, "Subnormal Serum Folate Due to Anticonvulsive Therapy. A Double-Blind Study of the Effect of Folic Acid Treatment in Patients with Drug-Induced Subnormal Serum Folates," *Arch. Neurol., 22*, 181 (1970).

(21) A. J. Ralston *et al.*, "Effects of Folic Acid on Fit-Frequency and Behaviour in Epileptics on Anticonvulsants," *Lancet, i*, 867 (1970).

(22) R. H. E. Grant and O. P. R. Stores, "Folic Acid in Folate-Deficient Patients with Epilepsy," *Brit. Med. J., 4*, 644 (1970).

(23) A. Richens, "Folic Acid in Epilepsy," *Brit. Med. J., 1*, 109 (1971).

(24) R. H. E. Grant *et al.*, "Folic Acid in Epilepsy," *Brit. Med. J., 1*, 728 (1971).

(25) S. J. Horwitz *et al.*, "Relation of Abnormal Folate Metabolism to Neuropathy Developing during Anticonvulsant Drug Therapy," *Lancet, i*, 563 (1968).

(26) J. Kariks *et al.*, "Serum Folic Acid and Phenytoin Levels in Permanently Hospitalized Epileptic Patients Receiving Anticonvulsant Drug Therapy," *Med. J. Aust., 2*, 368 (1971).

(27) C. Neubauer, "Mental Deterioration in Epilepsy Due to Folate Deficiency," *Brit. Med. J., 2*, 759 (1970).

(28) J. Preece *et al.*, "Relation of Serum to Red Cell Folate Concentrations in Drug-Treated Epileptic Patients," *Epilepsia, 12*, 335 (1971).

(29) "Use of Folic Acid in Pregnancy and in Clinical Disorders," *Med. Lett., 14*, 50 (1972).

[For additional information, see *Anticonvulsant Therapy*, p. 369.]

Nonproprietary and Trade Names of Drugs

Ethotoin—*Peganone*
Folic acid—*Various manufacturers*
Mephenytoin—*Mesantoin*

Phenobarbital—*Eskabarb, Luminal*
Phenytoin—*Dilantin*
Primidone—*Mysoline*

Prepared and evaluated by the Scientific Review Subpanel on Anticonvulsants and reviewed by Practitioner Panel I.

Phenytoin*—Halothane

Summary—Phenytoin may increase the hepatic toxicity of halothane, and halothane-induced hepatic dysfunction may increase the toxicity of phenytoin. However, the documentation for this drug interaction is limited and unreliable. Although more information is needed before the clinical significance of this drug interaction can be assessed, patients who show signs of hepatic toxicity following halothane anesthesia and who are receiving phenytoin should have serum phenytoin levels and clinical signs of toxicity closely monitored. If serum phenytoin levels are increased, the phenytoin dose should be decreased to avoid accumulation of the drug to levels above the therapeutic range.

Related Drugs—Two halogenated anesthetic agents, **fluroxene** (1) and halothane (2), have been suspected of interacting with phenytoin. Other halogenated anesthetic agents are **chloroform, enflurane, ethyl chloride, halopropane, methoxyflurane, trichloroethylene,** and **trichloromonofluoromethane,** although no interactions with phenytoin have been reported. Other hydantoin derivatives (*e.g.,* **ethotoin** and **mephenytoin)** and other anticonvulsants (*e.g.,* **primidone)** may interact with fluroxene or halothane, but supporting clinical evidence is lacking.

Pharmacological Effect and Mechanism—Hepatitis was reported in two patients receiving phenytoin and/or phenobarbital after fluroxene or halothane anesthesia. One patient who survived showed evidence of slow phenytoin metabolism attributed to the hepatic toxicity of halothane (2). In the other patient, the massive hepatic necrosis occurring after anesthesia and resulting in rapid death prompted the investigators to speculate that phenytoin increased the susceptibility of the liver to the toxicity of the anesthetic (1).

Evaluation of Clinical Data—Phenytoin (10 mg/kg/day po) was administered for an unspecified duration to a 10-year-old patient (2). While the dose was large, the only phenytoin side effects noted before surgery were nystagmus and gingival hyperplasia. Data on serum phenytoin levels after resolution of the halothane-induced hepatitis suggested that this dose was not excessive. The course after anesthesia was compatible with mild halothane-induced hepatic damage (3). Body temperature remained elevated for 3 days following a 90-min anesthesia with halothane. Serum glutamic oxaloacetic transaminase (SGOT) was elevated (observed, 120 units/ml; normal, 8–33 units/ml) 3 and 6 days after anesthesia while serum glutamic pyruvic transaminase (SGPT) remained normal. Phenytoin was continued intramuscularly after surgery at the same dose as given orally before admission. The intramuscular

---

* Phenytoin is the new official name for diphenylhydantoin.

route should have resulted in lower serum phenytoin levels (4, 5), but signs consistent with phenytoin toxicity (*e.g.*, nystagmus, blurring of vision, lethargy, and poor muscular tone) rapidly developed and the serum phenytoin concentration increased to a level (41 μg/ml) compatible with these symptoms. It was concluded that hepatic necrosis (diagnosed from histological examination) due to halothane had led to the phenytoin accumulation.

In the other report (1), severe hepatic necrosis resulted from fluroxene anesthesia in an elderly female treated with phenytoin (300 mg/day po) and phenobarbital (120 mg/day po) since early adulthood. In the week prior to anesthesia, the phenytoin dose was increased to 2400 mg/day po for control of left-sided seizures. The investigators questioned whether previous phenytoin administration had increased susceptibility to fluroxene toxicity but the presence of other enzyme-inducing agents (phenobarbital) precluded any conclusions on the effect of phenytoin.

■ Phenytoin may increase the hepatic toxicity of halothane, and halothane-induced hepatic dysfunction may increase phenytoin toxicity. However, the data concerning these effects are not reliable, and more information about this drug interaction is necessary before its clinical significance can be assessed.

Recommendations—When patients receiving phenytoin show signs of hepatitis (*i.e.*, fever and elevated SGOT), especially following anesthesia with fluorinated anesthetic agents, close monitoring of serum phenytoin levels and clinical signs of phenytoin toxicity (*e.g.*, nystagmus, blurring of vision, lethargy, and poor muscular tone) is indicated for possible reduction of dosage.

It is not clear if phenytoin increases the likelihood of halothane-induced liver necrosis. The cases presented raise this possibility but in no way document its occurrence. Neither changes in management nor additional precautions are warranted on the basis of these reports.

References

(1) E. S. Reynolds *et al.*, "Massive Hepatic Necrosis after Fluroxene Anesthesia—a Case of Drug Interaction?" *N. Engl. J. Med.*, *286*, 530 (1972).

(2) J. M. Karlin and H. Kutt, "Acute Diphenylhydantoin Intoxication following Halothane Anesthesia," *J. Pediat.*, *76*, 941 (1970).

(3) R. L. Peters *et al.*, "Hepatic Necrosis Associated with Halothane Anesthesia," *Amer. J. Med.*, *47*, 748 (1969).

(4) B. J. Wilder *et al.*, "A Method for Shifting from Oral to Intramuscular Diphenylhydantoin Administration," *Clin. Pharmacol. Ther.*, *16*, 507 (1974).

(5) E. E. Serrano *et al.*, "Plasma Diphenylhydantoin Values after Oral and Intramuscular Administration of Diphenylhydantoin," *Neurology*, *23*, 311 (1973).

[For additional information, see *Anesthetic Therapy*, p. 345, and *Anticonvulsant Therapy*, p. 369.]

Nonproprietary and Trade Names of Drugs

Chloroform—*Various manufacturers*
Enflurane—*Ethrane*
Ethotoin—*Peganone*
Ethyl chloride—*Various manufacturers*
Fluroxene—*Fluromar*
Halopropane—*Tebron*
Halothane—*Fluothane*

Mephenytoin—*Mesantoin*
Methoxyflurane—*Penthrane*
Phenytoin—*Dilantin*
Primidone—*Mysoline*
Trichloroethylene—*Trilene*
Trichloromonofluoromethane—*Various manufacturers*

> *Prepared and evaluated by the Scientific Review Subpanels on Anticonvulsants and Anesthetics and reviewed by Practitioner Panel II.*

Phenytoin*—Isoniazid

Summary—Patients who are genetically "slow" inactivators of isoniazid may experience phenytoin toxicity when receiving phenytoin and isoniazid concurrently. If toxicity occurs, phenytoin should be discontinued or the dosage should be reduced until toxic manifestations subside. Phenytoin should then be reinstituted or the dosage of the drug should be adjusted to achieve a therapeutically acceptable serúm phenytoin level.

Related Drugs—Other hydantoin derivatives (*e.g.*, **ethotoin** and **mephenytoin**) or anticonvulsants (*e.g.*, **primidone**) may interact with isoniazid, although supporting clinical evidence is not available.

Pharmacological Effect and Mechanism—In some instances, the concurrent administration of phenytoin and isoniazid will increase the serum phenytoin level significantly and may result in toxicity. This effect has been demonstrated in humans and animals (1, 2).

Phenytoin is metabolized primarily to 5-(*p*-hydroxyphenyl)-5-phenylhydantoin (3), with *para*-hydroxylation carried out by the microsomal system (1). Isoniazid inhibits *para*-hydroxylation of phenytoin, but the exact mechanism by which this is accomplished is not known (1). Studies of the microsomal system *in vitro* indicated that a noncompetitive inhibition by isoniazid may occur (1). *In vivo* animal studies showed that the inhibition of phenytoin metabolism is dependent on the dosage of isoniazid (1).

Folic acid may be necessary for the metabolism of phenytoin; antitubercular drugs may interact with folic acid, thus producing an inhibitory effect in this metabolic process. However, there is little evidence to support this hypothesis (2). In one patient, a decrease in the toxic serum level of phenytoin was associated with the administration of folic acid (15 mg/day po); reaccumulation occurred after folic acid was discontinued. Since aminosalicylic acid and isoniazid were administered concurrently, aminosalicylic acid was considered a contributing factor (2).

Evaluation of Clinical Data—The first report about this drug interaction discussed unexpected symptomatology (drowsiness and unsteadiness) in a group of 637 epileptic patients receiving isoniazid (300 mg/day po), phenytoin (100–400 mg/day po), and phenobarbital (4).

The drug interaction was later studied in 24 patients receiving phenytoin and isoniazid concurrently with either aminosalicylic acid or cycloserine (2). In one patient, aminosalicylic acid and isoniazid were each given alone without the occurrence of phenytoin toxicity or change in serum level; when given together, the serum phenytoin level increased from 20 μg/ml to a level of 30 μg/ml and the patient developed nystagmus and ataxia. On the basis of these data, it was concluded that aminosalicylic acid and isoniazid must be given concurrently to produce the inhibition of phenytoin metabolism.

In subsequent studies (5, 6), the interaction was correlated with the isoniazid inactivator phenotype of the individual. [The phenotype is a genetically determined characteristic, and each person can be classified as a "rapid" or "slow" inactivator of isoniazid (7).] Phenytoin (300 mg/day po) was administered for 3 weeks to 32 patients (18 rapid inactivators and 14 slow inactivators) who were also receiving aminosalicylic acid (15 g/day po) and isoniazid (300 mg/day po). Serum level measurements were carried out at weekly intervals (5). Six of the 32 patients (all slow inactivators) rapidly accumulated phenytoin and showed significantly higher mean serum levels than the remainder of the patients. The same patients developed

---

*Phenytoin is the new official name for diphenylhydantoin.

the typical signs and symptoms of phenytoin toxicity (*e.g.,* ataxia, drowsiness, and nystagmus) when serum levels rose above 20 μg/ml. The signs and symptoms subsided with a reduction of the dosage or with discontinuation of phenytoin. The other 26 patients did not develop signs of toxicity regardless of phenotype. Their serum levels plateaued within, or slightly higher than, the usual range (5–15 μg/ml) found in patients receiving long-term therapy (8). The same results were found in an almost identical group of 36 subjects (toxicity occurred in six subjects) (6).

■ Approximately 10–20% of a given group of patients receiving concurrent isoniazid–phenytoin or isoniazid–phenytoin–aminosalicylic acid therapy may develop phenytoin toxicity (4, 6, 8). Although slow isoniazid inactivators typically comprise about half of any patient group (5, 7), only the slowest inactivators exhibit clinically significant phenytoin toxicity, apparently irrespective of the other agents commonly used in such patients (*e.g.,* aminosalicylic acid or phenobarbital). In the remaining approximately 80–90% of a given group, the occurrence of some degree of isoniazid-induced decrease in phenytoin metabolism does not produce a significant elevation of phenytoin levels (2).

Recommendations—Patients receiving phenytoin and isoniazid concurrently should have periodic determinations of serum phenytoin levels and should be observed closely to detect early signs and symptoms of phenytoin intoxication (5). Patients known to be slow isoniazid inactivators should have their phenytoin dosage appropriately reduced when isoniazid is added to the treatment regimen.

Although considerable individual variation exists, nystagmus generally appears when the serum phenytoin level reaches 20 μg/ml or higher. Gait ataxia is observed at levels around 30 μg/ml with constant lethargy seen at levels approaching 40 μg/ml (8). If toxicity occurs, phenytoin should be discontinued or the dosage should be reduced until toxic signs and symptoms disappear. Then phenytoin can be reinstituted or the dosage can be adjusted until therapeutic levels are attained.

Two other antitubercular drugs, aminosalicylic acid and cycloserine, interact with phenytoin *in vitro,* although they are less potent than isoniazid in this regard (6).

References

(1) H. Kutt *et al.,* "Inhibition of Diphenylhydantoin Metabolism in Rats and Rat Liver Microsomes by Antitubercular Drugs," *Neurology, 18,* 706 (1968).

(2) H. Kutt *et al.,* "Depression of Parahydroxylation of Diphenylhydantoin by Antituberculosis Chemotherapy," *Neurology, 16,* 594 (1966).

(3) T. C. Butler, "The Metabolic Conversion of 5,5-Diphenyl Hydantoin to 5-(*p*-Hydroxyphenyl)-5-Phenyl Hydantoin," *J. Pharmacol. Exp. Ther., 119,* 1 (1957).

(4) F. J. Murray, "Outbreak of Unexpected Reactions among Epileptics Taking Isoniazid," *Amer. Rev. Resp. Dis., 86,* 729 (1962).

(5) R. W. Brennan *et al.,* "Diphenylhydantoin Intoxication Attendant to Slow Inactivation of Isoniazid," *Neurology, 20,* 687 (1970).

(6) H. Kutt *et al.,* "Diphenylhydantoin Intoxication. A Complication of Isoniazid Therapy," *Amer. Rev. Resp. Dis., 101,* 377 (1970).

(7) D. A. P. Evans *et al.,* "The Determination of the Isoniazid Inactivator Phenotype," *Amer. Rev. Resp. Dis., 82,* 853 (1960).

(8) H. Kutt and F. McDowell, "Management of Epilepsy with Diphenylhydantoin Sodium. Dosage Regulation for Problem Patients," *J. Amer. Med. Ass., 203,* 969 (1968).

[For additional information, see *Anticonvulsant Therapy,* p. 369.]

Nonproprietary and Trade Names of Drugs

Aminosalicylic acid—*Pamisyl, Parasal, Pasara Sodium, Rezipas*
Cycloserine—*Seromycin*
Ethotoin—*Peganone*

Isoniazid—*Various manufacturers*
Mephenytoin—*Mesantoin*
Phenytoin—*Dilantin*
Primidone—*Mysoline*

Prepared and evaluated by the Scientific Review Subpanel on Anticonvulsants and reviewed by Practitioner Panel III.

Phenytoin*—Methylphenidate

Summary—Methylphenidate raises serum phenytoin levels and may cause symptoms of phenytoin toxicity in some children, but these effects were not observed in controlled studies with adults. Although concurrent administration need not be avoided, the patient receiving these drugs should be observed closely for unexpected symptoms of phenytoin toxicity. If such symptoms occur, the phenytoin dose should be lowered and serum phenytoin levels should be determined.

Related Drugs—**Dextroamphetamine**, like methylphenidate, is used to treat hyperkinetic symptoms in children and to prevent drowsiness in adults (1), but it has not been reported to cause a rise in the serum level of any concurrently administered anticonvulsant drug. Related agents include **amphetamine** and **methamphetamine.**

Of the other anticonvulsants, only **primidone** (2) has been reported to interact with methylphenidate in a similar manner. Other hydantoin anticonvulsants are **ethotoin** and **mephenytoin.**

Pharmacological Effect and Mechanism—Although phenytoin and methylphenidate are used for their central nervous system effects, the increases in anticonvulsant levels are apparently due to methylphenidate-induced changes in hepatic phenytoin metabolism. *In vitro* studies (3, 4) showed that methylphenidate is a competitive inhibitor of the hepatic metabolism of phenytoin and other drugs. This effect is variable among species with humans being the most sensitive (2). Ritalinic acid, the major metabolite of methylphenidate in humans, was ineffective as an inhibitor (5).

Evaluation of Clinical Data—In a black male (age 5) receiving phenytoin (8.9 mg/kg/day po) and primidone (17.7 mg/kg/day po), the addition of methylphenidate (20–40 mg/day po) caused a rise in serum levels from 8 to 35 μg/ml for phenytoin, from 4 to 21 μg/ml for primidone, and from 23 to 39 μg/ml for phenobarbital (a metabolite of primidone) (2). These increases in anticonvulsant levels were associated with the development of ataxia. Drug levels reverted to control levels within 1 month after cessation of methylphenidate. However, in the same report, the serum anticonvulsant levels of two other hyperkinetic children were not elevated by methylphenidate. A report evaluating the clinical usefulness of serum anticonvulsant levels mentioned three cases of methylphenidate-induced phenytoin toxicity, but details of these cases were not given (6).

Two clinical studies (7, 8) failed to document the phenytoin–methylphenidate interaction. Both the elimination rate of phenytoin and the plateau phenytoin concentration were studied before and during methylphenidate administration (8), and no increase in the serum phenytoin level was found. All subjects or patients were over 15 years of age, and average doses were administered.

■ Methylphenidate has been associated with symptoms of phenytoin toxicity in a few children, but these effects were not observed in controlled studies in adults. Although the possibility exists that other factors were operant in one of the reported cases or that low metabolic capacity for phenytoin is required to see the effect, most patients taking these drugs concurrently will not show any evidence of a drug interaction.

Recommendations—Practitioners should not change doses of either methylphenidate or phenytoin or any other anticonvulsant when these drugs are used concurrently. However, if ataxia or other side effects indicative of anticonvulsant drug toxicity occur, serum levels of the anticonvulsant drug should be determined and doses should

---

*Phenytoin is the new official name for diphenylhydantoin.

be reduced to bring anticonvulsant levels into the therapeutic range. Although considerable individual variation exists, nystagmus generally appears when the serum phenytoin level reaches 20 μg/ml or higher. Gait ataxia is observed at levels around 30 μg/ml with constant lethargy seen at levels approaching 40 μg/ml (9).

References

(1) "The Pharmacological Basis of Thera-
    peutics," 5th ed., L. S. Goodman and
    A. Gilman, Eds., Macmillan, New York,
    NY 10022, 1975, p. 511.
(2) L. K. Garrettson *et al.*, "Methylpheni-
    date Interaction with Both Anticon-
    vulsants and Ethyl Biscoumacetate," *J.
    Amer. Med. Ass.*, *207*, 2053 (1969).
(3) J. M. Perel and N. Black, "*In Vitro*
    Metabolism Studies with Methylpheni-
    date," *Fed. Proc.*, *29*, 345 (1970).
(4) D. Hunninghake, "Studies of the In-
    hibition of Drug Metabolism by
    Methylphenidate," *Fed. Proc.*, *29*, 345
    (1970).
(5) P. G. Dayton *et al.*, "Physiological
    Disposition of Methylphenidate C^{14} in
    Man," *Fed. Proc.*, *29*, 345 (1970).
(6) E. B. Solow and J. B. Green, "The

Simultaneous Determination of Multiple Anticonvulsant Drug Levels by
Gas-Liquid Chromatography," *Neurology*, *22*, 540 (1972).
(7) B. L. Mirkin and F. Wright, "Drug
    Interactions: Effect of Methylpheni-
    date on the Disposition of Diphenyl-
    hydantoin in Man," *Neurology*, *21*,
    1123 (1971).
(8) H. J. Kupferberg *et al.*, "Effect of
    Methylphenidate on Plasma Anticon-
    vulsant Levels," *Clin. Pharmacol. Ther.*,
    13, 201 (1972).
(9) H. Kutt and F. McDowell, "Manage-
    ment of Epilepsy with Diphenylhydan-
    toin Sodium. Dosage Regulation for
    Problem Patients," *J. Amer. Med. Ass.*,
    203, 969 (1968).

[For additional information, see *Anticonvulsant Therapy*, p. 369.]

Nonproprietary and Trade Names of Drugs

Amphetamine complex—*Biphetamine*
Amphetamine sulfate—*Benzedrine*
Dextroamphetamine sulfate—*Dexedrine*
  and various combination products
Ethotoin—*Peganone*
Mephenytoin—*Mesantoin*

Methamphetamine hydrochloride—*Desoxyn,
  Norodin Hydrochloride, Syndrox*
Methylphenidate hydrochloride—*Ritalin
  Hydrochloride*
Phenytoin—*Dilantin*
Primidone—*Mysoline*

*Prepared and evaluated by the Scientific Review Subpanel
on Anticonvulsants and reviewed by Practitioner Panel IV.*

Phenytoin*—Phenobarbital

Summary—Phenobarbital may increase, decrease, or cause no change in phenytoin levels. Clinical reports of phenytoin toxicity due to this drug interaction are
rare and concurrent therapy need not be avoided. Serum phenytoin levels
should be determined periodically whenever phenobarbital is added to or withdrawn from the drug regimen to ascertain if an adjustment in the phenytoin
dosage is necessary.

Related Drugs—**Primidone,** a chemically related anticonvulsant, has been documented
to interact with phenobarbital in humans (1–3). Other hydantoin derivatives (*e.g.*,
ethotoin and **mephenytoin**) may also interact with phenobarbital, although clinical
documentation is lacking. Although not documented, other **barbiturates** also are
likely to interact with phenytoin.

Pharmacological Effect and Mechanism—Although contradictory evidence has been
published (4–10), sufficient animal (11, 12) and human (13–18) data indicate that

*Phenytoin is the new official name for diphenylhydantoin.

phenobarbital often reduces the serum levels and the serum half-life of phenytoin. Chronic administration of phenobarbital induces hepatic microsomal activity (13–17), which increases the rate of metabolism of phenytoin and decreases its half-life (4). Conversely, when large doses of phenobarbital are administered with phenytoin, the two drugs may compete for hepatic microsomal systems (4) and cause an increase in the phenytoin half-life.

Evaluation of Clinical Data—A study of 182 pediatric and adult seizure patients indicated that more patients experienced increased toxicity and seizures when phenytoin and phenobarbital were given concurrently than when either drug was given alone (19). Phenytoin toxicity also occurred in a patient after withdrawal of phenobarbital (4.16 mg/kg) from the drug regimen (18).

A single dose of phenytoin (10 mg/kg po) was administered to five nonepileptic children maintained on phenobarbital (5 mg/kg for 28 days). A 50% decrease in the mean serum phenytoin levels (when compared to mean serum levels obtained prior to phenobarbital administration) occurred (16).

The serum levels of phenobarbital and phenytoin in 73 epileptic patients receiving chronic phenobarbital (50–200 mg/day po) and phenytoin (100–300 mg/day po) therapy were much lower than the serum levels of either drug in patients receiving phenobarbital or phenytoin alone (17). The difference was statistically significant.

Other studies (13–15) also reported lower serum phenytoin levels occurring in most patients after concurrent phenobarbital administration.

However, some studies indicated that the effect of phenobarbital on the serum phenytoin levels is variable (4) or negligible (4–10). Some data suggest that this drug interaction also is less frequent in children (5, 7, 9), but low doses were used in these studies and correspondingly low serum levels occurred. It is possible that this drug interaction may be more pronounced in children at higher serum phenytoin levels.

■ Phenobarbital may increase (4), decrease (13–18), or cause no significant change (4–10) in serum phenytoin levels. Although the clinical outcome of concurrent administration of phenytoin and phenobarbital is unpredictable, phenytoin toxicity has occurred in at least one case when phenobarbital was withdrawn from the drug regimen (18). The variation of serum phenytoin levels reported during phenobarbital administration may be attributed to factors other than phenobarbital, *e.g.,* the patient's previous drug history (4), the patient's genetic predisposition (4), interpatient variation in the metabolism of phenytoin (14, 15), and the timing of phenobarbital administration (4).

Recommendations—Concurrent phenytoin and phenobarbital therapy need not be avoided when indicated. However, the unpredictable clinical outcome of the drug interaction requires that the serum phenytoin levels be determined when initiating concurrent therapy and periodically thereafter until the serum drug levels are stabilized. A determination of serum phenytoin and phenobarbital levels after 3 or 4 weeks of therapy may serve as a good indicator of the quality of the therapeutic regimen (20).

Serum drug levels should be determined at the first sign of phenytoin toxicity (*e.g.,* constant lethargy, gait ataxia, and nystagmus). The recommended serum level for phenytoin is 10–20 μg/ml (21, 22). Although considerable individual variation exists, nystagmus generally appears when the serum phenytoin level reaches 20 μg/ml or higher. Gait ataxia is observed at levels around 30 μg/ml with constant lethargy seen at levels approaching 40 μg/ml (21). If toxicity occurs, phenytoin should be discontinued or the dosage should be reduced until toxic signs and symptoms disappear. Then phenytoin can be reinstituted or the dosage can be adjusted until therapeutic levels are attained. The therapeutic serum range of phenobarbital is 10–30 μg/ml (20, 22).

References

(1) R. W. Fincham *et al.*, "The Influence of Diphenylhydantoin on Primidone Metabolism," *Arch. Neurol., 30,* 259 (1974).

(2) J. T. Wilson and G. R. Wilkinson, "Chronic and Severe Phenobarbital Intoxication in a Child Treated with Primidone and Diphenylhydantoin," *J. Pediat., 83,* 484 (1973).

(3) B. B. Gallagher *et al.*, "Primidone, Diphenylhydantoin and Phenobarbital. Aspects of Acute and Chronic Toxicity," *Neurology, 23,* 145 (1973).

(4) H. Kutt *et al.*, "The Effect of Phenobarbital on Plasma Diphenylhydantoin Level and Metabolism in Man and in Rat Liver Microsomes," *Neurology, 19,* 611 (1969).

(5) W. D. Diamond and R. A. Buchanan, "A Clinical Study of the Effect of Phenobarbital on Diphenylhydantoin Plasma Levels," *J. Clin. Pharmacol., 10,* 306 (1970).

(6) H. E. Booker *et al.*, "Concurrent Administration of Phenobarbital and Diphenylhydantoin: Lack of an Interference Effect," *Neurology, 21,* 383 (1971).

(7) N. Izumi, "Studies on Phenobarbital and Diphenylhydantoin in the Plasma and Phenobarbital in the Cerebrospinal Fluid. I. The Concurrent Determination of Phenobarbital and Diphenylhydantoin in the Plasma by Ultraviolet Spectrophotometry and Its Clinical Application," *Acta Paediat. Jap., 74,* 539 (1970).

(8) H. Vapaatalo and L. Lehtinen, "Variations of Serum Diphenylhydantoin Concentrations in Epileptic Outpatients," *Eur. Neurol., 5,* 303 (1971).

(9) R. A. Buchanan and R. J. Allen, "Diphenylhydantoin (Dilantin) and Phenobarbital Blood Levels in Epileptic Children," *Neurology, 21,* 866 (1971).

(10) C. F. Weiss and J. C. Heffelfinger, "Serial Dilantin Levels in Mentally Retarded Children," *Amer. J. Ment. Def., 73,* 826 (1968–1969).

(11) S. A. Cucinell *et al.*, "Stimulatory Effect of Phenobarbital on the Metabolism of Diphenylhydantoin," *J. Pharmacol. Exp. Ther., 141,* 157 (1963).

(12) H.-H. Frey *et al.*, "Study on Combined Treatment with Phenobarbital and Diphenylhydantoin," *Acta Pharmacol. Toxicol., 26,* 284 (1968).

(13) L. K. Garrettson and P. G. Dayton, "Disappearance of Phenobarbital and Diphenylhydantoin from Serum of Children," *Clin. Pharmacol. Ther., 11,* 674 (1970).

(14) M. Kristensen *et al.*, "The Influence of Phenobarbital on the Half-Life of Diphenylhydantoin in Man," *Acta Med. Scand., 185,* 347 (1969).

(15) S. A. Cucinell *et al.*, "Drug Interactions in Man. I. Lowering Effect of Phenobarbital on Plasma Levels of Bishydroxycoumarin (Dicumarol) and Diphenylhydantoin (Dilantin)," *Clin. Pharmacol. Ther., 6,* 420 (1965).

(16) R. Buchanan *et al.*, "The Effect of Phenobarbital on Diphenylhydantoin Metabolism in Children," *Pediatrics, 43,* 114 (1969).

(17) E. Sotaniemi *et al.*, "The Clinical Significance of Microsomal Enzyme Induction in the Therapy of Epileptic Patients," *Ann. Clin. Res., 2,* 223 (1970).

(18) P. L. Morselli *et al.*, "Interaction between Phenobarbital and Diphenylhydantoin in Animals and in Epileptic Patients," *Ann. N.Y. Acad. Sci., 179,* 88 (1971).

(19) H. Hooshmand, "Toxic Effects of Anticonvulsants: General Principles," *Pediatrics, 53,* 551 (1974).

(20) D. Svensmark and F. Buchthal, "Accumulation of Phenobarbital in Man," *Epilepsia, 4,* 199 (1963).

(21) H. Kutt and F. McDowell, "Management of Epilepsy with Diphenylhydantoin Sodium. Dosage Regulation for Problem Patients," *J. Amer. Med. Ass., 203,* 969 (1968).

(22) "To Each His Own Anticonvulsant Rx," *Medical World News,* May 21, 1971, pp. 15–16.

[For additional information, see *Anticonvulsant Therapy,* p. 369.]

Nonproprietary and Trade Names of Drugs

Ethotoin—*Peganone*

Mephenytoin—*Mesantoin*

Phenobarbital—*Eskabarb, Luminal*

Phenytoin—*Dilantin*

Primidone—*Mysoline*

Prepared and evaluated by the Scientific Review Subpanel on Anticonvulsants and reviewed by Practitioner Panel V.

Probenecid—Chlorothiazide

Summary—Long-term use of chlorothiazide and other thiazide diuretics frequently causes mild uric acid retention and diminishes some of the uricosuric effects of probenecid. Since the increase in serum urate levels is small and there is little correlation between these levels and clinical gout, more frequent monitoring of these levels is unnecessary. If feasible, baseline serum urate levels should be obtained when concurrent administration of these drugs is initiated to determine whether an initial increase in the dosage of probenecid is desirable.

Related Drugs—In addition to chlorothiazide, **bendroflumethiazide** (1), **hydrochloro-thiazide** (2–5), and **methyclothiazide** (6) have been reported to retain uric acid and could antagonize the uricosuric effects of probenecid. All other **thiazide diuretics** would be expected to act similarly.

Chlorthalidone (3, 4), **metolazone** (7), and **quinethazone** (8, 9) are chemically and pharmacologically related to thiazide diuretics and elevate serum urate levels. Therefore, these drugs may also interact with probenecid.

Many combination products containing a thiazide diuretic or related compounds are available.

Pharmacological Effect and Mechanism—Uricosuric doses of probenecid are thought to act predominantly by blocking the reabsorption of uric acid in the proximal renal tubules causing greatly enhanced urinary excretion of uric acid (10, 11). Hyperuricemia from chlorothiazide or other thiazide diuretic administration is probably caused either by competitive inhibition of uric acid secretion within the kidney (3, 12) or by indirect enhancement of renal reabsorption of uric acid through redistribution of renal blood flow (13, 14). Either mechanism results in more uric acid being retained and a decrease in the effects of probenecid.

Chlorothiazide and other thiazide diuretics cause a transient, but paradoxical, uricosuric response following the intravenous administration of therapeutic doses (2, 3, 12). This response is probably due to increased renal blood flow caused by the simultaneous intravenous administration of fluid and electrolytes with the thiazide diuretic, resulting in enhanced secretion instead of reabsorption of uric acid (13).

Evaluation of Clinical Data—Chlorothiazide-induced hyperuricemia has been documented (5, 15–18). Although increases in uric acid levels exceeding 6 mg% were produced with normal doses of chlorothiazide (18), most reports indicate that the usual uric acid evaluation is relatively minor, averaging 1.5–3.0 mg%. Most elevations occurred after administration of chlorothiazide for a period of 5 days to 10 months (2, 3, 12, 15). Single doses did not seem to induce any significant increase in serum uric acid levels (3).

■ Essentially all patients treated with chlorothiazide exhibit some degree of increase in serum urate. In patients with untreated or poorly controlled preexisting gouty arthritis, the evidence that gouty arthritis can be exacerbated by chlorothiazide is well documented (5, 15–17). Whether hyperuricemia is produced in a patient, however, is dependent on the pretreatment level of serum urates. Patients controlled on concurrent probenecid and chlorothiazide therapy may exhibit only minor elevations of serum urate levels which require no definitive action (2).

Recommendations—The long-term use of chlorothiazide with probenecid causes only a small increase in serum urate levels. Since the increase is small and there is little correlation between serum urate levels and clinical gout (19), more frequent monitoring of these levels is unnecessary. However, if feasible, baseline serum urate levels should be obtained when concurrent administration of these drugs is initiated. If serum urate levels are elevated from baseline values, an initial increase in the dosage of probenecid should be considered.

Other diuretics such as ethacrynic acid (13), furosemide (13, 20), mercurial diuretics (8) (rarely), and possibly triamterene (4) elevate serum urate levels and also may antagonize the actions of uricosuric drugs.

The uricosuric effects of sulfinpyrazone may be affected by chlorothiazide and similar acting diuretics.

References

(1) L. H. Feldman, "A New Antihypertensive Preparation Combining Rauwolfia, Bendroflumethiazide and Potassium," *N.C. Med. J.*, *23*, 248 (1962).

(2) E. D. Freis and R. F. Sappington, "Long-Term Effect of Probenecid on Diuretic-Induced Hyperuricemia," *J. Amer. Med. Ass.*, *198*, 127 (1966).

(3) J. M. Bryant *et al.*, "Hyperuricemia Induced by the Administration of Chlorthalidone and Other Sulfonamide Diuretics," *Amer. J. Med.*, *33*, 408 (1962).

(4) R. E. Spiekerman *et al.*, "Potassium-Sparing Effects of Triamterene in the Treatment of Hypertension," *Circulation*, *34*, 524 (1966).

(5) A. Aronoff and H. Barkum, "Hyperuricemia and Acute Gouty Arthritis Precipitated by Thiazide Derivatives," *Can. Med. Ass. J.*, *84*, 1181 (1961).

(6) F. H. Stern, "The Use of Methyclothiazide (Enduron) in Geriatric Patients," *J. Amer. Geriat. Soc.*, *10*, 256 (1962).

(7) "The Pharmacological Basis of Therapeutics," 5th ed., L. S. Goodman and A. Gilman, Eds., Macmillan, New York, NY 10022, 1975, pp. 829–830.

(8) A. N. Brest *et al.*, "Drug Control of Diuretic-Induced Hyperuricemia," *J. Amer. Med. Ass.*, *195*, 42 (1966).

(9) W. E. Parkes *et al.*, "Treatment of Hypertension with Quinethazone Alone or in Combination with Reserpine," *Practitioner*, *203*, 194 (1969).

(10) G. M. Fanelli, Jr. and I. M. Weiner, "Pyrazinoate Excretion in the Chimpanzee. Relation to Urate Disposition and the Actions of Uricosuric Drugs," *J. Clin. Invest.*, *52*, 1946 (1973).

(11) T. H. Steele and G. Boner, "Origins of the Uricosuric Response," *J. Clin. Invest.*, *52*, 1368 (1973).

(12) F. E. Demartini *et al.*, "Effect of Chlorothiazide on the Renal Excretion of Uric Acid," *Amer. J. Med.*, *32*, 572 (1962).

(13) T. H. Steele and S. Oppenheimer, "Factors Affecting Urate Excretion following Diuretic Administration in Man," *Amer. J. Med.*, *47*, 564 (1969).

(14) W. N. Suki *et al.*, "Mechanism of the Effect of Thiazide Diuretics on Calcium and Uric Acid," abstract, *J. Clin. Invest.*, *46*, 1121 (1967).

(15) B. G. Oren *et al.*, "Chlorothiazide (Diuril) as a Hyperuricacidemic Agent," *J. Amer. Med. Ass.*, *168*, 2128 (1958).

(16) L. J. Warshaw, "Acute Attacks of Gout Precipitated by Chlorothiazide-Induced Diuresis," *J. Amer. Med. Ass.*, *172*, 802 (1960).

(17) A. Aronoff, "Acute Gouty Arthritis Precipitated by Chlorothiazide," *N. Engl. J. Med.*, *262*, 767 (1960).

(18) J. H. Laragh *et al.*, "Effect of Chlorothiazide on Electrolyte Transport in Man. Its Use in the Treatment of Edema of Congestive Heart Failure, Nephrosis, and Cirrhosis," *J. Amer. Med. Ass.*, *166*, 145 (1958).

(19) J. B. Wyngarden, "Gout and Other Disorders of Uric Acid Metabolism," in "Principles of Internal Medicine," M. M. Wintrobe *et al.*, Eds., McGraw-Hill, New York, N.Y., 1970, p. 597.

(20) J. McSherry, "Acute Gout Complicating Frusemide Therapy," *Practitioner*, *201*, 809 (1968).

[For additional information, see *Uricosuric Therapy*, p. 447.]

Nonproprietary and Trade Names of Drugs

Bendroflumethiazide—*Naturetin*
Benzthiazide—*Aquatag, Exna*
Chlorothiazide—*Diuril*
Chlorthalidone—*Hygroton, Regroton*
Cyclothiazide—*Anhydron*

Ethacrynic acid—*Edecrin*
Flumethiazide—*Rautrax*
Furosemide—*Lasix*
Hydrochlorothiazide—*Esidrix, HydroDiuril, Oretic*

Continued on next page

Hydroflumethiazide—*Saluron*
Mercaptomerin sodium—*Thiomerin*
Methyclothiazide—*Aquatensen, Enduron*
Metolazone—*Zaroxolyn*
Polythiazide—*Renese*
Probenecid—*Benemid*
Quinethazone—*Hydromox*

Spironolactone—*Aldactone*
Sulfinpyrazone—*Anturane*
Triamterene—*Dyrenium*
Trichlormethiazide—*Metahydrin, Naqua*
Various combination products containing
a diuretic are available.

*Prepared and evaluated by the Scientific Review Subpanel on
Uricosuric Agents and reviewed by Practitioner Panel IV.*

Propoxyphene—Alcohol

Summary—Concurrent ingestion of propoxyphene and alcohol in large quantities may result in dangerous respiratory and central nervous system (CNS) depression attributable to their additive depressant effects. Despite reports of adverse effects resulting from propoxyphene–alcohol overdose, it is unlikely that such severe effects will occur after administration of therapeutic doses of propoxyphene and ingestion of moderate amounts of alcohol (90–120 ml of 100-proof whiskey). Patients ingesting both agents should be advised about the harmful CNS depressant effects of propoxyphene and alcohol and should be cautioned about driving an automobile and operating hazardous machinery.

Related Drugs—Other CNS depressants may interact in a manner similar to propoxyphene and alcohol.

Pharmacological Effect and Mechanism—Toxic doses of propoxyphene may cause coma, respiratory depression, and ultimately apnea and death (1–3). The minimum lethal dose of propoxyphene hydrochloride is considered to be 500–800 mg in adults (4). Near fatalities have been reported in infants with 200 mg (5), and one death occurred in a 12-month-old child who had ingested 650 mg of propoxyphene (6). Since propoxyphene is readily absorbed and bound by tissue in the brain, kidney, lung, and liver, serum levels cannot be accepted as a reliable measurement of the quantity of propoxyphene ingested (4). The toxic dose of propoxyphene napsylate has not been studied in humans.

The fatal quantity of alcohol for a 68.1 kg (150 lb) adult is 240 ml of 100% alcohol (480 ml of 100-proof whiskey) if consumed in less than 1 hr. Although the relationship between symptoms and blood alcohol levels cannot be stated conclusively, a blood alcohol level of 300–500 mg/100 ml is considered severe intoxication and can be fatal. Symptoms of toxicity include marked muscular incoordination, blurred vision, and approaching stupor. Severe hypoglycemia sometimes occurs with hypothermia, convulsions, and extensor rigidity of the extremities. If the blood alcohol level is at or above 500 mg/100 ml, coma and frequently death occur (7, 8).

Evaluation of Clinical Data—There are several reports of accidental or intentional death resulting from oral and parenteral propoxyphene administrations (9–12). One study (9) indicated that 12 fatalities were due to the concurrent use of propoxyphene and alcohol. In all cases, the deaths occurred in patients ingesting both propoxyphene and alcohol, one or both in excessive quantities.

■ An overdose of propoxyphene and concurrent ingestion of large amounts of alcohol (150–240 ml of 100-proof whiskey) may produce severe respiratory depression and death (9). However, despite reported adverse reactions and several deaths from propoxyphene–alcohol overdose, it is unlikely that administration of therapeutic doses of propoxyphene and ingestion of moderate amounts of alcohol (up to 120 ml of 100-proof whiskey) will cause similar effects.

Recommendations—Since concurrent ingestion of moderate amounts of alcohol and the administration of therapeutic doses of propoxyphene cause the same effects as the same amount of alcohol alone (*e.g.*, CNS depression), patients using both drugs should be cautioned about driving automobiles and operating hazardous machinery. Patients also should be advised about the dangers associated with concurrent ingestion of high doses of propoxyphene and large amounts of alcohol (*e.g.*, severe respiratory depression and death). If treatment of propoxyphene toxicity is necessary, naloxone has been used successfully to antagonize propoxyphene-induced toxic effects (13).

References

(1) E. B. Robbins, "The Pharmacologic Effects of a New Analgesic α-4-Dimethylamino-1,2-diphenyl-3-methyl-4-propionyloxybutane," *J. Amer. Pharm. Ass., Sci. Ed., 44*, 497 (1955).

(2) H. M. Cann and H. L. Verhulst, "Convulsions as a Manifestation of Acute Dextro Propoxyphene Intoxication," *Amer. J. Dis. Child., 99*, 380 (1960).

(3) S. D. Frasier *et al.*, "Dextropropoxyphene Hydrochloride Poisoning in Two Children," *J. Pediat., 63*, 158 (1963).

(4) R. L. Wolen *et al.*, "Concentration of Propoxyphene in Human Plasma following Oral, Intramuscular, and Intravenous Administration," *Toxicol. Appl. Pharmacol., 19*, 480 (1971).

(5) "Clinical Toxicology of Commercial Products," 3rd ed., M. N. Gleason *et al.*, Eds., Williams and Wilkins, Baltimore, Md., 1969, p. 120.

(6) "Darvon Products," National Clearinghouse for Poison Control Center.

(7) "Handbook of Poisoning," 7th ed., R. H. Dreisbach, Ed., Lange Medical Publications, Los Altos, Calif., 1971, p. 147.

(8) "Combined Effects of Alcohol and Other Drugs," R. B. Forney and F. W. Hughes, Eds., Charles C. Thomas, Springfield, Ill., 1968, pp. 11–41.

(9) W. Q. Sturner and J. C. Garriott, "Deaths Involving Propoxyphene. A Study of 41 Cases Over a Two-Year Period," *J. Amer. Med. Ass., 223*, 1125 (1973).

(10) J. S. Karliner, "Propoxyphene Hydrochloride Poisoning: Report of a Case Treated with Peritoneal Dialysis," *J. Amer. Med. Ass., 199*, 1006 (1967).

(11) L. J. Bogartz and W. C. Miller, "Pulmonary Edema Associated with Propoxyphene Intoxication," *J. Amer. Med. Ass., 215*, 259 (1971).

(12) Registry of Human Toxicology, 1970 and 1971, American Academy of Forensic Sciences, Dallas, Tex., 1971.

(13) P. M. Vlasses and T. Fraker, "Naloxone for Propoxyphene Overdosage," letter to the editor, *J. Amer. Med. Ass., 229*, 1167 (1974).

[For additional information, see *Analgesic Therapy (Nonnarcotic)*, p. 341.]

Nonproprietary and Trade Names of Drugs

Alcohol—*Various products and beverages*
Propoxyphene hydrochloride—*Darvon, Dolene, SK-65*

Propoxyphene napsylate—*Darvon-N*

Prepared and evaluated by the Scientific Review Subpanel on Analgesics and reviewed by Practitioner Panel IV.

Propoxyphene—Amphetamine

Summary—In toxic doses, propoxyphene can produce convulsions as well as central nervous system (CNS) depression. Amphetamines and other CNS stimulants should not be used in the treatment of propoxyphene poisoning because they may theoretically contribute to the onset of propoxyphene-induced convulsions.

Related Drugs—Although not documented, other CNS stimulants such as **dextroamphetamine, ephedrine, methamphetamine,** and **methylphenidate** may also interact similarly with propoxyphene.

Pharmacological Effect and Mechanism—Toxic doses of propoxyphene, in both animal studies and reported human cases, caused loss of consciousness, respiratory depression, and apnea (1–3). Convulsive seizures also have occurred (4, 5). Amphetamine produces CNS stimulation by indirectly increasing the release of norepinephrine and possibly by impeding its neuronal reuptake (6). Toxic doses of amphetamine result in convulsions and coma (7). There is evidence, from animal and human studies, that nalorphine and naloxone antagonize the respiratory depression and the convulsive disorder produced by a propoxyphene overdose (1, 8–10).

Evaluation of Clinical Data—There is ample clinical evidence that toxic doses of propoxyphene produce convulsions as well as CNS depression (2–5). There are no reported cases in which a CNS stimulant was administered to patients with propoxyphene poisoning. However, the use of such stimulants to overcome respiratory or cardiovascular collapse produced by a drug which may predispose the patient to convulsive seizures is contraindicated (11, 12).

■ Although there is no clinical evidence that the use of amphetamines increases the convulsive tendency in individuals with propoxyphene poisoning, the possible toxic effects that may occur indicate that concurrent use should be avoided.

Recommendations—Drug therapy for propoxyphene poisoning should include naloxone, which has been used with varying success in controlling both respiratory depression and convulsive seizures (2, 3, 9, 10). The use of amphetamines and other CNS stimulants is not recommended for the treatment of propoxyphene-induced CNS depression.

References

(1) E. B. Robbins, "The Pharmacologic Effects of a New Analgesic α-4-Dimethylamino-1,2-diphenyl-3-methyl-4-propionyloxybutane," *J. Amer. Pharm. Ass., Sci. Ed., 44,* 497 (1955).

(2) H. M. Cann and H. L. Verhulst, "Convulsions as a Manifestation of Acute Dextro Propoxyphene Intoxication," *Amer. J. Dis. Child., 99,* 380 (1960).

(3) S. D. Frasier et al., "Dextropropoxyphene Hydrochloride Poisoning in Two Children," *J. Pediat., 63,* 158 (1963).

(4) J. S. Karliner, "Propoxyphene Hydrochloride Poisoning: Report of a Case

Treated with Peritoneal Dialysis," *J. Amer. Med. Ass., 199,* 1006 (1967).

(5) W. H. McCarthy and R. L. Keenan, "Propoxyphene Hydrochloride Poisoning, Report of the First Fatality," *J. Amer. Med. Ass., 187,* 460 (1964).

(6) L. E. Hollister, "Clinical Use of Psychotherapeutic Drugs II: Antidepressant and Antianxiety Drugs and Special Problems in the Use of Psychotherapeutic Drugs," *Drugs, 4,* 361 (1972).

(7) "The Pharmacological Basis of Therapeutics," 5th ed., L. S. Goodman and A. Gilman, Eds., Macmillan, New York, NY 10022, 1975, pp. 498–499.

(8) J. E. Chapman and E. J. Walaszek, "Antagonism of Some Toxic Effects of Dextropropoxyphene by Nalorphine," *Toxicol. Appl. Pharmacol.*, *4*, 752 (1962).

(9) N. E. Gary *et al.*, "Acute Propoxyphene Hydrochloride Intoxication," *Arch. Intern. Med.*, *121*, 453 (1968).

(10) R. E. Fiut *et al.*, "Antagonism of Convulsive and Lethal Effects In-

duced by Propoxyphene," *J. Pharm. Sci.*, *55*, 1085 (1966).

(11) "Handbook of Poisoning," 7th ed., R. H. Dreisbach, Ed., Lange Medical Publications, Los Altos, Calif., 1971, p. 283.

(12) "Poisoning: Toxicology, Symptoms, Treatment," 3rd ed., J. M. Arena, Ed., Charles C. Thomas, Springfield, Ill., 1974, pp. 380–381.

[For additional information, see *Analgesic Therapy (Nonnarcotic)*, p. 341.]

Nonproprietary and Trade Names of Drugs

Amphetamine complex—*Biphetamine*
Amphetamine sulfate—*Benzedrine*
Dextroamphetamine sulfate—*Dexedrine and various combination products*
Ephedrine hydrochloride and sulfate—*Various manufacturers*

Methamphetamine hydrochloride—*Desoxyn, Norodin Hydrochloride, Syndrox*
Methylphenidate hydrochloride—*Ritalin Hydrochloride*
Propoxyphene hydrochloride—*Darvon, Dolene, SK-65*
Propoxyphene napsylate—*Darvon-N*

Prepared and evaluated by the Scientific Review Subpanel on Analgesics and reviewed by Practitioner Panel V.

Propranolol—Chlorpheniramine

Summary—Chlorpheniramine could theoretically prevent the β-adrenergic blocking effect of propranolol and enhance its quinidine-like effect. However, there are no reports of this drug interaction occurring in animals or in humans.

Related Drugs—**Brompheniramine, dexbrompheniramine,** and **dexchlorpheniramine** are structurally similar to chlorpheniramine and have many similar effects. They have not been studied for possible cardiac effects but have been shown to prevent amine uptake in experimental animals (1). **Diphenhydramine** (2), **pyrilamine** (3), and **tripelennamine** (4) are similar to chlorpheniramine in their actions. Other antihistamines include **chlorcyclizine, cyclizine, dimenhydrinate, methapyrilene, phenindamine,** and **promethazine.**

Pharmacological Effect and Mechanism—Propranolol is a competitive antagonist of catecholamines at β-adrenergic receptor sites. Chlorpheniramine acts at the adrenergic nerve terminal in a manner similar to cocaine by preventing uptake of catecholamines, thereby raising their concentration at β-adrenergic receptor sites (2, 4).

Both propranolol (5) and chlorpheniramine (6) have quinidine-like effects on myocardial conduction in high doses. The cocaine-like and quinidine-like effects of chlorpheniramine have been demonstrated only in experimental animals and a dose several times greater than that necessary for antihistaminic effect was used.

Evaluation of Clinical Data—Since no reports or studies have appeared, only speculation can be offered regarding the potential interaction. However, two mechanisms can be suggested. In the therapeutic situation, propranolol is often used in gradually increasing doses to find the level necessary to counteract an unknown amount of sympathetic activity. Concurrent administration of high doses of chlorpheniramine might decrease the effectiveness of propranolol, making higher doses of propranolol necessary. A second possibility is that the quinidine-like effect of propranolol is more evident at high doses of chlorpheniramine, leading to myocardial depression.

■ There would appear to be little likelihood of a clinically significant interaction between propranolol and chlorpheniramine in the doses normally used. Problems described may occur if large doses of either drug are used, but clinical data are not available.

Recommendations—The possibility of an interaction between propranolol and chlorpheniramine in high doses should be considered when administering both agents concurrently. However, until some clinical data about this drug interaction are reported, concurrent use of these drugs need not be avoided.

References

(1) S. Symchowicz *et al.*, "Inhibition of Dopamine Uptake into Synaptosomes of Rat Corpus Striatum by Chlorpheniramine and Its Structural Analogs," *Life Sci.*, *10*, 35 (1971).

(2) A. Carlsson and M. Lindqvist, "Central and Peripheral Monoaminergic Membrane-Pump Blockade by Some Addictive Analgesics and Antihistamines," *J. Pharm. Pharmacol.*, *21*, 460 (1969).

(3) R. E. Osterburg and T. Koppanyi, "Effects of Chlorpheniramine and Pyrilamine on the Atrial Actions of Acetylcholine, Tyramine, and Ephedrine," *J. Pharm. Sci.*, *58*, 1313 (1969).

(4) G. L. Johnson and J. B. Kahn, Jr., "Cocaine and Antihistaminic Compounds: Comparison of Effects of Some Cardiovascular Actions of Norepinephrine, Tyramine and Bretylium," *J. Pharmacol. Exp. Ther.*, *152*, 458 (1966).

(5) "The Pharmacological Basis of Therapeutics," 5th ed., L. S. Goodman and A. Gilman, Eds., Macmillan, New York, NY 10022, 1975, p. 699.

(6) M. W. Winbury and B. L. Alworth, "Suppression of Experimental Atrial Arrhythmias by Several Antihistamines," *Arch. Int. Pharmacodyn. Ther.*, *122*, 318 (1959).

[For additional information, see *Antiarrhythmia Therapy*, p. 350.]

Nonproprietary and Trade Names of Drugs

Brompheniramine maleate—*Dimetane and various combination products*
Chlorcyclizine hydrochloride—*Various combination products*
Chlorpheniramine maleate—*Chlor-Trimeton Maleate, Teldrin, and various combination products*
Cyclizine hydrochloride—*Marezine Hydrochloride*
Dexbrompheniramine maleate—*Disomer and various combination products*
Dexchlorpheniramine maleate—*Polaramine*

Dimenhydrinate—*Dramamine*
Diphenhydramine hydrochloride—*Benadryl*
Methapyrilene hydrochloride—*Histadyl*
Phenindamine tartrate—*Thephorin*
Promethazine hydrochloride—*Phenergan, Remsed*
Propranolol hydrochloride—*Inderal*
Pyrilamine maleate—*Various manufacturers*
Tripelennamine hydrochloride—*Pyribenzamine Hydrochloride*

Prepared and evaluated by the Scientific Review Subpanel on Antiarrhythmic Agents and reviewed by Practitioner Panel VI.

Propranolol—Desipramine

Summary—The anticholinergic activity of desipramine theoretically may antagonize the myocardial effects of propranolol, but clinical evidence for this interaction is lacking. Nevertheless, the use of propranolol alone or with other drugs requires caution.

Related Drugs—**Amitriptyline, doxepin, imipramine, nortriptyline,** and **protriptyline** are chemically and pharmacologically related to desipramine.

Pharmacological Effect and Mechanism—Theoretically, the anticholinergic effects of desipramine may antagonize the β-blocking effects of propranolol in myocardial tissue (1) and may counteract, to some degree, the bradycardia and decrease inotropic effects produced by propranolol. The tricyclic antidepressants inhibit the uptake of norepinephrine at the adrenergic nerve endings so that an increase in sympathomimetic response may occur (2). However, in the presence of propranolol, a slight decrease in pressor response may be produced because of the blockade of the cardiac action of norepinephrine (2).

Evaluation of Clinical Data—Reports concerning the effects of propranolol on pressor responses to norepinephrine have been limited largely to animal studies and the results in humans have been confusing and contradictory. In one study (3), prolonged infusion of levarterenol (norepinephrine) produced a slightly greater response after propranolol, but this effect was not observed by other investigators (4).

The possible antagonistic effects of desipramine on the myocardial effects of propranolol are probably more significant. Propranolol produces negative inotropic and chronotropic effects by β-adrenergic blockade. Drugs such as atropine that have significant anticholinergic activity may antagonize this propranolol-induced hemodynamic effect (5). This effect, however, is dependent on the existing degree of sympathetic tone present in the myocardium and the concentration of propranolol at the receptor site (1).

Propranolol has been used successfully to counteract the cardiotoxicity associated with tricyclic antidepressant poisoning (6, 7).

■ There is no substantial clinical evidence documenting an interaction between propranolol and desipramine. However, the indications for the use of propranolol, such as in the treatment of cardiac arrhythmias (paroxysmal atrial tachycardia and tachyarrhythmias associated with digitalis intoxication or anesthesia), warrant special precautions. Similar precautions also should be observed when desipramine is used concurrently.

Recommendations—Because substantial clinical evidence is lacking with respect to specific interactions of desipramine with propranolol, no additional precautions are necessary when these drugs are given concurrently. Precautions appropriate to the individual use of these drugs should be observed.

References

(1) D. G. Gibson, "Pharmacodynamic Properties of β-Adrenergic Receptor Blocking Drugs in Man," *Drugs, 7,* 8 (1974).

(2) "The Pharmacological Basis of Therapeutics," 5th ed., L. S. Goodman and A. Gilman, Eds., Macmillan, New York, NY 10022, 1975, pp. 548–549.

(3) W. E. Glover and K. J. Hutchison, "The Effect of a Beta-Receptor Antagonist (Propranolol) on the Cardiovascular Response to Intravenous Infusions of Noradrenaline in Man," *J. Physiol. (London), 177,* 59P (1965).

(4) I. Brick *et al.,* "Effects of Propranolol on Peripheral Vessels in Man," *Amer. J. Cardiol., 18,* 329 (1966).

(5) M. Stannard and G. Sloman, "Haemodynamic Effects of Propranolol," letter to the editor, *Brit. Med. J., 1,* 700 (1967).

(6) L. J. Marshall and V. A. Green, "Propranolol and Diazepam for Imipramine Poisoning," *Lancet,* ii, 1249 (1968).

(7) J. Vohra, "Cardiovascular Abnormalities following Tricyclic Antidepressant Drug Overdosage," *Drugs, 7,* 323 (1974).

[For additional information, see *Antidepressant Therapy,* p. 373.]

Nonproprietary and Trade Names of Drugs

Amitriptyline hydrochloride—*Elavil Hydrochloride and various combination products*
Desipramine hydrochloride—*Norpramin, Pertofrane*
Doxepin hydrochloride—*Adapin, Sinequan*
Imipramine hydrochloride—*Presamine, Tofranil, Tofranil PM*

Nortriptyline hydrochloride—*Aventyl Hydrochloride*
Propranolol hydrochloride—*Inderal*
Protriptyline hydrochloride—*Vivactil Hydrochloride*

Prepared and evaluated by the Scientific Review Subpanel on Autonomic Agents and reviewed by Practitioner Panel II.

Propranolol—Quinidine

Summary—Propranolol and quinidine have been found to have a beneficial effect when used together for the treatment of cardiac arrhythmias so that smaller doses of each drug may be employed. Concurrent administration may be used for conversion of atrial fibrillation to normal sinus rhythm and for prophylaxis of paroxysmal atrial arrhythmias in quinidine-resistant patients.

Related Drugs—The pharmacological effects of using quinidine with β-adrenergic blocking agents other than propranolol have not been studied, but the results may be similar to the response induced by propranolol and quinidine. **Cinchophen** and **quinine** are agents related to quinidine. The available salts of quinidine include the **gluconate, hydrochloride, polygalacturonate,** and **sulfate.**

Pharmacological Effect and Mechanism—Quinidine has a potent antiarrhythmic action, can accelerate or depress the heart rate through vagolytic and direct action, and has the following effects on the ECG: the PR interval is changed, the QRS complex is prolonged, and the QT interval is prolonged (1). Propranolol (10 mg iv) has the following effects: the heart rate is reduced, the QT interval is shortened, the amplitude of the T wave is increased, and the PR interval is usually unchanged (2). Both drugs reduce blood pressure in large doses and depress myocardial contractility but by different mechanisms. They both depress pacemaker activity, resting membrane potential, and conduction velocity and increase the refractory period (3). A nonspecific antiadrenergic blocking action also has been attributed to quinidine. Propranolol is generally classified as a β-adrenergic blocker (3), although in high doses propranolol produces a membrane-stabilizing action which is separate from its β-blocking action (4).

The mechanism of enhancement by combined drug effects is unclear but probably results from a reduced depolarization rate of the cardiac transmembrane action potential, an effect shared by both drugs. The effect is manifested by a decreased response of the myocardial tissue and a decreased rate of phase 4 diastolic depolarization.

Evaluation of Clinical Data—The original report (2) of this drug interaction involved two patients with atrial fibrillation who were resistant to toxic doses of quinidine but who were successfully converted and maintained with concurrent use of propranolol (80 mg/day po) and quinidine (1.2 g/day po). In a subsequent study (5), 17 patients with chronic atrial fibrillation were converted to normal sinus rhythm 15 out of 18 times by concurrent use of propranolol (30–60 mg/day po for 2–4 days) and quinidine

(0.6–1.2 g/day po). Several of these patients had been previously converted to normal sinus rhythm only by large doses of quinidine. After conversion, the patients were maintained by concurrent use of propranolol (usual dose, 30 mg/day po) and quinidine (usual dose, 1.0 g/day po). Sinus rhythm was maintained in 13 patients for up to 8 months.

Another report (6) described 10 cases of atrial fibrillation treated 5–17 days after open heart surgery for mitral valvular disease. In nine of the 10 patients, sinus rhythm was achieved by concurrent therapy with propranolol (30–60 mg/day po) and quinidine (1.2 g/day po).

Forty-eight patients (7) with paroxysmal (atrial, nodal, and ventricular) arrhythmias received propranolol (dose range, 15–160 mg/day po) and quinidine (dose range, 0.6–2.6 g/day po). Thirty-four patients showed significant improvement in the frequency of arrhythmias, and 26 of these patients remained in sinus rhythm while receiving these drugs. The use of propranolol and quinidine was no more successful than propranolol alone in the termination of atrial fibrillation or flutter. Concurrent therapy caused transient diarrhea in the majority of patients which was controlled by antidiarrheal drugs.

■ Successful conversion of chronic atrial arrhythmias is possible with propranolol and quinidine in patients who are resistant to high doses of either drug alone. Concurrent therapy reduces the likelihood of toxicity from either drug alone and has been recommended for the conversion of atrial fibrillation following surgical correction of mitral valvular disease (6). Additionally, concurrent propranolol and quinidine administration allows effective prophylaxis of atrial, nodal, and ventricular arrhythmias in quinidine-resistant patients (7). However, since the concurrent use of these drugs has not been compared to the use of propranolol alone in controlled studies, the advantages of concurrent therapy are not known.

Recommendations—Propranolol (10–15 mg po three or four times daily) followed by quinidine (300 mg po three or four times daily) may be useful for the conversion of atrial fibrillation to normal sinus rhythm (6). Although controlled studies are lacking, the treatment seems especially useful for arrhythmias resistant to quinidine alone and for atrial fibrillation following surgical procedures on the heart.

Conversion to sinus rhythm usually occurs in 3–5 days (6). Propranolol (40–160 mg/day po in divided doses) and quinidine (0.8–1.2 g/day po in divided doses) are recommended for prophylaxis of atrial, nodal, and ventricular arrhythmias in quinidine-resistant patients (7). The patient should be observed closely for any potential additive cardiodepressant effects.

References

(1) "The Pharmacological Basis of Therapeutics," 5th ed., L. S. Goodman and A. Gilman, Eds., Macmillan, New York, NY 10022, 1975, p. 686.

(2) S. Stern and S. Eisenberg, "The Effect of Propranolol (Inderal) on the Electrocardiogram of Normal Subjects," *Amer. Heart J.*, 77, 192 (1969).

(3) S. Stern, "Synergistic Action of Propranolol with Quinidine," *Amer. Heart J.*, 72, 569 (1966).

(4) J. E. Usubiaga, "Neuromuscular Effects of Beta-Adrenergic Blockers and Their Interaction with Skeletal Muscle Relaxants," *Anesthesiology*, 29, 484 (1968).

(5) S. Stern, "Conversion of Chronic Atrial Fibrillation to Sinus Rhythm with Combined Propranolol and Quinidine Treatment," *Amer. Heart J.*, 74, 170 (1967).

(6) S. Stern and J. B. Borman, "Early Conversion of Atrial Fibrillation after Open-Heart Surgery by Combined Propranolol and Quinidine Treatment," *Isr. J. Med. Sci.*, 5, 102 (1969).

(7) W. J. Fors, Jr., et al., "Evaluation of Propranolol and Quinidine in the Treatment of Quinidine-Resistant Arrhythmias," *Amer. J. Cardiol.*, 27, 190 (1971).

[For additional information, see *Antiarrhythmia Therapy*, p. 350.]

Nonproprietary and Trade Names of Drugs

Cinchophen—*Atophan*
Propranolol hydrochloride—*Inderal*
Quinidine gluconate—*Quinaglute*
Quinidine hydrochloride—*Various manufacturers*

Quinidine polygalacturonate—*Cardioquin*
Quinidine sulfate—*Quinidate, Quinidex*
Quinine—*Various manufacturers*

Prepared and evaluated by the Scientific Review Subpanel on Antiarrhythmic Agents and reviewed by Practitioner Panel III.

Quinidine—Aluminum Hydroxide

Summary—Aluminum hydroxide may delay the gastrointestinal absorption of quinidine in animals, but there is no clinical evidence that this drug interaction occurs in humans. Until clinical data are available, it may be prudent to avoid simultaneous administration of these drugs.

Related Drugs—Aluminum hydroxide is a common ingredient in many antacids. Quinidine is available as the **gluconate, hydrochloride, polygalacturonate,** or **sulfate; cinchophen** and **quinine** are related drugs.

Pharmacological Effect and Mechanism—Aluminum hydroxide is indicated in the treatment of hyperchlorhydria and peptic ulcer. Its effectiveness in these conditions is usually attributed to its adsorbent and neutralizing properties (1). Quinidine, an alkaloid derived from cinchona bark, is employed in the abolition and prevention of certain cardiac arrhythmias (1).

Aluminum hydroxide gel may delay intestinal absorption of other drugs by physical adsorption onto the gel surface (2). In addition, aluminum hydroxide may act by retarding gastric emptying (3, 4). In one study (4), delayed absorption of quinidine and its stereoisomer quinine in the rat was attributed to aluminum and magnesium hydroxides.

Evaluation of Clinical Data—There are no clinical reports in the literature specifically concerned with a quinidine–aluminum hydroxide interaction.

■ Since there are no published clinical data, no clinical significance can be ascribed to this interaction.

Recommendations—In view of the tendency of aluminum hydroxide to delay or reduce the absorption of various drugs, the practitioner should at least be aware of the potential disadvantage in administering quinidine with an aluminum-containing antacid. If possible, simultaneous use of these drugs should be avoided and the patient should be warned against self-medicating with aluminum-containing antacids.

References

(1) "The Pharmacological Basis of Therapeutics," 5th ed., L. S. Goodman and A. Gilman, Eds., Macmillan, New York, NY 10022, 1975, pp. 686–689.
(2) M. R. Gross, "The Adsorption of Some Anticholinergic Drugs by Various Antacids," Ph.D. Thesis, State University of Iowa, Ames, Iowa, 1962.

(3) A. Hurwitz and M. B. Sheehan, "The Effects of Antacids on the Absorption of Orally Administered Pentobarbital in the Rat," *J. Pharmacol. Exp. Ther.*, *179*, 124 (1971).
(4) A. Hurwitz, "The Effects of Antacids on Drug Absorption in Rats," *J. Lab. Clin. Med.*, *76*, 873 (1970).

[For additional information, see *Antiarrhythmia Therapy*, p. 350, and *Acid–Base Balance Therapy*, p. 327.]

Nonproprietary and Trade Names of Drugs

Aluminum-containing products—*Aludrox,*
  Alzinox, Amphojel, A-M-T, Camalox,
  Creamalin, Ducon, Gaviscon, Gelusil,
  Gelusil-M, Kolantyl Gel, Kudrox,
  Maalox, Malcogel, Mylanta, Oxaine-M,
  Phosphaljel, Robalate, Rolaids, Trisogel,
  WinGel

Cinchophen—*Atophan*
Quinidine gluconate—*Quinaglute*
Quinidine hydrochloride—*Various*
  manufacturers
Quinidine polygalacturonate—*Cardioquin*
Quinidine sulfate—*Quinidate, Quinidex*
Quinine—*Various manufacturers*

*Prepared and evaluated by the Scientific Review Subpanel on
Antiarrhythmic Agents and reviewed by Practitioner Panel IV.*

Quinidine—Reserpine

Summary—Clinical and experimental studies show that the antiarrhythmic and cardiodepressant effects of quinidine may be enhanced by the administration of reserpine. Although the data about the drug interaction are limited and unreliable, the possible adverse effects caused by concurrent administration of these drugs require that they be administered together cautiously.

Related Drugs—**Cinchophen** and **quinine** are agents related to quinidine. Several salts of quinidine are available including the **gluconate, hydrochloride, polygalacturonate,** and **sulfate.** In addition to reserpine, all of the other rauwolfia derivatives **alseroxylon, deserpidine, rescinnamine,** and **syrosingopine** can be expected to exhibit similar activity with quinidine.

Pharmacological Effect and Mechanism—Reserpine depletes myocardial tissue of 80–95% of its catecholamine stores (1–3) by causing the intraneuronal release of norepinephrine and by blocking the uptake of the neurotransmitter into the storage granules of the sympathetic nerve ending (4). This catecholamine depletion causes a decrease in the electrical automaticity and excitability of the myocardial tissue (4, 5), which results in decreased atrial and ventricular rates (1). This effect may enhance quinidine's direct myocardial tissue depressant activity (4, 5) and may result in the heart becoming still less excitable. These combined effects could result in quinidine toxicity, manifested as cardiac asystole or excessive bradycardia (4).

Experimental studies showed that the dose of quinidine required to produce atrioventricular blockade in guinea pigs was greatly reduced in reserpine-treated animals compared to animals not treated with reserpine. The effect was reversed when levarterenol (norepinephrine) was infused into the coronary circulation of the hearts of reserpine-treated animals (6). In another study (7), denervated cat hearts became increasingly sensitive to quinidine depression after reserpine pretreatment.

Evaluation of Clinical Data—Of 114 patients with atrial fibrillation treated with a combination product of reserpine (1.3 mg) and quinidine (1.3 g), 70% were converted to normal sinus rhythm (8). This effect was not observed in patients treated with digitalis therapy alone (8). However, this study was poorly controlled and the parameters used to measure the results were too subjective.

■ There is some clinical evidence that reserpine may enhance the cardiodepressant effects of quinidine. However, this evidence is not reliable. Because of the lack of reliable data, the clinical significance of this drug interaction cannot be determined.

Nevertheless, the potential adverse effects due to the concurrent use of these drugs require that these drugs be used together cautiously.

Recommendations—To minimize the possible toxic effects resulting from concurrent administration of quinidine and reserpine, treatment with these agents should not be initiated simultaneously. Treatment with reserpine should be initiated first and an interval of at least 24 hr should be allowed before introducing quinidine. (This interval allows reserpine to develop its cardiodepressant effect.) When quinidine is added to the regimen of a reserpine-treated patient, the dose should be increased cautiously and cardiac function should be monitored closely.

The actions of procainamide are similar to those of quinidine (9) and similar precautions should be taken when this antiarrhythmic drug is used concurrently with reserpine.

References

(1) J. Roberts et al., "Some Aspects of the Cardiac Actions of Reserpine and Pronethalol," Fed. Proc., 24, 1421 (1965).

(2) W. C. Lee and F. E. Shideman, "The Role of Myocardial Catecholamines in Cardiac Contractility," Science, 129, 967 (1959).

(3) M. K. Pasonen and O. Krayer, "The Release of Norepinephrine from the Mammalian Heart by Reserpine," J. Pharmacol. Exp. Ther., 123, 153 (1958).

(4) "The Pharmacological Basis of Therapeutics," 5th ed., L. S. Goodman and A. Gilman, Eds., Macmillan, New York, NY 10022, 1975, pp. 557–559, 690–691.

(5) "Drill's Pharmacology in Medicine," 4th ed., J. R. DiPalma, Ed., McGraw-Hill, New York, N.Y., 1971, pp. 566–569.

(6) G. Lorentz et al., "Influenza del Trattamento Reserpinico a Dosi 'Depletive' delle Catecolamine Tessutali Sulla Sensibilita Miocardica Alla Chinidina," Folia Cardiol., 26, 316 (1967).

(7) E. Nye and J. Roberts, "Effect of Reserpine on the Reactivity of Atrial and Ventricular Pacemakers to Quinidine," Nature, 210, 1376 (1966).

(8) P. Lampugani, "La Terapia della Fibrillazione Atriale con L'Associazione di Idrochinidina e Reserpina," Clin. Terape, 36, 491 (1966).

(9) D. T. Mason et al., "Antiarrhythmic Agents I: Mechanisms of Action and Clinical Pharmacology," Drugs, 5, 261 (1973).

[For additional information, see *Antiarrhythmia Therapy*, p. 350.]

Nonproprietary and Trade Names of Drugs

Alseroxylon—*Rautensin, Rauwiloid*
Cinchophen—*Atophan*
Deserpidine—*Harmonyl*
Procainamide hydrochloride—*Pronestyl*
Quinidine gluconate—*Quinaglute*
Quinidine hydrochloride—*Various manufacturers*
Quinidine polygalacturonate—*Cardioquin*

Quinidine sulfate—*Quinidate, Quinidex*
Quinine—*Various manufacturers*
Rauwolfia serpentina—*Raudixin and various combination products*
Rescinnamine—*Moderil*
Reserpine—*Reserpoid, Sandril, Serpasil, and various combination products*
Syrosingopine—*Singoserp*

Prepared and evaluated by the Scientific Review Subpanel on Antiarrhythmic Agents and reviewed by Practitioner Panel V.

Reserpine—Halothane

Summary—Contrary to earlier reports, patients receiving rauwolfia alkaloids tolerate well-managed anesthesia and surgery satisfactorily without an increased risk of hypotension. Discontinuing rauwolfia alkaloids 2 weeks prior to surgery, as previously recommended, is not clinically indicated. Nevertheless, patients should be observed closely for any unexpected hypotensive episodes.

Related Drugs—Although the occurrence of a drug interaction is doubtful, a decrease in blood pressure has been associated with the use of other general anesthetic agents and rauwolfia alkaloids. Such anesthetic agents include **cyclopropane** (1, 2), **ether** (2, 3), **methoxyflurane** (2), **nitrous oxide** (1, 3, 4), and **trichloroethylene** (1, 2). Anesthetic agents such as **chloroform, enflurane, ethyl chloride, fluroxene, halopropane,** and **trichloromonofluoromethane** have not been reported to interact with reserpine but could be expected to act similarly to other general anesthetics. Related rauwolfia compounds are **alseroxylon, deserpidine, rescinnamine,** and **syrosingopine.**

Pharmacological Effect and Mechanism—The rauwolfia alkaloids are known to lower or deplete stores of 5-hydroxytryptamine (serotonin) (5) and catecholamines (6–9) in the brain, heart, blood vessels, adrenal medulla, and other organs. Several explanations based primarily on animal studies have been given for the depressant effect of halothane on the heart. Halothane produces direct myocardial depression (10–12) and an increased parasympathetic nervous activity with a resultant reduction in heart rate and myocardial depression (13). In addition, halothane may also affect catecholamine activity through central nervous system depression of sympathetic activity (14), sympathetic blockade (15), or reduction of the effect of catecholamines on myocardial and vascular smooth muscle (16).

Therefore, concurrent administration of reserpine and halothane may cause enhanced depressant effects on the heart, resulting in decreased cardiac output and hypotension.

Evaluation of Clinical Data—Shortly after the introduction of the rauwolfia alkaloids, several reports were published which suggested that patients receiving these drugs tolerated anesthesia and surgery poorly and that they should not undergo surgery except in an emergency (1, 4, 17–19). The major problem encountered was said to be hypotension which responded poorly or not at all to vasopressors. For instances of elective surgery, it was suggested that rauwolfia alkaloids be discontinued 2 weeks prior to the operation.

As a result of these reports, rauwolfia alkaloid therapy was considered by many practitioners to be a contraindication to anesthesia and surgery. Ether and halothane were believed to be especially troublesome in these patients. However, the clinical experience of some anesthesiologists was that patients receiving rauwolfia alkaloids tolerated anesthesia and surgery satisfactorily if carefully managed (2, 3, 20).

The response to anesthesia and surgery was compared in two groups of hypertensive patients: one group was treated with rauwolfia alkaloids and the other was not (2). The incidence of hypotension in the rauwolfia-treated patients was less than in the untreated patients and was usually associated with blood loss, excessive speed of induction of anesthesia, surgical manipulation, position change, and excessive amounts of anesthetic agents. Ephedrine was found to be effective in treating hypotension in rauwolfia-treated patients. It was concluded that patients receiving rauwolfia alkaloids tolerate anesthesia and surgery satisfactorily and at least as well as hypertensive patients not treated with rauwolfia alkaloids. It was further concluded that elective surgery could be undertaken safely without discontinuing rauwolfia therapy. In this study (2), approximately half of each group was anesthetized with halothane.

Another study (3) found no differences in incidence of hypotension during surgery between hypertensive patients who continued on rauwolfia therapy and those who did not.

■ Hypertensive patients treated with rauwolfia alkaloids do not require discontinuation of this therapy prior to anesthesia and surgery. Although hypertensive patients receiving rauwolfia alkaloids are less prone to develop hypotension during surgery than untreated hypertensive patients, both types of patients are more prone to develop hypotension than normotensive patients (2, 21).

Recommendations—Clinical evidence indicates that long-term rauwolfia therapy is not a contraindication to anesthesia and surgery (2, 3). However, caution should be exercised during administration of halothane to patients receiving rauwolfia alkaloids. If vasopressors are indicated in the reserpine-treated patient, agents predominantly acting directly upon α-adrenergic receptors (e.g., dopamine, levarterenol, metaraminol, methoxamine, and phenylephrine) should be used rather than agents that depend primarily upon the release of catecholamines for their action (e.g., ephedrine and mephentermine) (21, 22).

References

(1) A. A. Smessaert and R. G. Hick, "Problems Caused by Rauwolfia Drugs during Anesthesia and Surgery," *N.Y. State J. Med.*, *61*, 2399 (1961).

(2) R. L. Katz et al., "Anesthesia, Surgery and Rauwolfia," *Anesthesiology*, *25*, 142 (1964).

(3) W. M. Munson and J. A. Jenicek, "Effect of Anesthetic Agents on Patients Receiving Reserpine Therapy," *Anesthesiology*, *23*, 741 (1962).

(4) C. H. Ziegler and J. B. Lovette, "Operative Complications after Therapy with Reserpine and Reserpine Compounds," *J. Amer. Med. Ass.*, *176*, 916 (1961).

(5) A. Pletscher et al., "Serotonin Release as a Possible Mechanism of Reserpine Action," *Science*, *122*, 374 (1955).

(6) B. B. Brodie, "Selective Release of Norepinephrine and Serotonin by Reserpine-like Compounds," *Dis. Nerv. Sys.*, *1*, suppl., 107 (1960).

(7) F. B. Orlans et al., "Pharmacological Consequences of the Selective Release of Peripheral Norepinephrine by Syrosingopine (Su 3118)," *J. Pharmacol. Exp. Ther.*, *128*, 131 (1960).

(8) J. H. Burn and M. J. Rand, "Norepinephrine in Artery Walls and Its Dispersal by Reserpine," *Brit. Med. J.*, *1*, 903 (1958).

(9) U. S. von Euler and F. Lishajko, "Effect of Reserpine on Release of Norepinephrine from Transmitter Granules in Adrenergic Nerves," *Science*, *132*, 351 (1960).

(10) W. Flacke and M. H. Alper, "Actions of Halothane and Norepinephrine in the Isolated Mammalian Heart," *Anesthesiology*, *23*, 793 (1962).

(11) A. H. Goldberg and W. C. Ullrick, "Effects of Halothane on Isometric Contractions of Isolated Heart

Muscle," *Anesthesiology*, *28*, 838 (1967).

(12) S. Shimosato and B. Etsten, "Performance of Digitalized Heart during Halothane Anesthesia," *Anesthesiology*, *24*, 41 (1963).

(13) M. B. Laver and H. Turndorf, "Atrial Activity and Systemic Blood Pressure during Anesthesia in Man," *Circulation*, *28*, 63 (1963).

(14) H. L. Price and M. L. Price, "Has Halothane a Predominant Circulatory Action?" *Anesthesiology*, *27*, 764 (1966).

(15) J. M. Garfield et al., "A Pharmacological Analysis of Ganglionic Actions of Some General Anesthetics," *Anesthesiology*, *29*, 79 (1968).

(16) M. L. Price and H. L. Price, "Effects of General Anesthetics on Contractile Responses of Rabbit Aortic Strips," *Anesthesiology*, *23*, 16 (1962).

(17) M. W. Foster, Jr., and R. F. Gayle, Jr., "Dangers in Combining Reserpine (Serpasil) with Electroconvulsive Therapy," *J. Amer. Med. Ass.*, *159*, 1520 (1955).

(18) C. S. Coakley et al., "Circulatory Responses during Anesthesia of Patients on Rauwolfia Therapy," *J. Amer. Med. Ass.*, *161*, 1143 (1956).

(19) S. Bracha and J. P. Hes, "Death Occurring during Combined Reserpine-Electroshock Treatment," *Amer. J. Psychiat.*, *113*, 257 (1956).

(20) M. H. Alper et al., "Pharmacology of Reserpine and Its Implications for Anesthesia," *Anesthesiology*, *24*, 524 (1963).

(21) A. J. Ominsky and H. Wollman, "Hazards of General Anesthesia in the Reserpinized Patient," *Anesthesiology*, *30*, 443 (1969).

(22) "The Pharmacological Basis of Therapeutics," 5th ed., L. S. Goodman and A. Gilman, Eds., Macmillan, New York, NY 10022, 1975, pp. 470–513.

[For additional information, see *Antihypertensive Therapy*, p. 381.]

Nonproprietary and Trade Names of Drugs

Alseroxylon—*Rautensin, Rauwiloid*
Chloroform—*Various manufacturers*
Cyclopropane—*Various manufacturers*
Deserpidine—*Harmonyl*
Dopamine hydrochloride—*Intropin*
Enflurane—*Ethrane*
Ether—*Various manufacturers*
Ethyl chloride—*Various manufacturers*
Fluroxene—*Fluromar*
Halopropane—*Tebron*
Halothane—*Fluothane*
Levarterenol bitartrate—*Levophed
Bitartrate*
Metaraminol bitartrate—*Aramine*
Methoxamine hydrochloride—*Vasoxyl*

Methoxyflurane—*Penthrane*
Nitrous oxide—*Various manufacturers*
Phenylephrine hydrochloride—*Neo-
Synephrine Hydrochloride and various
combination products*
Rauwolfia serpentina—*Raudixin and
various combination products*
Rescinnamine—*Moderil*
Reserpine—*Reserpoid, Sandril, Serpasil,
and various combination products*
Syrosingopine—*Singoserp*
Trichloroethylene—*Trilene*
Trichloromonofluoromethane—*Various
manufacturers*

*Prepared and evaluated by the Scientific Review Subpanel on
Antihypertensive Agents and reviewed by Practitioner Panel IV.*

Spironolactone—Aspirin

Summary—Aspirin reduced the natriuretic effects of spironolactone in normal subjects, but this drug interaction has not been reported in clinical practice. Aspirin did not affect spironolactone's antihypertensive action in a small group of low renin, hypertensive patients. Until more clinical data are available for evaluation, patients receiving spironolactone and aspirin concurrently should be monitored closely for symptoms of decreased clinical response to spironolactone.

Related Drugs—Although the clinical significance of this drug interaction has not been established, the relevant related drugs to aspirin would be all other oral **salicylates.**

Pharmacological Effect and Mechanism—The mechanism whereby aspirin inhibits the mineralocorticoid blocking properties of spironolactone is not established. Aspirin may displace spironolactone as a competitor with the mineralocorticoids for the receptor sites at the target tissue (1). The natriuretic response, however, also may be reduced by aspirin through a direct mineralocorticoid effect of aspirin, resulting in increased sodium- and chloride-ion reabsorption (2). In addition, aspirin may promote sodium- and chloride-ion reabsorption by reducing the conjugation of corticosteroids (3) or by enhancing the release of 17-hydroxycorticosteroids through pituitary–adrenal stimulation (3, 4).

Evaluation of Clinical Data—In a group of six normal subjects, the action of spironolactone (dose not reported) to increase urinary sodium excretion was reversed completely by subsequent administration (1.5 hr later) of aspirin (600 mg po) (1). When the order of drug administration was reversed, inhibition of sodium-ion excretion by aspirin was not as complete. These results are difficult to evaluate because of the short duration and the limited amount of information given about the study design.

In a well-controlled study (5), 10 healthy male subjects were utilized in a 6-week randomized, balanced, crossover study using a single dose (25, 50, or 100 mg) of spironolactone. Each subject was given fludrocortisone (1.0 mg po) to provide a constant mineralocorticoid stimulus against which the effects of acute or chronic administration of spironolactone could be assessed. This dose of fludrocortisone was followed in 2 hr by a dose of spironolactone. Aspirin (600 mg po) was administered 2 hr after spironolactone and reduced the natriuretic effect of single doses of spirono-lactone in 26 out of 30 doses (10 subjects × three dose levels) ($p<0.05$).

The second part of the study determined the effect of aspirin on chronic spirono-lactone administration. Seven of the 10 subjects were given spironolactone (25 mg four times daily for 7 days). A single dose of aspirin (600 mg po) reduced the natriuretic effectiveness of spironolactone in all subjects by a mean of 70% and reduced the mean overnight urine sodium content by 30% ($p<0.01$).

Five patients with low renin, essential hypertension were examined in a double-blind crossover study that lasted 22 weeks (6). Each patient had been maintained on spironolactone (100–300 mg/day po) for 4–18 months. Aspirin (3.6–4.8 g/day po for 6 weeks) did not alter the effect of spironolactone on blood pressure, serum electro-lytes, urea nitrogen, or plasma renin activity. However, two patients complained of gastric irritation by aspirin and may have not complied fully with the aspirin regimen.

■ Aspirin reduced the natriuretic effects of spironolactone in normal subjects, but this drug interaction has not been reported in clinical practice. Aspirin did not affect the antihypertensive action of spironolactone in a group of five patients, but two of these patients may not have complied with the aspirin dosage regimen and the patient sample size may have been too small. Therefore, since the clinical evidence about this drug interaction is not substantial, the clinical outcome cannot be predicted.

Recommendations—Until the clinical outcome of this drug interaction is established from additional data, the concurrent administration of spironolactone and aspirin need not be avoided. However, patients receiving these drugs should be monitored closely for symptoms of a possible decreased clinical response to spironolactone.

References

(1) H. C. Elliott, "Reduced Adrenocortical Steroid Excretion Rates in Man following Aspirin Administration," *Metabolism, 11*, 1015 (1962).

(2) A. G. Ramsay and H. C. Elliott, "Effect of Acetylsalicylic Acid on Ionic Reabsorption in the Renal Tubule," *Amer. J. Physiol., 213*, 323 (1967).

(3) A. K. Done et al., "Response of Plasma 17-Hydroxycorticosteroids to Salicylate Administration in Normal Human Subjects," *Metabolism, 4*, 129 (1955).

(4) A. K. Done et al., "Salicylates and the Pituitary-Adrenal System," *Metabolism, 7*, 52 (1958).

(5) M. G. Tweeddale and R. I. Ogilvie, "Antagonism of Spironolactone-Induced Natriuresis by Aspirin in Man," *N. Engl. J. Med., 289*, 198 (1973).

(6) J. W. Hollifield, "Failure of Aspirin to Antagonize Spironolactone's Antihyper-tensive Effect in Low-Renin Hypertension," *S. Med. J.*, in press.

[For additional information, see *Diuretic Therapy*, p. 414.]

Nonproprietary and Trade Names of Drugs

Aluminum aspirin—*Available in combination products*
Aspirin—*Available alone or as a fixed combination in many trade name products, especially over-the-counter preparations*
Calcium carbaspirin—*Calurin*
Carbethyl salicylate—*Sal-Ethyl Carbonate*
Choline salicylate—*Actasal, Arthropan*

Magnesium salicylate—*Various manufacturers*
Potassium salicylate—*Various manufacturers*
Salicylamide—*Various manufacturers*
Sodium salicylate—*Various manufacturers*
Spironolactone—*Aldactone and various combination products*

Prepared and evaluated by the Scientific Review Sub-panel on Diuretics and reviewed by Practitioner Panel I.

Succinylcholine—Dexpanthenol

Summary—Although one case report indicated that dexpanthenol may prolong the respiratory depression induced by succinylcholine, subsequent studies failed to verify this effect. Therefore, no additional precautions are necessary when these drugs are administered concurrently.

Related Drugs—There are no other neuromuscular blocking agents that will interact in the same manner with dexpanthenol.

Pharmacological Effect and Mechanism—Succinylcholine is a depolarizing skeletal muscle relaxant (1) whose duration of effect is dependent upon the rate of hydrolysis by pseudocholinesterase (2, 3).

Dexpanthenol is converted to pantothenic acid which, in turn, combines with some protein moiety to form coenzyme A, which then produces acetylcholine (4). It is used in surgery for postoperative and postpartum intestinal and ureteral atony (5).

If dexpanthenol-induced levels of acetylcholine become high enough to saturate the acetylcholinesterase enzyme system, the excess acetylcholine may then be hydrolyzed by pseudocholinesterase. Less pseudocholinesterase would be available to hydrolyze succinylcholine, possibly causing prolongation of its neuromuscular blockade.

Evaluation of Clinical Data—One case (6) reported temporary respiratory depression when dexpanthenol was initiated within 5 min after cessation of succinylcholine. However, this effect was not observed in six surgical patients who were given dexpanthenol followed immediately by succinylcholine (5).

■ Published evidence suggesting that dexpanthenol prolongs muscle relaxation when used with succinylcholine is based on only one case. Other factors and variables, such as an error in the administration technique (5) or an idiosyncratic reaction to succinylcholine (2, 7), may have caused the respiratory depression.

Recommendations—The possibility of an interaction occurring between succinylcholine and dexpanthenol under normal conditions appears to be minimal. Therefore, no additional precautions are necessary when these agents are used concurrently.

References

(1) "The Pharmacological Basis of Therapeutics," 5th ed., L. S. Goodman and A. Gilman, Eds., Macmillan, New York, NY 10022, 1975, p. 565.

(2) A. J. Gissen and W. L. Nastuk, "Succinylcholine and Decamethonium," *Anesthesiology, 33,* 611 (1970).

(3) D. J. Liddell, "Cholinesterase Variants and Suxamethonium Apnea," *Proc. Roy. Soc. Med., 61,* 10 (1968).

(4) H. Beckman, "Dilemmas in Drug Therapy," Saunders, Philadelphia, Pa., 1967, p. 271.

(5) R. Smith *et al.,* "Succinylcholine-Pantothenyl Alcohol: A Reappraisal," *Anesth. Analg., 48,* 205 (1969).

(6) P. Stewart, "Case Reports," *J. Amer. Ass. Nurse Anesth., 28,* 56 (1960).

(7) R. D. Kimbrough and J. E. Suggs, "Succinylcholine and Atypical Cholinesterase," *N. Engl. J. Med., 289,* 751 (1973).

[For additional information, see *Muscle Relaxant Therapy*, p. 435.]

Nonproprietary and Trade Names of Drugs

Dexpanthenol—*Ilopan*   Succinylcholine chloride—*Anectine, Quelicin Chloride*

Prepared and evaluated by the Scientific Review Subpanel on Muscle Relaxants and reviewed by Practitioner Panel III.

Sulfinpyrazone—Aspirin

Summary—Aspirin antagonizes sulfinpyrazone's ability to increase the renal excretion of uric acid and to reduce serum uric acid levels. Although the clinical effects of this drug interaction cannot be predicted, there are enough clinical data to recommend that the concurrent administration of sulfinpyrazone and aspirin should be avoided.

Related Drugs—All **salicylates** are metabolized to salicylic acid in the body (1) and should be expected to exert similar effects on the uricosuric activity of sulfinpyrazone. **Salicylamide,** although not metabolized to salicylic acid, is also excreted through the kidney (2) and may interact with sulfinpyrazone.

Oxyphenbutazone and **phenylbutazone** are chemically similar to sulfinpyrazone and possess mild uricosuric activity in high doses but are not used clinically for this purpose (1). Therefore, any effect aspirin would have on the uricosuric action of these drugs would be clinically unimportant.

Pharmacological Effect and Mechanism—Aspirin (4–6 g/day) and other salicylates, probenecid, and sulfinpyrazone promote the renal excretion of uric acid and its urate salts (3) and reduce serum urate levels. Uricosuric agents inhibit the renal tubular reabsorption of uric acid; the net uricosuria reflects the amount of renal uric acid filtered, and to a lesser extent, secreted by the kidneys (1, 4). Like other uricosurics (1), small doses of salicylates inhibit the tubular secretion of uric acid and thereby decrease urate elimination, whereas large doses (4–6 g) also inhibit tubular reabsorption to enhance uric acid excretion (3–5).

Sulfinpyrazone and salicylates may interact by multiple mechanisms. Sulfinpyrazone and salicylates compete for common binding sites on plasma proteins. Concurrent administration of these drugs decreases the binding capacity of sulfinpyrazone from 99 to 93% without altering the binding capacity of the salicylates.

Sulfinpyrazone and salicylates also compete for active tubular transport in the kidneys (1, 4). In the presence of sulfinpyrazone, the renal excretion of salicylates is reduced. The reduction is probably caused by preferential tubular secretion of sulfinpyrazone over salicylates and a pH-dependent, noncompetitive reabsorption of salicylates (4).

The salicylates appear to block the inhibitory effect of sulfinpyrazone on the tubular reabsorption of uric acid, causing uric acid retention in the body (4, 6).

Evaluation of Clinical Data—A pharmacokinetic study in which sulfinpyrazone and sodium salicylate were administered intravenously to humans and dogs provides the clinical evidence and suggests the mechanisms for this interaction (4). Nine gouty male patients received one drug for 1 hr and then both drugs for an additional 1 hr. In eight patients, the intravenous injections initially consisted of either 300 mg of sulfinpyrazone or 3 g of sodium salicylate as a priming dose, followed by constant rate infusions of 10 or 10–20 mg/min, respectively. The ninth patient's regimen differed only in that the initial intravenous dose contained 800 mg of sulfinpyrazone, followed by 3 g of sodium salicylate 1 hr later. The clinical data showed that the concurrent use of these agents abolished any uricosuric effect.

In another study (6), sodium salicylate (6 g) and sulfinpyrazone (0.6 g) administered to one patient resulted in the excretion of less urate than from the individual use of similar doses of these drugs or from no drugs at all.

■ The clinical data indicate that aspirin and other salicylates significantly reduce the uricosuric effects of sulfinpyrazone when these drugs are administered concurrently.

The dose of salicylate used in the studies was relatively high (>3 g) and the effect of lower doses of salicylates has not been studied. The clinical outcome of concurrent use of these drugs also has not been investigated.

Recommendations—Until more clinical data are reported, it is prudent for a patient receiving sulfinpyrazone to avoid concurrent use of salicylates, particularly in high doses (>3 g of sodium salicylate). The patient also should be cautioned about which nonprescription products contain aspirin so that such products can be avoided. This interaction is especially deleterious to individuals who are susceptible to gouty attacks, hyperuricemia, and urate stone formation.

Aspirin also reduces the effect of probenecid in humans (6, 7), and similar precautions should be followed when probenecid and aspirin are used concurrently.

References

(1) "The Pharmacological Basis of Therapeutics," 5th ed., L. S. Goodman and A. Gilman, Eds., Macmillan, New York, NY 10022, 1975, pp. 325–355.
(2) "Drill's Pharmacology in Medicine," 4th ed., J. R. DiPalma, Ed., McGraw-Hill, New York, N.Y., 1971, p. 401.
(3) A. B. Gutman, "Questions and Answers on 'Salicylates and Uric Acid'," *J. Amer. Med. Ass.*, *191*, 959 (1965).
(4) T.-F. Yu *et al.*, "Mutual Suppression of the Uricosuric Effects of Sulfinpyrazone and Salicylate: A Study on Inter-actions between Drugs," *J. Clin. Invest.*, *42*, 1330 (1963).
(5) M. L. Tainter and A. J. Ferris, "Aspirin in Modern Therapy," Bayer Company Division, Sterling Drug Inc., New York, N.Y., 1969, p. 23.
(6) J. E. Seegmiller and A. Grayzel, "Use of the Newer Uricosuric Agents in the Management of Gout," *J. Amer. Med. Ass.*, *173*, 1076 (1960).
(7) L. R. Pascale, "Inhibition of Uricosuric Action of Benemid by Salicylate," *J. Lab. Clin. Med.*, *45*, 771 (1955).

[For additional information, see *Uricosuric Therapy*, p. 447.]

Nonproprietary and Trade Names of Drugs

Aluminum aspirin—*Available in combination products*
Aspirin—*Available alone or as a fixed combination in many trade name products, especially over-the-counter preparations*
Calcium carbaspirin—*Calurin*
Carbethyl salicylate—*Sal-Ethyl Carbonate*
Choline salicylate—*Actasal, Arthropan*
Magnesium salicylate—*Various manufacturers*

Oxyphenbutazone—*Oxalid, Tandearil*
Phenylbutazone—*Azolid, Butazolidin*
Potassium salicylate—*Various manufacturers*
Probenecid—*Benemid*
Salicylamide—*Various manufacturers*
Sodium salicylate—*Various manufacturers*
Sulfinpyrazone—*Anturane*

Prepared and evaluated by the Scientific Review Subpanel on Uricosuric Agents and reviewed by Practitioner Panel V.

Tetracycline—Aluminum, Calcium, and Magnesium Ions

Summary—Simultaneous administration of aluminum, calcium, or magnesium ions significantly decreases the gastrointestinal (GI) absorption of tetracycline. This drug interaction may be clinically significant in severe infections where high doses of tetracycline are necessary. Simultaneous use of products containing these ions (*e.g.*, antacids and laxatives) or ingestion of foods containing calcium (*e.g.*, cottage cheese and milk) should be avoided in patients receiving tetracycline compounds.

Related Drugs—**Demeclocycline** (1, 2) and **oxytetracycline** (2, 3) have been reported to interact with aluminum ions and dairy products containing calcium (*e.g.,* cottage cheese and milk). **Doxycycline** has been reported to interact with aluminum hydroxide (2) but may not interact with dairy products (2, 3). **Chlortetracycline** has been reported to interact with aluminum ions (4) and **methacycline** has been reported to interact with dairy products (3). The manufacturer of **minocycline** claims that this tetracycline analog is unaffected by nondairy food and dairy products (5, 6), but this claim is based on unpublished data and cannot be evaluated. All other **tetracyclines** are expected to interact with these ions in a similar manner.

Aluminum, calcium, or magnesium ions are the major ingredients of most commercial antacid products (7), and any antacid product containing these ions can be expected to interact with the tetracyclines. Magnesium ions also are a major ingredient of many laxative products (*e.g.,* milk of magnesia and citrate of magnesia) (7).

Pharmacological Effect and Mechanism—Tetracycline is incompletely absorbed from the intestines (8) and forms relatively insoluble chelates with metallic ions (8, 9). Aluminum ions form the most stable complexes while magnesium and calcium ions form much weaker complexes (10–12). Tetracycline is probably absorbed through passive diffusion (13), and the formation of the metallic chelate may depress this diffusion significantly (9, 14). The ability to form these chelates is dependent upon the pH of the system: at low pH there is little chelate formation while at high pH there is significant chelate formation (9).

Evaluation of Clinical Data—The effect of aluminum-containing antacids on the absorption of tetracycline compounds is well documented in clinical studies. In one study (4), the serum levels of chlortetracycline (500 mg po every 6 hr) were determined in six normal subjects and five hospitalized patients after simultaneous administration of aluminum hydroxide gel (30 ml) for 3 days. After 48 hr of simultaneous administration, the serum chlortetracycline level decreased from 5.9 to less than 1 μg/ml in four of the five hospitalized patients. The fifth patient maintained a level of 5 μg/ml in spite of aluminum hydroxide administration. One patient suffered a recurrence of a urinary tract infection on the third day of concurrent treatment which promptly subsided when aluminum hydroxide was discontinued. The addition of aluminum hydroxide gel was followed by a sharp drop in the serum chlortetracycline level in each of the six normal subjects. The average serum chlortetracycline level before aluminum hydroxide gel administration was 4.2 μg/ml while the average serum level after simultaneous administration was 0.49 μg/ml.

In separate treatments, five subjects were given either oxytetracycline (1 g) or chlortetracycline (1 g) for 4 days (15). The subjects received aluminum hydroxide gel (30 ml) simultaneously on 2 days. Antacid administration caused a marked depression (>50% in most cases) in serum antibiotic levels in these subjects.

Simultaneous administration of aluminum hydroxide (15 ml) resulted in an almost 100% reduction in the serum antibiotic concentration of four subjects who had received single doses of demeclocycline (300 mg) and four subjects who had received single doses of doxycycline (100 mg) when compared to controls (2).

The clinical studies involving the interaction between calcium ions and tetracycline compounds involved simultaneous administration of calcium as an excipient present in tetracycline capsules or in dairy products (*e.g.,* buttermilk, cottage cheese, or whole milk). In 43 healthy subjects (16), use of tetracycline capsules containing elemental calcium (11–35 mg) resulted in a 20–60% lower serum tetracycline level than the use of tetracycline capsules without calcium. In another study (17), 24 patients received tetracycline (250 mg) with dicalcium phosphate (40 mg of calcium) and 27 patients received tetracycline preparations containing citric acid or lactose. In all cases, the serum levels produced by the tetracycline product containing calcium were 25–50% less than the serum levels resulting from products without calcium.

The simultaneous use of dairy products (*e.g.,* cottage cheese and milk) also decreases the GI absorption of tetracycline. These dairy products contain calcium (in amounts ranging from 90 to 133 mg/100 g) (18) in sufficient quantities to interact with the tetracycline product. In one study (1), 12 volunteers were given a single dose of demeclocycline (300 mg) with either fresh pasteurized buttermilk (240 ml), cottage cheese (240 g), or fresh pasteurized whole milk (240 ml). Serum demeclocycline levels decreased an average of 60–70% when compared to a control group of six patients who received demeclocycline (300 mg) with water. Four other patients received aluminum hydroxide (20 ml) simultaneously with demeclocycline and showed 76% lower serum antibiotic levels than the control group.

In four subjects in a crossover study (2), single doses of demeclocycline (300 mg) and doxycycline (100 mg) were given simultaneously with either food and homogenized milk (480 ml), with food and no dairy products, or with skim milk. An average decrease of 45–70% in serum demeclocycline levels occurred in all three groups when compared to a control group of subjects receiving this antibiotic with water. A 19–34% decrease in the serum doxycycline levels occurred in subjects receiving dairy products, but there was no decrease in the serum doxycycline levels in those subjects taking the antibiotic simultaneously with nondairy food.

Five subjects were given fresh whole milk (300 ml) simultaneously with single doses of doxycycline (200 mg po), methacycline (300 mg po), oxytetracycline (500 mg po), or tetracycline (500 mg po) (3). There was a 63–67% decrease in the peak serum antibiotic level when compared with control values for all tetracyclines except doxycycline, which was unaffected. There was a similar decrease in the serum tetracycline level when whole milk was ingested 30 min prior to tetracycline administration. Simultaneous administration of curdled milk caused a 35% decrease in the serum tetracycline level, indicating less interference than fresh milk with tetracycline absorption.

The only clinical investigation of the interaction between magnesium ions and tetracycline involved eight healthy adults (19). Oral doses of 500 or 1000 mg of tetracycline were given alone and then with 50% magnesium sulfate solution (30 ml) or castor oil (30 ml). Simultaneous administration of tetracycline with 50% magnesium sulfate resulted in tetracycline levels 75% lower than those attained when castor oil was given. When 15 ml of the 50% magnesium sulfate solution was given simultaneously with tetracycline in one patient, there was no decrease observed in the serum tetracycline level.

■ Based on published data, simultaneous administration of aluminum-containing antacids and tetracycline or its analogs probably results in a significant reduction in the serum antibiotic levels. Although there are no investigations concerning simultaneous administration of calcium-containing antacids and tetracycline compounds, the amount of calcium contained in commercially available antacid products [57–400 mg/5 ml or tablet (7)] is sufficient to decrease serum tetracycline levels significantly. Moreover, simultaneous use of the tetracyclines with dairy products such as cottage cheese and milk should be avoided.

The evidence supporting a similar interaction with magnesium-containing products is not as conclusive. In the only clinical study (19), the dose of magnesium used (15 g) was much larger than the amount normally present in magnesium-containing products (7) (except citrate of magnesia and magnesium sulfate solution). In fact, there was no interaction in one patient at half the dose of magnesium sulfate (7.5 g). However, since most antacids containing magnesium also contain aluminum (7), magnesium-containing antacids may still decrease tetracycline absorption.

Since most studies utilized healthy subjects, the therapeutic outcome of this drug interaction is unknown. Nevertheless, in certain severe infections where high serum tetracycline levels are desirable, this drug interaction may be therapeutically significant.

Recommendations—Simultaneous use of antacids containing aluminum, calcium, or magnesium ions or dairy products containing calcium (*e.g.*, cottage cheese and milk) with tetracycline or its analogs should be avoided. Laxative products containing magnesium in amounts equal to or greater than 15 g/dose (*e.g.*, citrate of magnesia) should also be avoided.

If antacids are indicated, they should be administered at least 3 hr after tetracycline administration to allow the maximum amount of tetracycline to be absorbed (20). Because there are no data to predict the appropriate time interval between administration of these drugs, administration of the antacid before tetracycline should be avoided.

Simultaneous ingestion of food with tetracycline or its analogs may delay the rate (1, 2) or the extent (1, 2, 21) of absorption of the antibiotic. The difference in the results may be due to the presence of calcium-containing foods in some of the meals, the type of tetracycline analog used, or the use of single or multiple doses of the antibiotic. Simultaneous ingestion of food and tetracycline or its analogs (with the exception of doxycycline and perhaps minocycline) should be avoided whenever possible.

Food or milk does not affect the absorption of doxycycline significantly and can be given simultaneously with this antibiotic (2, 3). The evidence that minocycline is unaffected by food or milk (5, 6) has not been published and cannot be evaluated. Therefore, until some clinical data have been published to support this claim, it is prudent to avoid simultaneous administration of milk with minocycline. Sodium bicarbonate antacids also affect the absorption of tetracycline by altering GI pH and should be avoided (22).

References

(1) J. Scheiner and W. A. Altemeier, "Experimental Study of Factors Inhibiting Absorption and Effective Therapeutic Levels of Declomycin," *Surg. Gynecol. Obstet.*, *114*, 9 (1962).

(2) J. E. Rosenblatt *et al.*, "Comparison of In Vitro Activity and Clinical Pharmacology of Doxycycline with Other Tetracyclines," *Antimicrob. Ag. Chemother.*, 134 (1966).

(3) M. J. Mattila *et al.*, "Interference of Iron Preparations and Milk with the Absorption of Tetracyclines," *Excerpta Medica Int. Cong. Ser.*, *254*, 128 (1971).

(4) B. A. Waisbren and J. S. Hueckel, "Reduced Absorption of Aureomycin Caused by Aluminum Hydroxide Gel (Amphojel)," *Proc. Soc. Exp. Biol. Med.*, *73*, 73 (1950).

(5) Minocin Package Insert, Lederle Laboratories, Pearl River, N.Y., Sept. 1974.

(6) "Minocin, Minocycline," Medical Advisory Department, Lederle Laboratories, American Cyanamid Co., Pearl River, NY 10965, 1975, pp. 10–11.

(7) "Handbook of Non-Prescription Drugs," G. B. Griffenhagen and L. Hawkins, Eds., American Pharmaceutical Association, Washington, D. C., 1973, pp. 7, 62.

(8) C. M. Kunin and M. Finland, "Clinical Pharmacology of the Tetracycline Antibiotics," *Clin. Pharmacol. Ther.*, *2*, 51 (1961).

(9) T. F. Chin and J. L. Lach, "Drug Diffusion and Bioavailability: Tetracycline Metallic Chelation," *Amer. J. Hosp. Pharm.*, *32*, 625 (1975).

(10) A. Albert, "Avidity of Terramycin and Aureomycin for Metallic Cations," *Nature*, *172*, 201 (1953).

(11) A. Albert and C. W. Rees, "Avidity of the Tetracyclines for the Cations of Metals," *Nature*, *177*, 433 (1956).

(12) K. W. Kohn, "Mediation of Divalent Metal Ions in the Binding of Tetracycline to Macromolecules," *Nature*, *191*, 1156 (1961).

(13) J. L. Colaizzi and P. R. Klink, "pH-Partition Behavior of Tetracyclines," *J. Pharm. Sci.*, *58*, 1184 (1969).

(14) K. Kakemi *et al.*, "Absorption and Excretion of Drugs. XXXVI. Effect of Ca^{2+} on the Absorption of Tetracycline from the Small Intestine (1)," *Chem. Pharm. Bull.*, *16*, 2200 (1968).

(15) J. C. Michel *et al.*, "Effect of Food and Antacids on Blood Levels of Aureomycin and Terramycin," *J. Lab. Clin. Med., 36*, 632 (1950).

(16) W. M. Sweeney *et al.*, "Absorption of Tetracycline in Human Beings as Affected by Certain Excipients," *Antibiot. Med. Clin. Ther., 4*, 642 (1957).

(17) W. P. Boger and J. J. Gavin, "An Evaluation of Tetracycline Preparations," *N. Engl. J. Med., 261*, 827 (1959).

(18) "Scientific Tables," 7th ed., K. Diem and C. Lentner, Eds., Ciba-Geigy Ltd., Basel, Switzerland, 1970, pp. 510–511.

(19) R. S. Harcourt and M. Hamburger,

"The Effect of Magnesium Sulfate in Lowering Tetracycline Blood Levels," *J. Lab. Clin. Med., 50*, 464 (1957).

(20) "The Pharmacological Basis of Therapeutics," 5th ed., L. S. Goodman and A. Gilman, Eds., Macmillan, New York, NY 10022, 1975, p. 1185.

(21) W. M. M. Kirby *et al.*, "Comparison of Two New Tetracyclines with Tetracycline and Demethylchlortetracycline," *Antimicrob. Ag. Chemother., 1*, 286 (1961).

(22) W. H. Barr *et al.*, "Decrease of Tetracycline Absorption in Man by Sodium Bicarbonate," *Clin. Pharmacol. Ther., 12*, 779 (1971).

[For additional information, see *Anti-Infective Therapy*, p. 388.]

Nonproprietary and Trade Names of Drugs

Aluminum-, calcium-, and magnesium-containing products—*Aludrox, Alzinox, Amphojel, A-M-T, Camalox, Creamalin, Dicarbosil, DiGel, Ducon, Gaviscon, Gelusil, Gelusil-M, Kolantyl Gel, Kudrox, Maalox, Malcogel, Mylanta, Oxaine-M, Phosphaljel, Robalate, Rolaids, Titralac, Trisogel, Tums, WinGel*

Chlortetracycline hydrochloride—*Aureomycin*

Demeclocycline—*Declomycin*

Doxycycline monohydrate—*Doxy-II Monohydrate, Doxychel, Vibramycin Monohydrate*

Methacycline hydrochloride—*Rondomycin*

Minocycline hydrochloride—*Minocin, Vectrin*

Oxytetracycline—*Dalimycin, Terramycin*

Oxytetracycline hydrochloride—*Oxy-Kesso-Tetra, Oxy-Tetrachel, Terramycin Hydrochloride*

Rolitetracycline—*Syntetrin*

Tetracycline—*Achromycin, Panmycin, Panmycin KM, Sumycin, Tetracyn, Tetrex-S*

Tetracycline hydrochloride—*Achromycin, Bristacycline, Cyclopar, Panmycin, Robitet, Steclin, Sumycin, Tetracyn*

Tetracycline phosphate complex—*Tetrex*

Prepared and evaluated by the Scientific Review Subpanel on Anti-Infectives and reviewed by Practitioner Panel II.

Tetracycline—Ferrous Sulfate

Summary—The oral administration of ferrous sulfate (200–600 mg) interferes with the absorption of tetracycline from the gastrointestinal (GI) tract and vice versa, leading to decreased serum levels of the antibiotic and the iron salt, respectively. If simultaneous administration is necessary, patients should receive tetracycline 3 hr after or 2 hr before iron administration.

Related Drugs—Of the tetracycline analogs, **doxycycline** (1, 2), **methacycline** (1), and **oxytetracycline** (1) have demonstrated a similar interaction with iron. Although there is no documentation, other **tetracycline analogs** theoretically can be expected to behave similarly.

Other salts of iron such as **ferrous fumarate** (3) and **ferrous gluconate** (3) have been shown to interact with tetracycline. Since the interaction between tetracycline and iron appears to be due to the ferrous or ferric ion, preparations such as **ferro-cholinate** and **ferrous lactate** can also be expected to inhibit the absorption of tetracycline. Most commercial iron preparations are in the ferrous form.

Pharmacological Effect and Mechanism—The oral administration of ferrous ion, like other polyvalent cations, decreases the GI absorption of tetracycline (1, 4) and tetracycline derivatives (1). The precise mechanism by which iron impairs tetracycline absorption is unclear. Since tetracycline binds with several divalent cations (5–7), two possible mechanisms have been proposed: tetracyclines may form chelates with ferrous ions, causing inhibition of absorption; or in the presence of ferrous ion, tetracyclines may bind to protein residues present in the intestine (8).

Evaluation of Clinical Data—In a controlled study (1), five healthy subjects received either doxycycline (200 mg po), methacycline (300 mg po), oxytetracycline (500 mg po), or tetracycline (500 mg po). A similar group received the same dose of antibiotic plus ferrous sulfate (200 mg po). Concurrent iron administration decreased the maximum serum concentrations of tetracycline and oxytetracycline by approximately 50%. The effect of concurrent iron administration on the serum levels of doxycycline and methacycline was even greater, producing more than an 80% reduction in the serum level.

The effect of the time interval between tetracycline and iron administration was investigated in a second controlled study using a group of 38 healthy subjects (4). During the first phase of the study, 20 subjects received tetracycline (500 mg po) while ingesting ferrous sulfate (600 mg po) either simultaneously or 0.5, 1, 2, or 3 hr before the antibiotic. In the second phase of the investigation, ferrous sulfate (600 mg po) was administered to 15 subjects 1, 2, or 3 hr after tetracycline (500 mg po). In the final phase, 10 subjects received tetracycline (500 mg po) every 12 hr for 4 days and ferrous sulfate (400 mg po) at the same time or 2 hr after the antibiotic. Control groups in each phase received tetracycline (500 mg po) only.

When tetracycline was ingested 0.5, 1, and 2 hr after the iron, significant ($p<0.001$, $p<0.01$, and $p<0.05$, respectively) reductions in serum antibiotic levels were seen. When iron was administered 3 hr before or 2 hr after tetracycline administration, the results (4) indicated that satisfactory serum tetracycline levels were obtained. Simultaneous oral administration of the drugs twice daily for 4 days failed to reduce the effects of the interaction. After 4 days of simultaneous administration of tetracycline–ferrous sulfate, serum antibiotic levels in several subjects were substantially below the commonly accepted minimum inhibitory concentration of 0.6 μg/ml. Moreover, the mean serum level for the group was only slightly above (0.86 ± 0.19 μg/ml) the minimum inhibitory concentration. When ferrous sulfate was administered 2 hr after the antibiotic, adequate serum tetracycline levels were obtained.

In a double-blind crossover study in seven patients (2), ferrous sulfate (400 mg po) was given 3, 7, and 11 hr after a daily dose of doxycycline (200 mg/day po on the first day, 100 mg/day po for an additional 4 days). The serum doxycycline levels were 20–45% lower with simultaneous treatment than with doxycycline and placebo treatment. The difference was statistically significant ($p<0.05$). The half-life of a single intravenous dose of doxycycline (100 mg) was significantly shortened ($p<0.02$) from 16.6 ± 0.07 to 11.0 ± 0.4 hr in four patients treated concurrently with ferrous sulfate (400 mg po). Because the half-life of doxycycline given intravenously was shortened by oral iron administration, the investigators concluded that iron may chelate with doxycycline during its intestinal secretion phase.

The inhibitory effect of various iron salts, all containing elemental iron (40 mg), on the simultaneous absorption of tetracycline (500 mg po) was investigated in a double-blind crossover study of six healthy subjects (3). The salts used were ferric sodium edetate, ferrous fumarate, ferrous gluconate, ferrous succinate, ferrous sulfate, and ferrous tartrate. Ferrous sulfate caused the largest reduction in serum tetracycline levels (80–90%), followed by ferrous fumarate, ferrous gluconate, and ferrous succinate (all 70–80%), ferrous tartrate (50%), and ferric sodium edetate (30%). All results were highly statistically significant. The difference in ability of the iron salts to interfere with tetracycline absorption appeared to be related to the amount of iron normally absorbed from each salt.

The effect of tetracycline on iron absorption in humans has not been clearly defined. In a single-blind, randomized crossover study (8), 10 volunteers were given a ferrous sulfate–ascorbic acid combination (400 mg po) with placebo or with tetracycline (1 g po). The subjects served as their own controls. The amount of iron absorbed, measured by indirect means, was not significantly different in either group. However, in a study (9) of 11 patients with normal or depleted iron stores, tetracycline (500 mg po) inhibited the absorption of ferrous sulfate solution or capsules (containing 50 mg of ferrous ion) from 32 to 78% in subjects with depleted iron stores. The investigators concluded that the difference of the results obtained from this study (9) compared to previous results (8) were related to improved techniques.

■ Based on these reports, the concurrent administration of tetracycline or its analogs and ferrous sulfate results in a statistically significant reduction in the serum levels of the antibiotic and in the amount of iron absorbed. The amount of the reduction is dependent on many factors: formulation differences among ferrous sulfate dosage forms (10), type of iron salt used (3), the type of tetracycline compound used (1, 2), and the time interval between administration of these drugs (4). The drug interaction may be therapeutically significant in certain severe infections where high serum levels of tetracycline are desirable or in certain patients with depleted body stores of iron (*e.g.*, anemic patients).

Recommendations—Ferrous sulfate should not be given simultaneously with tetracycline or tetracycline analogs. In those situations in which it is necessary for patients to receive both iron and tetracycline therapy orally, this interaction may be avoided by administering the ferrous sulfate not less than 3 hr before or 2 hr after tetracycline.

References

(1) P. J. Neuvonen *et al.*, "Interference of Iron with the Absorption of Tetracyclines in Man," *Brit. Med., J., 4,* 532 (1970).

(2) P. J. Neuvonen and O. Penttila, "Effect of Oral Ferrous Sulphate on the Half-Life of Doxycycline in Man," *Eur. J. Clin. Pharmacol., 7,* 361 (1974).

(3) P. J. Neuvonen and H. Turakka, "Inhibitory Effect of Various Iron Salts on the Absorption of Tetracycline in Man," *Eur. J. Clin. Pharmacol., 7,* 357 (1974).

(4) G. Gothoni *et al.*, "Iron–Tetracycline Interaction: Effect of Time Interval between the Drugs," *Acta Med. Scand., 191,* 409 (1972).

(5) K. W. Kohn, "Mediation of Divalent Metal Ions in the Binding of Tetra-

cycline to Macromolecules," *Nature, 191,* 1156 (1961).

(6) A. Albert and C. W. Rees, "Avidity of the Tetracyclines for the Cations of Metals," *Nature, 177,* 433 (1956).

(7) A. Albert, "Avidity of Terramycin and Aureomycin for Metallic Cations," *Nature, 172,* 201 (1953).

(8) N. J. Greenberger, "Absorption of Tetracyclines: Interference by Iron," *Ann. Intern. Med., 74,* 792 (1971).

(9) H. C. Heinrich and K. H. Oppitz, "Tetracycline Inhibits Iron Absorption in Man," *Naturwissenschaften, 60,* 524 (1973).

(10) C. E. Blezek *et al.*, "Some Dissolution Aspects of Ferrous Sulfate Tablets," *Amer. J. Hosp. Pharm., 27,* 533 (1970).

[For additional information, see *Anti-Infective Therapy*, p. 388.]

Nonproprietary and Trade Names of Drugs

Chlortetracycline hydrochloride—
  Aureomycin
Demeclocycline—*Declomycin*
Doxycycline monohydrate—*Doxy-II
  Monohydrate, Doxychel, Vibramycin
  Monohydrate*
Ferrocholinate—*Chel-Iron, Ferrolip*
Ferrous fumarate, gluconate, lactate, and
  sulfate—*Various manufacturers,
  available alone or as a fixed
  combination*
Methacycline hydrochloride—*Rondomycin*
Minocycline hydrochloride—*Minocin,
  Vectrin*

Oxytetracycline—*Dalimycin, Terramycin*
Oxytetracycline hydrochloride—
  *Oxy-Kesso-Tetra, Oxy-Tetrachel,
  Terramycin Hydrochloride*
Rolitetracycline—*Syntetrin*
Tetracycline—*Achromycin, Panmycin,
  Panmycin KM, Sumycin, Tetracyn,
  Tetrex-S*
Tetracycline hydrochloride—*Achromycin,
  Bristacycline, Cyclopar, Panmycin,
  Robitet, Steclin, Sumycin, Tetracyn*
Tetracycline phosphate complex—*Tetrex*

*Prepared and evaluated by the Scientific Review Subpanel
on Anti-Infectives and reviewed by Practitioner Panel III.*

Tetracycline—Methoxyflurane

Summary—Prerenal azotemia and drug toxicity may arise when tetracyclines are administered to patients with decreased renal function. Methoxyflurane is associated with a dose-related impairment of renal function, so the potential for tetracycline toxicity may be increased following methoxyflurane anesthesia. It has been suggested, but not documented, that tetracycline may enhance the nephrotoxicity of methoxyflurane. Until more is known concerning the possible combined effects of tetracycline administration and methoxyflurane anesthesia on renal function, concurrent use of these drugs should be avoided.

Related Drugs—All **tetracyclines** except **doxycycline** may exhibit the same pattern of toxicity (1).

The only general anesthetic implicated as a causative agent of renal toxicity is methoxyflurane. Other halogenated anesthetic agents are **chloroform, enflurane, ethyl chloride, fluroxene, halopropane, halothane, trichloroethylene,** and **trichloromonofluoromethane,** although no interactions with tetracycline have been reported.

Pharmacological Effect and Mechanism—Tetracyclines prevent polypeptide synthesis by blocking attachment of amino acid–transfer-RNA complexes to ribosomes (2). This blockade produces a surplus of intracellular amino acids which are metabolized into urea and other end-products, resulting in an increased plasma nitrogen load to the kidneys. If renal function is impaired, elevated blood urea nitrogen occurs (3). In addition to other routes, tetracyclines are excreted through the kidneys. With impaired renal function, standard doses of tetracyclines may result in high serum drug concentrations. At serum levels above 20 μg/ml, symptoms of toxicity occur, including weakness, malaise, vomiting, fever, muscle twitching, and shock. Very high tetracycline doses produce renal tubular degeneration in rabbits (4). Another report in dogs suggests that tetracyclines might accelerate methoxyflurane biotransformation and/or impair renal excretion of potential nephrotoxic metabolites (5). No similar effect has been seen in other experimental animals or in humans.

Methoxyflurane nephrotoxicity appears to be dose related (6) and is associated with renal oxalosis (7) and with an increase in serum inorganic fluoride (8). High serum levels of inorganic fluoride may render the distal tubule unresponsive to anti-diuretic hormone (9), producing polyuria. The renal oxalosis occurs in some patients and appears to be associated with anuria. It is most likely that the increase in serum inorganic fluoride is responsible for methoxyflurane nephrotoxicity (6).

Evaluation of Clinical Data—Prerenal azotemia caused by tetracyclines has been demonstrated (10) and it has been suggested, although with little clinical documentation, that tetracyclines in high doses (>1 g/day) may be nephrotoxic (11).

The nephrotoxic potential of methoxyflurane (administered in high doses) is well established (12). One report (13) suggested that tetracycline (1–2 g/day po or iv) exaggerated the renal toxicity of methoxyflurane in seven patients undergoing major abdominal or thoracic surgery. However, the data also could indicate a simple addition of the known toxic effects of tetracycline and methoxyflurane to the already complicated clinical disorders. None of the patients had polyuria, and the three who died had renal oxalosis. Another patient (14) who died after tetracycline (2 g/day iv) and methoxyflurane had both renal oxalosis and polyuria.

Two additional case reports suggest that tetracycline may augment the nephrotoxicity of methoxyflurane. In one case (15), a patient received methoxyflurane on five occasions but developed renal failure only on the one occasion when tetracycline was administered (total dose, 3.5 g iv). In another case (16), a patient developed "polyuric acute renal failure" subsequent to methoxyflurane anesthesia and tetracycline therapy (100 mg im four times daily). The investigators attributed the high serum and urinary oxalate levels seen in this patient to the effect of tetracycline.

■ Nephrotoxicity may result in patients receiving high doses of methoxyflurane (17). In patients with impaired renal function, tetracycline elimination is decreased, and toxic accumulation may occur. Tetracycline itself is toxic and also contributes to elevation of blood urea nitrogen (11, 12). Although no clinical data are available, tetracycline possibly may induce or enhance methoxyflurane nephrotoxicity.

Recommendations—Until more is known concerning the possible effects of concurrent tetracycline administration and methoxyflurane anesthesia on renal function, these agents should not be used together. When alternative therapy is not possible, concurrent use of tetracycline and methoxyflurane should be approached with great caution. Adequate monitoring of the patient's renal function should be provided. Doxycycline apparently has few prerenal effects (1) and might be a safe alternative to tetracycline.

Gentamicin and kanamycin also have been associated with methoxyflurane nephropathy and should be used with care in methoxyflurane-anesthetized patients (18).

References

(1) P. J. Little et al., "Tetracyclines and Renal Failure," N. Z. Med. J., 72, 183 (1970).

(2) V. Lorain, "The Mode of Action of Antibiotics on Gram-Negative Bacilli," Arch. Intern. Med., 128, 623 (1971).

(3) M. E. Shils, "Some Metabolic Aspects of Tetracyclines," Clin. Pharmacol. Ther., 3, 321 (1962).

(4) S. M. Farhat et al., "Clinical Toxicity of Antibiotics Correlated with Animal Studies," Arch. Surg. (Chicago), 76, 762 (1958).

(5) R. K. Stoelting and P. S. Gibbs, "Effect of Tetracycline Therapy on Renal Function after Methoxyflurane Anesthesia," Anesth. Analg., 52, 431 (1973).

(6) R. I. Mazze et al., "Dose-Related Methoxyflurane Nephrotoxicity in Rats: A Biochemical and Pathologic Correlation," Anesthesiology, 36, 571 (1972).

(7) J. A. Frascino et al., "Renal Oxalosis and Azotemia after Methoxyflurane," N. Engl. J. Med., 283, 676 (1970).

(8) R. I. Mazze et al., "Methoxyflurane Metabolism and Renal Dysfunction: Clinical Correlation in Man," Anesthesiology, 35, 247 (1971).

(9) Committee on Anesthesia, National Academy of Sciences–National Research Council, "Statement Regarding the Role of Methoxyflurane in the Production of Renal Dysfunction," Anesthesiology, 34, 505 (1971).

(10) M. E. Shils, "Renal Disease and the Metabolic Effects of Tetracycline," *Ann. Intern. Med., 58*, 389 (1963).

(11) R. B. Breitenbucher *et al.*, "Hepatorenal Toxicity of Tetracycline," *Minn. Med., 53*, 949 (1970).

(12) R. I. Mazze *et al.*, "Renal Dysfunction Associated with Methoxyflurane Anesthesia. A Randomized Prospective Clinical Evaluation," *J. Amer. Med. Ass., 216*, 278 (1971).

(13) E. Y. Kuzucu, "Methoxyflurane, Tetracycline, and Renal Failure," *J. Amer. Med. Ass., 211*, 1162 (1970).

(14) B. J. Panner *et al.*, "Toxicity following Methoxyflurane Anesthesia. I. Clinical and Pathological Observations in Two Fatal Cases," *J. Amer. Med. Ass., 214*, 86 (1970).

(15) D. D. Albers *et al.*, "Renal Failure following Prostatovesiculectomy Related to Methoxyflurane Anesthesia and Tetracycline—Complicated by Candida Infection," *J. Urol., 106*, 348 (1971).

(16) E. A. Proctor and F. L. Barton, "Polyuric Acute Renal Failure after Methoxyflurane and Tetracycline," *Brit. Med. J., 4*, 661 (1971).

(17) W. B. Crandall *et al.*, "Nephrotoxicity Associated with Methoxyflurane Anesthesia," *Anesthesiology, 27*, 591 (1966).

(18) M. J. Cousins and R. I. Mazze, "Tetracycline, Methoxyflurane Anesthesia and Renal Dysfunction," *Lancet, i*, 751 (1972).

[For additional information, see *Anti-Infective Therapy*, p. 388.]

Nonproprietary and Trade Names of Drugs

Chloroform—*Various manufacturers*
Chlortetracycline hydrochloride—*Aureomycin*
Demeclocycline—*Declomycin*
Doxycycline monohydrate—*Doxy-II Monohydrate, Doxychel, Vibramycin Monohydrate*
Enflurane—*Ethrane*
Ethyl chloride—*Various manufacturers*
Fluroxene—*Fluoromar*
Gentamicin sulfate—*Garamycin*
Halopropane—*Tebron*
Halothane—*Fluothane*
Kanamycin sulfate—*Kantrex*
Methacycline hydrochloride—*Rondomycin*
Methoxyflurane—*Penthrane*
Minocycline hydrochloride—*Minocin, Vectrin*

Oxytetracycline—*Dalimycin, Terramycin*
Oxytetracycline hydrochloride—*Oxy-Kesso-Tetra, Oxy-Tetrachel, Terramycin Hydrochloride*
Rolitetracycline—*Syntetrin*
Tetracycline—*Achromycin, Panmycin, Panmycin KM, Sumycin, Tetracyn, Tetrex-S*
Tetracycline hydrochloride—*Achromycin, Bristacycline, Cyclopar, Panmycin, Robitet, Steclin, Sumycin, Tetracyn*
Tetracycline phosphate complex—*Tetrex*
Trichloroethylene—*Trilene*
Trichloromonofluoromethane—*Various manufacturers*

Prepared and evaluated by the Scientific Review Subpanels on Anti-Infectives and Anesthetics and reviewed by Practitioner Panel V.

Thiopental—Reserpine

Summary—Reserpine may enhance the central nervous system (CNS) depression caused by barbiturates prior to surgery, resulting in hypotension and bradycardia. Although clinical reports about the drug interaction are inconclusive, the anesthesiologist should be aware that the patient has been treated with reserpine in order that possible hypotension and bradycardia may be anticipated. Reserpine also blocked the anticonvulsant effects of barbiturates in animals, but reports of the drug interaction in humans are lacking.

Related Drugs—**Pentobarbital** (1, 2) and **thiamylal** (3, 4) are reported to interact with reserpine in animals. Although not documented, other **barbiturates** can be expected to interact with reserpine due to their similar pharmacological effects.

Because of similarity of action, all other rauwolfia alkaloids (**alseroxylon, deser-pidine, rescinnamine,** and **syrosingopine**) have the potential for interacting with thiopental or other barbiturates.

Pharmacological Effect and Mechanism—Reserpine causes a depletion of catecholamines and 5-hydroxytryptamine (serotonin) in the central and peripheral nervous systems and cardiovascular tissue. Reserpine interferes with the binding of 5-hydroxytryptamine at the receptor sites, decreases the synthesis of norepinephrine and epinephrine by depleting their precursor dopamine, and competitively inhibits uptake of catecholamines into storage vesicles (5). Human subjects receiving reserpine are more relaxed and tend to be less alert but are easily aroused even when large doses are given (6).

The action of barbiturates on the CNS is not fully understood, but they can produce hypnosis and anesthesia, anticonvulsant effects, and other effects such as autonomic nervous system depression and respiratory depression (7).

Two interactions between reserpine and barbiturates have been demonstrated in animals: prevention of the anticonvulsant action of barbiturates and enhancement of CNS depression. In studies with experimental animals (3, 8, 9), reserpine antagonized the ability of barbiturates and anticonvulsants to increase the electroshock convulsive threshold. Severe reactions (confusion, lethargy, and severe hypotension) and deaths resulted from electroshock therapy in patients pretreated with reserpine (10–12). Reserpine also prolongs barbiturate-induced sleeping times (1, 13, 14).

In a study using barbital-sedated dogs, reserpine produced a gradual and persistent blood pressure and respiratory depression (15). This effect is believed to be due to a central inhibition of the sympathetic nervous system, possibly through specific hypothalamic depression.

Evaluation of Clinical Data—Clinical reports relating to the antagonism by reserpine of the anticonvulsant effects of barbiturates in humans are lacking, although reserpine has been reported to lower the seizure threshold in electroshock therapy (10–12).

Several studies (2, 4) reported bradycardia and hypotension after thiopental-induced anesthesia of patients treated with reserpine; however, these studies were uncontrolled, and the effects were never conclusively attributed to the concurrent administration of thiopental and reserpine. In addition, the studies were complicated by the fact that premedications such as meperidine, morphine, or pentobarbital were administered with atropine or scopolamine in addition to an inhalation anesthetic. In one study (4), circulatory changes did not occur until 1.5 mg of decamethonium bromide was administered; in the other study (2), the number of cases (five) was too small to draw valid conclusions.

In a controlled study, approximately 50% of both a control group (16 patients) and a group treated with reserpine (42 patients) developed bradycardia and hypotension after thiopental-induced anesthesia using various preoperative medications and gaseous anesthetics (16). However, in a similar controlled study (17), no differences in sleeping time or apnea were found between 30 reserpine-treated patients and 102 patients in the control group with an equal number from each group developing severe hypotension. Other studies (18, 19) also demonstrated that reserpine-treated patients tolerate anesthesia and surgical procedures well.

■ The reserpine-induced decrease in anticonvulsant activity of barbiturates appears to be of little clinical concern. Of greater importance is the development of hypotension and bradycardia during anesthesia, but clinical evidence about this effect is inconclusive.

Recommendations—Withdrawal of reserpine prior to surgery is not mandatory; however, the anesthesiologist should be aware that the patient has been receiving rauwolfia alkaloids and that hypotension and bradycardia may occur. If vasopressors are indicated in the reserpine-treated patient, agents predominantly acting directly upon α-adrenergic receptors (*e.g.*, dopamine, levarterenol, metaraminol, methoxamine, and phenylephrine) should be used rather than agents that depend primarily upon the release of catecholamines for their action (*e.g.*, ephedrine and mephentermine) (5, 20).

References

(1) S. Garattini *et al.*, "Reserpine Derivatives with Specific Hypotensive or Sedative Activity," *Nature, 183*, 1273 (1959).

(2) C. H. Ziegler and J. B. Lovette, "Operative Complications after Therapy with Reserpine and Reserpine Compounds," *J. Amer. Med. Ass., 176*, 916 (1961).

(3) W. D. Gray and C. E. Rauh, "The Anticonvulsant Action of Inhibitors of Carbonic Anhydrase: Relation to Endogenous Amines in Brain," *J. Pharmacol. Exp. Ther., 155*, 127 (1967).

(4) C. S. Coakley *et al.*, "Circulatory Responses during Anesthesia of Patients on Rauwolfia Therapy," *J. Amer. Med. Ass., 161*, 1143 (1956).

(5) "The Pharmacological Basis of Therapeutics," 5th ed., L. S. Goodman and A. Gilman, Eds., Macmillan, New York, NY 10022, 1975, pp. 470–513, 557.

(6) "Drill's Pharmacology in Medicine," 4th ed., J. R. DiPalma, Ed., McGraw-Hill, New York, N.Y., 1971, pp. 463–488.

(7) *Ibid.*, pp. 250–274.

(8) W. D. Gray *et al.*, "The Mechanism of the Antagonistic Action of Reserpine on the Anticonvulsant Effect of Inhibitors of Carbonic Anhydrase," *J. Pharmacol. Exp. Ther., 139*, 350 (1963).

(9) G. Chen and C. R. Ensor, "Antagonism Studies on Reserpine and Certain CNS Depressants," *Proc. Soc. Exp. Biol. Med., 87*, 602 (1954).

(10) M. W. Foster and R. F. Gayle, Jr., "Dangers in Combining Reserpine (Serpasil) with Electroconvulsive Therapy," *J. Amer. Med. Ass., 159*, 1520 (1955).

(11) S. Berg *et al.*, "Comparative Evaluation of the Safety of Chlorpromazine and Reserpine Used in Conjunction with ECT," *J. Neuropsychiat., 1*, 104 (1959).

(12) L. Kalinowsky, "The Danger of Various Types of Medication during Electric Convulsive Therapy," *Amer. J. Psychiat., 112*, 745 (1955).

(13) B. B. Brodie *et al.*, "Potentiating Action of Chlorpromazine and Reserpine," *Nature, 175*, 1133 (1955).

(14) V. H. Sethy *et al.*, "Potentiation of Barbital Sodium Hypnosis as a Screening Method for Central Nervous System Depressants," *Indian J. Med. Sci., 21*, 32 (1967).

(15) J. H. Trapold *et al.*, "Cardiovascular and Respiratory Effects of Serpasil, A New Crystalline Alkaloid from Rauwolfia Serpentina Benth, in the Dog," *J. Pharmacol. Exp. Ther., 110*, 205 (1954).

(16) W. M. Munson and J. A. Jenicek, "Effect of Anesthetic Agents on Patients Receiving Reserpine Therapy," *Anesthesiology, 23*, 741 (1962).

(17) T. Tammisto *et al.*, "The Effect of Reserpine, Chlordiazepoxide and Imipramine Treatment on the Potency of Thiopental in Man," *Ann. Chir. Gynaecol. Fen., 56*, 323 (1967).

(18) R. L. Katz *et al.*, "Anesthesia, Surgery and Rauwolfia," *Anesthesiology, 25*, 142 (1964).

(19) M. H. Alper *et al.*, "Pharmacology of Reserpine and Its Implications for Anesthesia," *Anesthesiology, 24*, 524 (1963).

(20) A. J. Ominsky and H. Wollman, "Hazards of General Anesthesia in the Reserpinized Patient," *Anesthesiology, 30*, 443 (1969).

[For additional information, see *Sedative–Hypnotic Therapy*, p. 442.]

Nonproprietary and Trade Names of Drugs

Allobarbital—*Diadol*
Alseroxylon—*Rautensin, Rauwiloid*
Amobarbital—*Amytal and various combination products*
Aprobarbital—*Alurate*
Barbital—*Neurondia*
Butabarbital sodium—*Butisol Sodium*
Butalbital—*Available in combination products*
Deserpidine—*Harmonyl*

Dopamine hydrochloride—*Intropin*
Ephedrine hydrochloride and sulfate—*Various manufacturers*
Hexobarbital—*Sombulex*
Levarterenol bitartrate—*Levophed Bitartrate*
Mephentermine—*Wyamine*
Mephobarbital—*Mebaral, Mebroin*
Metaraminol bitartrate—*Aramine*
Metharbital—*Gemonil*

Methohexital sodium—*Brevital Sodium*
Methoxamine hydrochloride—*Vasoxyl*
Pentobarbital—*Nembutal and various
  combination products*
Phenobarbital—*Eskabarb, Luminal*
Phenylephrine hydrochloride—*Neo-
  Synephrine Hydrochloride and various
  combination products*
Rauwolfia serpentina—*Raudixin and
  various combination products*

Rescinnamine—*Moderil*
Reserpine—*Reserpoid, Sandril, Serpasil,
  and various combination products*
Secobarbital—*Seconal and various
  combination products*
Syrosingopine—*Singoserp*
Talbutal—*Lotusate*
Thiamylal sodium—*Surital Sodium*
Thiopental sodium—*Pentothal Sodium*

*Prepared and evaluated by the Scientific Review Subpanel on
Sedative–Hypnotics and reviewed by Practitioner Panel III.*

Thyroid—Cholestyramine

Summary—Cholestyramine may cause a clinically significant decrease in the absorption of thyroid hormone when these drugs are given simultaneously. To avoid this effect, the time interval between thyroid hormone and cholestyramine administration should be as far apart as possible (optimally 5 hr). Additionally, any patient receiving these drugs concurrently should be observed for signs or symptoms of hypothyroidism.

Related Drugs—Since all thyroid compounds are basically the same, they would be expected to interact with cholestyramine in a similar manner. This conclusion is supported by the clinical evidence that **levothyroxine sodium** (1) and **thyroxine** (a compound in thyroid extract) (2) interact with cholestyramine.

   Colestipol and **polyamine-methylene resin** are other anion-exchange resins similar to cholestyramine that might also bind thyroid if administered concurrently.

Pharmacological Effect and Mechanism—Cholestyramine reportedly forms very strong ionic bonds with thyroid in the gastrointestinal tract which results in decreased absorption of orally administered thyroid. A significant amount of thyroxine (3000 mg) can be bound by a small amount of cholestyramine (50 mg) (1). Thyroid is excreted in the bile and reabsorbed into the enterohepatic circulation. Cholestyramine may bind thyroxine in the gut and prevent its enterohepatic recirculation, which would enhance the excretion of thyroxine into the feces (2).

Evaluation of Clinical Data—A clinical study of this drug interaction was performed in two subjects with hypothyroidism and five healthy subjects (1). One hypothyroid patient was given thyroid extract (60 mg/day po) and the other patient was given levothyroxine sodium (100 μg/day po). The dose of cholestyramine was 4 g four times daily. Each study period was 7 days. Thyroxine I 131 was also used to determine the patients' retention of thyroid. The results showed a nearly twofold increase in cumulative stool radioactivity as compared to control studies. There was correspondingly less thyroxine isotope absorbed as determined by measuring the amount of isotope in the urine and remaining in the body.

   The effect of the time interval between the administration of a dose of cholestyramine resin and a subsequent dose of thyroxine I 131 was studied in five healthy volunteers. Equal doses of thyroxine I 131 were given orally either simultaneously with cholestyramine or at intervals of either 1, 2, 2.5, 4, or 5 hr after cholestyramine. The results showed that the shorter the time interval between the ingestion of cholestyramine and the time of ingestion of thyroxine I 131, the greater was the interaction with cholestyramine. In three of the five patients, thyroxine absorption was normal when 5 hr had elapsed between the doses of cholestyramine and thyroxine I 131.

■ On the basis of the published clinical evidence, the interaction between cholestyramine and thyroid hormone may cause a clinically significant decrease in the amount of thyroid hormone absorbed in the body during concurrent administration.

Recommendations—Thyroxine and cholestyramine should be administered as far apart as possible (optimally 5 hr). When these drugs are used concurrently, the patient should be observed for symptoms of hypothyroidism [e.g., weakness, fatigue, cold intolerance, and dry, puffy skin (3)].

If possible, before cholestyramine is added to the drug regimen of a patient maintained on a thyroid preparation, baseline thyroid status should be determined by measuring serum liothyronine (triiodothyronine, t_3), thyroxine (t_4), and thyroid-stimulating hormone (TSH) levels. Periodic evaluation of these levels should be performed to detect changes in thyroid response.

References

(1) R. C. Northcutt et al., "The Influence of Cholestyramine on Thyroxine Absorption," J. Amer. Med. Ass., 208, 1857 (1969).
(2) F. Bergman et al., "Influence of Cholestyramine on Absorption and Excretion of Thyroxine in Syrian Hamster," Acta Endocrinol., 53, 256 (1966).

(3) "Current Diagnosis and Treatment," M. A. Krupp and M. J. Chatton, Eds., Lange Medical Publications, Los Altos, Calif., 1972, p. 611.

[For additional information, see Hypolipidemic Therapy, p. 428.]

Nonproprietary and Trade Names of Drugs

Cholestyramine resin—Cuemid, Questran
Colestipol hydrochloride—Colestid
Dextrothyroxine sodium—Choloxin
Levothyroxine sodium—Letter, Synthroid
Liothyronine sodium—Cytomel
Liotrix—Euthroid, Thyrolar

Polyamine-methylene resin—Resinat
Thyroglobulin—Proloid
Thyroid—Thyrar
Thyroxine fraction—Various manufacturers

Prepared and evaluated by the Scientific Review Subpanel on Hypolipidemic Agents and reviewed by Practitioner Panel V.

Tolbutamide—Alcohol

Summary—Tolbutamide and alcohol interact by multiple mechanisms and cause unpredictable fluctuations in serum glucose levels. The most serious effects are symptoms of severe hypoglycemia. Alcohol ingestion may also precipitate a disulfiram-like reaction (e.g., flushing, headache, palpitations, and a feeling of breathlessness) in patients stabilized on a sulfonylurea (particularly chlorpropamide). Diabetic patients receiving sulfonylureas should abstain from drinking alcohol. If abstinence is not feasible, the patient should avoid ingesting large amounts of alcohol and should be cautioned about the potentially severe effects caused by concurrent ingestion of these agents.

Related Drugs—**Chlorpropamide** (1–3) also interacts similarly with alcohol. There is no documentation for the other sulfonylureas, **acetohexamide** and **tolazamide,** but they can be expected to interact with alcohol in a similar manner.

Pharmacological Effect and Mechanism—The interaction between tolbutamide and alcohol occurs by several different mechanisms. Alcohol intensifies the effect of the tolbutamide enhancement of the acute phase release of insulin from the pancreatic β-cells (4). This effect has been referred to as the "alcohol priming" of insulin release and probably only affects the immediate supply of insulin present, not the amount being manufactured (5).

Short-term administration of large amounts of alcohol (170–200 mg/kg/hr iv for 6 hr) to normal nonalcoholic subjects increased the tolbutamide half-life, probably by decreasing its metabolism in the liver (6). Conversely, chronic alcohol ingestion caused a significant decrease in the tolbutamide half-life (6–8), most likely by increasing its metabolic transformation in the liver. The half-life of tolbutamide in the alcoholic subject returns to normal after a month or more of abstinence from alcohol (6–8).

Alcohol, in amounts as small as 0.5 g/kg (70 ml of 100-proof whiskey), inhibits gluconeogenesis in the liver of alcoholic and nonalcoholic subjects whenever that homeostatic mechanism is required to respond to tolbutamide-induced hypoglycemia (9–12). However, alcoholic beverages, particularly beer, may increase serum glucose levels because of their high carbohydrate content (13).

Chlorpropamide and, to a lesser extent, other sulfonylureas cause a disulfiram-like reaction (*e.g.,* flushing, headache, palpitations, and a feeling of breathlessness) in patients a short time after alcohol is ingested (equal to amounts as small as 50 ml of 100-proof whiskey) (2, 3, 14). This reaction to alcohol is attributed to an abnormal response of small blood vessels induced by chlorpropamide; this response is not related to an excessive accumulation of acetaldehyde (3).

Evaluation of Clinical Data—There are many reports of a drug interaction between tolbutamide and alcohol in nonalcoholic diabetic or normal subjects. In one study (6), six healthy subjects received tolbutamide (1 g po) while alcohol was infused (170–200 mg/kg/hr iv for 6 hr); the tolbutamide half-life was prolonged with an average increase of 39.8%. In another study (1), 14 patients who received either chlorpropamide (0.5–3 g po) or tolbutamide (0.5–3 g po) experienced a hypoglycemic reaction after concurrent use of alcohol (amount not reported). However, in a later study of four patients taking sulfonylureas (type and dose not reported), concurrent use of alcohol (35 ml of 100% alcohol, equal to 70 ml of 100-proof whiskey) did not cause any significant difference in the mean glucose levels (13). Two additional patients treated with insulin experienced severe hypoglycemic episodes after ingestion of the same quantities of alcohol.

An altered effect of tolbutamide metabolism in alcoholic subjects also was reported (6–8). In these patients (who all had a history of consuming at least 200 g of alcohol/day), the tolbutamide half-life was decreased significantly. When alcohol was withheld from these patients, the half-life slowly increased to normal after a month or more.

A disulfiram-like response to therapeutic doses of chlorpropamide was reported in patients ingesting moderate amounts of alcohol (25 ml of 100% alcohol, equal to 50 ml of 100-proof whiskey) (2, 3, 14). The onset of symptoms (flushing with an intense feeling of facial warmth, pounding headache, palpitations, and a feeling of breathlessness) occurred almost immediately (3–15 min) after alcohol ingestion (even in small amounts). The symptoms lasted for about 1 hr or longer. It has been reported (3, 14) that 13–63% of patients receiving chlorpropamide and ingesting alcohol experience these symptoms. This reaction to alcohol is limited primarily to patients receiving chlorpropamide, although it could occur with other sulfonylureas (15, 16).

■ Concurrent ingestion of alcohol and tolbutamide or other sulfonylureas results in unpredictable and potentially dangerous alterations in the effects of the sulfonylureas. The most dangerous effects are symptoms of severe hypoglycemia. Factors such as the particular hypoglycemic agent used, amount and type of alcoholic beverage ingested, pattern of alcohol use, and the patient's hepatic status influence the clinical outcome of this drug interaction. Additionally, alcohol ingestion may precipitate a disulfiram-like reaction (*e.g.*, flushing, headache, palpitations, and a feeling of breathlessness) in patients receiving a sulfonylurea (particularly chlorpropamide).

Recommendations—There are significant differences of opinion about whether to advise diabetic patients to avoid alcohol intake (13). Although complete abstinence from alcohol may be desirable, this recommendation is not practical for all patients.

If a patient desires an occasional drink, small amounts of low alcoholic content wines should be suggested (13). Since moderate quantities of alcohol (equal to 50 ml of 100-proof whiskey) can precipitate a disulfiram-like response in patients receiving chlorpropamide (2, 3), patients receiving this drug must either abstain from alcohol or should be switched to another sulfonylurea or to insulin (16).

Insulin-dependent diabetic patients should be discouraged from excessive alcohol intake because of the possibility of precipitating a life-threatening hypoglycemic crisis. The concurrent use of insulin and alcohol by alcoholic patients has led to two deaths and three instances of permanent mental impairment (9). In each case, patients stabilized on insulin were found comatose or semiconscious from hypoglycemia caused by consumption of excessive amounts of alcohol. Chronic alcoholic patients being withdrawn from alcohol should have their doses of tolbutamide adjusted downward periodically to compensate for the expected increase in the tolbutamide half-life (6).

Any diabetic patient, particularly one who drinks alcohol, should be cautioned to avoid undernourishment. The patient also should be informed that a diabetic who becomes hypoglycemic after ingesting alcohol may be thought to be inebriated and deprived of the necessary emergency treatment (13). Additionally, the mental confusion of alcoholism is frequently accompanied by dietary indiscretion, a failure to eat, and use of inadequate or excessive doses of insulin or other hypoglycemic agents (9, 17).

References

(1) E. Schulz, "Severe Hypoglycemic Reactions after Tolbutamide, Carbutamide, and Chlorpropamide," *Arch. Klin. Med.*, *214*, 135 (1968).

(2) D. D. Klink *et al.*, "Disulfiram-Like Reaction to Chlorpropamide (Diabinese)," *Wis. Med. J.*, 134 (March 1969).

(3) M. G. Fitzgerald *et al.*, "Alcohol Sensitivity in Diabetics Receiving Chlorpropamide," *Diabetes*, *11*, 40 (1962).

(4) A. M. Siegal *et al.*, "Some Aspects of 'Acute Phase' Insulin Release in Healthy Subjects," *Diabetes*, *21*, 157 (1972).

(5) R. Freidenberg *et al.*, "Differential Plasma Insulin Response to Glucose and Glucagon Stimulation following Ethanol Priming," *Diabetes*, *20*, 397 (1971).

(6) N. Carulli *et al.*, "Alcohol-Drugs Interaction in Man: Alcohol and Tolbutamide," *Eur. J. Clin. Invest.*, *1*, 421 (1971).

(7) R. M. H. Kater *et al.*, "Increased Rate of Tolbutamide Metabolism in Alcoholic Patients," *J. Amer. Med. Ass.*, *207*, 363 (1969).

(8) M. N. Shah *et al.*, "Comparison of Blood Clearance of Ethanol and Tolbutamide and the Activity of Hepatic Ethanol-Oxidizing and Drug-Metabolizing Enzymes in Chronic Alcoholic Subjects," *Amer. J. Clin. Nutr.*, *25*, 135 (1972).

(9) R. A. Arky *et al.*, "Irreversible Hypoglycemia, A Complication of Alcohol and Insulin," *J. Amer. Med. Ass.*, *206*, 575 (1968).

(10) A. Dornhorst and A. Ouyang, "Effect of Alcohol on Glucose Tolerance," *Lancet, iii,* 957 (1971).

(11) G. B. Phillips and H. F. Safrit, "Alcoholic Diabetes: Induction of Glucose Intolerance with Alcohol," *J. Amer. Med. Ass., 217,* 1513 (1971).

(12) M. C. DeMoura *et al.,* "Clinical Alcohol Hypoglycemia," *Ann. Intern. Med., 66,* 893 (1967).

(13) C. H. Walsh *et al.,* "Effect of Moderate Alcohol Intake on Control of Diabetes," *Diabetes, 23,* 440 (1974).

(14) E. N. Wardle and G. O. Richardson, "Alcohol and Glibenclamide," *Brit. Med. J., 3,* 309 (1971).

(15) J. M. Stowers, "Alcohol and Glibenclamide," *Brit. Med. J., 3,* 533 (1971).

(16) S. Signorelli, "Tolerance for Alcohol in Patients on Chlorpropamide," *Ann. N.Y. Acad. Sci., 74,* 900 (1959).

(17) "Alcohol and Hypoglycemic Coma," *J. Amer. Med. Ass., 206,* 639 (1968).

[For additional information, see *Hypoglycemic Therapy*, p. 422, and *Phenformin–Alcohol*, p. 177.]

Nonproprietary and Trade Names of Drugs

Acetohexamide—*Dymelor*
Alcohol—*Various products and beverages*
Chlorpropamide—*Diabinese*

Insulin—*Iletin*
Tolazamide—*Tolinase*
Tolbutamide—*Orinase*

Prepared and evaluated by the Scientific Review Subpanels on Hypoglycemic Agents and Sedative–Hypnotics and reviewed by Practitioner Panel I.

Tolbutamide—Chloramphenicol

Summary—Initiation of chloramphenicol therapy in diabetic patients controlled with tolbutamide or a related sulfonylurea may prolong the pharmacological action of the oral hypoglycemic agent, possibly resulting in symptoms of severe hypoglycemia. Frequent determinations of the serum glucose levels are recommended to ascertain if a reduction of the dose of tolbutamide or other sulfonylurea is indicated. If serum glucose levels vary in an erratic manner with tolbutamide therapy, insulin therapy should be substituted.

Related Drugs—In addition to tolbutamide, the hypoglycemic effect of **chlorpropamide** also has been reported to be prolonged by concurrent administration of chloramphenicol (1). **Tolazamide** is metabolized to six metabolites, three of which exhibit only slight hypoglycemic activity (2), and therefore can be considered functionally inactivated by metabolism. Although there is no documentation, tolazamide may theoretically be expected to interact with chloramphenicol in a manner similar to tolbutamide. **Acetohexamide** is metabolized to hydroxyhexamide, which is 2–3 times more potent and has a half-life that is approximately 4 times longer than the parent compound (2, 3). Since acetohexamide disappears from the body faster than its active metabolite, the amount of the more potent metabolite present in the body should be decreased by inhibition of acetohexamide metabolism. Therefore, the combined pharmacological action of acetohexamide and its metabolite would decrease (rather than increase) after inhibition of acetohexamide's metabolism by chloramphenicol. There is, however, no documentation of this interaction occurring.

Pharmacological Effect and Mechanism—The short-term effect of tolbutamide and other sulfonylureas is to stimulate release of endogenous insulin from the islet tissue of the pancreas. However, by unknown mechanisms, long-term use of the sulfonylureas causes a decrease in serum glucose levels in the presence of reduced insulin levels (2).

Tolbutamide is metabolized to butyl-*p*-carboxyphenylsulfonylurea, the major excretory product (4). It is thought that chloramphenicol may inhibit this metabolism, thereby prolonging the half-life and pharmacological effect of tolbutamide (5).

Evaluation of Clinical Data—A retrospective analysis (5) was made on a case report (6) of a 76-year-old male who had experienced a severe hypoglycemic episode 3 days after tolbutamide (0.5 g/day po) was initiated. It was discovered that 4 days prior to this hypoglycemic episode, chloramphenicol (2 g/day) was administered to treat a urinary tract infection. Based on this observation, the serum tolbutamide levels were measured in two sets of three patients who had been receiving tolbutamide and chloramphenicol concurrently. In the first three patients, the serum tolbutamide levels were measured after chloramphenicol (2 g/day po) was given for 10 days. The serum levels almost doubled in all three patients. In one subject, the serum level increased from approximately 7.5 mg/100 ml to approximately 14 mg/100 ml during this 10-day period.

In the second set of patients (5), the serum half-life of tolbutamide was measured after chloramphenicol (2 g/day iv) was given for 10 days. The half-life increased from an average of 5.4 hr to an average of 14.7 hr. In one patient, chloramphenicol (3 g iv) caused a rapid increase in the tolbutamide half-life from 5 to 8.75 hr. A similar increase in the tolbutamide half-life (from 4.75 to 7 hr) occurred in another patient given chloramphenicol (1.5 g iv).

In a similar study (5), the tolbutamide half-life increased in patients also receiving chloramphenicol.

The chlorpropamide half-life in subjects with normal renal function was shown to be about 36 hr (2). However, in a study (1) of five patients with normal renal function, the chlorpropamide half-life increased to 40, 60, 82, 116, and 146 hr with concurrent chloramphenicol administration (1.5–3.0 g).

■ When administered concurrently, chloramphenicol may prolong the tolbutamide half-life significantly. Since the reported cases occurred within the therapeutic dose range of each drug (5, 6), it can be surmised that concurrent use of these agents may increase the pharmacological effect of tolbutamide, possibly resulting in a hypoglycemic crisis.

Recommendations—Because chloramphenicol probably would be used only for a short period, frequent determinations of serum glucose levels should be performed to ascertain if a reduction in the dose of tolbutamide is necessary. If the situation arises where the serum glucose levels cannot be effectively controlled by tolbutamide, insulin therapy may be utilized. An increased dose of tolbutamide will probably be necessary when chloramphenicol is withdrawn.

References

(1) B. Petitpierre and J. Fabre, "Chlorpropamide and Chloramphenicol," *Lancet, i*, 789 (1970).

(2) "Diabetes Mellitus," 11th ed., A. Marble *et al.*, Eds., Lea and Febiger, Philadelphia, Pa., 1971, p. 305.

(3) "The Pharmacological Basis of Therapeutics," 5th ed., L. S. Goodman and A. Gilman, Eds., Macmillan, New York, NY 10022, 1975, p. 1521.

(4) R. C. Thomas and G. J. Ikeda, "The Metabolic Fate of Tolbutamide in Man and in the Rat," *J. Med. Chem., 9*, 507 (1966).

(5) L. K. Christensen and L. Skovsted, "Inhibition of Drug Metabolism by Chloramphenicol," *Lancet, ii*, 1397 (1969).

(6) J. M. Hansen and M. Kristensen, "Tolbutamide in the Treatment of Parkinson's Disease, A Double Blind Trial," *Dan. Med. Bull., 12*, 181 (1965).

[For additional information, see *Hypoglycemic Therapy*, p. 422.]

Nonproprietary and Trade Names of Drugs

Acetohexamide—*Dymelor*   Chlorpropamide—*Diabinese*
Chloramphenicol—*Amphicol, Chloromycetin,*   Tolazamide—*Tolinase*
  Mychel   Tolbutamide—*Orinase*

*Prepared and evaluated by the Scientific Review Subpanels on Hypogly-
cemic Agents and Anti-Infectives and reviewed by Practitioner Panel II.*

Tolbutamide—Dicumarol

Summary—Dicumarol increases the serum half-life of tolbutamide and may cause symptoms of hypoglycemia. This effect usually occurs 3–4 days after initiating dicumarol therapy. If dicumarol and a hypoglycemic drug must be given concurrently, insulin, which has not been reported to interact with dicumarol, may be substituted for tolbutamide. Otherwise, the tolbutamide dose should be adjusted accordingly whenever dicumarol is added to or withdrawn from the drug regimen.

Related Drugs—The serum half-life of **chlorpropamide** is increased by concurrent dicumarol administration, suggesting inhibition of chlorpropamide metabolism (1). **Tolazamide** is metabolized to six metabolites, three of which exhibit slight hypoglycemic activity (2), and therefore can be considered functionally inactivated by metabolism. Although there is no documentation, tolazamide may theoretically be expected to interact with dicumarol in a manner similar to tolbutamide.

Hydroxyhexamide, the metabolite of **acetohexamide,** is 2–3 times more potent (2) and its half-life in serum is approximately 4 times longer than the parent compound (3). Since acetohexamide disappears from the body faster than its active metabolite, the amount of the more potent metabolite present in the body should be' decreased by inhibition of acetohexamide metabolism. Therefore, the combined pharmacological action of acetohexamide and its metabolite would be decreased (rather than increased) after inhibition of acetohexamide's metabolism by dicumarol. However, there is no documentation in support of this theory.

Of the coumarin anticoagulants, **phenprocoumon** interacts with tolbutamide in animals (4). Chlorpropamide may interact with **acenocoumarol** (5), but the evidence is not conclusive. There are no reports of **warfarin** affecting the action of the sulfonylureas, although tolbutamide displaces warfarin from protein binding sites *in vitro* (6). Of the indandione derivatives, **phenindione** does not affect the metabolism of tolbutamide (7), and the possibility of an interaction between a sulfonylurea and any other indandione derivative (*e.g.*, **anisindione** and **diphenadione)** cannot be predicted.

Pharmacological Effect and Mechanism—Tolbutamide is almost completely metabolized in humans to two inactive metabolites that are excreted in the urine (3, 8). Chlorpropamide is the longest acting sulfonylurea and as much as 80% of it may be metabolized to inactive metabolites that are excreted in the urine (9, 10). At normal clinical serum levels, chlorpropamide and tolbutamide are 87 and 97% bound to plasma proteins, respectively (11).

Based on indirect evidence, it has been suggested that dicumarol inhibits the metabolism of chlorpropamide (1) and tolbutamide (7, 12), resulting in the prolongation of their half-lives. However, a retrospective study of 143 cases failed to establish any effect of dicumarol or warfarin on the action of tolbutamide or insulin (13). Warfarin was displaced from human serum albumin by tolbutamide in *in vitro* experiments (6), but the clinical significance of this observation has not been demonstrated.

Evaluation of Clinical Data—In an early report of this drug interaction, four elderly adult diabetic patients receiving tolbutamide (500 mg/day po) were given dicumarol (in doses adjusted to give a prothrombin–proconvertin level of 30%) (7). Beginning 3 days after initiation of anticoagulant therapy, the average peak serum tolbutamide concentration in the patients rose from 4 to 13.6 mg/100 ml. In three patients, dicumarol was withdrawn after 8 days of treatment and within 1 week tolbutamide levels returned to preanticoagulant levels. There was also a corresponding decrease in the fasting serum glucose level during concurrent administration of tolbutamide and dicumarol.

In the same study (7), eight healthy subjects received tolbutamide (1 g iv) before and after 1 week of treatment with dicumarol (dose not reported). The average tolbutamide half-life was increased from 4.9 to 17.5 hr after dicumarol administration. No change in the average peak serum level or the half-life of tolbutamide was found in two patients who received tolbutamide and phenindione concurrently.

A patient treated with chlorpropamide (375 mg/day po for 2 years) for parkinsonism experienced signs and symptoms of hypoglycemia shortly after dicumarol (dose not reported) was added to the treatment regimen (1). The serum chlorpropamide level increased to 18.4 mg/100 ml (expected serum level, 12 mg/100 ml) and the chlorpropamide half-life increased to 80 hr (normal, 32–38 hr). After dicumarol was withdrawn, the signs and symptoms of hypoglycemia disappeared and the chlorpropamide half-life decreased to 30 hr.

The same investigators subsequently reported on three diabetic patients receiving chlorpropamide (250 mg/day po) and dicumarol (titrated to achieve a plasma proconvertin level of 40%) (1). The serum chlorpropamide level increased from 7.6 to 13.3 mg/100 ml 3–4 days after concurrent therapy was initiated. In one of these patients, the serum chlorpropamide level did not return to predicumarol levels until approximately 17 days after the withdrawal of the anticoagulant. Two nondiabetic volunteers were given ^{35}S-labeled chlorpropamide (450 mg iv) before and after 6 days of treatment with dicumarol (dose not reported). Before treatment with dicumarol, chlorpropamide half-lives in these patients were 38 and 35 hr. During treatment with dicumarol, the half-lives increased to 94 and 84 hr, respectively (1).

Three healthy adults (12) were given tolbutamide (1.08 g iv) after a 1-week treatment with dicumarol (50 mg/day po). The mean tolbutamide half-life increased from 7 to 24 hr during a 7-hr period, and the mean serum tolbutamide level increased from 11.1 to 19.4 mg/100 ml.

Two patients stabilized on dicumarol experienced a prolongation of prothrombin time when tolbutamide (1–2 g/day po) was initiated (14). Subsequent studies in three additional patients and *in vitro* observations failed to verify this association. The lack of effect by tolbutamide also was observed in a retrospective analysis of 143 cases of diabetic patients (13). The patients received either insulin and warfarin, insulin and dicumarol, tolbutamide and warfarin, or tolbutamide and dicumarol. A statistical analysis failed to demonstrate any difference between tolbutamide and insulin in their effects on anticoagulant therapy when compared with controls.

■ Dicumarol may significantly increase the half-life of chlorpropamide and tolbutamide, beginning within 4 days after initiating concurrent therapy. It is difficult to determine if this increase will result in a clinically significant hypoglycemic crisis. The only patient who actually experienced a hypoglycemic crisis while taking these drugs concurrently had previously reduced his dietary intake of carbohydrates (1).

Recommendations—If dicumarol is the anticoagulant of choice in patients receiving oral sulfonylureas, the patient may be switched to insulin. If dicumarol and a sulfonylurea must be given concurrently, the sulfonylurea dose should be adjusted accordingly when dicumarol is added to or withdrawn from the drug regimen. Serum glucose levels should be monitored for several days, during and after concurrent therapy.

References

(1) M. Kristensen and J. M. Hansen, "Accumulation of Chlorpropamide Caused by Dicoumarol," *Acta Med. Scand., 183,* 83 (1968).

(2) "Diabetes Mellitus," 11th ed., A. Marble *et al.,* Eds., Lea and Febiger, Philadelphia, Pa., 1971, p. 307.

(3) "The Pharmacological Basis of Therapeutics," 5th ed., L. S. Goodman and A. Gilman, Eds., Macmillan, New York, NY 10022, 1975, p. 1520.

(4) M. Mahfouz *et al.,* "Potentiation of the Hypoglycaemic Action of Tolbutamide by Different Drugs," *Arzneim.-Forsch., 20,* 120 (1970).

(5) B. Petitpierre *et al.,* "Behavior of Chlorpropamide in Renal Insufficiency and under the Effect of Associated Drug Therapy," *Int. J. Clin. Pharmacol. Ther. Toxicol., 6,* 120 (1972).

(6) H. M. Solomon *et al.,* "The Displacement of Phenylbutazone-¹⁴C and Warfarin-¹⁴C from Human Albumin by Various Drugs and Fatty Acids," *Biochem. Pharmacol., 17,* 143 (1968).

(7) M. Kristensen and J. M. Hansen, "Potentiation of the Tolbutamide Effect by Dicumarol," *Diabetes, 16,* 211 (1967).

(8) R. C. Thomas and G. J. Ikeda, "The Metabolic Fate of Tolbutamide in Man and in the Rat," *J. Med. Chem., 9,* 507 (1966).

(9) P. M. Brotherton *et al.,* "A Study of the Metabolic Fate of Chlorpropamide in Man," *Clin. Pharmacol. Ther., 10,* 505 (1969).

(10) J. A. Taylor, "Pharmacokinetics and Biotransformation of Chlorpropamide in Man," *Clin. Pharmacol. Ther., 13,* 710 (1972).

(11) H. Wishinsky *et al.,* "Protein Interactions of Sulfonylurea Compounds," *Diabetes, 11,* suppl., 18 (1962).

(12) H. M. Solomon and J. J. Schrogie, "Effect of Phenyramidol and Bishydroxycoumarin on the Metabolism of Tolbutamide in Human Subjects," *Metabolism, 16,* 1029 (1967).

(13) R. L. Poucher and T. J. Vecchio, "Absence of Tolbutamide Effect on Anticoagulant Therapy," *J. Amer. Med. Ass., 197,* 1069 (1966).

(14) H. Chaplin and M. Cassell, "Studies on the Possible Relationship of Tolbutamide to Dicumarol in Anticoagulant Therapy," *Amer. J. Med. Sci., 235,* 706 (1958).

[For additional information, see *Hypoglycemic Therapy,* p. 422.]

Nonproprietary and Trade Names of Drugs

Acenocoumarol—*Sintrom*
Acetohexamide—*Dymelor*
Anisindione—*Miradon*
Chlorpropamide—*Diabinese*
Dicumarol—*Various manufacturers*
Diphenadione—*Dipaxin*
Insulin—*Iletin*

Phenindione—*Hedulin*
Phenprocoumon—*Liquamar*
Tolazamide—*Tolinase*
Tolbutamide—*Orinase*
Warfarin potassium—*Athrombin-K*
Warfarin sodium—*Coumadin Sodium, Panwarfin*

Prepared and evaluated by the Scientific Review Subpanels on Hypoglycemic Agents and Anticoagulants and reviewed by Practitioner Panel VI.

Tolbutamide—Phenylbutazone

Summary—The hypoglycemic activity of tolbutamide may be enhanced by the concurrent administration of phenylbutazone, and downward adjustment of the tolbutamide dosage may be indicated.

Related Drugs—In addition to tolbutamide, **acetohexamide** (1) and **chlorpropamide** (2, 3) may be expected to interact with phenylbutazone. Similarities in chemical structure and mode of action suggest that the effects of **tolazamide** also may be increased by phenylbutazone. Although not documented, **oxyphenbutazone** and possibly **sulfinpyrazone** can be expected to interact similarly to phenylbutazone.

Pharmacological Effect and Mechanism—Acetohexamide is metabolized *in vivo* to hydroxyhexamide which also possesses hypoglycemic activity. Phenylbutazone may interfere with the renal excretion of this active metabolite, thereby increasing the hypoglycemic response to acetohexamide (2). Phenylbutazone apparently also inhibits the renal clearance of chlorpropamide (1).

Phenylbutazone was originally thought to increase the hypoglycemic response of tolbutamide by inhibiting the conversion of tolbutamide to its inactive metabolite, thereby increasing the hypoglycemic effect (2). However, the results of a recent study suggest that phenylbutazone may inhibit tolbutamide excretion in a manner similar to the other sulfonylureas (4). Unfortunately, these results are questionable because of the small number of patients tested and the fact that the investigator could not measure the serum levels of the metabolite of tolbutamide. Moreover, the results were not statistically analyzed.

Evaluation of Clinical Data—In one study (3), phenylbutazone (dose and route not reported) enhanced the hypoglycemia caused by chlorpropamide (0.5–3 g po) and tolbutamide (0.5–3 g po) in 14 diabetic patients.

An increase in the signs and symptoms of hypoglycemia after concurrent administration of tolbutamide and phenylbutazone was also observed in separate case reports. In one report (5), a 64-year-old diabetic patient had been taking tolbutamide (1 g/day po) and phenylbutazone (800 mg/day po) at the same time and had experienced a severe hypoglycemic crisis for 2 days. It was later found that the patient had preexisting liver dysfunction which may have contributed to the toxic reaction to tolbutamide (6). In the other report (7), a diabetic patient stabilized on tolbutamide suffered an acute hypoglycemic attack after 4 days of concurrent administration of phenylbutazone (600 mg/day po).

In two normal subjects, the half-life of tolbutamide increased from 4 to 4.25 to 8.5 and 6.5 hr, respectively, after phenylbutazone (600 mg/day po) was administered (8). The serum tolbutamide level in a diabetic patient increased from 8.6 to 12.9 mg/100 ml after initiation of therapy with phenylbutazone (600 mg/day po).

The development of hypoglycemic coma in a patient receiving both acetohexamide and phenylbutazone led to a study (1) involving nine patients to determine the nature and significance of this interaction. Pretreatment with phenylbutazone (100 mg po four times daily for 1 week) caused a greater and more prolonged lowering of the serum glucose level following intravenous administration of acetohexamide than in patients not pretreated. The serum half-life of acetohexamide was not altered by phenylbutazone; however, the half-life of hydroxyhexamide was prolonged considerably.

A decreased (rather than increased) half-life resulting from phenylbutazone was observed in three diabetic patients previously stabilized on tolbutamide (9). In each case, the fasting serum glucose level of each patient rose significantly after therapy with phenylbutazone (600 mg/day po) was begun. Since these patients were all non-white Africans, it was hypothesized that the paradoxical behavior of phenylbutazone was due to a differing metabolic action in different races.

■ The available evidence indicates a definite possibility that phenylbutazone can enhance the hypoglycemic activity of tolbutamide or other sulfonylurea derivatives. This response may develop when the usual recommended doses of these agents are employed. Loss of control of the diabetic state may result, which could lead to the development of severe hypoglycemia. More studies would be desirable to clarify whether the enhanced hypoglycemic activity is to be expected routinely when these drugs are administered concurrently or whether it is only likely to occur under certain selected circumstances. Moreover, some studies should attempt to elucidate the possible different effects concurrent use of these drugs would have in patients of different ethnic backgrounds.

Recommendations—In most cases, the enhanced hypoglycemic activity of the sulfonylureas produced by phenylbutazone may be overcome by reducing the dose of the oral hypoglycemic agent. The agents can continue to be given concurrently; however, the therapy should be supervised closely, and the dosage should be adjusted if necessary. Since phenylbutazone is often given for only a short period, it may be necessary to change the sulfonylurea dose when phenylbutazone is discontinued. Serum glucose levels should be monitored closely during the time period that the drugs are administered concurrently.

Oxyphenbutazone is likely to alter the response to hypoglycemic agents in the same manner as phenylbutazone; therefore, it would offer no advantage in these situations. Indomethacin, which might be an alternative to phenylbutazone in certain situations, has not been reported to interact with hypoglycemic agents. However, indomethacin does possess certain properties (*e.g.*, it is highly protein bound) that suggest a possible interaction. Therefore, if it is used concurrently with a hypoglycemic agent, appropriate caution should be exercised.

Phenylbutazone has not been reported to influence the activity of phenformin, and, in some patients, this agent might be a suitable alternative to tolbutamide. However, phenformin and tolbutamide differ in some of their properties, and the difficulties encountered in changing hypoglycemic agents may present a greater problem than the initial interaction.

If short-term phenylbutazone therapy is indicated, insulin may be considered as a possible alternative to tolbutamide. The fact that the opposite effect (decreased activity of tolbutamide) may occur in the non-Caucasian patients, particularly in Africans (9), should be considered when concurrent tolbutamide and phenylbutazone therapy is indicated for such patients.

References

(1) J. B. Field *et al.*, "Potentiation of Acetohexamide Hypoglycemia by Phenylbutazone," *N. Engl. J. Med.*, *277*, 889 (1967).

(2) M. Dalgas *et al.*, "Hypoglycemic Episodes Induced by Phenylbutazone in Diabetic Patients Treated with Chlorpropamide," *Ugesk. Laeger.*, *127*, 834 (1965); through H. M. Solomon, "Clinical Disorders of Drug Interaction," *Advan. Intern. Med.*, *16*, 285 (1970).

(3) E. Schulz, "Severe Hypoglycemic Reactions after Tolbutamide, Carbutamide, and Chlorpropamide," *Arch. Klin. Med.*, *214*, 135 (1968).

(4) K. F. Ober, "Mechanism of Interaction of Tolbutamide and Phenylbutazone in Diabetic Patients," *Eur. J. Clin. Pharmacol.*, *7*, 291 (1974).

(5) H. Tannenbaum *et al.*, "Phenylbutazone–Tolbutamide Drug Interaction," *N. Engl. J. Med.*, *290*, 344 (1974).

(6) H. Ueda *et al.*, "Disappearance Rate of Tolbutamide in Normal Subjects and in Diabetes Mellitus, Liver Cirrhosis and Renal Disease," *Diabetes*, *12*, 414 (1963).

(7) M. Mahfouz *et al.*, "Potentiation of the Hypoglycaemic Action of Tolbutamide by Different Drugs," *Arzneim.-Forsch.*, *20*, 120 (1970).

(8) L. K. Christensen *et al.*, "Sulphaphenazole-Induced Hypoglycaemic Attacks in Tolbutamide-Treated Diabetics," *Lancet*, *ii*, 1298 (1963).

(9) S. K. Owusu and K. Ocran, "Paradoxical Behaviour of Phenylbutazone in African Diabetics," *Lancet*, *i*, 440 (1972).

[For additional information, see *Hypoglycemic Therapy*, p. 422.]

Nonproprietary and Trade Names of Drugs

Acetohexamide—*Dymelor*
Chlorpropamide—*Diabinese*
Indomethacin—*Indocin*
Insulin—*Iletin*
Oxyphenbutazone—*Oxalid, Tandearil*

Phenformin hydrochloride—*DBI, Meltrol*
Phenylbutazone—*Azolid, Butazolidin*
Sulfinpyrazone—*Anturane*
Tolazamide—*Tolinase*
Tolbutamide—*Orinase*

*Prepared and evaluated by the Scientific Review Subpanels on Hypogly-
cemic Agents and Analgesics and reviewed by Practitioner Panel II.*

Tolbutamide—Sulfaphenazole

Summary—Sulfaphenazole enhances the action of tolbutamide and may cause symptoms of severe hypoglycemia in diabetic patients. It is unclear whether this interaction also occurs with other sulfonamides or sulfonylurea compounds. Nevertheless, serum glucose levels should be obtained for diabetic patients taking sulfonylureas and sulfonamides concurrently to determine if alternative drugs should be used or if a reduction in the dose of the sulfonylurea is required.

Related Drugs—The hypoglycemic effect of **chlorpropamide** (1, 2) has also been reported to be prolonged by sulfonamides. The sulfonylureas, **acetohexamide** and **tolazamide,** are metabolized differently than tolbutamide (3) and may possibly interact differently with the sulfonamides. However, since the interactions between these drugs have not been studied, it is possible that the sulfonamides may interact with them in a manner similar to tolbutamide.

Sulfamethazine (1), **sulfamethizole** (4), and **sulfisoxazole** (2, 5) have been reported to interact with the sulfonylureas in a manner similar to sulfaphenazole. However, sulfamethizole has also been shown not to prolong the tolbutamide half-life (6). **Sulfadiazine** (7), **sulfadimethoxine** (7), and **sulfamethoxypyridazine** (7) appear not to produce hypoglycemic episodes similar to those caused by sulfaphenazole. Because of the variations in response to different sulfonamides, it is difficult to predict if other **sulfonamides** such as **sulfameter** and **sulfamethoxazole** will interact with the sulfonylureas.

Pharmacological Effect and Mechanism—The degree to which sulfonamides interact with sulfonylureas is dependent upon various factors including protein binding, metabolism, and renal excretion. Results from one study (7) led to the conclusion that sulfaphenazole significantly enhances the hypoglycemic response in tolbutamide-treated diabetic patients by displacing tolbutamide from its plasma protein binding sites. Sulfaphenazole also was reported to inhibit the carboxylation of tolbutamide by some as yet unexplained mechanism. Other studies (1, 2) indicated that when sulfonamides are administered in addition to a sulfonylurea, the latter will be displaced from its plasma protein binding sites. This displacement may result in severe hypoglycemia. Another study (8) concluded that diminished hepatic metabolism or renal clearance could be responsible for the prolonged effect of tolbutamide.

Evaluation of Clinical Data—Most evidence about this drug interaction is from case reports in which symptoms of severe hypoglycemia occurred when a sulfonamide was added to the regimen of patients stabilized on chlorpropamide or tolbutamide.

Symptoms of severe hypoglycemia were observed in an 81-year-old diabetic patient and a 47-year-old diabetic patient receiving tolbutamide (2 g/day po) and sulfisoxazole (2 g/day po) concurrently (5). The symptoms of hypoglycemia occurred 1 and 11 days after sulfisoxazole therapy was initiated in the 81- and 47-year-old patients, respectively. When tolbutamide was discontinued in these patients, the symptoms subsided. Although the investigators suggested that the hypoglycemia was caused by enhancement of the hypoglycemic effect of tolbutamide by sulfisoxazole, other causative factors, such as the administration of chloramphenicol (see *Tolbutamide–Chloramphenicol*, p. 243) concurrently in one patient and the presence of renal disease in the other (8), could not be ruled out.

Severe hypoglycemic symptoms also have been attributed to concurrent administration of chlorpropamide and a sulfonamide. In the first case (1), a 67-year-old diabetic patient stabilized on chlorpropamide (250 mg/day po) experienced symptoms of severe hypoglycemia 2 days after beginning sulfamethazine therapy (dose not reported). Although renal dysfunction was considered as the possible cause of this hypoglycemia, the patient had a normal blood urea nitrogen level and showed no signs of renal impairment. In the second report (2), symptoms of severe hypoglycemia occurred in a 77-year-old diabetic patient 1 day after sulfisoxazole (4 g/day po) was added to the drug regimen of chlorpropamide (500 mg/day po) and phenformin (50 mg/day po). However, the hypoglycemic symptoms may have been caused by the concurrent administration of phenformin and chlorpropamide. The patient was stabilized after discontinuation of the hypoglycemic agents.

A comprehensive study of possible drug interactions between tolbutamide and the sulfonamides was initiated after three diabetic patients experienced severe hypoglycemic episodes when sulfaphenazole (2 g/day po) was added to their drug regimens which included tolbutamide (1–2 g/day po) (7). The onset of hypoglycemic symptoms occurred from 2 to 11 days after initiation of sulfaphenazole therapy. The age of the patients ranged from 75 to 82 years and all three may have had some renal damage. Five additional patients treated with tolbutamide (1–2 g/day po) also were studied and all experienced severe hypoglycemic episodes a few days after sulfaphenazole was administered concurrently. When sulfaphenazole was withdrawn, the serum glucose values returned to the original levels in 24–48 hr. Sulfaphenazole (2 g/day po) also was administered to three diabetic patients who were not being treated with tolbutamide and there was no resultant decrease in their serum glucose levels. Four other sulfonamides (sulfadiazine, sulfadimethoxine, sulfamethoxypyridazine, and sulfisoxazole) were tested in the five patients and no hypoglycemic episodes occurred.

The effects of various sulfonamides on the half-life of tolbutamide were measured in 14 healthy subjects (6). Various doses of each sulfonamide and tolbutamide were given intravenously. Only sulfaphenazole increased the half-life of tolbutamide significantly (five- or sixfold increase in the half-life). The other sulfonamides tested were sulfamethizole, sulfadimethoxine, and sulfisoxazole. In a later study (4), sulfamethizole (4 g/day po) increased the half-life of tolbutamide from 5.2 to 9.2 hr in six patients.

■ While there is some evidence that a clinically significant interaction occurs between some sulfonamides (particularly sulfaphenazole) and chlorpropamide or tolbutamide, this evidence is not conclusive. In two cases (2, 5), the presence of phenformin or chloramphenicol in the drug regimens could have enhanced the effect of tolbutamide and caused the subsequent hypoglycemic episodes. Moreover, most patients studied were elderly, a group known to be prone to renal dysfunction (9), a condition which could allow toxic accumulation of tolbutamide in the body (8).

If a clinically significant drug interaction occurs between the sulfonamides and tolbutamide or chlorpropamide, it is more likely to occur with sulfaphenazole than any other sulfonamide. Sulfamethazine also has been reported to interact (1), but the evidence supporting the likelihood of sulfamethizole and sulfisoxazole interacting with tolbutamide or chlorpropamide is contradictory (2, 4–7). The other sulfonamides tested that did not demonstrate a drug interaction were sulfadiazine, sulfadimethoxine, and sulfamethoxypyridazine (6, 7).

There is not a definite correlation between duration of action of the sulfonamide and the potential for a drug interaction. Sulfamethazine and sulfaphenazole are intermediate-acting sulfonamides and have been shown to interact with chlorpropamide and tolbutamide, but the intermediate-acting sulfonamide sulfadiazine has not demonstrated a similar effect. The short-acting sulfonamides sulfamethizole and sulfisoxazole reportedly have been shown to interact with tolbutamide and chlorpropamide (2, 4–6), although these observations are controversial. However, the long-acting sulfonamides sulfadimethoxine and sulfamethoxypyridazine have been shown not to affect the half-life or the hypoglycemic action of tolbutamide.

If a drug interaction occurs between chlorpropamide or tolbutamide and a sulfonamide, it will probably occur a few days after the addition of the sulfonamide to the chlorpropamide or tolbutamide drug regimen and will occur with normal therapeutic doses of each drug.

Recommendations—Serum glucose levels should be determined prior to and shortly after the addition of a sulfonamide (particularly sulfaphenazole) to a tolbutamide or chlorpropamide drug regimen to ascertain if a reduction in the dose of the hypoglycemic drug is required. Depending upon the length of therapy with the sulfonamide, the determination of periodic serum glucose levels should be considered. If the serum glucose levels cannot be controlled when the patient is taking these drugs concurrently, then an alternative anti-infective or insulin should be used.

References

(1) J. L. C. Dall *et al.*, "Hypoglycaemia Due to Chlorpropamide," *Scot. Med. J.*, *12*, 403 (1967).

(2) H. St. George Tucker and J. I. Hirsch, "Sulfonamide-Sulfonylurea Interaction," *N. Engl. J. Med.*, *286*, 110 (1972).

(3) "Diabetes Mellitus," 11th ed., A. Marble *et al.*, Eds., Lea and Febiger, Philadelphia, Pa., 1971, p. 305.

(4) B. Lumholtz *et al.*, "Sulfamethizole-Induced Inhibition of Diphenylhydantoin, Tolbutamide, and Warfarin Metabolism," *Clin. Pharmacol. Ther.*, *17*, 731 (1975).

(5) J. S. Soeldner and J. Steinke, "Hypoglycemia in Tolbutamide-Treated Diabetics: Report of Two Cases with Measurement of Serum Insulin," *J. Amer. Med. Ass.*, *193*, 398 (1965).

(6) U. C. Dubach *et al.*, "Influence of Sulfonamides on the Blood Sugar Decreasing Effect of Oral Antidiabetics," *Schweiz. Med. Wochenscher.*, *96*, 1483 (1966).

(7) L. K. Christensen *et al.*, "Sulphaphenazole-Induced Hypoglycaemic Attacks in Tolbutamide-Treated Diabetics," *Lancet*, *ii*, 1298 (1963).

(8) H. Ueda *et al.*, "Disappearance Rate of Tolbutamide in Normal Subjects and in Diabetes Mellitus, Liver Cirrhosis and Renal Disease," *Diabetes*, *12*, 414 (1963).

(9) M. R. P. Hall, "Drug Therapy in the Elderly," *Brit. Med. J.*, *14*, 582 (1973).

[For additional information, see *Hypoglycemic Therapy*, p. 422.]

Nonproprietary and Trade Names of Drugs

Acetohexamide—*Dymelor*
Chlorpropamide—*Diabinese*
Insulin—*Iletin*
Sulfadiazine—*Various manufacturers*
Sulfameter—*Sulla*
Sulfamethazine—*Various combination products*
Sulfamethizole—*Thiosulfil*

Sulfamethoxazole—*Bactrim, Gantanol, Septra*
Sulfamethoxypyridazine—*Midicel*
Sulfaphenazole—*Orisul, Sulfabid*
Sulfisoxazole—*Gantrisin, SK-Soxazole*
Tolazamide—*Tolinase*
Tolbutamide—*Orinase*

Prepared and evaluated by the Scientific Review Subpanels on Hypoglycemic Agents and Anti-Infectives and reviewed by Practitioner Panel III.

Tubocurarine—Chlorothiazide

Summary—Chlorothiazide may enhance the neuromuscular blockade produced by tubocurarine by causing hypokalemia. This drug interaction is not supported by any clinical evidence, but plasma potassium levels should be determined in all patients, including those not taking chlorothiazide, before administering tubocurarine.

Related Drugs—If the potential exists for a drug interaction between tubocurarine and chlorothiazide, it may also occur with other potassium-depleting diuretics such as **chlorthalidone, ethacrynic acid, furosemide, mercurial diuretics, metolazone, quinethazone,** and other **thiazide diuretics** or other neuromuscular blocking agents such as **decamethonium, gallamine triethiodide, pancuronium,** and **succinylcholine.**

Pharmacological Effect and Mechanism—Chlorothiazide enhanced the neuromuscular blocking effect of tubocurarine in *in vitro* experiments on cat muscle strips (1). Although no mechanism of action has been established, hypokalemia may intensify the action of the neuromuscular blocking agents (2). Chlorothiazide and other potassium-depleting diuretics are known to cause hypokalemia (3) and may enhance this effect (4).

Evaluation of Clinical Data—There are no clinical reports of a significant drug interaction occurring between tubocurarine or other neuromuscular blocking agents and chlorothiazide or other diuretics. There have been a number of unsupported statements in the scientific literature suggesting that this drug interaction may be clinically significant (4–6).

■ No clinical significance can be ascribed to this interaction.

Recommendations—Since there is no clinical documentation and little animal data to support the significance of this drug interaction, there appears little need for additional precautions in patients receiving these drugs concurrently. However, prior to administering a neuromuscular blocking agent, plasma potassium levels should be determined in all patients even if they are not receiving chlorothiazide concurrently (5, 6).

References

(1) G. L. Gessa and W. Ferrari, "Influence of Chlorothiazide, Hydrochlorothiazide and Acetazolamide on Neuromuscular Transmission in Mammals," *Arch. Int. Pharmacodyn. Ther., 144,* 258 (1963).

(2) A. P. McLaughlin *et al.,* "Hazards of Gallamine Administration in Patients with Renal Failure," *J. Urol., 108,* 515 (1972).

(3) J. L. Katsikas and C. Goldsmith, "Disorders of Potassium Metabolism,"

Med. Clin. N. Amer., 55, 503 (1971).

(4) R. B. Clark and E. S. Maier, "Effects of Previous and Concomitant Drug Therapy on Surgery and Anesthesia," *GP, 29,* 106 (1964).

(5) J. H. Moyer *et al.,* "Medical Considerations in the Hypertensive Patient Undergoing Surgery," *Amer. J. Cardiol., 12,* 286 (1963).

(6) L. F. Prescott, "Clinically Important Drug Interactions," *Drugs, 5,* 161 (1973).

[For additional information, see *Muscle Relaxant Therapy,* p. 435.]

Nonproprietary and Trade Names of Drugs

Bendroflumethiazide—*Naturetin*
Benzthiazide—*Aquatag, Exna*
Chlorothiazide—*Diuril*
Chlorthalidone—*Hygroton, Regroton*

Cyclothiazide—*Anhydron*
Decamethonium bromide—*Syncurine*
Ethacrynic acid—*Edecrin*
Flumethiazide—*Rautrax*

Continued on next page

Furosemide—*Lasix*
Gallamine triethiodide—*Flaxedil*
Hydrochlorothiazide—*Esidrix, HydroDiuril, Oretic*
Hydroflumethiazide—*Saluron*
Mercaptomerin sodium—*Thiomerin*
Metolazone—*Zaroxolyn*
Methyclothiazide—*Aquatensen, Enduron*
Metocurine (Dimethyl tubocurarine) chloride—*Mecostrin*
Metocurine (Dimethyl tubocurarine) iodide —*Metubine*

Pancuronium bromide—*Pavulon*
Polythiazide—*Renese*
Quinethazone—*Hydromox*
Spironolactone—*Aldactone*
Succinylcholine chloride—*Anectine, Quelicin Chloride*
Triamterene—*Dyrenium*
Trichlormethiazide—*Metahydrin, Naqua*
Tubocurarine chloride—*Tubarine*
Various combination products containing a diuretic are available.

Prepared and evaluated by the Scientific Review Subpanel on Muscle Relaxants and reviewed by Practitioner Panel IV.

Tubocurarine—Neomycin

Summary—Neomycin and some related antibiotics produce a neuromuscular transmission failure which may cause prolonged respiratory depression or apnea in surgical patients treated concurrently with tubocurarine and other neuromuscular depressants. Concurrent use of these drugs should be avoided, and antibiotics that do not block neuromuscular transmission should be utilized. If these drugs must be used together, the patient should be observed closely for any unexpected prolongation of respiratory depression.

Related Drugs—In addition to neomycin, respiratory depression has been reported with chemically and pharmacologically related antibiotics such as **colistin** (1, 2), **dihydrostreptomycin** (1, 2), **gentamicin** (3), **kanamycin** (1, 2), **streptomycin** (1, 2), and **viomycin** (1).

In addition to tubocurarine, an additive neuromuscular depression has been reported to occur with **decamethonium** (4), **gallamine triethiodide** (1), and **succinylcholine** (1). **Pancuronium** also may interact with neomycin and related antibiotics, but no documentation is available.

Pharmacological Effect and Mechanism—Early laboratory data indicated that some antibiotics produced death by respiratory failure (5). This antibiotic apnea was subsequently shown for neomycin and some related agents to be due to a peripheral neuromuscular failure rather than central depression. The failure is the partial result of a competitive postjunctional anticholinergic action at the neuroeffector site since the transmission blockade is partially reversed by neostigmine (6–9).

Clinical data and the efficacy of calcium in reversing antibiotic-induced muscular weakness (7, 8, 10) indicate that neomycin also may produce a presynaptic acetylcholine release deficit.

Calcium is more effective than neostigmine in reversing neomycin-induced transmission failure in cats, especially when the failure is complete (8, 10). Antibiotic transmission blockade is intensified by hypocalcemia and by drugs that competitively antagonize neuromuscular transmission. The latter is produced consistently with tubocurarine in animals (7, 9). Intensification of antibiotic-induced neuromuscular blockade by other curare-like neuromuscular blockers has not been evaluated experimentally but could also be expected to occur with gallamine triethiodide (11, 12).

Interactions between some antibiotics and the depolarizing, noncompetitive neuro-muscular depressants also occur in humans when the latter are given prior to the antibiotic (13, 14). Enhancement of neuromuscular activity, in this case, may be due to the increase in sensitivity of the postsynaptic membrane to competitive blockers which follows recovery from the depolarizing blockade produced by decamethonium (15) or succinylcholine (15).

Evaluation of Clinical Data—More than 100 cases of antibiotic-induced respiratory depression have been reported since the correlation of respiratory weakness or failure with neomycin administration was first described (1, 2, 16). Most cases involved a sudden onset of dyspnea which progressed rapidly to a prolonged apnea immediately after surgery when these antibiotics were used in doses of from 2 to 5 g (13). The depression observed is characterized by a prolonged and, at times, irreversible failure of respiratory function (13, 16, 17). The respiratory depression has occurred at all doses and has followed intraperitoneal, intravenous, intramuscular, oral, intraluminal, intrapleural, and irrigation administrations of these antibiotics (3, 18–27).

For those cases occurring during or immediately following surgery, the antibiotic-induced neuromuscular blockade was thought to be enhanced by ether anesthesia or by the presence of another neuromuscular depressant (13, 17–21, 24). Antibiotic-induced muscle weakness can occur in the absence of anesthetics, especially if renal disease with hypocalcemia is present. In these patients, the weakness extends to muscles of the head, neck, and extremities and follows a distribution similar to myasthenia gravis (2, 5).

■ Neomycin and related antibiotics produce a profound neuromuscular blockade in humans. Use of these antibiotics with neuromuscular blocking agents could lead to a prolonged and an irreversible respiratory failure.

Recommendations—Neomycin and related antibiotics should be used with caution in patients in whom tubocurarine and other neuromuscular depressants have been used. This therapeutic precaution also includes patients with existing muscle weakness or renal disease in which serum levels of the antibiotics remain high in the presence of hypocalcemia. Caution should be exercised in the use of these antibiotics in pre-surgical preparation regimens.

Neuromuscular weakness also has been reported after concurrent administration of bacitracin, clindamycin, lincomycin, polymyxin, and tetracycline (1, 2, 28). Anti-biotic alternatives that have not been reported to produce neuromuscular weakness include chloramphenicol, erythromycin, oleandomycin, penicillin, ristocetin, and vancomycin (1, 2).

Reversal of antibiotic-induced muscle weakness and respiratory arrest has been attempted using calcium (23, 27), edrophonium (14), and neostigmine (14, 23, 27). In general, the success has been variable and dependent on the severity of the depression. In a few cases in which patients were studied electromyographically, there appeared to be a curare-like neuromuscular blockade and, in agreement with animal studies, a presynaptic defect (25). Neostigmine would be capable of reversing only the curare-like portion of the transmission failure and should not be used for treating toxic reactions caused by depolarizing agents such as succinylcholine (29).

References

(1) C. B. Pittinger and R. Adamson, "Antibiotic Blockade of Neuromuscular Function," *Ann. Rev. Pharmacol., 12,* 169 (1972).

(2) C. B. Pittinger *et al.,* "Antibiotic-Induced Paralysis," *Anesth. Analg., 49,* 487 (1970).

(3) A. W. Warner and E. Sanders, "Neuromuscular Blockade Associated with Gentamicin Therapy," *J. Amer. Med. Ass., 215,* 1153 (1971).

(4) K. Iwatsuke *et al.,* "Effects of Strep-tomycin on the Action of Muscle Re-laxants," *Med. J. Shinshu Univ., 3,* 299 (1958).

(5) H. J. Robinson and H. Molitor, "Some Toxicological and Pharmacological Properties of Gramicidin, Tyrocidine and Tyrothricin," *J. Pharmacol. Exp. Ther.*, *74*, 75 (1941).

(6) O. V. Brazil and A. P. Corrado, "The Curariform Action of Streptomycin," *J. Pharmacol. Exp. Ther.*, *120*, 452 (1957).

(7) A. P. Corrado et al., "Neuro-muscular Blockade by Neomycin, Potentiation by Ether Anesthesia and *d*-Tubocurarine and Antagonism by Calcium and Prostigmine," *Arch. Int. Pharmacodyn. Ther.*, *121*, 380 (1959).

(8) D. Elmqvist and J.-O. Josefsson, "The Nature of the Neuromuscular Block Produced by Neomycine," *Acta Physiol. Scand.*, *54*, 105 (1962).

(9) J. C. Timmerman et al., "Neuromuscular Blocking Properties of Various Antibiotic Agents," *Toxicol. Appl. Pharmacol.*, *1*, 299 (1959).

(10) V. F. Stanley et al., "Neomycin-Curare Neuromuscular Block and Reversal in Cats," *Anesthesiology*, *31*, 228 (1969).

(11) R. Bryce-Smith and H. D. O'Brien, "Fluothane: A Non-Explosive Volatile Anaesthetic Agent," *Brit. Med. J.*, *2*, 969 (1956).

(12) F. F. Foldes, "The Pharmacology of Neuromuscular Blocking Agents in Man," *Clin. Pharmacol. Ther.*, *1*, 345 (1960).

(13) F. F. Foldes et al., "Prolonged Respiratory Depression Caused by Drug Combinations. Muscle Relaxants and Intraperitoneal Antibiotics as Etiologic Agents," *J. Amer. Med. Ass.*, *183*, 672 (1963).

(14) H. G. Benz et al., " 'Recurarization' by Intraperitoneal Antibiotics," *Brit. Med. J.*, *2*, 241 (1961).

(15) S. Thesleff, "The Mode of Neuromuscular Block Caused by Acetylcholine, Nicotine, Decamethonium and Succinylcholine," *Acta Physiol. Scand.*, *34*, 218 (1955).

(16) J. E. Pridgen, "Respiratory Arrest Thought to be Due to Intraperitoneal Neomycin," *Surgery*, *40*, 571 (1956).

(17) B. W. Webber, "Respiratory Arrest following Intraperitoneal Administration of Neomycin," *Arch. Surg.*, *75*, 174 (1957).

(18) B. E. Ferrara and R. D. Phillips, "Respiratory Arrest following Administration of Intraperitoneal Neomycin," *Amer. Surg.*, *23*, 710 (1957).

(19) "Case Report No. 203," *American Society of Anesthesiology News Letter*, *22*, 33 (1958).

(20) W. P. Doremus, "Respiratory Arrest following Intraperitoneal Use of Neomycin," *Ann. Surg.*, *149*, 546 (1959).

(21) O. Stechishin et al., "Neuromuscular Paralysis and Respiratory Arrest Caused by Intrapleural Neomycin," *Can. Med. Ass. J.*, *81*, 32 (1959).

(22) E. A. Cooper and R. de G. Hanson, "Oral Neomycin and Anaesthesia," *Brit. Med. J.*, *2*, 1527 (1963).

(23) C. R. Ream, "Respiratory and Cardiac Arrest after Intravenous Administration of Kanamycin with Reversal of Toxic Effects by Neostigmine," *Ann. Intern. Med.*, *59*, 384 (1963).

(24) G. A. Small, "Respiratory Paralysis after a Large Dose of Intraperitoneal Polymyxin B and Bacitracin," *Anesth. Analg.*, *43*, 137 (1964).

(25) M. P. McQuillen et al., "Myasthenic Syndrome Associated with Antibiotics," *Arch. Neurol.*, *18*, 402 (1968).

(26) W. P. G. Jones, "Calcium Treatment for Ineffective Respiration Resulting from Administration of Neomycin," *J. Amer. Med. Ass.*, *170*, 943 (1959).

(27) R. G. Oriscello and N. P. Depasquele, "Neomycin Wound Irrigation: Report of a Case Associated with Massive Absorption with Nephro and Neurotoxicity," *Amer. J. Ther. Clin. Rep.*, *1*, 1 (1975).

(28) R. P. Fogdall and R. D. Miller, "Prolongation of a Pancuronium Induced Neuromuscular Blockade by Clindamycin," *Anesthesiology*, *41*, 407 (1974).

(29) "The Pharmacological Basis of Therapeutics," 5th ed., L. S. Goodman and A. Gilman, Eds., Macmillan, New York, NY 10022, 1975, p. 584.

[For additional information, see *Muscle Relaxant Therapy*, p. 435.]

Nonproprietary and Trade Names of Drugs

Amoxicillin—*Amoxil*
Ampicillin—*Alpen, Amcill, Omnipen, Penbritin, Polycillin, Principen, Totacillin*
Bacitracin—*Various manufacturers*
Carbenicillin disodium—*Geopen, Pyopen*
Chloramphenicol—*Amphicol, Chloromycetin, Mychel*
Chlortetracycline hydrochloride—*Aureomycin*

Clindamycin hydrochloride—*Cleocin Hydrochloride*
Cloxacillin sodium monohydrate—*Tegopen*
Colistin sulfate—*Coly-Mycin S*
Decamethonium bromide—*Syncurine*
Demeclocycline—*Declomycin*
Dicloxacillin sodium monohydrate—*Dynapen, Pathocil, Veracillin*
Dihydrostreptomycin sulfate—*Various manufacturers*

Diphenicillin sodium—*Ancillin*
Doxycycline monohydrate—*Doxy-II Monohydrate, Doxychel, Vibramycin Monohydrate*
Edrophonium chloride—*Tensilon*
Erythromycin—*E-Mycin, Erythrocin, Ilotycin*
Erythromycin estolate—*Ilosone*
Erythromycin ethylsuccinate—*Erythrocin Ethyl Succinate, Pediamycin*
Erythromycin gluceptate—*Ilotycin Gluceptate*
Erythromycin stearate—*Bristamycin, Erythrocin Stearate, Ethril*
Gallamine triethiodide—*Flaxedil*
Gentamicin sulfate—*Garamycin*
Kanamycin sulfate—*Kantrex*
Lincomycin hydrochloride—*Lincocin*
Methacycline hydrochloride—*Rondomycin*
Methicillin sodium—*Staphcillin*
Metocurine (Dimethyl tubocurarine) chloride—*Mecostrin*
Metocurine (Dimethyl tubocurarine) iodide—*Metubine*
Minocycline hydrochloride—*Minocin, Vectrin*
Nafcillin sodium—*Unipen*
Neomycin sulfate—*Mycifradin Sulfate, Myciguent, Neobiotic*
Neostigmine methylsulfate—*Prostigmin Methylsulfate*
Oleandomycin phosphate—*Various manufacturers*
Oxacillin sodium—*Bactocill, Prostaphlin*
Oxytetracycline—*Dalimycin, Terramycin*

Oxytetracycline hydrochloride—*Oxy-Kesso-Tetra, Oxy-Tetrachel, Terramycin Hydrochloride*
Pancuronium bromide—*Pavulon*
Penicillin G benzathine—*Bicillin, Permapen*
Penicillin G potassium—*Dramcillin, G-Recillin, Hyasorb, Kesso-Pen, Palocillin S-10, Pedacillin, Pentids, Pfizerpen, Sugracillin*
Penicillin G procaine—*Crysticillin AS, Diurnal-Penicillin, Duracillin A.S., Pentids-P, Pfizerpen-AS, Wycillin*
Penicillin V benzathine—*Pen-Vee*
Penicillin V potassium—*Compocillin-VK, Ledercillin VK, Robicillin VK, Uticillin VK, V-Cillin K, Veetids*
Phenethicillin potassium—*Darcil, Maxipen, Syncillin*
Polymyxin B sulfate—*Various manufacturers*
Propicillin potassium—*Brocillin, Ultrapen*
Ristocetin—*Spontin*
Rolitetracycline—*Syntetrin*
Streptomycin sulfate—*Various manufacturers*
Succinylcholine chloride—*Anectine, Quelicin Chloride*
Tetracycline—*Achromycin, Panmycin, Panmycin KM, Sumycin, Tetracyn, Tetrex-S*
Tetracycline hydrochloride—*Achromycin, Bristacycline, Cyclopar, Panmycin, Robitet, Steclin, Sumycin, Tetracyn*
Tetracycline phosphate complex—*Tetrex*
Tubocurarine chloride—*Tubarine*
Vancomycin hydrochloride—*Vancocin Hydrochloride*

Prepared and evaluated by the Scientific Review Subpanel on Muscle Relaxants and reviewed by Practitioner Panel I.

Tubocurarine—Propranolol

Summary—The neuromuscular blockade produced by tubocurarine was prolonged in two thyrotoxic patients receiving high doses (120 mg/day for 14 days) of propranolol. Although the drug interaction occurred in a small number of patients receiving high doses of propranolol, each patient receiving propranolol should be observed closely for an unexpected prolonged neuromuscular blockade (*e.g.*, respiratory depression and apnea) from tubocurarine.

Related Drugs—The depolarizing muscle relaxants **decamethonium** (1) and **succinylcholine** (1–3) have been shown to interact with propranolol in a similar manner to tubocurarine in animals. Although there is no documentation, the nondepolarizing muscle relaxants **gallamine triethiodide** and **pancuronium** also should interact with propranolol.

Pharmacological Effect and Mechanism—Tubocurarine administration results in a blockade of neuromuscular transmission of the nondepolarizing type. Tubocurarine occupies receptors on the postjunctional membrane and interferes with the ability of acetylcholine to depolarize the postjunctional membrane (4).

Propranolol enhances the tubocurarine-induced neuromuscular blockade by two possible mechanisms. Propranolol depresses posttetanic repetitive activity that is thought to be localized at the motor nerve terminal and therefore may enhance the depression of motor nerve terminal activity of tubocurarine (3, 4). Propranolol also may render the postjunctional membrane insensitive to acetylcholine (3, 5). Administration of a membrane stabilizer, such as propranolol, and tubocurarine may result in synergism inhibiting the depolarizing actions of acetylcholine. This effect probably does not occur with depolarizing muscle relaxants such as succinylcholine.

Although not documented in humans or animals, the hypotensive effect of tubocurarine (6–8) theoretically may be augmented by blockade of the β-adrenergic receptors in the heart by propranolol.

Evaluation of Clinical Data—Two thyrotoxic patients were given propranolol (120 mg/day po for 14 days) to reduce their heart rates prior to a thyroidectomy (9). When tubocurarine (30 or 42 mg) was administered during surgery, the patients experienced an unexpected prolongation of the effect of tubocurarine. One patient also was given succinylcholine (75 mg). In both patients, repeated doses of neostigmine (2.5 mg/dose) and atropine (0.6–1.2 mg) were given until improvement in respiratory function was observed. Tubocurarine was used without propranolol in a subsequent operation in one patient without recurrence of prolongation from tubocurarine.

■ When administered preoperatively, propranolol may prolong the neuromuscular blocking effects of tubocurarine. Because this drug interaction was observed only in patients receiving large doses of propranolol, patients receiving normal or low doses may not experience a similar effect with tubocurarine.

Recommendations—Patients receiving propranolol should be observed closely for any unexpected prolongation of the neuromuscular blockade from tubocurarine administration (*e.g.*, respiratory depression and apnea). When this prolongation occurs, neostigmine (1–3 mg) with atropine (0.6–1.2 mg) may be given (9, 10).

Using too large a dose of tubocurarine in patients receiving propranolol could be avoided by gauging the dose of tubocurarine according to their response to peripheral nerve stimulation (11).

References

(1) L. Wislicki and I. Rosenblum, "Effects of Propranolol on the Action of Neuromuscular Blocking Drugs," *Brit. J. Anaesth.*, *39*, 939 (1967).

(2) L. Wislicki and I. Rosenblum, "The Effects of Propranolol on Normal and Denervated Muscle," *Arch. Int. Pharmacodyn. Ther.*, *170*, 117 (1967).

(3) J. E. Usubiaga, "Neuromuscular Effects of Beta Adrenergic Blockers and Their Interaction with Skeletal Muscle Relaxants," *Anesthesiology*, *29*, 484 (1968).

(4) F. G. Standaert and J. E. Adams, "The Actions of Succinylcholine on the Mammalian Motor Nerve Terminal," *J. Pharmacol. Exp. Ther.*, *149*, 113 (1965).

(5) E. W. Gill and E. M. Vaughn-Williams, "Local Anesthetic Activity of Beta Receptor Antagonist Pronethalol," *Nature*, *201*, 199 (1964).

(6) R. K. Stoelting, "Blood-Pressure Responses to *d*-Tubocurarine and Its Preservatives in Anesthetized Patients," *Anesthesiology*, *35*, 315 (1971).

(7) N. T. Smith and C. E. Whitcher, "Hemodynamic Effects of Gallamine and Tubocurarine Administered during Halothane Anesthesia," *J. Amer. Med. Ass.*, *199*, 704 (1967).

(8) W. L. Munger *et al.*, "The Dependence of *d*-Tubocurarine-Induced Hypotension on Alveolar Concentration of Halothane, Dose of *d*-Tubocurarine, and Nitrous Oxide," *Anesthesiology*, *40*, 442 (1974).

(9) M. S. Rozen and F. Whan, "Prolonged Curarization Associated with Propranolol," *Med. J. Aust.*, *1*, 467 (1972).

(10) "The Pharmacological Basis of Ther-
apeutics," 5th ed., L. S. Goodman and
A. Gilman, Eds., Macmillan, New York,
NY 10022, 1975, pp. 575–588.

(11) H. C. Churchill-Davidson, "A Port-
able Peripheral Nerve Stimulator,"
Anesthesiology, 26, 224 (1965).

[For additional information, see *Muscle Relaxant Therapy,* p. 435, and *Antiarrhythmia Therapy,* p. 350.]

Nonproprietary and Trade Names of Drugs

Decamethonium bromide—*Syncurine*
Gallamine triethiodide—*Flaxedil*
Metocurine (Dimethyl tubocurarine)
  chloride—*Mecostrin*
Metocurine (Dimethyl tubocurarine) iodide
  —*Metubine*

Pancuronium bromide—*Pavulon*
Propranolol hydrochloride—*Inderal*
Succinylcholine chloride—*Anectine, Quelicin
  Chloride*
Tubocurarine chloride—*Tubarine*

*Prepared and evaluated by the Scientific Review Subpanel
on Muscle Relaxants and reviewed by Practitioner Panel V.*

Tubocurarine—Quinidine

Summary—Quinidine, administered parenterally shortly after or simultaneously with tubocurarine, may enhance or cause recurrent neuromuscular effects of tubocurarine, resulting in a prolongation or intensification of respiratory depression and apnea. Although the evidence to support this drug interaction consists only of case reports, the potential hazards resulting from concurrent therapy require that the patient be observed closely for any unexpected increases in the intensity or duration of the neuromuscular blockade from tubocurarine.

Related Drugs—**Gallamine triethiodide** (1), a nondepolarizing muscle relaxant similar to tubocurarine, has been shown to interact with quinidine in animals. **Pancuronium** is a nondepolarizing skeletal muscle relaxant and, although not studied, should interact with quinidine in a similar manner. The depolarizing muscle relaxants **decamethonium** (1, 2) and **succinylcholine** (1–3) also have been shown to interact with quinidine in animals. **Succinylcholine** also has been reported to interact with quinidine in humans (4).

Although no drug interaction has been documented, other cinchona alkaloids (*e.g.*, **cinchophen** and **quinine**) may also interact with tubocurarine. Quinidine is available as the **gluconate, hydrochloride, polygalacturonate,** and **sulfate.**

Pharmacological Effect and Mechanism—Tubocurarine and related agents cause neuromuscular blockade by competing with acetylcholine for the cholinergic receptor located in the postjunctional membrane (5). Tubocurarine blockade is antagonized by edrophonium and neostigmine. Succinylcholine causes neuromuscular blockade by inducing an initial depolarization followed by desensitization of the postjunctional membrane to acetylcholine.

Quinidine, used mainly in the therapy of atrial fibrillation and certain other cardiac arrhythmias, increases the refractory period of cardiac and skeletal muscle and reduces the responses to repetitive nerve stimulation and acetylcholine.

When quinidine is used with neuromuscular blockers, an increased intensity and prolongation of the curariform effects on respiratory muscles occur, which may result in respiratory depression and apnea. Evidence for this combined action was derived from animal studies employing nerve-muscle preparations and using the rabbit head-drop method. In these studies (1–3), quinidine increased the intensity and duration of the neuromuscular blockade of decamethonium, gallamine triethiodide, succinylcholine, and tubocurarine.

Evaluation of Clinical Data—The clinical data that support this drug interaction consist of case reports (2, 4, 6, 7). In three case reports (2, 6, 7), tubocurarine was given concurrently with quinidine while in the other report (4) succinylcholine was used. In the cases where quinidine (200–300 mg im) and tubocurarine (7.2–36 mg im) were given concurrently, quinidine injected shortly after recovery from the muscular blockade caused recurarization, increased respiratory impairment, and ultimately resulted in apnea in the patient. In two cases, the administration of edrophonium and neostigmine successfully revived the patients (2, 7). In the other case (6), no improvement was noted with the administration of these drugs.

In the other report (4), the investigator observed two patients in whom quinidine (300 mg), slowly administered intravenously, caused a return of the paralysis induced by succinylcholine (40 mg iv).

■ Quinidine may enhance or cause a recurrence of the neuromuscular effects of tubocurarine. Although the clinical documentation for this drug interaction is limited to case reports, the potential hazards that may result from concurrent therapy (*e.g.*, apnea and respiratory depression) require that the patient be observed closely for any unexpected increases in the intensity or duration of the respiratory depression caused by tubocurarine.

Recommendations—Because of the serious consequences of this drug interaction, close observation of the patient's respiration is required. If prolonged muscle paralysis causes respiratory depression, neostigmine (1–3 mg iv) administered with atropine sulfate (0.6–1.2 mg iv) may be used to antagonize the action of tubocurarine (5). These drugs have been reported to be ineffective in one case (6) and are not recommended for treating toxic reactions of the depolarizing agents such as succinylcholine (5).

References

(1) R. D. Miller *et al.*, "The Potentiation of Neuromuscular Blocking Agents by Quinidine," *Anesthesiology*, *28*, 1036 (1967).

(2) J. L. Schmidt *et al.*, "The Effect of Quinidine on the Action of Muscle Relaxants," *J. Amer. Med. Ass.*, *183*, 669 (1963).

(3) M. F. Cuthbert, "The Effect of Quinidine and Procainamide on the Neuromuscular Blocking Action of Suxamethonium," *Brit. J. Anaesth.*, *38*, 775 (1966).

(4) A. W. Grogono, "Anaesthesia for Atrial Defibrillation," *Lancet, ii*, 1039 (1963).

(5) "The Pharmacological Basis of Therapeutics," 5th ed., L. S. Goodman and A. Gilman, Eds., Macmillan, New York, NY 10022, 1975, pp. 575–588.

(6) W. L. Way *et al.*, "Recurarization with Quinidine," *J. Amer. Med. Ass.*, *200*, 163 (1967).

(7) L. A. Boere, "Fehler und Gefahren. Recurarisation nach Chinindinsulfat," *Anaesthesist, 13*, 368 (1964).

[For additional information, see *Muscle Relaxant Therapy*, p. 435, and *Antiarrhythmia Therapy*, p. 350.]

Nonproprietary and Trade Names of Drugs

Cinchophen—*Atophan*
Decamethonium bromide—*Syncurine*
Gallamine triethiodide—*Flaxedil*
Metocurine (Dimethyl tubocurarine) chloride—*Mecostrin*
Metocurine (Dimethyl tubocurarine) iodide—*Metubine*
Pancuronium bromide—*Pavulon*
Quinidine gluconate—*Quinaglute*

Quinidine hydrochloride—*Various manufacturers*
Quinidine polygalacturonate—*Cardioquin*
Quinidine sulfate—*Quinidate, Quinidex*
Quinine—*Various manufacturers*
Succinylcholine chloride—*Anectine, Quelicin Chloride*
Tubocurarine chloride—*Tubarine*

Prepared and evaluated by the Scientific Review Subpanel on Muscle Relaxants and reviewed by Practitioner Panel VI.

Vitamin D—Phenytoin*

Summary—Phenytoin increases the metabolic inactivation of vitamin D and decreases the half-life of vitamin D in the body, possibly resulting in hypocalcemia and, in debilitated patients, clinical osteomalacia or rickets. These effects are more severe when phenytoin is used with other anticonvulsants (particularly phenobarbital). Patients receiving phenytoin should have adequate nutrition and exposure to sunlight. When indicated, periodic serum calcium level determinations and radiological examination of bone changes should be performed in patients receiving anticonvulsants.

Related Drugs—Other hydantoin derivatives (*e.g.*, **ethotoin** and **mephenytoin)** and other anticonvulsants (*e.g.*, **primidone**) also may interact with vitamin D (dihydrotachysterol, ergocalciferol, and cholecalciferol).

Pharmacological Effect and Mechanism—Phenytoin decreases serum calcium levels and increases serum alkaline phosphatase levels in humans (1–3). Phenytoin also decreases bone mineral mass (3–5), probably through a decrease in serum 25-hydroxycholecalciferol (1).

Because phenytoin induces hepatic enzymes (6, 7), its effect on vitamin D may result from the following: (*a*) induction of the hepatic microsomal oxidative enzyme system, causing an increase in the hydroxylation of cholecalciferol and 25-hydroxycholecalciferol to more polar inactive metabolites (1, 8), and (*b*) an increase in hepatic glucuronidation of cholecalciferol, which is excreted as an inactive glucuronide (3, 9).

Phenytoin inhibits parathyroid-induced mobilization of bone calcium *in vitro* (10), suggesting that vitamin D-independent factors may play a role in phenytoin-induced hypocalcemia and metabolic bone disease.

There is no evidence regarding a direct effect of phenytoin on intestinal calcium absorption (11).

Evaluation of Clinical Data—Only a few cases of phenytoin-induced rickets have been reported (12–14), but there have been several case reports of osteomalacia and rickets associated with phenytoin used concurrently with other anticonvulsants (15–22).

In one study (5), 23 epileptic patients (1–13 years of age) treated with phenytoin (3.3–6.6 mg/kg/day po) alone were compared with 20 matched control subjects. The phenytoin-treated subjects showed a significant decrease in bone mineral mass as determined by direct photon absorption. This reduction was reversed by calcium lactate (390 mg/day po) and vitamin D (2000 units/day po) but not by calcium lactate and placebo.

In another report (3), 91 epileptic adults, 19 of whom were being treated with phenytoin alone, were studied for radiological evidence of decreased trabeculation of the proximal end of the femur. The phenytoin-treated patients had lower serum calcium levels, higher serum alkaline phosphatase levels, and more trabecular loss (46% compared to 6%) than controls ($p = 0.005$). The effect was even more profound in those patients receiving several anticonvulsants concurrently. No correlation was found between duration of phenytoin therapy and the changes in the blood and in the bone.

The effect of phenytoin and phenobarbital on serum 25-hydroxycalciferol levels was studied in 48 patients receiving phenytoin (289 $\pm$ 11 mg/day po) and phenobarbital (111 $\pm$ 13 mg/day po) (1). Thirty-five percent of these patients had significantly decreased serum 25-hydroxycalciferol levels and 19% had significant hypocalcemia (serum calcium levels, <9 mg%) as compared to controls. The alkaline phosphatase level in the test group was higher than in the control group and the

---

'* Phenytoin is the new official name for diphenylhydantoin.

serum phosphatase and serum albumin levels were similar. Patients receiving phenytoin alone exhibited similar but less marked changes.

Fifty-six epileptic children receiving chronic therapy with phenobarbital (average dose, 72–76 mg/day po) and/or phenytoin (average dose, 136–160 mg/day po) were compared to 51 patient controls to determine the effects of anticonvulsant therapy on mineral vitamin D and bone metabolism (23). The results showed that concurrent anticonvulsant therapy was associated with the greatest reduction in serum calcium and serum 25-hydroxycalciferol levels and bone mass. Phenobarbital and phenytoin alone had comparable effects on the serum measurements and on the bone density and were additive when used together. No correlation was found between the duration of therapy with either or both anticonvulsants and any of the changes observed.

■ The occurrence of rickets and osteomalacia due to phenytoin has not been well established. Other causes were not ruled out and no chemical and radiological studies were done before initiating therapy. Moreover, a review of approximately 15,000 patients with severe epilepsy of some type failed to show any cause and effect relationship between osteomalacia or rickets and the administration of phenytoin (24, 25). Nevertheless, there does appear to be a clinically significant effect of phenytoin on bone structure and serum calcium levels, particularly with high doses and/or when administered with other anticonvulsants (particularly phenobarbital). However, no correlation has been found between duration of therapy and the occurrence of biochemical or bone changes (3, 23). Even in the absence of clinical rickets or osteomalacia, weakened skeletal structure in a patient subject to convulsions can be hazardous (26). Hypocalcemia contributes to an increase in seizure frequency, making the management of epilepsy more difficult (27). Black patients are potentially more susceptible to alterations in vitamin D metabolism because of less penetration of solar UV irradiation to the stratum granulosum layer of the skin where 7-dehydrocholesterol is activated (1, 8, 28).

Recommendations—Whenever feasible, patients receiving phenytoin who are predisposed to development of osteomalacia and rickets [*i.e.*, Blacks, children, patients taking several anticonvulsants concurrently (particularly phenobarbital), patients who are very inactive or have limited exposure to sunlight, and patients with marginal dietary intake] should be monitored periodically for decreased serum calcium levels and bone demineralization. Adequate nutrition by ingestion of food rich in vitamin D (*e.g.*, fish and eggs) and sufficient exposure to sunlight are necessary for all patients receiving anticonvulsants. Vitamin D therapy (dosage must be individualized) also may be required in some patients to prevent development of osteomalacia and rickets.

References

(1) T. J. Hahn *et al.*, "Effect of Chronic Anticonvulsant Therapy on Serum 25-Hydroxycalciferol Levels in Adults," *N. Engl. J. Med.*, *287*, 900 (1972).

(2) A. Richens and D. J. F. Rowe, "Disturbance of Calcium Metabolism by Anticonvulsant Drugs," *Brit. Med. J.*, *4*, 73 (1970).

(3) E. Sotaniemi *et al.*, "Radiologic Bone Changes and Hypocalcemia with Anticonvulsant Therapy in Epilepsy," *Ann. Intern. Med.*, *77*, 389 (1972).

(4) C. Christiansen *et al.*, "Latent Osteomalacia in Epileptic Patients on Anticonvulsants," *Brit. Med. J.*, *3*, 738 (1972).

(5) C. Christiansen *et al.*, "Effect of Vitamin D on Bone Mineral Mass in Normal Subjects and in Epileptic Patients on Anticonvulsants: A Controlled Therapeutic Trial," *Brit. Med. J.*, *2*, 208 (1973).

(6) A. H. Conney, "Pharmacological Implications of Microsomal Enzyme Induction," *Pharmacol. Rev.*, *19*, 317 (1967).

(7) R. Kuntzman, "Drugs and Enzyme Induction," *Ann. Rev. Pharmacol.*, *9*, 21 (1969).

(8) T. J. Hahn, "Anticonvulsant Therapy and Vitamin D.," *Ann. Intern. Med.*, *78*, 308 (1973).

(9) J. Hunter *et al.*, "Altered Calcium Metabolism in Epileptic Children on Anticonvulsants," *Brit. Med. J.*, *4*, 202 (1971).

(10) M. V. Jenkins *et al.*, "The Effect of Anticonvulsant Drugs *in vitro* on Bone Calcium Mobilization by Parathyroid Hormone," *Clin. Sci. Mol. Med.*, *45*, 1p (1973)

(11) M. Villareale *et al.*, "Diphenylhydantoin: Effects on Calcium Metabolism in the Chick," *Science*, *183*, 671 (1974).

(12) N. Matsuo *et al.*, "Diphenylhydantoin Associated Rickets," *Pediat. Res.*, *6*, 400 (1972).

(13) J. Mace *et al.*, "Diphenylhydantoin and Rickets," *Lancet*, i, 1119 (1973).

(14) K. G. Tolman *et al.*, "Rickets Associated with Anticonvulsant Medications," *Clin. Res.*, *20*, 414 (1972).

(15) A. Borgstedt *et al.*, "Long-Term Administration of Antiepileptic Drugs and the Development of Rickets," *J. Pediat.*, *81*, 9 (1972).

(16) N. R. Dennis, "Rickets following Anticonvulsant Therapy," *Proc. Roy. Soc. Med.*, *65*, 730 (1972).

(17) C. E. Dent *et al.*, "Osteomalacia with Long-Term Anticonvulsant Therapy in Epilepsy," *Brit. Med. J.*, *4*, 69 (1970).

(18) R. Greenlaw *et al.*, "Osteomalacia (OM) from Anticonvulsant (ACV) Drugs: Therapeutic Implications," *Clin. Res.*, *20*, 56 (1972).

(19) R. Kruse, "Osteopathien Bei Antiepileptischer Langzeittherapie (Vorlaufige Mitteilung)," *Mschr. Kinderheilk.*, *116*, 378 (1968).

(20) H. L. Medlinsky, "Rickets Associated with Anticonvulsant Medication," *Pediatrics*, *53*, 91 (1974).

(21) M. Teotia and S. P. Teotia, "Rickets Precipitated by Anticonvulsant Drugs in a Child Receiving Prophylactic Vitamin D," *Amer. J. Dis. Child.*, *125*, 850 (1973).

(22) C. Christiansen *et al.*, "Incidence of Anticonvulsant Osteomalacia and Effect of Vitamin D: Controlled Therapeutic Trial," *Brit. Med. J.*, *4*, 695 (1973).

(23) T. J. Hahn *et al.*, "Serum 25-Hydroxycalciferol Levels and Bone Mass in Children on Chronic Anticonvulsant Therapy," *N. Engl. J. Med.*, *292*, 550 (1975).

(24) S. Livingston *et al.*, "Anticonvulsant Drugs and Vitamin D Metabolism," *J. Amer. Med. Ass.*, *224*, 1634 (1973).

(25) S. Livingston and W. Berman, "Antiepileptic Drugs and the Development of Rickets," *J. Pediat.*, *82*, 347 (1973).

(26) L. V. Gould, "Anticonvulsant Drugs and Vitamin D Metabolism," *J. Amer. Med. Ass.*, *225*, 995 (1973).

(27) B. Frame, "Hypocalcemia and Osteomalacia Associated with Anticonvulsant Therapy," *Ann. Intern. Med.*, *74*, 294 (1971).

(28) W. F. Loomis, "Skin-Pigment Regulation of Vitamin-D Biosynthesis in Man," *Science*, *157*, 501 (1967).

[For additional information, see *Anticonvulsant Therapy*, p. 369.]

Nonproprietary and Trade Names of Drugs

Ethotoin—*Peganone*
Mephenytoin—*Mesantoin*
Phenobarbital—*Eskabarb, Luminal*
Phenytoin—*Dilantin*

Primidone—*Mysoline*
Vitamin D—*Available alone and in various combination products*

Prepared and evaluated by the Scientific Review Subpanels on Anticonvulsants and Vitamins and reviewed by Practitioner Panel II.

Warfarin—Acetaminophen

Summary—In therapeutic doses, acetaminophen produces only slight increases, if any, in the hypoprothrombinemic response to warfarin. In patients treated with anticoagulants, acetaminophen is preferable to aspirin when antipyretic or analgesic action is desired.

Related Drugs—Other related coumarin anticoagulants include **acenocoumarol, dicumarol,** and **phenprocoumon** and the related indandione anticoagulants are **anisindione, diphenadione,** and **phenindione.**

Pharmacological Effect and Mechanism—Since the significance of this interaction is still unconfirmed, the mechanism by which acetaminophen may enhance the hypoprothrombinemic effect of warfarin has not been investigated.

Evaluation of Clinical Data—Changes in the one-stage prothrombin time were studied (1) in 62 patients who had been receiving maintenance doses of oral anticoagulants (anisindione, dicumarol, phenprocoumon, and warfarin sodium) concurrently with acetaminophen (650 mg po four times daily). These patients were divided into groups of 12, 25, and 25. In the group of 12, warfarin and acetaminophen were administered for 4 weeks. The other two groups were given acetaminophen for 2 weeks, followed or preceded by administration of a placebo for 2 weeks. In the group of 12 patients, there was a statistically significant 5.3-sec increase in the one-stage prothrombin time after the third week, necessitating a reduction (from 5.8 to 4.4 mg) in the warfarin dose. In the two groups of 25 patients, there was a 3.6-sec increase (both statistically significant) during the 2-week administration of acetaminophen.

To evaluate the immediate effect of acetaminophen on prothrombin time in patients receiving oral anticoagulant therapy, 10 patients previously maintained on oral anticoagulants (phenprocoumon and warfarin sodium) were also given acetaminophen (650 mg po) at 8 a.m. and 12 noon. Another 10 patients were given a placebo at 8 a.m. and 12 noon. The baseline prothrombin time was taken at 8 a.m. of the morning in which the anticoagulant was administered. In no instance was there a statistically significant difference in the prothrombin times of these patients (2).

A third study (3) showed a statistically insignificant 1.2-sec increase in the prothrombin time in 10 patients who had received a total of 3.25 g/day po of acetaminophen for 2 weeks concurrently with maintenance doses of warfarin.

■ On the basis of reported clinical data, acetaminophen does not cause therapeutically significant increases in prothrombin time in patients receiving maintenance doses of warfarin. Although one study (1) showed a statistically significant enhancement of the effects of warfarin by acetaminophen, this increase was relatively small and not substantiated by subsequent studies (2, 3).

Recommendations—Any enhancement of the hypoprothrombinemic action of warfarin by acetaminophen appears to be minor. The use of acetaminophen is preferable to aspirin as an antipyretic or analgesic in patients receiving oral anticoagulants (4, 5). However, this does not preclude the need for close attention to the patient's response to anticoagulant therapy when acetaminophen is added to the drug regimen.

References

(1) A. M. Antlitz et al., "Potentiation of Oral Anticoagulant Therapy by Acetaminophen," Curr. Ther. Res., 10, 501 (1968).

(2) A. M. Antlitz and L. F. Awalt, "A Double Blind Study of Acetaminophen Used in Conjunction with Oral Anticoagulant Therapy," Curr. Ther. Res., 11, 360 (1969).

(3) J. A. Udall, "Drug Interference with Warfarin Therapy," Clin. Med., 77(8), 20 (1970).

(4) J. Koch-Weser and E. M. Sellers, "Drug Interactions with Coumarin Anticoagulants," N. Engl. J. Med., 285, 547 (1971).

(5) C. H. Mielke et al., "Hemostasis, Antipyretics, and Mild Analgesics: Acetaminophen vs Aspirin," J. Amer. Med. Ass., 235, 613 (1976).

[For additional information, see Anticoagulant Therapy, p. 358.]

Nonproprietary and Trade Names of Drugs

Acenocoumarol—*Sintrom*
Acetaminophen—*Datril, Nebs, SK-APAP, Tempra, Tenlap, Tylenol, Valadrol, and various combination products*
Anisindione—*Miradon*
Dicumarol—*Various manufacturers*

Diphenadione—*Dipaxin*
Phenindione—*Hedulin*
Phenprocoumon—*Liquamar*
Warfarin potassium—*Athrombin-K*
Warfarin sodium—*Coumadin Sodium, Panwarfin*

Prepared and evaluated by the Scientific Review Subpanel on Anticoagulants and reviewed by Practitioner Panel I.

Warfarin—Alcohol

Summary—The incidental use of small or moderate amounts of alcohol (<120 ml of 100-proof whiskey) by patients receiving warfarin is not contraindicated. However, in chronic heavy alcohol users with liver dysfunction, warfarin activity may be altered. In these patients, frequent determinations of prothrombin time are necessary, and sudden changes in alcohol consumption should be avoided.

Related Drugs—Alcohol might be expected to interact with other oral anticoagulants such as **acenocoumarol, anisindione, dicumarol, diphenadione, phenindione,** and **phenprocoumon.**

Pharmacological Effect and Mechanism—Warfarin depresses plasma prothrombin activity by interfering with the synthesis of coagulation factors II, VII, IX, and X in the liver *via* the vitamin K pathway (1). Alcohol has been suggested to influence warfarin activity by one or both of the following mechanisms: (*a*) by initially increasing, but then decreasing, the levels of coagulation factors II, VII, and X (2); or (*b*) by stimulating the hepatic enzymes responsible for the metabolism of warfarin (3). These actions may result in a variable and unpredictable response to warfarin therapy in patients ingesting alcohol, particularly in alcoholics with or without signs of liver dysfunction.

Evaluation of Clinical Data—Clinical reports on the effects of alcohol on anticoagulant therapy are conflicting. One study (4) in five healthy male volunteers who received blended brandy in soda water in amounts equivalent to 109–367 ml of 100% alcohol over 2.5–4 hr demonstrated an increase in erythrocyte aggregation attributable to alcohol ingestion. However, investigations of the effects of alcohol on the prothrombin time of these subjects (who were not receiving anticoagulants) yielded no conclusive results.

In a subsequent study (5) designed to determine the effects of alcohol on anticoagulant therapy, three groups of subjects received either 250 ml of gin over 1 hr, 180–200 ml of brandy over 1 hr, or an intravenous infusion of alcohol (500 ml of a 10% by volume solution over 45 min). All subjects also received phenprocoumon (dosage not reported). Very few changes in the prothrombin time could be attributed to the effects of alcohol; the investigator concluded that alcohol produces no acute effects on the liver cells which would affect significantly the response to anticoagulant therapy.

The ingestion of 300–800 ml of wine and/or 160 or 250 ml of whiskey over 30–90 min by 12 patients (2) receiving anticoagulant therapy resulted in an initially slight increase in factors II, VII, and X, followed by a pronounced decrease in factors VII and X and a less pronounced decrease in factor II.

Effects of long-term alcohol ingestion on warfarin removal were also studied (3) by determining the rate of warfarin clearance from the circulation in 15 alcoholic and 11 control patients, none of whom had any signs of liver dysfunction. Although the half-life of warfarin in the alcoholic patients (26.5 hr) was significantly shorter than the 41.1 hr warfarin half-life in the controls, there was no corresponding difference in the prothrombin times of the two groups.

Hepatic dysfunction due to chronic alcoholism has been identified as the cause for the loss of anticoagulant control in one patient (6) who had been ingesting large amounts of alcohol (2.12 liters of vodka/weekend). Another patient who had been a moderate user of alcohol (50 ml of whiskey/day) stopped consuming alcohol after being stabilized on warfarin (7). Forty days later, the patient began to take the same amount of alcohol which caused a rapid change of anticoagulant control and a significant increase in serum warfarin levels. After the alcohol ingestion was discontinued, anticoagulant control and serum warfarin levels returned to the previous levels.

■ Although conflicting, the clinical data indicate that most patients receiving anticoagulants and ingesting small to moderate quantities of alcohol (not more than 120 ml of 100-proof whiskey) would not be expected to experience adverse effects. However, in patients who are chronic alcoholics with liver dysfunction or who ingest large quantities of alcohol over short periods, the response to warfarin therapy may be altered.

Recommendations—The intermittent use of moderate amounts of alcohol (<120 ml of 100-proof whiskey) by patients receiving warfarin anticoagulant therapy is not contraindicated. When warfarin therapy is used in alcoholic subjects, close observation of plasma prothrombin activity must be maintained, particularly if hepatic dysfunction also exists. Sudden changes in alcohol intake or erratic consumption of alcohol should be avoided since this may alter the patient's response to warfarin.

References

(1) "The Pharmacological Basis of Therapeutics," 5th ed., L. S. Goodman and A. Gilman, Eds., Macmillan, New York, NY 10022, 1975, p. 1356.

(2) G. Reidler, "Einfluss des Alkohols auf die Antikoagulantientherapie," *Thromb. Diath. Haemorrh.*, *16*, 613 (1966).

(3) R. M. H. Kater *et al.*, "Increased Rate of Clearance of Drugs from the Circulation of Alcoholics," *Amer. J. Med. Sci.*, *258*, 35 (1969).

(4) O. Forsander and H. Suomalainen, "Alcohol Intake and Erythrocyte Aggregation," *Quart. J. Stud. Alc.*, *16*, 614 (1955).

(5) E. Waris, "Effect of Ethyl Alcohol on Some Coagulation Factors in Man during Anticoagulant Therapy," *Ann. Med. Int. Fenn.*, *41*, 45 (1963).

(6) J. A. Udall, "Drug Interference with Warfarin Therapy," *Clin. Med.*, *77*(8), 20 (1970).

(7) A. Breckenridge and M. Orme, "Clinical Implications of Enzyme Induction," *Ann. N.Y. Acad. Sci.*, *179*, 421 (1971).

[For additional information, see *Anticoagulant Therapy*, p. 358.]

Nonproprietary and Trade Names of Drugs

Acenocoumarol—*Sintrom*
Alcohol—*Various products and beverages*
Anisindione—*Miradon*
Dicumarol—*Various manufacturers*
Diphenadione—*Dipaxin*

Phenindione—*Hedulin*
Phenprocoumon—*Liquamar*
Warfarin potassium—*Athrombin-K*
Warfarin sodium—*Coumadin Sodium, Panwarfin*

Prepared and evaluated by the Scientific Review Subpanel on Anticoagulants and reviewed by Practitioner Panel II.

Warfarin—Aluminum and Magnesium Ions

Summary—The interaction between warfarin and aluminum or magnesium hydroxide is based upon theoretical considerations, and recent clinical studies indicate that this interaction may not be clinically significant. Although it might be prudent to avoid simultaneous administration of these two drugs whenever possible, the patient should not be denied the benefits of either drug when simultaneous administration is unavoidable.

Related Drugs—In theory, aluminum or magnesium hydroxide may interfere with the absorption of warfarin by alkalinizing the gastrointestinal contents (1). If this hypothesis is valid, any antacid substance that produces an alkaline pH at the site of warfarin absorption may be equally implicated. Additional antacid substances include other **aluminum salts** and **calcium-, magnesium-,** and **sodium-containing antacid preparations.**

Dicumarol is chemically related to warfarin and is used similarly in clinical practice. However, its interaction with antacids has been shown to differ from that proposed for warfarin (1). While magnesium hydroxide does not influence the absorption of warfarin (2), it has been demonstrated that a magnesium hydroxide suspension actually enhances the absorption of dicumarol, resulting in higher peak serum levels in humans (1) and dogs (3). This enhancement was attributed to complex formation between magnesium and dicumarol which changes the solubility characteristics of dicumarol.

The effects of aluminum or magnesium products on other coumarin (*e.g.,* **acenocoumarol** and **phenprocoumon)** or indandione (*e.g.,* **anisindione, diphenadione,** and **phenindione)** anticoagulants have not been evaluated.

Pharmacological Effect and Mechanism—Warfarin is a weak acid. In an alkaline medium, it exists predominantly in the poorly absorbed, ionized form. It is proposed that antacids, such as aluminum or magnesium hydroxide, produce an alkaline pH at the warfarin site of absorption and thus may promote the formation of the ionized moiety. There is no suggestion that aluminum or magnesium hydroxide binds warfarin directly.

A significant decrease in the absorption of warfarin due to the antacid properties of aluminum or magnesium hydroxide would have a deleterious effect on the ability of warfarin to increase prothrombin time (1, 2).

Evaluation of Clinical Data—Although many early reviews stated that this drug interaction is theoretically possible (4–6), subsequent clinical studies failed to confirm that it is clinically significant.

In six normal subjects tested over 48 hr (2), an aluminum–magnesium hydroxide mixture (30 ml po) administered initially with a single dose of warfarin (40 mg po) and then at 2-hr intervals without warfarin for four subsequent doses failed to alter serum warfarin levels or prothrombin time significantly. These subjects served as their own controls.

In another study (1), 12 normal subjects were divided into two groups. One group received a single dose of warfarin (75 mg po) and the other received a single dose of dicumarol (300 mg po). Aluminum hydroxide gel (15 ml po), magnesium hydroxide suspension (15 ml po), or water was given concurrently and 3 hr later to each subject. The concurrent administration of aluminum hydroxide gel with warfarin or dicumarol had no effect on mean serum anticoagulant levels or prothrombin times. The magnesium hydroxide suspension did not affect the serum levels or prothrombin activity of warfarin, but it increased the mean peak serum dicumarol levels. However, the effect on the prothrombin activity of dicumarol was minimal, and there was large intersubject variation in serum dicumarol levels.

■ The clinical evidence indicates that a clinically significant drug interaction does not occur between aluminum hydroxide and dicumarol or warfarin. Simultaneous administration of magnesium hydroxide suspension does not affect warfarin but may increase the serum dicumarol levels. However, because of the wide intersubject variability of serum dicumarol levels and the lack of observed clinical effects, the therapeutic significance of this drug interaction is not known.

Recommendations—Generally, the addition of any drug to the regimen of a patient receiving coumarin anticoagulants necessitates monitoring the patient closely. The addition of an antacid containing aluminum or magnesium hydroxide or a laxative containing magnesium hydroxide is no exception. Although the potential for dicumarol or warfarin to interact with aluminum or magnesium hydroxide seems remote, it would be prudent to instruct the patient to avoid taking these products within 1–2 hr of taking dicumarol or warfarin. This recommendation could be accomplished without seriously compromising the effectiveness of antacid or laxative therapy or inconveniencing the patient. However, the patient should not be denied the benefits of these drugs when their simultaneous administration is unavoidable.

References

(1) J. J. Ambre and L. J. Fisher, "The Effect of Coadministration of Aluminum and Magnesium Hydroxides on Absorption of Anticoagulants in Man," *Clin. Pharmacol. Ther.*, *14*, 231 (1973).

(2) D. S. Robinson *et al.*, "Interaction of Warfarin and Nonsystemic Gastrointestinal Drugs," *Clin. Pharmacol. Ther.*, *12*, 491 (1971).

(3) M. J. Akers *et al.*, "Alterations in Absorption of Dicumarol by Various Excipient Materials," *J. Pharm. Sci.*, *62*, 391 (1973).

(4) K. L. Melmon *et al.*, "Drug Interactions that Can Affect Your Patients," *Patient Care*, *1*, 32 (1967).

(5) D. A. Hussar, "Tabular Compilation of Drug Interactions," *Amer. J. Pharm.*, *141*, 109 (1969).

(6) E. Hartshorn, "Drug Interaction," *Drug Intel.*, *2*, 174 (1968).

[For additional information, see *Anticoagulant Therapy*, p. 358.]

Nonproprietary and Trade Names of Drugs

Acenocoumarol—*Sintrom*
Aluminum-, calcium-, or magnesium-containing products—*Aludrox, Alzinox, Amphojel, A-M-T, Camalox, Creamalin, Dicarbosil, DiGel, Ducon, Gaviscon, Gelusil, Gelusil-M, Kolantyl Gel, Kudrox, Maalox, Malcogel, Mylanta, Oxaine-M, Phosphaljel, Robalate, Rolaids, Titralac, Trisogel, Tums, WinGel*

Anisindione—*Miradon*
Dicumarol—*Various manufacturers*
Diphenadione—*Dipaxin*
Phenindione—*Hedulin*
Phenprocoumon—*Liquamar*
Warfarin potassium—*Athrombin-K*
Warfarin sodium—*Coumadin Sodium, Panwarfin*

Prepared and evaluated by the Scientific Review Subpanel on Anticoagulants and reviewed by Practitioner Panel II.

Warfarin—Ascorbic Acid

Summary—Several reports suggest that large doses of ascorbic acid may counteract the hypoprothrombinemic effect of warfarin, but no clinical study supports this observation. However, the practitioner should be aware of this potential drug interaction and should inquire about ascorbic acid intake in anticoagulant-treated patients who respond erratically.

Related Drugs—There are no drugs chemically related to ascorbic acid. Related oral anticoagulants are other coumarin derivatives, **acenocoumarol, dicumarol,** and **phenprocoumon,** and indandione derivatives, **anisindione, diphenadione,** and **phenindione.**

Pharmacological Effect and Mechanism—Ascorbic acid has no known effect on clotting factors or the clotting reaction. A lack of ascorbic acid (which can be manifested clinically as scurvy) is associated with bleeding problems related to structural defects in the vascular wall. Coumarin and indandione drugs affect clotting by antagonizing the action of vitamin K, which is responsible for the synthesis of factors II, VII, IX, and X in the liver (1). There are no studies showing that ascorbic acid affects this action of the anticoagulants or the metabolism of the anticoagulants. However, ascorbic acid has been reported to alter blood coagulation by its role in improving blood vessel wall structure and/or promoting proper metabolism of fat (2).

Another theory is that large doses of ascorbic acid may cause diarrhea, resulting in decreased absorption of warfarin from the gastrointestinal (GI) tract (3).

Animal studies are conflicting and have provided little additional information; ascorbic acid decreased the anticoagulant effect in two studies (4, 5) and had no effect in three other reports (6–8).

Evaluation of Clinical Data—There are two case reports of a diminished hypoprothrombinemic effect of warfarin when ascorbic acid was also administered (6, 9), but various controlled investigations of this effect showed conflicting results. Five patients receiving long-term warfarin therapy were also given ascorbic acid (1 g/day po) for 14 days; no significant changes were found in the blood coagulability test after ascorbic acid therapy (10). These findings have been questioned (2, 11). An increase of thrombotic episodes was observed in a small number of patients receiving ascorbic acid (200 mg po) (11) while the other study (2) reported a decreased incidence of thrombosis in a larger sample of selected patients who had been given ascorbic acid (1 g/day po). Both studies were double blind and the observed patients were thought to be especially susceptible to thrombotic episodes.

High doses of ascorbic acid (up to 10 g) failed to show a clinically significant antagonism of the hypoprothrombinemic action of warfarin in 19 patients (3). One group of 14 patients received ascorbic acid in doses of 3 g/day po for 1 week and 5 g/day po for 1 week. Another group of five patients received 10-g/day po doses of ascorbic acid for 1 week. Each patient served as his or her own control, and all had been stabilized on warfarin previously.

No clinically important change was observed in the prothrombin ratios of any patient receiving ascorbic acid. There was a significant fall in the serum warfarin level (mean of 17.5%) in each patient, but it apparently was too small to antagonize the hypoprothrombinemic action of warfarin. The five patients given the larger doses of ascorbic acid (10 g/day) had diarrhea, and all patients had some looseness in the stool. It was concluded that the GI effects of ascorbic acid may have decreased warfarin absorption, resulting in lower serum warfarin levels.

■ Although there are two reports associating ascorbic acid with increased blood coagulation, subsequent controlled studies (3, 10) failed to confirm this earlier finding with large doses of ascorbic acid. The fact that it occurred in high doses (9) or in patients with a history of venous thrombosis (2, 11) may explain the variable results reported. Nevertheless, based on the available evidence, this drug interaction appears to be clinically insignificant.

Recommendations—Because of the isolated reports of ascorbic acid interference with anticoagulant therapy, practitioners should be aware of this possible interaction and should inquire about ascorbic acid intake in anticoagulant-treated patients who respond erratically. No other additional precautions are needed when these drugs are used concurrently.

References

(1) "The Pharmacological Basis of Therapeutics," 5th ed., L. S. Goodman and A. Gilman, Eds., Macmillan, New York, NY 10022, 1975, pp. 1356, 1453, 1667.

(2) C. R. Spittle, "Vitamin C and Deep-Vein Thrombosis," *Lancet, ii,* 199 (1973).

(3) C. L. Feetam et al., "Lack of a Clinically Important Interaction between Warfarin and Ascorbic Acid," *Toxicol. Appl. Pharmacol., 31,* 544 (1975).

(4) L. T. Sigell and H. C. Flessa, "Drug Interactions with Anticoagulants," *J. Amer. Med. Ass., 214,* 2035 (1970).

(5) W. R. Sullivan et al., "Studies on the Hemorrhagic Sweet Clover Disease XII: The Effect of *l*-Ascorbic Acid on the Hypoprothrombinemia Induced by 3,3'-Methylenebis(4-hydroxycoumarin) in the Guinea Pig," *J. Biol. Chem., 151,* 477 (1943).

(6) G. Rosenthal, "Interaction of Ascorbic Acid and Warfarin," *J. Amer. Med. Ass., 215,* 1671 (1971).

(7) F. W. Deckert, "Ascorbic Acid and Warfarin," *J. Amer. Med. Ass., 223,* 440 (1973).

(8) C. A. Bauman et al., "Studies on the Hemorrhagic Sweet Clover Disease X: Induced Vitamin C Excretion in the Rat and Its Effect on the Hypoprothrombinemia Caused by 3,3'-Methylenebis(4-hydroxycoumarin)," *J. Biol. Chem., 146,* 7 (1942).

(9) E. C. Smith et al., "Interaction of Ascorbic Acid and Warfarin," *J. Amer. Med. Ass., 221,* 1166 (1972).

(10) R. Hume et al., "Interaction of Ascorbic Acid and Warfarin," *J. Amer. Med. Ass., 219,* 1479 (1972).

(11) C. T. Andrews and T. S. Wilson, "Vitamin C and Thrombotic Episodes," *Lancet, ii,* 39 (1973).

[For additional information, see Anticoagulant Therapy, p. 358.]

Nonproprietary and Trade Names of Drugs

Acenocoumarol—*Sintrom*
Anisindione—*Miradon*
Ascorbic acid—*Available alone and in combination products*
Dicumarol—*Various manufacturers*
Diphenadione—*Dipaxin*

Phenindione—*Hedulin*
Phenprocoumon—*Liquamar*
Warfarin potassium—*Athrombin-K*
Warfarin sodium—*Coumadin Sodium, Panwarfin*

Prepared and evaluated by the Scientific Review Subpanel on Anticoagulants and reviewed by Practitioner Panel III.

Warfarin—Aspirin

Summary—Aspirin (moderate to large doses, 3 g or more/day po) may enhance the hypoprothrombinemic effect of warfarin and other anticoagulants when given concurrently. In lower doses (<3 g/day po), aspirin may not affect anticoagulant-induced hypoprothrombinemia but it may inhibit platelet aggregation and cause undesirable bleeding episodes. Concurrent administration of warfarin and aspirin should be avoided and a suitable alternative to aspirin (e.g., acetaminophen or ibuprofen) should be used.

Related Drugs—The coumarin anticoagulant **acenocoumarol** has interacted with aspirin in a manner similar to warfarin (1). **Dicumarol** is unaffected by low doses of aspirin (2), but the effect of high doses of aspirin on its hypoprothrombinemic action has not been studied. **Phenprocoumon** would probably interact with aspirin, but clinical documentation is lacking.

The indandione anticoagulants (e.g., **anisindione, diphenadione,** and **phenindione**) may also interact with aspirin, although phenindione was unaffected by low doses of aspirin (2).

Sodium salicylate enhances the hypoprothrombinemic effect of oral anticoagulants (3) but possibly to a lesser extent than aspirin (4). Sodium salicylate (enteric coated) is less likely to produce gastrointestinal (GI) bleeding, but it is also less likely to be absorbed properly.

The liberation of salicylic acid is probably necessary for the hypoprothrombinemic effect of aspirin and other **salicylates.** **Salicylamide,** which is not hydrolyzed to salicylic acid, has little influence on prothrombin time (5).

Pharmacological Effect and Mechanism—Aspirin may enhance the hypoprothrombinemic action of warfarin or other anticoagulants by multiple mechanisms. Aspirin depresses gastric acid secretion and mucus production in the gastric mucosa and breaks the gastric mucosal barrier to hydrogen and other ions by acting locally on the human mucosa (6). Fecal blood loss (0.2–13.5 ml/day) often occurs after aspirin administration (7). GI hemorrhage also has been associated with aspirin administration (8).

Aspirin, in doses as low as 300 mg/day po, increased the cutaneous bleeding time by inhibiting platelet aggregation (9–11). Inhibition of platelet aggregation probably occurs because aspirin interferes with the release of adenosine diphosphate from platelets (12). The acetyl group is apparently necessary for the effects on platelet aggregation since agents such as sodium salicylate do not share this effect (12, 13).

Agents that are hydrolyzed to salicylic acid such as aspirin cause dose-related increases in plasma prothrombin time (5). At moderate to high doses (1.3–6 g/day po), aspirin increases slightly the prothrombin time ($\sim$ 3 sec over control values) (3, 5). At higher doses (6–8 g/day po), aspirin-induced increases in prothrombin times are larger (5–31 sec above control values) (4).

Aspirin is protein bound (70%) (14) and the chronic use of aspirin, but not other salicylates, alters the structure of the serum albumin molecule (15, 16). Therefore, aspirin may either displace warfarin or prevent it from binding with the serum albumin. However, there is no evidence that this mechanism is clinically important.

Evaluation of Clinical Data—Clinical data are conflicting regarding the enhancement of the hypoprothrombinemic effect of anticoagulants by salicylate compounds. In one study (1), 11 of 17 patients required a reduction (average decrease of $\sim$ 30%) in their anticoagulant (acenocoumarol) dose when aspirin was administered concurrently. Unfortunately, patient responses to the anticoagulant varied considerably prior to aspirin administration and may be responsible for the required reduction in anticoagulant dose. Since there was no information provided about possible changes in the patients' prothrombin times, a causal relationship between aspirin administration and the enhanced anticoagulant effect cannot be established.

In another study (17), aspirin (3 g/day po for 14 days) did not prolong the prothrombin time in 10 patients stabilized on warfarin. Warfarin was instituted 2 weeks prior to aspirin administration and each patient served as his or her own control.

Two other reports (10, 18) indicated that the effect of aspirin on a patient's response to an anticoagulant may be dose related. Administration of aspirin (1.95 g/day po) to eight patients receiving an anticoagulant (anticoagulant not specified) did not prolong the undiluted one-stage prothrombin time (18). When aspirin (3.9 g) was administered to five of the same subjects, two showed a marked prolongation of the prothrombin time.

In a later study (10), the same investigators used the same doses of aspirin in 11 healthy subjects receiving warfarin. The prothrombin time was prolonged significantly in four of the 11 subjects receiving the low doses (1.95 g/day po) of aspirin and in all four subjects receiving the higher doses (3.9 g/day po) of aspirin. At the lower doses of aspirin, mild signs of hemorrhage developed in two patients, neither of whom showed a decrease in prothrombin activity. At the higher doses, all four patients had signs of hemorrhage and demonstrated an enhancement of the hypoprothrombinemic effect of warfarin. The cutaneous bleeding time was unaffected by warfarin, slightly prolonged by aspirin alone, and markedly prolonged by concurrent warfarin and aspirin.

Based on the data generated from the two reports (10, 18), the investigators concluded that aspirin does not augment the prothrombin effect of anticoagulants at low doses (<3 g) but does so significantly at moderate to high doses (>3 g). However, they observed that aspirin will still cause bleeding at lower doses, but through its direct effects on platelet aggregation and on the gastric mucosa.

■ Aspirin, in moderate to large doses (>3 g/day po) may enhance the hypoprothrombinemic effect of anticoagulants when given concurrently. At lower doses (<3 g/day po), aspirin probably will not affect anticoagulant-induced hypoprothrombinemia but may independently cause undesirable bleeding episodes. However, the clinical data about this drug interaction are derived from poorly controlled studies and may not be reliable. Therefore, the clinical outcome of concurrent use of these drugs cannot be predicted.

Recommendations—Concurrent administration of aspirin and warfarin or other anticoagulants should be avoided. Acetaminophen does not prolong the prothrombin time significantly (see *Warfarin–Acetaminophen*, p. 263) and may be a useful alternative to aspirin for analgesia and antipyresis in anticoagulant-treated patients (19). Ibuprofen does not interact with oral anticoagulants (20–22) but does affect platelet aggregation and causes GI irritation (23, 24). Although the drug may be a safer alternative to aspirin in anticoagulant-treated patients, it should still be used cautiously.

If warfarin and aspirin must be used concurrently, the lowest effective dose of aspirin should be used. Prothrombin times should be determined frequently to ascertain if an adjustment in the anticoagulant dose is necessary, particularly after aspirin is added to or withdrawn from the patient's drug regimen.

Since many nonprescription drug combination products contain aspirin (25), patients should be advised to consult a pharmacist or physician before using such products.

References

(1) R. M. Watson and R. N. Pierson, "Effect of Anticoagulant Therapy upon Aspirin-Induced Gastrointestinal Bleeding," *Circulation, 24,* 613 (1961).

(2) S. Jarnum, "Cinchophen and Acetylsalicylic Acid in Anticoagulant Treatment," *Scand. J. Lab. Clin. Invest.,* 6, 91 (1954).

(3) O. O. Meyer and B. Howard, "Production of Hypoprothrombinemia and Hypocoagulability of the Blood with Salicylates," *Proc. Soc. Exp. Biol. Med., 53,* 251 (1943).

(4) S. Shapiro et al., "Studies on Prothrombin: IV. The Prothrombinopenic Effect of Salicylate in Man," *Proc. Soc. Exp. Biol. Med., 53,* 251 (1943).

(5) A. J. Quick and L. Clesceri, "Influence of Acetylsalicylic Acid and Salicylamide on the Coagulation of Blood," *J. Pharmacol. Exp. Ther., 128,* 95 (1960).

(6) M. G. Geall et al., "Profile of Gastric Potential Difference in Man. Effects of Aspirin, Alcohol, Bile and Endogenous Acid," *Gastroenterology, 58,* 437 (1970).

(7) K. K. Matsumoto and M. I. Grossman, "Quantitative Measurement of Gastrointestinal Blood Loss during Ingestion of Aspirin," *Proc. Soc. Exp. Biol. Med., 102,* 517 (1959).

(8) O. D. Needham et al., "Aspirin and Alcohol in Gastrointestinal Haemorrhage," *Gut, 12,* 819 (1971).

(9) R. K. Stuart, "Platelet Function Studies in Human Beings Receiving 300 mg of Aspirin per Day," *J. Lab. Clin. Med., 75,* 463 (1970).

(10) R. A. O'Reilly, "Impact of Aspirin and Chlorthalidone on the Pharmacodynamics of Oral Anticoagulant Drugs in Man," *Ann. N.Y. Acad. Sci., 179,* 173 (1971).

(11) C. H. Mielke, Jr., and A. F. Britten, "Use of Aspirin or Acetaminophen in Hemophilia," *N. Engl. J. Med., 282,* 1270 (1970).

(12) A. J. Marcus, "Platelet Function," *N. Engl. J. Med., 280,* 1278 (1969).

(13) H. J. Weiss, "Platelet Physiology and Abnormalities of Platelet Function," *N. Engl. J. Med., 293,* 580 (1975).

(14) M. R. McDougal, "Interactions of Drugs with Aspirin," *J. Amer. Pharm. Ass., NS10,* 83 (1970).

(15) R. S. Farr, "The Need to Re-Evaluate Acetylsalicylic Acid (Aspirin)," *J. Allergy, 45,* 321 (1970).

(16) D. Hawkins *et al.*, "Structural Changes Human Serum Albumin Induced by Ingestion of Acetylsalicylic Acid," *J. Clin. Invest.*, *48*, 536 (1969).

(17) J. A. Udall, "Drug Interference with Warfarin Therapy," *Clin. Med.*, *77* (8), 20 (1970).

(18) R. A. O'Reilly and P. M. Aggeler, "Determinants of the Response to Oral Anticoagulant Drugs in Man," *Pharmacol. Rev.*, *22*, 35 (1970).

(19) C. H. Mielke *et al.*, "Hemostasis, Antipyretics, and Mild Analgesics: Acetaminophen vs Aspirin," *J. Amer. Med. Ass.*, *235*, 613 (1976).

(20) D. Thilo *et al.*, "A Study of the Effects of the Anti-Rheumatic Drug Ibuprofen on Patients Being Treated with the Oral Anticoagulant Phenprocoumon," *J. Intern. Med. Res.*, *2*, 276 (1974).

(21) M. J. Boekhout-Mussert and E. A. Loeliger, "Influence of Ibuprofen on Oral Anticoagulation with Phenprocoumon," *J. Intern. Med. Res.*, *2*, 279 (1974).

(22) L. Goncalves, "Influence of Ibuprofen on Homeostasis in Patients on Anticoagulant Therapy," *J. Intern. Med. Res.*, *1*, 180 (1973).

(23) J. R. Lewis, "Evaluation of Ibuprofen (Motrin)," *J. Amer. Med. Ass.*, *233*, 364 (1975).

(24) E. F. Davies and G. S. Avery, "Ibuprofen: A Review of Its Pharmacological Properties and Therapeutic Efficacy in Rheumatic Disorders," *Drugs*, *2*, 416 (1971).

(25) "Handbook of Non-Prescription Drugs," G. B. Griffenhagen and L. Hawkins, Eds., American Pharmaceutical Association, Washington, D.C., 1973, p. 36.

[For additional information, see *Anticoagulant Therapy*, p. 358.]

Nonproprietary and Trade Names of Drugs

Acetaminophen—*Datril, Nebs, SK-APAP, Tempra, Tenlap, Tylenol, Valadol, and various combination products*
Acenocoumarol—*Sintrom*
Aluminum aspirin—*Available in combination products*
Anisindione—*Miradon*
Aspirin—*Available alone or as a fixed combination in many trade name products, especially over-the-counter preparations*
Calcium carbaspirin—*Calurin*
Carbethyl salicylate—*Sal-Ethyl Carbonate*
Choline salicylate—*Actasal, Arthropan*
Dicumarol—*Various manufacturers*

Diphenadione—*Dipaxin*
Ibuprofen—*Motrin*
Magnesium salicylate—*Various manufacturers*
Phenindione—*Hedulin*
Phenprocoumon—*Liquamar*
Potassium salicylate—*Various manufacturers*
Salicylamide—*Various manufacturers*
Sodium salicylate—*Various manufacturers*
Warfarin potassium—*Athrombin-K*
Warfarin sodium—*Coumadin Sodium, Panwarfin*

Prepared and evaluated by the Scientific Review Subpanel on Anticoagulants and reviewed by Practitioner Panel III.

Warfarin—Chloral Hydrate

Summary—Concurrent administration of warfarin and chloral hydrate may result in a transient, but slight, increase in the hypoprothrombinemic response to warfarin. However, there have been no reports of hemorrhagic complications due to concurrent use of these drugs, and the drug interaction does not appear to be clinically significant. Nevertheless, precautions appropriate to the individual use of these drugs should still be exercised.

Related Drugs—The coumarin anticoagulants are **acenocoumarol, dicumarol,** and **phenprocoumon.** The indandione derivatives are **anisindione, diphenadione,** and phenindione. **Chloral betaine** (1, 2) and **triclofos** (3) are slowly hydrolyzed in the stomach to yield chloral hydrate and have been shown to decrease the warfarin half-life by increasing the amount of unbound warfarin available for metabolism.

Pharmacological Effect and Mechanism—Although chloral hydrate was originally thought to accelerate the metabolism of anticoagulants (4), subsequent studies (5) indicated that a metabolite of chloral hydrate displaces warfarin from its protein binding site, causing more unbound warfarin to be available for metabolism and resulting in an increased hypoprothrombinemic effect.

Chloral hydrate reportedly decreased the hypoprothrombinemic action of dicumarol in two patients by induction of the coumarin-metabolizing enzymes (4). The enzyme-inducing effect of chloral hydrate has been shown not to occur in animals (6) and has not been demonstrated in subsequent clinical studies (1, 2, 7–11).

Repeated administration of chloral hydrate to human subjects shortened the serum half-life of dicumarol (4) and warfarin (1, 7, 8), although not that of the less protein-bound ethyl biscoumacetate (9). If these shortened half-lives were due to enzyme induction by chloral hydrate, they should be accompanied by a decreased hypoprothrombinemic effect. Actually, administration of a single dose of warfarin to volunteers produced the same mean one-stage prothrombin time prolongation before and after treatment with chloral hydrate (8) or chloral betaine (1).

In three volunteers and in hospitalized patients stabilized on warfarin, the hypo-prothrombinemic effect was increased by 50–100% after concurrent administration of chloral hydrate (7, 8). This enhancement was accompanied by a return of total serum warfarin to normal levels (1, 7, 8, 10, 11).

A major metabolite of chloral hydrate, trichloroacetic acid, is highly bound to serum albumin, accumulates in blood to concentrations greater than 100 mg/liter during chloral hydrate therapy (7, 8), and displaces warfarin from binding sites on albumin *in vitro* (8) and *in vivo* (8, 10). Since only 3% of warfarin is present in the unbound form at typical clinical levels of the drug (12), displacement of even small additional amounts of drug represents a large percentage increase in the level of unbound drug.

Displacement of warfarin from protein binding sites has two major consequences. First, the concentration of unbound drug in equilibrium with the site of warfarin action is greater; hence, there will be a greater inhibition of the synthesis of vitamin K-sensitive clotting factors (II, VII, IX, and X). Second, the fractions of drug available for metabolism and for glomerular filtration are greater, accounting for the shortened serum half-life of the drug.

Evaluation of Clinical Data—Of 500 warfarin-treated patients monitored prospectively, 237 were given chloral hydrate while receiving warfarin (7). Fifty-two of the patients did not receive chloral hydrate for at least 3 consecutive days before and after a period of 3 consecutive days of chloral hydrate therapy in order that their responses during chloral hydrate therapy could be compared to the responses while not taking chloral hydrate. Thirteen of these 52 patients (25%) showed clearcut enhanced anticoagulant effect but none developed bleeding as a consequence of this additional prothrombin time prolongation. The remaining patients were too unstable clinically to analyze or the anticoagulant effect was not altered. Inhibition of the hypoprothrombinemic action of warfarin by chloral hydrate did not appear in any of the 52 patients.

In a retrospective study, 32 patients who received warfarin and chloral hydrate (500–1000 mg/day po) concurrently received less warfarin during the first 4 days of therapy than in a control group of 67 patients (13). The difference was small (<2 mg/patient) and there was no difference between the two groups after the fifth day of therapy.

Triclofos (22 mg/kg/day po) was administered to seven healthy volunteers stabilized on warfarin (3). Three patients required a 30–50% reduction in their daily warfarin dosage during the first days of triclofos administration to prevent excessive prothrombin time prolongation.

Ten patients with cardiovascular disorders and four healthy volunteers were tested for the short-term and long-term effects of concurrent administration of warfarin and chloral hydrate (14). There was a statistically, but not clinically, significant enhancement of prothrombin activity (measured by an increase in prothrombin time) in five subjects receiving short-term anticoagulant therapy and receiving chloral hydrate (1 g/day po). No statistically significant effects were found in 10 patients receiving long-term anticoagulant therapy concurrently with long-term administration of chloral hydrate (500 mg).

Other clinical reports (9–11) provided no evidence of an increase in warfarin activity by chloral hydrate (1–1.5 g/day po). These reports show that the period after concurrent warfarin–chloral hydrate therapy is associated with lower total serum warfarin levels and no change in prothrombin complex activity.

Another study (2) found no significant differences in prothrombin times, serum warfarin levels, or daily warfarin requirements of patients treated with chloral betaine (850 mg/day po) and placebo treatment in 16 patients receiving long-term warfarin therapy. It was suggested (15) that this study (2) did not carefully examine the short-term effects of chloral hydrate on warfarin, but this suggestion has been refuted (16).

■ In healthy volunteers under well-controlled experimental conditions, chloral hydrate caused a slight transient increase in the hypoprothrombinemic effect of warfarin. This effect is limited to the first few days of concurrent therapy. There have been no reports of hemorrhagic complications attributed to concurrent administration of these drugs, and this drug interaction appears not to be clinically significant. However, the usual clinical setting of anticoagulant use is complex. Often many other drugs are being given concurrently, and it is difficult to ascribe a particular change in prothrombin time to a specific drug.

Recommendations—Concurrent administration of chloral hydrate and warfarin or other anticoagulants need not be avoided, but precautions appropriate to the individual use of these drugs should still be exercised.

References

(1) M. G. MacDonald *et al.*, "The Effects of Phenobarbital, Chloral Betaine, and Glutethimide Administration on Warfarin Plasma Levels and Hypoprothrombinemic Responses in Man," *Clin. Pharmacol. Ther.*, *10*, 80 (1969).

(2) P. F. Griner *et al.*, "Chloral Hydrate and Warfarin Interaction: Clinical Significance," *Ann. Intern. Med.*, *74*, 540 (1971).

(3) E. M. Sellers *et al.*, "Enhancement of Warfarin-Induced Hypoprothrombinemia by Triclofos," *Clin. Pharmacol. Ther.*, *13*, 911 (1972).

(4) S. A. Cucinell *et al.*, "The Effect of Chloral Hydrate on Bishydroxycoumarin Metabolism; a Fatal Outcome," *J. Amer. Med. Ass.*, *197*, 366 (1966).

(5) J. Koch-Weser and E. M. Sellers, "Drug Interactions with Coumarin Anticoagulants," *N. Engl. J. Med.*, *285*, 487, 547 (1971).

(6) M. Weiner, "Species Differences in the Effect of Chloral Hydrate on Coumarin Anticoagulants," *Ann. N.Y. Acad. Sci.*, *179*, 226 (1971).

(7) E. M. Sellers and J. Koch-Weser, "Kinetics and Clinical Importance of Displacement of Warfarin from Albumin by Acidic Drugs," *Ann. N.Y. Acad. Sci.*, *179*, 213 (1971).

(8) E. M. Sellers and J. Koch-Weser, "Potentiation of Warfarin-Induced Hypoprothrombinemia by Chloral Hydrate," *N. Engl. J. Med.*, *283*, 827 (1970).

(9) I. E. Van Dam and M. J. H. Gribnau-Overkamp, "The Effect of Some Sedatives (Phenobarbital, Glutethimide, Chlordiazepoxide, Chloral Hydrate) on the Rate of Disappearance of Ethyl Biscoumacetate from the Plasma," *Folia Med. Neerl.*, *10*, 141 (1967).

(10) A. Breckenridge et al., "Drug Interactions with Warfarin: Studies with Dichloralphenazone, Chloral Hydrate and Phenazone (Antipyrine)," Clin. Sci., 40, 351 (1971).

(11) A. Breckenridge and M. Orme, "Clinical Implications of Enzyme Induction," Ann. N.Y. Acad. Sci., 179, 421 (1971).

(12) H. M. Solomon and J. J. Schrogie, "The Effect of Various Drugs on the Binding of Warfarin-^{14}C to Human Albumin," Biochem. Pharmacol., 16, 1219 (1967).

(13) "Interaction between Chloral Hydrate and Warfarin," N. Engl. J. Med., 286, 53 (1972).

(14) J. A. Udall, "Warfarin-Chloral Hydrate Interaction. Pharmacological Activity and Clinical Significance," Ann. Intern. Med., 81, 341 (1974).

(15) J. Koch-Weser et al., "Chloral Hydrate and Warfarin Therapy," Ann. Intern. Med., 75, 141 (1971).

(16) P. F. Griner et al., "Chloral Hydrate and Warfarin Interaction: Clinical Significance," Ann. Intern. Med., 75, 141 (1971).

[For additional information, see Anticoagulant Therapy, p. 358.]

Nonproprietary and Trade Names of Drugs

Acenocoumarol—Sintrom
Anisindione—Miradon
Chloral betaine—Beta-Chlor
Chloral hydrate—Kessodrate, Noctec, Somnos
Dicumarol—Various manufacturers
Diphenadione—Dipaxin

Phenindione—Hedulin
Phenprocoumon—Liquamar
Triclofos sodium—Triclos
Warfarin potassium—Athrombin-K
Warfarin sodium—Coumadin Sodium, Panwarfin

Prepared and evaluated by the Scientific Review Subpanel on Anticoagulants and reviewed by Practitioner Panel IV.

Warfarin—Chlordiazepoxide

Summary—Clinical studies have produced no convincing data that chlordiazepoxide significantly alters patient response to warfarin, although one case report indicated that an interaction may occur. Therefore, no additional precautions are necessary when these drugs are given concurrently.

Related Drugs—Other benzodiazepine compounds studied include **diazepam** (1–4), **flurazepam** (5), and **nitrazepam** (2, 4, 6). Other benzodiazepine drugs are **clonazepam, clorazepate,** and **oxazepam.**

Although most studies have involved the use of warfarin sodium, **phenprocoumon** (6) also has been shown not to interact with benzodiazepine compounds. **Dicumarol** has been reported to interact with diazepam in one case report (7). The other coumarin anticoagulant is **acenocoumarol,** and the indandione anticoagulants are **anisindione, diphenadione,** and **phenindione.**

Pharmacological Effect and Mechanism—Chlordiazepoxide stimulated hepatic microsomal drug-metabolizing enzymes in the rat (8). However, the dosage employed was substantially higher than that usually employed in humans. While stimulation of hepatic microsomal enzymes may be a property of this class of drugs, there is no evidence that this effect is significant when usual therapeutic dosages are employed (1–4, 6, 9, 10).

Evaluation of Clinical Data—The drug interaction between benzodiazepines and oral anticoagulants is based on a case report of a 63-year-old patient who had been receiving dicumarol (150 mg/day po) for 2.5 years (7). The patient exhibited subcutaneous bleeding in the upper and lower extremities and an increase in prothrombin time (amount not reported) after receiving diazepam (20 mg/day po for 14 days) concurrently. The patient's only other medications were pentaerythritol tetranitrate and nitroglycerin. Based on the information provided about the case, there was a strong association between diazepam administration and the increased hypoprothrombinemic effect of dicumarol. However, not enough information was provided to establish a causal relationship. Moreover, this reported drug interaction was not observed in controlled clinical studies.

Chlordiazepoxide (30 mg/day po) did not effect routine coagulation tests significantly in 10 normal patients or in patients with ischemic or rheumatic heart disease receiving long-term warfarin therapy (9). Daily administration of chlordiazepoxide (50 mg po) 21 days between loading doses of warfarin caused no significant change either in the biological half-life or in the hypoprothrombinemic response to warfarin in another study of eight subjects (10). Similar results were reported in a study of patients stabilized on warfarin given both diazepam (5 mg/day po) and chlordiazepoxide (30 mg/day po) (1).

Subsequent well-controlled studies of concurrent use of chlordiazepoxide, diazepam, or nitrazepam with phenprocoumon or warfarin confirmed these observations (2, 4, 6).

■ The clinical evidence indicates that it is not likely that chlordiazepoxide has a significant effect on the hypoprothrombinemic action of the oral anticoagulants.

Recommendations—Chlordiazepoxide and other benzodiazepine compounds appear to have no significant effect on the hypoprothrombinemic action of the oral anticoagulants. Their preferential use, instead of several sedative–hypnotic agents known to interact with anticoagulants, is recommended (2, 6, 10). For patients receiving oral anticoagulants, flurazepam is a suitable and safe hypnotic agent and usually is given at a dose of 15–30 mg at bedtime (11).

References

(1) H. M. Solomon *et al.*, "Mechanisms of Drug Interactions," *J. Amer. Med. Ass.*, *216*, 1997 (1971).

(2) M. Orme *et al.*, "Interactions of Benzodiazepines with Warfarin," *Brit. Med. J.*, *3*, 611 (1972).

(3) P. Ristola and K. Pyorala, "Determinants of the Response to Coumarin Anticoagulants in Patients with Acute Myocardial Infarction," *Acta Med. Scand.*, *192*, 183 (1972).

(4) J. B. Whitefield *et al.*, "Change in Plasma Gamma-Glutamyl Transpeptidase Activity and Altered Drug Metabolism in Man," *Brit. Med. J.*, *1*, 316 (1973).

(5) "Benzodiazepines in Clinical Practice," D. J. Greenblatt and R. I. Shader, Eds., Raven, New York, NY 10024, 1974, pp. 248–250.

(6) R. Bieger *et al.*, "Influence of Nitrazepam on Oral Anticoagulation with Phenprocoumon," *Clin. Pharmacol. Ther.*, *13*, 361 (1972).

(7) P. J. Taylor, "Hemorrhage while on Anticoagulant Therapy Precipitated by Drug Interaction," *Ariz. Med.*, *24*, 697 (1967).

(8) D. R. Hoogland *et al.*, "Metabolism and Tolerance Studies with Chlordiazepoxide-2-^{14}C in the Rat," *Toxicol. Appl. Pharmacol.*, *9*, 116 (1966).

(9) H. Lackner and V. E. Hunt, "The Effect of Librium on Hemostasis," *Amer. J. Med. Sci.*, *256*, 368 (1968).

(10) D. S. Robinson and D. Sylwester, "Interaction of Commonly Prescribed Drugs and Warfarin," *Ann. Intern. Med.*, *72*, 853 (1970).

(11) "A Clinical Evaluation of Flurazepam," *J. Clin. Pharm. New Drugs*, *12*, 217 (1972).

[For additional information, see *Anticoagulant Therapy*, p. 358.]

Nonproprietary and Trade Names of Drugs

Acenocoumarol—*Sintrom*
Anisindione—*Miradon*
Chlordiazepoxide—*Libritabs*
Chlordiazepoxide hydrochloride—*Librium*
 and various combination products
Clonazepam—*Clonopin*
Clorazepate dipotassium—*Tranxene*
Diazepam—*Valium*
Dicumarol—*Various manufacturers*

Diphenadione—*Dipaxin*
Flurazepam hydrochloride—*Dalmane*
Nitrazepam—*Mogadon*
Oxazepam—*Serax*
Phenindione—*Hedulin*
Phenprocoumon—*Liquamar*
Warfarin potassium—*Athrombin-K*
Warfarin sodium—*Coumadin Sodium,*
 Panwarfin

*Prepared and evaluated by the Scientific Review Subpanel
on Anticoagulants and reviewed by Practitioner Panel V.*

Warfarin—Cholestyramine

Summary—The binding of warfarin to cholestyramine has been demonstrated in experimental systems and appears to be related to pH, pKa, and sequence of administration. In the presence of cholestyramine, reductions in serum warfarin levels and an associated reduced hypoprothrombinemic effect have been statistically demonstrated in normal subjects. However, the data are insufficient to predict the clinical outcome of this drug interaction. Concurrent administration of these drugs should be avoided when possible. If these drugs are used concurrently, the effect of the drug interaction may be minimized by administering cholestyramine as long as possible (at least 3 hr but preferably 6 hr) after warfarin.

Related Drugs—Other coumarin derivatives (*e.g.*, **acenocoumarol, dicumarol,** and **phenprocoumon)** have not been studied but may be expected to interact with cholestyramine in a similar manner. The indandione derivatives (*e.g.*, **anisindione, diphenadione,** and **phenindione)** are nonionic and are not likely to interact with cholestyramine, although specific data are lacking.

Pharmacological Effect and Mechanism—Cholestyramine is an insoluble chloride salt of a basic ion-exchange resin. It exchanges chloride ions for bile acid salts in the intestine where it binds the bile acid salts into insoluble complexes. This binding prevents reabsorption and reexcretion of the bile acid salts in the bile, facilitating their fecal excretion (1–5). Cholestyramine binds to other anionic substances and the extent of its binding appears to depend on the pKa of the anionic agent and the environmental pH.

Warfarin inhibits synthesis of prothrombin and other clotting factors through a series of biochemical mechanisms affecting vitamin K utilization (6, 7). Warfarin is an anionic compound with a functional enol group that binds to cholestyramine *in vitro* (8) and *in vivo* (9). The proposed mechanism of interaction involves a decrease in warfarin absorption due to its binding to cholestyramine, resulting in reduced serum warfarin levels and a subsequent reduction in the hypoprothrombinemic effect. Cholestyramine also has been reported to decrease vitamin K absorption, resulting in an enhanced hypoprothrombinemic response to warfarin. However, the clinical significance of this effect has not been established (10).

Evaluation of Clinical Data—Cholestyramine (4 g po) was administered simultaneously, 3 hr before, or 6 hr after a single dose of warfarin (40 mg po) in six normal subjects (9). A statistically significant decrease (when compared to controls) in serum warfarin levels occurred at 6 and 48 hr after warfarin administration. The decrease in serum warfarin levels occurred with all administration intervals. A statistically significant decrease was also noted when prothrombin times were determined 48 hr after warfarin administration.

Two patients previously maintained on warfarin experienced large fluctuations in prothrombin times after cholestyramine therapy was begun. One patient suffered more frequent cerebral ischemic attacks soon after the addition of cholestyramine to the dosage regimen (personal communication, D. W. Bilheimer, Southwestern Medical School, Dallas, Tex.) (11). Cholestyramine was discontinued in this patient after attempts to stabilize the effect of warfarin were unsuccessful. The patient's prothrombin time subsequently was controlled and the ischemic attacks were fewer. However, since additional information about the two patients is lacking, a causal relationship between decreased warfarin effect and cholestyramine administration cannot be established.

■ Cholestyramine decreased serum levels and the hypoprothrombinemic effect of warfarin in normal subjects and has been implicated as a possible causative factor for decreased warfarin response in two patients. However, the data are insufficient to determine the clinical outcome of long-term concurrent administration of these drugs. In the only major study done to investigate the effect of cholestyramine on the action of warfarin (9), the patient population studied was limited and normal and only single, large doses of warfarin were used. Moreover, determinations of the prothrombin time 48 hr after a single dose of warfarin may be unrelated to the chronic prothrombin time stabilization required during prolonged warfarin therapy. In the only other report of adverse effects due to this drug interaction (11), there were insufficient controls for a causal relationship between cholestyramine administration and warfarin effect to be established. Additionally, the ability of cholestyramine to decrease vitamin K absorption also may be a factor influencing the effects of the interaction (10).

Recommendations—Until the clinical significance of this drug interaction is more carefully assessed, concurrent administration of warfarin and cholestyramine should be avoided if possible. When these drugs must be used concurrently, the interaction can be minimized by administering cholestyramine as long as possible (at least 3 hr but preferably 6 hr) after warfarin. The anticoagulant effect (prothrombin times) should always be monitored in both acute and chronic patients.

References

(1) J. B. Carey and G. Williams, "Relief of the Pruritis of Jaundice with a Bile-Acid Sequestering Resin," *J. Amer. Med. Ass.*, *176*, 432 (1961).

(2) J. T. Garbutt and T. J. Kenney, "Effect of Cholestyramine on Bile Acid Metabolism in Normal Man," *J. Clin. Invest.*, *51*, 2781 (1972).

(3) S. M. Grundy, "Treatment of Hypercholesterolemia by Interference with Bile Acid Metabolism," *Arch. Intern. Med.*, *130*, 638 (1972).

(4) "An Antipruritic Agent for Primary Biliary Cirrhosis and Cholestatic Jaundice," *J. Amer. Med. Ass.*, *197*, 261 (1966).

(5) D. J. Nazir *et al.*, "Mechanisms of Action of Cholestyramine in the Treatment of Hypercholesterolemia," *Circulation*, *46*, 95 (1972).

(6) R. G. Bell *et al.*, "Mechanism of Action of Warfarin. Warfarin and Metabolism of Vitamin K_1," *Biochemistry*, *11*, 1959 (1972).

(7) I. L. Woolf and B. M. Babior, "Vitamin K and Warfarin. Metabolism, Function and Interaction," *Amer. J. Med.*, *53*, 261 (1972).

(8) D. G. Gallo *et al.*, "The Interaction between Cholestyramine and Drugs," *Proc. Soc. Exp. Biol. Med.*, *120*, 60 (1965).

(9) D. S. Robinson *et al.*, "Interaction of Warfarin and Nonsystemic Gastrointestinal Drugs," *Clin. Pharmacol. Ther., 12,* 491 (1971).

(10) L. Gross and M. Brotman, "Hypoprothrombinemia and Hemorrhage Asso-

ciated with Cholestyramine Therapy," *Ann. Intern. Med., 72,* 95 (1970).

(11) R. I. Levy *et al.*, "Dietary and Drug Treatment of Primary Hyperlipoproteinemia," *Ann. Intern. Med., 77,* 267 (1972).

[For additional information, see *Anticoagulant Therapy*, p. 358.]

Nonproprietary and Trade Names of Drugs

Acenocoumarol—*Sintrom*
Anisindione—*Miradon*
Cholestyramine resin—*Cuemid, Questran*
Dicumarol—*Various manufacturers*
Diphenadione—*Dipaxin*

Phenindione—*Hedulin*
Phenprocoumon—*Liquamar*
Warfarin potassium—*Athrombin-K*
Warfarin sodium—*Coumadin Sodium, Panwarfin*

Prepared and evaluated by the Scientific Review Subpanel on Anticoagulants and reviewed by Practitioner Panel V.

Warfarin—Clofibrate

Summary—Clofibrate enhances the effect of warfarin in patients receiving these drugs concurrently; this enhancement may lead to severe hemorrhage and possibly death. To determine if a decrease in the dosage of warfarin is necessary when these drugs are used concurrently, frequent prothrombin time determinations are necessary.

Related Drugs—The coumarin anticoagulant **dicumarol** (1) and the indandione anticoagulant **phenindione** (2, 3) are reported to interact with clofibrate in the same manner as warfarin.

Although there is no documentation, the other coumarin anticoagulants **(acenocoumarol** and **phenprocoumon**) and indandione anticoagulants **(anisindione** and **diphenadione**) could also interact with clofibrate.

Pharmacological Effect and Mechanism—Clofibrate is used to reduce serum lipoproteins (mostly the very low density type) and serum triglycerides in patients in whom the levels of these compounds are elevated. Although the mechanism of this action is unclear, clofibrate appears to inhibit cholesterol synthesis and the transfer of triglycerides from the liver to the serum and to promote the renal excretion of neutral sterols (4).

Clofibrate increases the response to oral anticoagulants in animals (5, 6) and humans (1–3, 6–12). The exact mechanism of this interaction is not known, but clofibrate appears to displace warfarin competitively and noncompetitively from binding to the plasma albumin molecule (1, 13, 14), depending on the concentration of clofibrate in the plasma.

One study (7) reported that clofibrate prolonged the warfarin half-life in dogs from 28.5 to 44 hr. It was suggested that clofibrate may somehow interfere with the metabolism of warfarin, thereby enhancing its effect.

Other studies (9, 15, 16) suggested that the hypolipidemic effect of clofibrate also reduces the vitamin K stores in the liver, leading to further suppression of factors II, VII, IX, and X, which are also decreased by warfarin.

Evaluation of Clinical Data—Clofibrate (1.5 g/day po) caused an increased response to anticoagulants in 14 patients with high cholesterol levels (12). These patients had been receiving long-term anticoagulant therapy, the majority with phenindione. Six of the 14 patients also experienced bleeding episodes, with one death occurring that may have been due to a pulmonary hemorrhage.

A statistically significant decrease in the requirements of warfarin was observed in 11 patients treated with clofibrate (30 mg/kg po) (10). These patients had high serum lipid levels and a history of myocardial infarction.

Another report (6) noted that about one-third less warfarin was required for 13 patients after clofibrate (1.25–2 g/day po) was begun. Initially, all but one patient had elevated cholesterol levels.

In an extensive investigation (2), the responses of 42 patients receiving clofibrate and an anticoagulant (warfarin or phenindione) concurrently were monitored in three separate hospitals. In 30 of the 42 patients, a reduction in the requirements for warfarin was observed after clofibrate therapy was begun. At least five patients had bleeding episodes; in at least 14 other patients, bleeding was probably avoided by adjusting the dose. All patients had either hypercholesterolemia or evidence of previous myocardial infarction. The clofibrate dosage was not reported.

This interaction was reported to occur infrequently in a study (9) of 10 patients receiving both warfarin and clofibrate (2 g/day po). Only two of the 10 patients showed any enhancement of the anticoagulant effect, and no bleeding episodes were reported. Since these patients were not picked on the basis of high serum lipid levels, the difference in results from the previous studies might be related to the reduction of hyperlipidemia caused by clofibrate. However, this conclusion is not consistent with enhancement of the effects of warfarin observed in six healthy patients also receiving clofibrate (2 g/day po) (8).

Massive hemorrhage and death were reported in a patient receiving warfarin (2.5 mg/day po) and clofibrate (2 g/day po) for 3 years (5). Although other causative factors such as possible liver or renal dysfunction or vitamin K deficiency could not be ruled out, the sequence of events leading to this patient's death suggested deficiencies in blood coagulation factors II, VII, and X, all of which may be influenced by concurrent warfarin–clofibrate therapy.

■ Enhancement of the effects of warfarin and subsequent hypoprothrombinemia may be expected to occur in most patients receiving warfarin and clofibrate concurrently if no adjustments in anticoagulant doses are made. The hypoprothrombinemia resulting from this interaction can cause severe hemorrhage and sometimes death (7, 12). The onset of this effect is unpredictable; it may be immediate or delayed (7).

Recommendations—Because the concurrent use of these two drugs can result in hemorrhage and possibly death, frequent prothrombin time determinations should be made whenever warfarin and clofibrate are used together and the warfarin dosage should be reduced accordingly. Although the manufacturer of clofibrate has recommended an automatic reduction in the dose of the anticoagulant by approximately one-half (17), there is no published scientific documentation to support this action. Moreover, since each patient responds differently to an anticoagulant, the automatic reduction in dose may be inadequate to prevent excessive hypoprothrombinemia caused by the drug interaction or the adjusted dose may be too low to maintain adequate anticoagulation.

References

(1) J. J. Schrogie and H. M. Solomon, "The Anticoagulant Response to Bishydroxycoumarin II. The Effect of D-Thyroxine, Clofibrate, and Norethandrolone," *Clin. Pharmacol. Ther.*, *8*, 70 (1967).

(2) M. F. Oliver et al., "Effect of Atromid and Ethyl Chlorophenoxyisobutyrate on Anticoagulant Requirements," Lancet, i, 143 (1963).

(3) G. M. McAndrew and H. W. Fullerton, "The Effect of Atromid on the Recalcified Plasma Clotting Time after High-Fat Meals," J. Atheroscler. Res., 3, 634 (1963).

(4) "The Pharmacological Basis of Therapeutics," 5th ed., L. S. Goodman and A. Gilman, Eds., Macmillan, New York, NY 10022, 1975, p. 747.

(5) R. B. Solomon and F. Rosner, "Massive Hemorrhage and Death during Treatment with Clofibrate and Warfarin," N.Y. State J. Med., 73, 2002 (1973).

(6) T. B. Counihan and P. Keelan, "Atromid in High Cholesterol States," J. Atheroscler. Res., 3, 580 (1963).

(7) D. B. Hunninghake and D. L. Azarnoff, "Drug Interactions with Warfarin," Arch. Intern. Med., 121, 349 (1968).

(8) K. Pyorala et al., "Warfarin Metabolism during Ethyl Chlorophenoxyisobutyrate Treatment," Ann. Med. Int. Fenn., 75, 157 (1968).

(9) J. A. Udall, "Drug Interference with Warfarin Therapy," Clin. Med., 77(8), 20 (1970).

(10) S. D. Roberts and J. F. Pantridge, "Effect of Atromid on Requirements of Warfarin," J. Atheroscler. Res., 3, 655 (1963).

(11) G. E. Owen Williams et al., "Atromid and Anticoagulant Therapy," J. Atheroscler. Res., 3, 658 (1963).

(12) A. S. Rogen and J. C. Ferguson, "Clinical Observations on Patients Treated with Atromid and Anticoagulants," J. Atheroscler. Res., 3, 671 (1963).

(13) H. M. Solomon et al., "The Displacement of Phenylbutazone-^{14}C and Warfarin-^{14}C from Human Albumin by Various Drugs and Fatty Acids," Biochem. Pharmacol., 17, 143 (1968).

(14) H. M. Solomon and J. J. Schrogie, "The Effect of Various Drugs on the Binding of Warfarin-^{14}C to Human Albumin," Biochem. Pharmacol., 16, 1219 (1967).

(15) R. H. Furman et al., "Serum-Lipid Reducing Agents and Anticoagulant Requirements," Lancet, i, 893 (1963).

(16) E. A. Nikkila and R. Pelkonen, "Serum-Lipid-Reducing Agents and Anticoagulant Requirements," Lancet, i, 332 (1963).

(17) "Physicians' Desk Reference," 29th ed., Medical Economics, Inc., Oradell, NJ 07649, 1975, p. 580.

[For additional information, see Anticoagulant Therapy, p. 358.]

Nonproprietary and Trade Names of Drugs

Acenocoumarol—Sintrom
Anisindione—Miradon
Clofibrate—Atromid-S
Dicumarol—Various manufacturers
Diphenadione—Dipaxin

Phenindione—Hedulin
Phenprocoumon—Liquamar
Warfarin potassium—Athrombin-K
Warfarin sodium—Coumadin Sodium, Panwarfin

Prepared and evaluated by the Scientific Review Subpanel on Anticoagulants and reviewed by Practitioner Panel IV.

Warfarin—Diphenhydramine

Summary—Although frequently discussed in the scientific literature, no clinically significant interactions between warfarin and diphenhydramine have been reported. Therefore, no additional precautions other than those normally employed are necessary when these drugs are given concurrently.

Related Drugs—Related antihistamines include **brompheniramine, chlorcyclizine, chlorpheniramine, cyclizine, dexbrompheniramine, dexchlorpheniramine, dimenhydrinate, methapyrilene, phenindamine, promethazine, pyrilamine,** and **tripelennamine.**

   Other anticoagulants are **acenocoumarol, anisindione, dicumarol, diphenadione, phenindione,** and **phenprocoumon.**

Pharmacological Effect and Mechanism—In animals, chlorcyclizine, chlorpheniramine, cyclizine, diphenhydramine, and hydroxyzine induce hepatic microsomal

enzymes that metabolize certain drugs. An increased rate of metabolism of carisoprodol, hexobarbital, meprobamate, pentobarbital, and zoxazolamine occurred in liver
microsomal preparations of rats pretreated with these antihistamines. The effect on
anticoagulant drug metabolism was not tested (1–3).

In vitro tests showed that antihistamines can impair platelet function, but this
effect is probably not clinically significant (4, 5).

Evaluation of Clinical Data—Several reviews briefly mentioned that antihistamines
interfere with anticoagulant therapy (4, 6–8); however, no documentation was presented. No case reports of anticoagulation problems caused by antihistamines have
appeared.

■ Because of the lack of clinical data, there does not appear to be any clinically
important effect on anticoagulant therapy by diphenhydramine or other antihistamines.

Recommendations—No additional precautions other than those normally employed
appear necessary when warfarin and diphenhydramine or other antihistamines are
used concurrently.

References

(1) R. Kato *et al.*, "Further Studies on
the Inhibition and Stimulation of
Microsomal Drug-Metabolizing Enzymes of Rat Liver by Various Compounds," *Biochem. Pharmacol., 13,* 69
(1964).
(2) A. H. Conney *et al.*, "Adaptive Increases in Drug-Metabolizing Enzymes
Induced by Phenobarbital and Other
Drugs," *J. Pharmacol. Exp. Ther.,
130,* 1 (1960).
(3) D. B. Hunninghake and D. L. Azarnoff,
"Drug Interactions with Warfarin,"
Arch. Intern. Med., 121, 349 (1968).
(4) D. Deykin, "Warfarin Interaction,"
Drug Ther., 1, 20 (1971).
(5) J. F. Mustard and M. A. Packham,

"Factors Influencing Platelet Function:
Adhesion, Release, and Aggregation,"
Pharmacol. Rev., 22, 97 (1970).
(6) R. A. Elias, in "Anticoagulant Therapy
in Ischemic Heart Disease," International Anticoagulant Symposium,
Miami Beach, Fla., 1964, Grune and
Stratton, New York, N.Y., 1965, pp.
443–448.
(7) N. Formiller and M. S. Cohon, "Coumarin and Indandione Anticoagulants:
Potentiators and Antagonists," *Amer.
J. Hosp. Pharm., 26,* 574 (1969).
(8) E. A. Hartshorn, "Drug Interactions.
III. Classes of Drugs and Their Interactions. Antihistamines," *Drug Intel.,
2,* 198 (1968).

[For additional information, see *Anticoagulant Therapy,* p. 358.]

Nonproprietary and Trade Names of Drugs

Acenocoumarol—*Sintrom*
Anisindione—*Miradon*
Brompheniramine maleate—*Dimetane and
  various combination products*
Chlorcyclizine hydrochloride—*Various
  combination products*
Chlorpheniramine maleate—*Chlor-Trimeton
  Maleate, Teldrin, and various
  combination products*
Cyclizine hydrochloride—*Marezine
  Hydrochloride*
Dexbrompheniramine maleate—*Disomer
  and various combination products*
Dexchlorpheniramine maleate—*Polaramine*
Dicumarol—*Various manufacturers*
Dimenhydrinate—*Dramamine*

Diphenadione—*Dipaxin*
Diphenhydramine hydrochloride—*Benadryl*
Methapyrilene hydrochloride—*Histadyl*
Phenindamine tartrate—*Thephorin*
Phenindione—*Hedulin*
Phenprocoumon—*Liquamar*
Promethazine hydrochloride—*Phenergan,
  Remsed*
Pyrilamine maleate—*Various
  manufacturers*
Tripelennamine hydrochloride—
  Pyribenzamine Hydrochloride
Warfarin potassium—*Athrombin-K*
Warfarin sodium—*Coumadin Sodium,
  Panwarfin*

*Prepared and evaluated by the Scientific Review Subpanel
on Anticoagulants and reviewed by Practitioner Panel V.*

Warfarin—Glutethimide

Summary—Glutethimide stimulates the metabolism of warfarin and reduces its effect when these drugs are given concurrently. The addition of glutethimide to the drug regimen of a patient receiving warfarin necessitates an upward adjustment in the warfarin dose to maintain adequate anticoagulation. Conversely, the withdrawal of glutethimide from the regimen of persons concurrently receiving warfarin could lead to severe hemorrhage.

Related Drugs—There are no reports implicating the chemical analog of glutethimide, **methyprylon,** as an interacting substance with oral anticoagulants.

Although most studies have involved the use of warfarin, other coumarin anticoagulants, **acenocoumarol, dicumarol,** and **phenprocoumon,** as well as the indandione derivatives, **anisindione, diphenadione,** and **phenindione,** may interact with glutethimide in a manner similar to warfarin.

Pharmacological Effect and Mechanism—Glutethimide is capable of increasing the activity of the hepatic microsomal enzymes involved in drug metabolism (1, 2). This effect can appear from several days to 1 week after initiation of glutethimide and may continue for several weeks after its withdrawal (1). When administered to dogs for 12 days, glutethimide (80 mg/kg/day) reduced the serum warfarin half-life by approximately 50% (3).

Evaluation of Clinical Data—In a double-blind study, a 15% decrease in the average hypoprothrombinemic response was observed in 10 healthy male volunteers to whom a single dose of warfarin (40–60 mg po) was administered after 3 weeks of pretreatment with glutethimide (1.0 g/day po) (1). When compared to control values, glutethimide caused a marked reduction in the serum warfarin level and reduced the serum warfarin half-life by nearly 50%.

Similar effects of glutethimide in decreasing the warfarin half-life were observed in a study of hospitalized patients (4). In this study, 13 patients receiving warfarin therapy given glutethimide (625 mg/day po for 7 days) showed a 33% reduction in the warfarin half-life.

■ The clinical data indicate that glutethimide reduces the activity of oral anticoagulants when administered at therapeutic dosage levels. Its effects of decreasing both the serum half-life and hypoprothrombinemic response to oral anticoagulants appear similar in magnitude to barbiturates (1).

Recommendations—Glutethimide should not be initiated or discontinued in a patient receiving oral anticoagulants without close attention to possible readjustment of the anticoagulant dosage. The use of a benzodiazepine compound as a substitute for glutethimide should be considered, since these compounds do not significantly affect the prothrombin time achieved with anticoagulants (see *Warfarin–Chlordiazepoxide*, p. 276).

References

(1) M. G. MacDonald *et al.*, "The Effects of Phenobarbital, Chloral Betaine, and Glutethimide Administration on Warfarin Plasma Levels and Hypoprothrombinemic Responses in Man," *Clin. Pharmacol. Ther.*, *10*, 80 (1969).

(2) A. H. Conney, "Pharmacological Implications of Microsomal Enzyme Induction," *Pharmacol. Rev.*, *19*, 317 (1967).

(3) D. B. Hunninghake and D. L. Azarnoff, "Drug Interactions with Warfarin," *Arch. Intern. Med.*, *121*, 349 (1968).

(4) M. Corn, "Effect of Phenobarbital and Glutethimide on Biological Half-Life of Warfarin," *Thromb. Diath. Haemorrh.*, *16*, 606 (1966).

[For additional information, see *Anticoagulant Therapy*, p. 358.]

Nonproprietary and Trade Names of Drugs

Acenocoumarol—*Sintrom*
Anisindione—*Miradon*
Dicumarol—*Various manufacturers*
Diphenadione—*Dipaxin*
Glutethimide—*Doriden*
Methyprylon—*Noludar*

Phenindione—*Hedulin*
Phenprocoumon—*Liquamar*
Warfarin potassium—*Athrombin-K*
Warfarin sodium—*Coumadin Sodium,*
   Panwarfin

*Prepared and evaluated by the Scientific Review Subpanel
on Anticoagulants and reviewed by Practitioner Panel VI.*

Warfarin—Griseofulvin

Summary—Griseofulvin (1 g/day po) may decrease the hypoprothrombinemic effects of warfarin in some, but not all, patients receiving these drugs concurrently. Since the drug interaction occurs in only a few patients, concurrent administration need not be avoided. Close monitoring of prothrombin time is required when griseofulvin is added to or withdrawn from the anticoagulant drug regimen.

Related Drugs—Other coumarin anticoagulants **acenocoumarol, dicumarol,** and **phenprocoumon** might be expected to interact with griseofulvin in a manner similar to warfarin, although no interactions have been reported. The indandione anticoagulants **anisindione, diphenadione,** and **phenindione** also may have the potential for interacting with griseofulvin, although there have been no such reports.

Pharmacological Effect and Mechanism—Griseofulvin decreases the hypoprothrombinemic effect of warfarin probably by inducing liver microsomal enzymes (1) and increasing the metabolic biotransformation of warfarin. It also has been suggested that griseofulvin may interfere with the absorption of warfarin (2).

Evaluation of Clinical Data—A decrease in the anticoagulant effect of warfarin was observed in three patients who had received microcrystalline griseofulvin (1 g/day po) (1). In one patient, the plasma prothrombin activity increased from 20 to 68% of normal and in another patient it increased from 30 to 100%. The third patient experienced only a slight increase (from 17 to 25%). No change was noted in a healthy subject receiving warfarin therapy who was given microcrystalline griseofulvin (4 g/day po).

Four of 10 patients stabilized on warfarin showed a small decrease (average, 4.2 sec) in prothrombin time during and after 2 weeks of griseofulvin (1.0 g/day, apparently *not* microcrystallized) (3).

■ Griseofulvin (1 g/day po) may decrease significantly the hypoprothrombinemic effects of warfarin, but the data are limited to reports of two patients (1). A clinically significant drug interaction was not observed in a controlled study of 10 patients (3) nor in two additional subjects (1). Therefore, the clinical outcome of this drug interaction cannot be predicted, but the interaction appears limited to a few patients.

Recommendations—This interaction should be considered when warfarin and griseofulvin are administered concurrently. Prothrombin time should be determined two or three times weekly until a stable level is attained. The warfarin dosage may need to be increased in some patients receiving griseofulvin to attain therapeutic serum warfarin levels. Upon discontinuation of griseofulvin, the anticoagulant dosage should be reduced and prothrombin time should be monitored to prevent potential hemorrhage. Many patients require no adjustment of anticoagulant dosage, since the interaction occurs only in some patients.

References

(1) S. I. Cullen and P. M. Catalano, "Griseofulvin–Warfarin Antagonism," *J. Amer. Med. Ass.*, *199*, 582 (1967).
(2) J. Koch-Weser and E. M. Sellers, "Drug Interactions with Coumarin

Anticoagulants," *N. Engl. J. Med.*, *285*, 487, 547 (1971).
(3) J. A. Udall, "Drug Interference with Warfarin Therapy," *Clin. Med.*, *77* (8), 20 (1970).

[For additional information, see *Anticoagulant Therapy*, p. 358.]

Nonproprietary and Trade Names of Drugs

Acenocoumarol—*Sintrom*
Anisindione—*Miradon*
Dicumarol—*Various manufacturers*
Diphenadione—*Dipaxin*
Griseofulvin—*Fulvin U/F, Grifulvin V, Grisactin, Gris-PEG*

Phenindione—*Hedulin*
Phenprocoumon—*Liquamar*
Warfarin potassium—*Athrombin-K*
Warfarin sodium—*Coumadin Sodium, Panwarfin*

Prepared and evaluated by the Scientific Review Subpanel on Anticoagulants and reviewed by Practitioner Panel VI.

Warfarin—Indomethacin

Summary—Contrary to statements in published reviews, indomethacin does not enhance the hypoprothrombinemic effect of warfarin or other oral anticoagulants when these drugs are administered concurrently. However, indomethacin causes gastric ulceration and hemorrhage and inhibits platelet aggregation and should be used cautiously in patients receiving warfarin or other anticoagulants.

Related Drugs—There are no other drugs chemically related to indomethacin. The coumarin derivatives **acenocoumarol** (1), **dicumarol** (2), and **phenprocoumon** (3, 4) do not interact with indomethacin. All indandione derivatives (*e.g.*, **anisindione, diphenadione,** and **phenindione**) also would not be expected to interact with indomethacin.

Pharmacological Effect and Mechanism—Indomethacin displaces phenylbutazone from albumin *in vitro* by competing for the same binding site (5). Since phenylbutazone is more strongly bound to albumin than is warfarin, indomethacin may also decrease the albumin binding of anticoagulants (2, 5). It has been suggested that indomethacin may have a transient enhancing effect on oral anticoagulants (2) in chronically treated patients, but this effect has not been demonstrated clinically.

Evaluation of Clinical Data—Several reviews indicated that indomethacin increases the activity of oral anticoagulants (6–8). It has been speculated that indomethacin is likely to enhance the hypoprothrombinemic action of oral anticoagulants because of *in vitro* evidence that indomethacin displaces oral anticoagulants from protein binding sites (2). However, results from seven studies (1, 3, 5, 9–12) indicate that indomethacin (75–100 mg/day po) has no enhancing effect on the activity of oral anticoagulants.

Two double-blind, placebo-controlled, randomized studies demonstrated the lack of a clinically significant interaction between warfarin and indomethacin (12). In the first study, 16 volunteers received oral warfarin for 11 days and were stabilized at a prothrombin time 1.5–2.5 times normal. Indomethacin (100 mg/day po) or placebo was then administered for 5 days. No statistically significant change in prothrombin time occurred in either the placebo or indomethacin group. The second study compared the effects of placebo and indomethacin on the half-life of warfarin and the duration of its hypoprothrombinemic effect. No significant differences in either parameter were noted between the placebo and the indomethacin-treated groups.

The failure of indomethacin to interact with warfarin was also noted in one case study (10) in which the administration of indomethacin (75 mg/day po) did not effect the anticoagulant control of a patient stabilized on warfarin.

■ The clinical evidence indicates that indomethacin has little, if any, direct influence on the effects of oral anticoagulants.

Recommendations—Although all available data indicate that indomethacin causes no significant enhancement of oral anticoagulant activity, it does cause gastric ulceration and hemorrhage and may inhibit platelet aggregation (13). Thus, it must be used with caution in patients receiving anticoagulants. The patient should be monitored for possible gastric ulceration and hemorrhage because such effects could be serious in a patient maintained on oral anticoagulants.

Other anti-inflammatory drugs such as aspirin (see *Warfarin–Aspirin*, p. 270), phenylbutazone (see *Warfarin–Phenylbutazone*, p. 295), or steroids (14, 15) affect the oral anticoagulant response to a greater degree than indomethacin. There are no reports that gold salts or ibuprofen affects anticoagulant drugs.

References

(1) G. Gaspardy *et al.*, "Effect of Combination of Indomethacin and Syncumar (Acenocoumarol) on the Prothrombin Level in the Blood Plasma," *Z. Rheumaforsch.*, *26*, 332 (1967).

(2) J. Koch-Weser and E. M. Sellers, "Drug Interactions with Coumarin Anticoagulants," *N. Engl. J. Med.*, *285*, 547 (1971).

(3) K. H. Muller and K. Herrmann, "Is a Simultaneous Treatment with Anticoagulants and Indomethacin Compatible," *Med. Welt.*, *29*, 1553 (1966).

(4) H. Frost and H. Hess, "Concomitant Administration of Indomethacin and Anticoagulants," International Symposium on Inflammation, Friedburg im Breisgau, Germany, May 4-6, 1966, R. Heister and H. F. Hofmann, Eds., Urban and Schwarzenberg, Munich, Germany, 1966.

(5) H. M. Solomon *et al.*, "The Displacement of Phenylbutazone-¹⁴C and Warfarin-¹⁴C from Human Albumin by Various Drugs and Fatty Acids," *Biochem. Pharmacol.*, *17*, 143 (1968).

(6) H. F. Morrelli and K. L. Melmon, "The Clinician's Approach to Drug Interactions," *Calif. Med.*, *109*, 380 (1968).

(7) M. Lubran, "The Effects of Drugs on Laboratory Values," *Med. Clin. N. Amer.*, *53*, 211 (1969).

(8) F. H. Meyers *et al.*, "Review of Medical Pharmacology," Lange Medical Publications, Los Altos, Calif., 1972, p. 651.

(9) G. Muller and W. Zollinger, "Indomethacin Influence on Blood Clotting with Particular Respect to the Interference of Anticoagulants," *Praxis*, *55*, 1462 (1966).

(10) B. I. Hoffbrand and D. A. Kininmonth, "Potentiation of Anticoagulants," *Brit. Med. J.*, *2*, 838 (1967).

(11) C. B. Hobbs *et al.*, "Potentiation of Anticoagulant Therapy by Oxyphenylbutazone: (A Probable Case)," *Postgrad. Med. J.*, *41*, 563 (1965).

(12) E. S. Vesell *et al.*, "Failure of Indomethacin and Warfarin to Interact in Normal Human Volunteers," *J. Clin. Pharmacol.*, *15*, 486 (1975).

(13) J. R. O'Brien *et al.*, "A Comparison of an Effect of Different Anti-inflammatory Drugs on Human Platelets," *J. Clin. Pathol.*, *23*, 522 (1970).

(14) H. Van Cauwenberge and L. B. Jaques, "Haemorrhagic Effect of ACTH with Anticoagulants," *Can. Med. Ass. J.*, *79*, 536 (1958).

(15) J. B. Chatterjea and L. Salomon,

"Antagonistic Effect of A.C.T.H. and Cortisone on the Anticoagulant Activity of Ethyl Biscoumacetate," *Brit. Med. J.*, *2*, 790 (1954).

[For additional information, see *Anticoagulant Therapy*, p. 358.]

Nonproprietary and Trade Names of Drugs

Acenocoumarol—*Sintrom*
Anisindione—*Miradon*
Dicumarol—*Various manufacturers*
Diphenadione—*Dipaxin*
Ibuprofen—*Motrin*
Indomethacin—*Indocin*

Phenindione—*Hedulin*
Phenprocoumon—*Liquamar*
Warfarin potassium—*Athrombin-K*
Warfarin sodium—*Coumadin Sodium, Panwarfin*

Prepared and evaluated by the Scientific Review Subpanel on Anticoagulants and reviewed by Practitioner Panel VI.

Warfarin—Meprobamate

Summary—Meprobamate is capable of inducing the hepatic microsomal enzymes that metabolize warfarin in animals. However, clinical evidence for this antagonism using normally prescribed meprobamate doses is lacking, and concurrent use of these drugs does not need to be avoided.

Related Drugs—Chemically related analogs of the simple aliphatic compound, meprobamate, in clinical use include **carisoprodol, chlormezanone, chlorphenesin, methocarbamol,** and **tybamate.** Other coumarin anticoagulants include **acenocoumarol, dicumarol,** and **phenprocoumon.** The indandione anticoagulants include **anisindione, diphenadione,** and **phenindione.**

Pharmacological Effect and Mechanism—Meprobamate is capable of inducing the hepatic microsomal enzymes involved in drug metabolism in animals (1). Therefore, it may accelerate the metabolic inactivation of the large number of drugs metabolized by this enzyme system. Meprobamate was reported to have accelerated its own metabolism in humans when given for prolonged periods (1) and reduced the serum warfarin half-life in dogs when administered (~ 100 mg/kg) for 12 days (2).

Evaluation of Clinical Data—Meprobamate (1.6 g/day po) was administered for 2 weeks (3) to nine patients stabilized on long-term warfarin therapy. Meprobamate was then withdrawn but observation of the patients continued for 2 weeks. The one-stage prothrombin time decreased slightly in five patients, increased slightly in three, and remained constant in one (3).

In a controlled study (4), 10 patients stabilized on long-term anticoagulant therapy received meprobamate (2.4 g/day po) for 4 weeks. The prothrombin time was studied for 7 weeks, starting 1 week prior to administration of meprobamate and ending 2 weeks after meprobamate was discontinued. A control group of 11 patients stabilized on long-term warfarin therapy was given a placebo during this period. The addition of meprobamate to the regimen showed a tendency to reduce prothrombin time when compared with the placebo group. However, the difference was not sufficient to warrant additional caution in monitoring these patients, and there was no demonstrated difference in the two groups after meprobamate and the placebo were withdrawn.

■ The clinical data indicate that concurrent administration of meprobamate and warfarin causes little, if any, change in the prothrombin time. If there is any effect on the prothrombin time, it is not clinically significant.

Recommendations—Since the data indicate that a clinically significant drug interaction does not occur, concurrent use of warfarin and meprobamate need not be avoided.

References

(1) A. H. Conney, "Pharmacological Implications of Microsomal Enzyme Induction," *Pharmacol. Rev.*, *19*, 317 (1967).

(2) D. B. Hunninghake and D. L. Azarnoff, "Drug Interactions with Warfarin," *Arch. Intern. Med.*, *121*, 349 (1968).

(3) J. A. Udall, "Warfarin Therapy not Influenced by Meprobamate. A Controlled Study in Nine Men," *Curr. Ther. Res.*, *12*, 724 (1970).

(4) L. Gould *et al.*, "Prothrombin Levels Maintained with Meprobamate and Warfarin," *J. Amer. Med. Ass.*, *220*, 1460 (1972).

[For additional information, see *Anticoagulant Therapy*, p. 358.]

Nonproprietary and Trade Names of Drugs

Acenocoumarol—*Sintrom*
Anisindione—*Miradon*
Carisoprodol—*Rela, Soma*
Chlormezanone—*Trancopal*
Chlorphenesin carbamate—*Maolate*
Dicumarol—*Various manufacturers*
Diphenadione—*Dipaxin*
Meprobamate—*Equanil, Meprospan, Miltown, and various combination products*

Methocarbamol—*Robaxin*
Phenindione—*Hedulin*
Phenprocoumon—*Liquamar*
Tybamate—*Solacen, Tybatran*
Warfarin potassium—*Athrombin-K*
Warfarin sodium—*Coumadin Sodium, Panwarfin*

Prepared and evaluated by the Scientific Review Subpanel on Anticoagulants and reviewed by Practitioner Panel I.

Warfarin—Methandrostenolone

Summary—Methandrostenolone and other C-17-alkylated androgens in therapeutic doses increase the hypoprothrombinemic action of warfarin significantly. Reduction of the anticoagulant dosage is probably necessary when these drugs are used concurrently.

Related Drugs—In theory, all C-17-alkylated androgens should be capable of causing this type of interaction. There is clinical evidence that **norethandrolone** (1) and **oxymetholone** (2) can do so. Other C-17-alkylated androgens are **fluoxymesterone, methyltestosterone, oxandrolone,** and **stanozolol.**

The activity of the coumarin anticoagulants **acenocoumarol** (3) and **dicumarol** (1) and the indandione anticoagulant **phenindione** (4) have also been enhanced by the C-17-alkylated androgens. Other coumarin (*e.g.*, **phenprocoumon**) or indandione (*e.g.*, **anisindione** and **diphenadione)** anticoagulants may interact with the C-17-alkylated androgens.

Pharmacological Effect and Mechanism—Methandrostenolone (5) and other C-17-alkylated androgens produce a significant decrease in the anticoagulant requirement of patients receiving oral anticoagulants. Despite adequate documentation, however, a satisfactory explanation for the decreased tolerance produced by these agents has not been found. None of the C-17-alkylated androgens causes an alteration of metabolism of warfarin (1, 6).

There is no evidence of a change in prothrombin complex activity due to the drugs (5, 6). Alternative suggestions as to the mode of action include a possible increase in the rate of decay of clotting proteins or a decrease in the availability of vitamin K to receptor sites in the liver (1). Another suggestion (1) was the enhancement of the anticoagulant effect by an increase in the affinity of receptor sites for warfarin. Because these drugs are known to produce minor changes in liver function, there is a possibility that the hepatic synthesizing capacity for vitamin K-sensitive clotting factors is altered. However, in the absence of anticoagulants, prothrombin time prolongation by androsterone has not been noted. The precise mechanism of action, therefore, remains unclear.

Evaluation of Clinical Data—In seven patients receiving warfarin, methandrostenolone (10 mg/day po) produced a significant decrease (~ 38%) in anticoagulant dosage requirements after 2 weeks (5). Similar data were provided when norethandrolone (10 mg/day po) was administered to 10 patients stabilized on anticoagulants (1). A case (7) was reported with clinical hemorrhage when methandrostenolone (5 mg/day po) was given to a patient who had previously been under good anticoagulant control.

The anticoagulant effect was increased after the addition of oxymetholone (2 mg/kg po) to five patients receiving anticoagulants and undergoing chronic hemodialysis (2). Each of these patients developed clinical bleeding episodes in addition to prolongation of the prothrombin time. Enhancement of the anticoagulant effect was reported (4) in six cases when oxymetholone (15 mg/day po) was given to patients stabilized on warfarin. Two of these cases resulted in significant bleeding episodes.

In 11 patients (3, 8–10) who received either methandrostenolone (5–9 mg/day po) or oxymetholone (30–200 mg/day po) concurrently with acenocoumarol or warfarin, the anticoagulant dose had to be reduced significantly. In four cases, moderate to severe hemorrhage occurred and one patient was switched and maintained on a non-C-17-alkylated androgen with no similar adverse effects.

■ Enhancement of the activity of anticoagulant drugs occurs frequently in individuals who also receive methandrostenolone or other C-17-alkylated androgens. The effect is clinically significant and may produce serious hemorrhagic complications. Non-C-17-alkylated androgens may not cause a similar effect, but there are insufficient data to support this conclusion.

Recommendations—While there is no contraindication to the concurrent use of warfarin or other oral anticoagulants and methandrostenolone, the practitioner must be aware that enhancement of the anticoagulant effect frequently occurs with C-17-alkylated androgens and must be prepared to reduce the oral anticoagulant dosage as indicated by changes in the prothrombin time.

Although documentation is limited (8), the non-C-17-alkylated androgens (such as nandrolone) may not affect anticoagulant response significantly and may be considered as alternative drugs to the C-17-alkylated androgens.

References

(1) J. J. Schrogie and H. M. Solomon, "The Anticoagulant Response to Bis-hydroxycoumarin II. The Effect of D-Thyroxine, Clofibrate, and Nor-ethandrolone," *Clin. Pharmacol. Ther.,* 8, 70 (1967).
(2) B. H. B. Robinson *et al.,* "Decreased

Anticoagulant Tolerance with Oxymetholone," *Lancet, i,* 1356 (1971).
(3) J. C. De Oya *et al.,* "Decreased Anticoagulant Tolerance with Oxymetholone in Paroxysmal Nocturnal Haemoglobinuria," *Lancet, ii,* 259 (1971).

(4) R. G. M. Longridge *et al.*, "Decreased Anticoagulant Tolerance with Oxymetholone," *Lancet, ii,* 90 (1971).

(5) K. Pyorala and M. Kekki, "Decreased Anticoagulant Tolerance during Methandrostenolone Therapy," *Scand. J. Clin. Lab. Invest., 15,* 367 (1963).

(6) J. Koch-Weser and E. M. Sellers, "Drug Interactions with Coumarin Anticoagulants," *N. Engl. J. Med., 285,* 547 (1971).

(7) G. E. McLaughlin *et al.*, "Hemarthrosis Complicating Anticoagulant

Therapy: Report of Three Cases," *J. Amer. Med. Ass., 196,* 1020 (1966).

(8) M. S. Edwards and J. R. Curtis, "Decreased Anticoagulant Tolerance with Oxymetholone," *Lancet, ii,* 221 (1971).

(9) F. C. Dresdale and J. C. Hayes, "Potential Dangers in the Combined Use of Methandrostenolone and Sodium Warfarin," *J. Med. Soc. N.J., 64,* 609 (1967).

(10) M. Murakami *et al.*, "Effects of Anabolic Steroids on Anticoagulant Requirements," *Jap. Circ. J., 29,* 243 (1965).

[For additional information, see *Anticoagulant Therapy,* p. 358.]

Nonproprietary and Trade Names of Drugs

Acenocoumarol—*Sintrom*
Anisindione—*Miradon*
Dicumarol—*Various manufacturers*
Diphenadione—*Dipaxin*
Fluoxymesterone—*Halotestin, Ora-Testryl, Ultradren*
Methandrostenolone—*Dianabol*
Methyltestosterone—*Metandren, Oreton Methyl, and various combination products*
Nandrolone decanoate—*Deca-Durabolin*

Nandrolone phenpropionate—*Durabolin*
Norethandrolone—*Various manufacturers*
Oxandrolone—*Anavar*
Oxymetholone—*Adroyd, Anadrol*
Phenindione—*Hedulin*
Phenprocoumon—*Liquamar*
Stanozolol—*Winstrol*
Warfarin potassium—*Athrombin-K*
Warfarin sodium—*Coumadin Sodium, Panwarfin*

Prepared and evaluated by the Scientific Review Subpanel on Anticoagulants and reviewed by Practitioner Panel II.

Warfarin—Phenobarbital

Summary—The anticoagulant effect of warfarin can be decreased in patients receiving phenobarbital concurrently, and it may be necessary to increase the warfarin dose to achieve the desired anticoagulant activity. However, if phenobarbital is then subsequently discontinued, it probably will be necessary to decrease the warfarin dosage accordingly.

Related Drugs—Although most reports of barbiturate–anticoagulant interactions involved the use of phenobarbital with warfarin or **dicumarol** (1–4), the other commercially available coumarin anticoagulants, **acenocoumarol** (4) and **phenprocoumon** (5), are influenced similarly. Similar caution also is indicated with the indandione anticoagulants, **anisindione, diphenadione,** and **phenindione,** although no interactions have been reported.

Other barbiturates, **amobarbital** (6, 7), **aprobarbital** (8), **barbital** (9, 10), **butabarbital** (5), **pentobarbital** (11), and **secobarbital** (6, 7), also interact with the coumarin anticoagulants. All other **barbiturates** may act in a manner similar to that of phenobarbital in reducing anticoagulant activity, although there are no specific reports.

Pharmacological Effect and Mechanism—Phenobarbital increases the synthesis and activity of the liver microsomal enzymes involved in the metabolism of many drugs, including anticoagulants such as warfarin (2, 12). Although warfarin exists as two isomers, the barbiturates increase the biotransformation of both comparably (13). The result of this interaction is a decreased response to the anticoagulant due to more rapid metabolism and excretion.

Factors other than enzyme induction may be involved in the barbiturate-induced decrease in anticoagulant activity. One report (1) indicated that heptabarbital may decrease the absorption of dicumarol from the gastrointestinal (GI) tract. Another study (2) suggested that the decreased effect of warfarin after heptabarbital treatment is attributable only to the induction of liver enzymes and that there is no evidence that heptabarbital affects the distribution of warfarin in the body, the synthesis or degradation of clotting factors, or the affinity between warfarin and its receptors. In contrast to the other coumarins, the GI absorption of dicumarol is incomplete. Therefore, the different findings of these two studies (1, 2) (as to the mechanisms involved in producing a decreased anticoagulant effect) suggest that differences may exist depending on the particular anticoagulant used.

Evaluation of Clinical Data—Chronic phenobarbital administration (65–120 mg/day po) significantly lowered the serum dicumarol levels (by ~ 30%) in eight patients (3). A decrease in the warfarin half-life (of >20%) also was noted in 13 of 21 patients receiving phenobarbital concurrently (210 mg/day po) (14). There was no apparent explanation why some patients experienced this effect and others did not. Phenobarbital did not notably affect the GI absorption of warfarin, and the altered activity was attributed to enzyme induction.

A decreased warfarin effect (by ~ 25%) was observed in 15 of 16 patients who were receiving phenobarbital (~ 2 mg/kg/day po) (15). The effect became evident after the first week of concurrent therapy. After phenobarbital was discontinued, warfarin activity gradually returned to the control values, but satisfactory control was not achieved in most cases until at least 2 weeks after phenobarbital was discontinued.

In a review of the records of 52 patients treated with anticoagulants, 40 patients also received a barbiturate (16). The control of the anticoagulant effect was more erratic in the patients also receiving a barbiturate and increased doses of the anticoagulant also were required (sometimes up to three times greater than prebarbiturate requirements). Discontinuation of the barbiturate may have precipitated hemorrhage that resulted in two deaths (16).

In 10 healthy subjects, phenobarbital (120 mg/day po) lowered the serum warfarin level and reduced the warfarin half-life by nearly 50% (17). This study involved a determination of serum warfarin levels and prothrombin times after a single warfarin dose (40–60 mg po) given prior to and immediately following 3 weeks of phenobarbital administration.

Barbiturates other than phenobarbital also decrease anticoagulant activity. Butabarbital (15–30 mg po four times daily) altered significantly (by ~ 38%) the amount of warfarin (in five patients) and phenprocoumon (in seven patients) necessary for optimum prothrombin activity (5). This effect was seen as early as 2 weeks after initiation of butabarbital therapy and the decrease in anticoagulant activity persisted for about 6 weeks after withdrawal of butabarbital.

There have been conflicting reports concerning the activity of secobarbital. Secobarbital did not have a noticeable effect on drug metabolism in one study (18), but other observations indicate that secobarbital may decrease anticoagulant activity. In eight healthy subjects, usual hypnotic doses (100–200 mg po) of secobarbital accelerated the metabolism of warfarin significantly, causing a decrease in anticoagulant activity (7). In another study (6) of three subjects, secobarbital caused a significant decrease in serum warfarin levels with an accompanying change in anticoagulant control. Administration of secobarbital (100 mg po at night) to six patients for 33 nights caused a reduction in the steady-state concentration that ranged from 5 to 64.5% (19).

Studies with amobarbital demonstrated that this agent also is likely to decrease the anticoagulant activity of warfarin (6, 7).

■ When phenobarbital (or another barbiturate) is given concurrently with warfarin (or another coumarin anticoagulant), it is likely that there will be a resultant decrease in anticoagulant activity. This interaction is probably related to the dose of the barbiturate used (19). The lowest dose of phenobarbital causing enzyme induction in these studies was 65 mg/day (3).

The amount of decrease in warfarin activity is difficult to predict because of individual variation in response to the anticoagulant, but it has been estimated to be as high as 50% (12). Because of this decrease, the patient may be deprived of adequate anticoagulant therapy and may be exposed to an increased risk of thrombus formation. Even if the interaction is recognized and the warfarin dose is increased to compensate for the loss of activity, serious problems can still occur. If phenobarbital is discontinued, the warfarin dose will probably have to be reduced. Otherwise, the higher dosage that is necessary when phenobarbital is given concurrently may be excessive when it is withdrawn and may result in hemorrhage.

The sequence of administration of the two drugs also may be an important factor in the development of an interaction. If phenobarbital therapy is initiated in a patient stabilized on a particular dose of warfarin, it is likely that the anticoagulant effect will be decreased, necessitating an increase in dosage. Conversely, if warfarin therapy is initiated in a patient already receiving phenobarbital, the enzyme induction effect already will be present and the dose of warfarin will be established initially at a time when liver enzyme activity is increased. In either case, if phenobarbital is discontinued, the therapy should be monitored closely and the need for reducing the anticoagulant dosage must be considered.

All barbiturates may cause enzyme induction and it is likely that their individual capacities to produce this effect are similar. It is difficult to anticipate the rate of onset and the extent of enzyme induction or how rapidly the enzyme activity will return to normal levels when the barbiturate is discontinued. These factors vary with the individual and also depend on the dosage and the duration of treatment with the barbiturate. Several studies (1, 2, 14, 16) indicated that the effect of barbiturates in decreasing anticoagulant activity is evident within 2–5 days and it is likely that barbiturate administration for 1 week or longer will produce this effect in almost all patients (12). There is considerable variation in the extent of this effect from one patient to another. There have been varying reports about how rapidly enzyme activity returns to pretreatment levels when the barbiturate is discontinued. However, it is probable that normal enzyme activity will be restored in 2–3 weeks in most situations (12).

Recommendations—Although warfarin therapy must be monitored closely even if other drugs are not given concurrently, particular caution must be exercised when phenobarbital is administered concurrently. If possible, it is best to avoid the concurrent use of warfarin and phenobarbital, although appropriate dosage adjustments could be made if such therapy is necessary.

The benzodiazepines have not been shown to interact with anticoagulants (see *Warfarin–Chlordiazepoxide*, p. 276) and one of these agents might be a useful alternative to a barbiturate in patients for whom a barbiturate might be prescribed.

When coumarin anticoagulant therapy is employed, particular caution is warranted when any drug is added to or withdrawn from the drug regimen. Patients should be advised to contact their physician or pharmacist before initiating, changing, or discontinuing any drug including their nonprescription medications.

The practitioner should also be aware that many combination products contain phenobarbital in quantities sufficient to affect warfarin activity.

References

(1) P. M. Aggeler and R. A. O'Reilly, "Effect of Heptabarbital on the Response to Bishydroxycoumarin in Man," *J. Lab. Clin. Med., 74,* 229 (1969).

(2) G. Levy *et al.*, "Pharmacokinetic Analysis of the Effect of Barbiturate on the Anticoagulant Action of Warfarin in Man," *Clin. Pharmacol. Ther., 11,* 372 (1970).

(3) S. A. Cucinell *et al.*, "Drug Interactions in Man I. Lowering Effect of Phenobarbital on Plasma Levels of Bishydroxycoumarin (Dicumarol) and Diphenylhydantoin (Dilantin)," *Clin. Pharmacol. Ther., 6,* 420 (1965).

(4) P. G. Dayton *et al.*, "The Influence of Barbiturates on Coumarin Plasma Levels and Prothrombin Response," *J. Clin. Invest., 40,* 1797 (1961).

(5) A. M. Antlitz *et al.*, "Effect of Butabarbital on Orally Administered Anticoagulants," *Curr. Ther. Res., 10,* 70 (1968).

(6) A. Breckenridge and M. Orme, "Clinical Implications of Enzyme Induction," *Ann. N.Y. Acad. Sci., 179,* 421 (1971).

(7) D. S. Robinson and D. Sylwester, "Interaction of Commonly Prescribed Drugs and Warfarin," *Ann. Intern. Med., 72,* 853 (1970).

(8) S. Johansson, "Apparent Resistance to Oral Anticoagulant Therapy and Influence of Hypnotics on Some Coagulation Factors," *Acta Med. Scand., 184,* 297 (1968).

(9) R. M. Welch *et al.*, "An Experimental Model in Dogs for Studying Interactions of Drugs with Bishydroxycoumarin," *Clin. Pharmacol. Ther., 10,* 817 (1969).

(10) M. Weiner, "Effect of Centrally Active Drugs on the Action of Coumarin Anticoagulants," *Nature, 212,* 1599 (1966).

(11) O. N. Lucas, "Study of the Interaction of Barbiturates and Dicumarol and Their Effect on Prothrombin Activity, Hemorrhage, and Sleeping Time in Rats," *Can. J. Physiol. Pharmacol., 45,* 905 (1967).

(12) J. Koch-Weser and E. M. Sellers, "Drug Interactions with Coumarin Anticoagulants," *N. Engl. J. Med., 285,* 547 (1971).

(13) A. Breckenridge *et al.*, "Increased Rates of Drug Oxidation in Man," in "Drug Interaction," P. L. Morselli and S. Garattini, Eds., Raven, New York, N.Y., 1974, p. 223.

(14) M. Corn, "Effect of Phenobarbital and Glutethimide on Biological Half-Life of Warfarin," *Thromb. Diath. Haemorrh., 16,* 606 (1966).

(15) D. S. Robinson and M. G. MacDonald, "The Effect of Phenobarbital Administration on the Control of Coagulation Achieved during Warfarin Therapy," *Hosp. Form. Management, 2,* 43 (April 1967).

(16) M. G. MacDonald and D. S. Robinson, "Clinical Observations of Possible Barbiturate Interference with Anticoagulation," *J. Amer. Med. Ass., 204,* 97 (1968).

(17) M. G. MacDonald *et al.*, "The Effects of Phenobarbital, Chloral Betaine, and Glutethimide Administration on Warfarin Plasma Levels and Hypoprothrombinemic Responses in Man," *Clin. Pharmacol. Ther., 10,* 80 (1969).

(18) S. A. Cucinell *et al.*, "The Effect of Chloral Hydrate on Bishydroxycoumarin Metabolism. A Fatal Outcome," *J. Amer. Med. Ass., 197,* 366 (1966).

(19) A. Breckenridge *et al.*, "Dose-Dependent Enzyme Induction," *Clin. Pharmacol. Ther., 14,* 514 (1973).

[For additional information, see *Anticoagulant Therapy,* p. 358.]

Nonproprietary and Trade Names of Drugs

Acenocoumarol—*Sintrom*
Allobarbital—*Diadol*
Amobarbital—*Amytal and various combination products*
Anisindione—*Miradon*
Aprobarbital—*Alurate*
Barbital—*Neurondia*
Butabarbital sodium—*Butisol Sodium*
Butalbital—*Available in combination products*
Dicumarol—*Various manufacturers*
Diphenadione—*Dipaxin*
Hexobarbital—*Sombulex*
Mephobarbital—*Mebaral, Mebroin*

Metharbital—*Gemonil*
Methohexital sodium—*Brevital Sodium*
Pentobarbital—*Nembutal and various combination products*
Phenindione—*Hedulin*
Phenobarbital—*Eskabarb, Luminal*
Phenprocoumon—*Liquamar*
Secobarbital—*Seconal and various combination products*
Talbutal—*Lotusate*
Thiopental sodium—*Pentothal Sodium*
Warfarin potassium—*Athrombin-K*
Warfarin sodium—*Coumadin Sodium, Panwarfin*

Prepared and evaluated by the Scientific Review Subpanel on Anticoagulants and reviewed by Practitioner Panel III.

Warfarin—Phenylbutazone

Summary—Phenylbutazone enhances the hypoprothrombinemic effect of warfarin and causes serious bleeding episodes. Concurrent use of these drugs should be avoided.

Related Drugs—The coumarin anticoagulants **acenocoumarol** (1) and **phenprocoumon** (2) also have been reported to interact with phenylbutazone or its analogs. There has been no report about an interaction between **dicumarol** and phenylbutazone, but this anticoagulant would probably interact with phenylbutazone in a manner similar to warfarin.

Enhanced anticoagulant effect of indandiones such as **phenindione** has been attributed to phenylbutazone in two patients (3). However, *in vitro* studies using human plasma indicated that phenylbutazone does not alter the plasma binding of phenindione (1). Other indandiones are **anisindione** and **diphenadione.**

Oxyphenbutazone, a metabolite of phenylbutazone, also interacted with the coumarin anticoagulants in two humans (4, 5).

Pharmacological Effect and Mechanism—About 97% of warfarin in the blood is bound to plasma albumin (6). A comparable level of binding occurs with other coumarin and indandione drugs. Acidic drugs, such as phenylbutazone, can displace warfarin from its binding site on the albumin molecule, resulting in a greater concentration of unbound warfarin in the plasma. As more unbound warfarin becomes available to react with its specific sites of biological activity in the liver, the hypoprothrombinemic effect increases. At the same time, more unbound warfarin is available for metabolism by the hepatic drug-metabolizing enzymes, increasing the rates of warfarin degradation and elimination. Although the serum half-life of warfarin is decreased, the increase in unbound warfarin is the prominent effect (7).

In vitro tests (6–8) clearly demonstrated the displacing action of phenylbutazone on albumin-bound warfarin. Phenylbutazone markedly diminished the albumin–warfarin association constant by competing for binding sites on the albumin molecule (4, 6–8). The amount displaced increases with increasing serum concentrations of phenylbutazone (6). The effect of phenylbutazone on warfarin occurs at average therapeutic doses of phenylbutazone (300 mg/day po). In one experimental trial (9), enhancement of warfarin's action occurred soon after phenylbutazone therapy was started, and it can occur as early as 1 day (10, 11).

The interaction of phenylbutazone with warfarin is not the only cause of hemorrhagic complications. Phenylbutazone treatment produces an increase in gastric ulceration, and gastrointestinal (GI) hemorrhage has been a dangerous side effect. In patients treated with anticoagulants, the threat from such hemorrhage is even greater (10).

Experimentally, phenylbutazone diminishes collagen-induced platelet aggregation, and this reduction might contribute to bleeding episodes (12). In certain animal species, phenylbutazone induces hepatic microsomal drug-metabolizing enzymes, decreasing the anticoagulant effect of warfarin (13). Phenylbutazone has an enzyme-inducing effect in humans (14), but this effect on warfarin anticoagulation in humans has not been adequately studied.

This interaction might be influenced by the stereochemical structure of warfarin. Studies in humans indicated that phenylbutazone affects the plasma clearance of the two isomers of warfarin differently (15). The plasma clearance was slowed with one isomer while the plasma clearance increased with the other isomer. The rate of clearance of racemic warfarin was unaffected by phenylbutazone.

Evaluation of Clinical Data—Several case reports (4, 5, 16–18) implicate phenylbutazone and oxyphenbutazone as causing hypoprothrombinemia and bleeding in patients receiving anticoagulants. In a controlled study, a significant increase in the anticoagulant effect of warfarin was observed when phenylbutazone (300 mg/day po for 7 days) was given to 10 normal subjects (9).

■ The enhancement of the hypoprothrombinemic action of warfarin by phenylbutazone or its congeners can be expected to occur in almost all patients to whom these drugs are given (9). The effect can occur as early as 1 day after phenylbutazone is given to patients receiving anticoagulants and, quite predictably, in almost all patients within the first week of concurrent therapy (10, 11).

Recommendations—Concurrent warfarin and phenylbutazone therapy poses serious hemorrhagic threats to all patients in whom it is used and should be avoided. If it must be used, daily prothrombin determinations and close observation for episodes of bleeding are mandatory.

Alternatives to phenylbutazone should be used whenever possible. Aspirin interacts with warfarin and should not be used (see *Warfarin–Aspirin*, p. 270). Although indomethacin does not prolong prothrombin time (19), it does have side effects including gastric ulceration and bleeding that make it unsuitable for concurrent use with warfarin (see *Warfarin–Indomethacin*, p. 286). Ibuprofen does not enhance the hypoprothrombinemic effect of warfarin (20–22), but it does affect platelet function and cause gastric irritation (23, 24). Although it may be the most suitable alternative to phenylbutazone in anticoagulant-treated patients, it should still be used cautiously.

Excessive hypoprothrombinemia can be treated with phytonadione (vitamin K_1) (5–10 mg im or po) and by omission of the anticoagulant until prothrombin levels return to the proper range. Larger doses of vitamin K do not hasten response and will make the patient resistant to subsequent warfarin therapy. Evidence of hemorrhage requires immediate return of prothrombin levels to normal ranges, attention to blood volume restoration, and other medical and surgical treatments as indicated. If hemorrhage is severe, fresh frozen plasma may be given to supply clotting factors (25).

Antipyrine (*in vivo*) and sulfinpyrazone (*in vitro*) have been reported to interact with warfarin (26, 27) and should be used cautiously in patients receiving anticoagulants.

References

(1) J. P. Tillement *et al.*, "Effect of Phenylbutazone on the Binding of Vitamin K Antagonists to Albumin," *Eur. J. Clin. Pharmacol.*, *6*, 15 (1973).

(2) K. Seiler and F. Duckert, "Properties of 3-(1-Phenyl-Propyl)-4-Oxycoumarin (Marcoumar) in the Plasma When Tested in Normal Cases and Under the Influence of Drugs," *Thromb. Diath. Haemorrh.*, *19*, 89 (1968).

(3) A. Kindermann, "Vascular Allergis due to Butalidon and Hazards of Its Combined Use with Athrombon (Phenylindandione)," *Dermatol. Wochenschr.*, *143*, 172 (1961).

(4) C. B. Hobbs *et al.*, "Potentiation of Anticoagulant Therapy by Oxyphenylbutazone: (A Probable Case)," *Postgrad. Med. J.*, *41*, 563 (1965).

(5) S. Fox, "Potentiation of Anticoagulants Caused by Pyrazole Compounds," *J. Amer. Med. Ass.*, *188*, 320 (1964).

(6) H. M. Solomon and J. J. Schrogie, "The Effect of Various Drugs on the Binding of Warfarin-^{14}C to Human Albumin," *Biochem. Pharmacol.*, *16*, 1219 (1967).

(7) R. A. O'Reilly and G. Levy, "Pharmacokinetic Analysis of Potentiating Effect of Phenylbutazone on Anticoagulant Action of Warfarin in Man," *J. Pharm. Sci.*, *59*, 1258 (1970).

(8) P. M. Aggeler *et al.*, "Potentiation of Anticoagulant Effect of Warfarin by Phenylbutazone," *N. Engl. J. Med.*, *276*, 496 (1967).

(9) J. A. Udall, "Drug Interference with Warfarin Therapy," *Clin. Med.*, *77* (8), 20 (1970).

(10) J. Koch-Weser and E. M. Sellers, "Drug Interactions with Coumarin Anticoagulants," *N. Engl. J. Med.*, *285*, 487, 547 (1971).

(11) E. M. Sellers and J. Koch-Weser, "Kinetics and Clinical Importance of Displacement of Warfarin from Albumin by Acidic Drugs," *Ann. N.Y. Acad. Sci., 179*, 213 (1971).

(12) R. A. O'Reilly and P. M. Aggeler, "Determinants of the Response to Oral Anticoagulant Drugs in Man," *Pharmacol. Rev., 22*, 35 (1970).

(13) R. M. Welch *et al.*, "An Experimental Model in Dogs for Studying Interactions of Drugs with Bishydroxycoumarin," *Clin. Pharmacol. Ther., 10*, 817 (1969).

(14) A. H. Conney, "Pharmacological Implications of Microsomal Enzyme Induction," *Pharmacol. Rev., 19*, 317 (1967).

(15) R. J. Lewis *et al.*, "Warfarin: Stereochemical Aspects of Its Metabolism and the Interaction with Phenylbutazone," *J. Clin. Invest., 53*, 1607 (1974).

(16) M. J. Eisen, "Combined Effect of Sodium Warfarin and Phenylbutazone," *J. Amer. Med. Ass., 189*, 64 (1964).

(17) B. I. Hoffbrand and D. A. Kininmonth, "Potentiation of Anticoagulants," *Brit. Med. J., 2*, 838 (1967).

(18) J. Bull and J. Mackinnon, "Phenylbutazone and Anticoagulant Control," *Practitioner, 215*, 767 (1975).

(19) E. S. Vesell *et al.*, "Failure of Indomethacin and Warfarin to Interact in Normal Human Volunteers," *J. Clin. Pharmacol., 15*, 486 (1975).

(20) L. J. Davis, "Ibuprofen," *Drug Intel., 9*, 501 (1975).

(21) L. Goncalves, "Influence of Ibuprofen on Homeostasis in Patients on Anticoagulant Therapy," *J. Intern. Med. Res., 1*, 180 (1973).

(22) D. Thilo and F. Duckert, "A Study of the Effects of the Anti-Rheumatic Drug Ibuprofen (Brufen) on Patients Being Treated with the Oral Anticoagulant Phenprocoumon (Marcoumin)," *J. Intern. Med. Res., 2*, 276 (1974).

(23) J. R. Lewis, "Evaluation of Ibuprofen (Motrin)," *J. Amer. Med. Ass., 233*, 364 (1975).

(24) E. F. Davies and G. S. Avery, "Ibuprofen: A Review of Its Pharmacological Properties and Therapeutic Efficacy in Rheumatic Disorders," *Drugs, 2*, 416 (1971).

(25) W. W. Coon and P. W. Willis, "Some Aspects of the Pharmacology of Oral Anticoagulants," *Clin. Pharmacol. Ther., 11*, 312 (1970).

(26) A. Breckenridge *et al.*, "Drug Interactions with Warfarin: Dichloralphenazone, Chloral Hydrate and Phenazone (Antipyrine)," *Clin. Sci., 40*, 351 (1971).

(27) K. Seiler and F. Duckert, "Intoxication with Phenprocoumon (Marcoumar). Pharmacokinetics and Side Effects," *Thromb. Diath. Haemorrh., 21*, 320 (1969).

[For additional information, see *Anticoagulant Therapy*, p. 358.]

Nonproprietary and Trade Names of Drugs

Acenocoumarol—*Sintrom*
Anisindione—*Miradon*
Antipyrine—*Various manufacturers*
Dicumarol—*Various manufacturers*
Diphenadione—*Dipaxin*
Ibuprofen—*Motrin*
Oxyphenbutazone—*Oxalid, Tandearil*
Phenindione—*Hedulin*

Phenprocoumon—*Liquamar*
Phenylbutazone—*Azolid, Butazolidin*
Phytonadione—*AquaMephyton, Konakion*
Sulfinpyrazone—*Anturane*
Warfarin potassium—*Athrombin-K*
Warfarin sodium—*Coumadin Sodium, Panwarfin*

Prepared and evaluated by the Scientific Review Subpanel on Anticoagulants and reviewed by Practitioner Panel IV.

Warfarin—Quinidine

Summary—Quinidine and its analogs exert a mild direct hypoprothrombinemic effect which enhances the hypoprothrombinemic action of warfarin in some patients and may cause hemorrhage. Concurrent therapy should be avoided whenever possible; in those situations where both drugs are necessary, appropriate caution must be exercised.

Related Drugs—The other cinchona alkaloids, **cinchophen** and **quinine,** apparently exert a direct hypoprothrombinemic effect by depressing the hepatic enzyme system that synthesizes the vitamin K-dependent factors II, VII, IX, and X (1–3) and could interact with warfarin also. Quinidine is available as the **gluconate, hydrochloride, polygalacturonate,** and **sulfate.**

The coumarin anticoagulant **dicumarol** and the indandione anticoagulant **phenindione** have been reported to be similar to warfarin with respect to an interaction with quinidine (2).

The other coumarin anticoagulants, **acenocoumarol** and **phenprocoumon,** and the indandione anticoagulants, **anisindione** and **diphenadione,** are also expected to behave similarly.

Pharmacological Effect and Mechanism—The cinchona alkaloids are capable of depressing vitamin K-dependent clotting factor production by a direct effect on the liver enzyme system (1–3). Therefore, certain patients, whose synthesis of these clotting factors is already depressed by warfarin, may develop excessive hypoprothrombinemia with bleeding when quinidine is administered concurrently (3).

Evaluation of Clinical Data—There are at least two reports (3, 4) of four patients stabilized on warfarin who developed severe hypoprothrombinemia and, in three cases, hemorrhage when quinidine (600–1200 mg/day po) was administered. Although the addition of quinidine to the regimen was not positively identified as the causative factor of the hypoprothrombinemia, it was the only common factor. Moreover, the prothrombin activity returned to normal levels after quinidine was discontinued. A survey of 1500 patients treated with anticoagulants noted that quinidine had been responsible for hemorrhage in many cases, but no data were given (5).

However, a well-controlled study of 10 patients stabilized on warfarin did not show any statistically significant change in prothrombin time when quinidine (800 mg/day po) was added to the drug regimen (6).

■ The clinical evidence indicates that this drug interaction probably does not occur in all patients. Nevertheless, the severity of the outcome of using these drugs together is sufficient to recommend extreme caution when these drugs are given concurrently.

Recommendations—The concurrent administration of warfarin and quinidine is not recommended; but, if necessary, it should be undertaken cautiously with frequent monitoring of prothrombin times and clinical symptoms of warfarin overdose (*e.g.,* hematuria, melena, and bruising). Use of an alternative antiarrhythmic agent that does not interact with warfarin (*e.g.,* procainamide) may be preferable to the use of quinidine.

References

(1) L. A. Pirk and R. Engelberg, "Hypoprothrombinemic Action of Quinidine Sulfate," *J. Amer. Med. Ass., 128,* 1093 (1945).

(2) S. Jarnum, "Cinchophen and Acetylsalicylic Acid in Anticoagulant Treatment," *Scand. J. Clin. Lab. Invest., 6,* 91 (1954).

(3) J. Koch-Weser, "Quinidine-Induced Hypoprothrombinemic Hemorrhage in Patients on Chronic Warfarin Therapy," *Ann. Intern. Med., 68,* 511 (1968).

(4) A. B. Gazzaniga and D. R. Stewart, "Possible Quinidine-Induced Hemorrhage in a Patient on Warfarin Sodium," *N. Engl. J. Med., 280,* 711 (1969).

(5) J. L. Beaumont and A. Tarrit, "Les Accidents Hemorragiques Survenus au Cours de 1500 Traitements Anticoagulants," *Sang., 26,* 680 (1955).

(6) J. A. Udall, "Drug Interference with Warfarin Therapy," *Clin. Med., 77* (8), 20 (1970).

[For additional information, see *Anticoagulant Therapy,* p. 358.]

Nonproprietary and Trade Names of Drugs

Acenocoumarol—*Sintrom*
Anisindione—*Miradon*
Cinchophen—*Atophan*
Dicumarol—*Various manufacturers*
Diphenadione—*Dipaxin*
Phenindione—*Hedulin*
Phenprocoumon—*Liquamar*
Procainamide hydrochloride—*Pronestyl*
Quinidine gluconate—*Quinaglute*

Quinidine hydrochloride—*Various manufacturers*
Quinidine polygalacturonate—*Cardioquin*
Quinidine sulfate—*Quinidate, Quinidex*
Quinine—*Various manufacturers*
Warfarin potassium—*Athrombin-K*
Warfarin sodium—*Coumadin Sodium, Panwarfin*

*Prepared and evaluated by the Scientific Review Subpanel
on Anticoagulants and reviewed by Practitioner Panel I.*

Warfarin—Tetracycline

Summary—There is a theoretical possibility that tetracycline may interfere with warfarin activity, but there is no direct clinical evidence that this effect occurs. Until more clinical data are published, no additional precautions other than those normally utilized for these drugs are necessary.

Related Drugs—Various **tetracycline analogs** are available. Other coumarin anticoagulants include **acenocoumarol, dicumarol,** and **phenprocoumon.** Indandione anticoagulants include **anisindione, diphenadione,** and **phenindione.**

Pharmacological Effect and Mechanism—Tetracycline is a broad spectrum antibiotic that prevents bacterial cell polypeptide synthesis by blocking attachment of amino acid–transfer-RNA complexes to ribosomes (1).

Warfarin produces its anticoagulant effect by inhibiting the vitamin K-dependent synthesis of factors II, VII, IX, and X in the liver (1). Theoretically, tetracycline may enhance warfarin activity by reducing intestinal bacteria and decreasing the availability of vitamin K produced by the bacteria. However, vitamin K availability is not dependent solely on bacterial synthesis but is also dependent on dietary intake. Therefore, when bacterial synthesis of vitamin K is decreased, hypoprothrombinemia occurs only if the dietary intake of vitamin K is also restricted (2, 3). Another postulated mechanism (4) suggests that the tetracycline antibiotics themselves may act as anticoagulants by preventing the conversion of prothrombin to thrombin.

Evaluation of Clinical Data—Although references to alterations of warfarin therapy induced by tetracycline have appeared (5, 6), there is no adequate documentation for this interaction. In one study (4), 25 randomly selected patients treated with tetracycline (or an analog) were observed to ascertain if tetracycline influenced the blood coagulation process. The patients were receiving intravenous infusions of the antibiotics (0.5–1.0 g/liter). In most cases, the patients had received the antibiotics for several days prior to the study. No baseline coagulation studies were done. Plasma prothrombin activity in 14 patients was slightly to markedly diminished when it was determined by the Quick technique. However, when determined using the more specific, modified one-stage test, prothrombin activity was not as markedly depressed. Plasma prothrombin utilization appeared to be impaired in six of these patients. The results suggested that tetracycline may impair the utilization of prothrombin during the blood coagulation process. Upon investigation of plasma thromboplastin generation in two healthy subjects and five patients receiving intensive tetracycline therapy, it was postulated that tetracycline might prevent the conversion of antihemophilic globulin to its active form (4).

There have been three reports of gastrointestinal hemorrhage following tetracycline administration (oral and intramuscular). However, in these cases, it is impossible to rule out causative factors other than the antibiotic itself (7).

■ No direct evidence indicates that the oral administration of tetracycline has a significant effect on the hypoprothrombinemic activity of oral anticoagulants. Moreover, the one study investigating the hypoprothrombinemic effects of tetracycline was poorly designed (4). Since no baseline coagulation tests were performed on these patients prior to tetracycline administration, the results may be due to individual patient variation or to laboratory error.

Recommendations—The possibility of enhanced warfarin activity by orally administered tetracycline appears to be slight when dietary intake of vitamin K is maintained at adequate levels. Therefore, the concurrent use of these drugs in patients with adequate dietary intake of vitamin K would not be expected to result in adverse effects. Nevertheless, close monitoring of prothrombin activity is warranted when the two drugs are administered concurrently as it generally is whenever any drug is added to or deleted from the regimen of any patient receiving an anticoagulant.

References

(1) "The Pharmacological Basis of Therapeutics," 5th ed., L. S. Goodman and A. Gilman, Eds., Macmillan, New York, NY 10022, 1975, pp. 1184, 1355.
(2) R. A. O'Reilly and P. M. Aggeler, "Determinants of the Response to Oral Anticoagulant Drugs in Man," *Pharmacol. Rev.*, *22*, 35 (1970).
(3) J. A. Udall, "Human Sources and Absorption of Vitamin K in Relation to Anticoagulation Stability," *J. Amer. Med. Ass.*, *194*, 127 (1965).
(4) R. L. Searcy *et al.*, "Evaluation of the Blood-Clotting Mechanism in Tetracycline-Treated Patients," *Antimicrob. Ag. Chemother.*, *4*, 179 (1964).
(5) D. Bernstein, "Drugs Known to Interact with Coumarin-Type Anticoagulants," *Drug Intel.*, *5*, 276 (1971).
(6) I. H. Stockley, "Interactions with Anti-Infective Agents," *Pharm. J.*, *210*, 36 (1973).
(7) A. P. Klippel and B. Pitsinger, "Hypoprothombinemia Secondary to Antibiotic Therapy and Manifested by Massive Gastrointestinal Hemorrhage," *Arch. Surg.*, *96*, 226 (1968).

[For additional information, see *Anticoagulant Therapy*, p. 358.]

Nonproprietary and Trade Names of Drugs

Acenocoumarol—*Sintrom*
Anisindione—*Miradon*
Chlortetracycline hydrochloride—*Aureomycin*
Demeclocycline—*Declomycin*
Dicumarol—*Various manufacturers*
Diphenadione—*Dipaxin*
Doxycycline monohydrate—*Doxy-II Monohydrate, Doxychel, Vibramycin Monohydrate*
Methacycline hydrochloride—*Rondomycin*
Minocycline hydrochloride—*Minocin, Vectrin*
Oxytetracycline—*Dalimycin, Terramycin*
Oxytetracycline hydrochloride—*Oxy-Kesso-Tetra, Oxy-Tetrachel, Terramycin Hydrochloride*

Phenindione—*Hedulin*
Phenprocoumon—*Liquamar*
Rolitetracycline—*Syntetrin*
Tetracycline—*Achromycin, Panmycin, Panmycin KM, Sumycin, Tetracyn, Tetrex-S*
Tetracycline hydrochloride—*Achromycin, Bristacycline, Cyclopar, Panmycin, Robitet, Steclin, Sumycin, Tetracyn*
Tetracycline phosphate complex—*Tetrex*
Warfarin potassium—*Athrombin-K*
Warfarin sodium—*Coumadin Sodium, Panwarfin*

Prepared and evaluated by the Scientific Review Subpanel on Anticoagulants and reviewed by Practitioner Panel II.

Warfarin—Thyroid

Summary—Thyroid compounds increase the hypoprothrombinemic effect of warfarin and other anticoagulants. Close monitoring of the prothrombin time is required when these drugs are given concurrently to determine if a reduction in the warfarin dose is needed.

Related Drugs—The coumarin anticoagulants **acenocoumarol** (1) and **dicumarol** (2) and the indandione anticoagulant **phenindione** (1) have been shown to interact with a thyroid compound. Although clinical evidence is lacking, all other coumarin (**phenprocoumon**) and indandione (**anisindione** and **diphenadione**) anticoagulants may be expected to interact in a similar manner with thyroid compounds.

Since all thyroid compounds are basically alike (3), they all should be expected to interact with anticoagulants similarly. This conclusion is supported by the clinical evidence that **liothyronine** (1) and **thyroid extract** (4) (which contains thyroxine and liothyronine) have enhanced the effects of oral anticoagulants.

Pharmacological Effect and Mechanism—In mice, large doses of both dextrothyroxine and levothyroxine inhibited the metabolism of dicumarol (2). It has been demonstrated in rats that the activity level of the thyroid affects the prothrombin time response to warfarin (5). Rats made hypothyroid by the administration of methimazole had a decreased response to warfarin while rats made hyperthyroid by the administration of levothyroxine had an increased response to warfarin with a significant increase in hypoprothrombinemia.

In humans, therapeutic doses of dextrothyroxine enhance the anticoagulant effect of dicumarol but do not affect its rate of metabolism. The concentration of the vitamin K-dependent clotting factors has not been demonstrated to be affected by treatment with dextrothyroxine. Absorption and distribution of dicumarol are not affected since its serum levels are not altered by treatment with dextrothyroxine (2, 6).

At therapeutic levels, dextrothyroxine does not displace warfarin from human albumin binding sites (6) but does increase the affinity of the warfarin receptor site for warfarin by a factor of 2.4 (7). This increase in receptor site affinity for the oral anticoagulants is thought to be responsible for the increased anticoagulant effect observed in patients treated with both coumarin and indandione anticoagulants.

However, there are other possible explanations for the enhancement of the effect of the oral anticoagulants by thyroid compounds, including the enhancement of anticoagulant action by a decrease in serum lipids with a reduction in the availability of vitamin K (8). Thyroid compounds that produce a hypermetabolic state (liothyronine and thyroxine) increase the rate of decay of the vitamin K-dependent clotting factors and, in the presence of oral anticoagulants, normal compensation by increased synthesis is prevented (9, 10).

Evaluation of Clinical Data—Seven of 11 patients receiving dextrothyroxine (4–8 mg/day po) required a reduction in the dose of warfarin ranging from 2.5 to 30 mg during the first 4 weeks of therapy (11). A hemorrhagic episode occurred in one patient.

A patient receiving long-term anticoagulant therapy developed myxedema and required an approximately threefold increase in the acenocoumarol dose (1). Following treatment with liothyronine (16 mg/day po) and restoration to a normal metabolic state, the anticoagulant requirement returned to premyxedematous levels. A second myxedematous patient required phenindione (200 mg/day po) to maintain the prothrombin time in the therapeutic range. Following treatment with liothyronine (dose not reported), the requirement for phenindione decreased to 75 mg/day.

■ Several reports (1, 11) demonstrate that the interaction of thyroid preparations and the oral anticoagulants is clinically significant. Many patients with atherosclerosis have hypercholesterolemia and are receiving long-term anticoagulant therapy. Since it has become popular to reduce serum cholesterol levels with various pharmacological agents including dextrothyroxine (3), the enhancement of the response to oral anticoagulants by dextrothyroxine is important.

Recommendations—Patients treated concurrently with oral anticoagulants and thyroid compounds may require a reduction in the dose of anticoagulant to maintain the prothrombin time in the therapeutic range. Since serum levels of anticoagulants are not altered by thyroid compounds, measurements of these serum levels are not useful. A decrease in the anticoagulant requirement usually develops within 1–4 weeks after starting therapy with thyroid compounds (11).

Close monitoring of the prothrombin time during this period is mandatory, with appropriate reduction in the dose of the anticoagulant. Since hyperthyroidism may increase patient sensitivity to warfarin (12), individuals undergoing unexplained changes in anticoagulant requirements should have an evaluation of thyroid function.

References

(1) M. B. Walters, "The Relationship between Thyroid Function and Anticoagulant Therapy," *Amer. J. Cardiol.*, *11*, 112 (1963).

(2) J. J. Schrogie and H. M. Solomon, "The Anticoagulant Response to Bishydroxycoumarin II. The Effect of D-Thyroxine, Clofibrate, and Norethandrolone," *Clin. Pharmacol. Ther.*, *8*, 70 (1967).

(3) R. I. Levy *et al.*, "Treatment of Hyperlipidemia," *N. Engl. J. Med.*, *290*, 1295 (1974).

(4) C. Dufault *et al.*, "Influence of Dextrothyroxine and Androsterone on Blood Clotting Factors and Serum Cholesterol in Patients with Atherosclerosis," *Can. Med. Ass. J.*, *85*, 1025 (1961).

(5) J. Lowenthal and L. M. Fisher, "The Effect of Thyroid Function on the Prothrombin Time Response to Warfarin in Rats," *Experientia*, *13*, 253 (1957).

(6) H. M. Solomon and J. J. Schrogie, "The Effect of Various Drugs on the Binding of Warfarin-^{14}C to Human Albumin," *Biochem. Pharmacol.*, *16*, 1219 (1967).

(7) H. M. Solomon and J. J. Schrogie, "Change in Receptor Site Affinity: A Proposed Explanation for the Potentiating Effect of D-Thyroxine on the Anticoagulant Response to Warfarin," *Clin. Pharmacol. Ther.*, *8*, 797 (1967).

(8) J. Koch-Weser and E. M. Sellers, "Drug Interactions with Coumarin Anticoagulants," *N. Engl. J. Med.*, *285*, 487, 547 (1971).

(9) E. A. Loeliger *et al.*, "The Biological Disappearance Rate of Prothrombin Factors VII, IX, and X from Plasma in Hypothyroidism, Hyperthyroidism and during Fever," *Thromb. Diath. Haemorrh.*, *10*, 267 (1964).

(10) M. Weintraub *et al.*, "The Effects of Dextrothyroxine on the Kinetics of Prothrombin Activity: Proposed Mechanism of the Potentiation of Warfarin by D-Thyroxine," *J. Lab. Clin. Med.*, *81*, 273 (1973).

(11) J. C. Owens *et al.*, "Effect of Sodium Dextrothyroxine in Patients Receiving Anticoagulants," *N. Engl. J. Med.*, *266*, 76 (1962).

(12) T. Self *et al.*, "Warfarin-Induced Hypoprothrombinemia, Potentiation by Hyperthyroidism," *J. Amer. Med. Ass.*, *231*, 1165 (1975).

[For additional information, see *Anticoagulant Therapy*, p. 358.]

Nonproprietary and Trade Names of Drugs

Acenocoumarol—*Sintrom*
Anisindione—*Miradon*
Dextrothyroxine sodium—*Choloxin*
Dicumarol—*Various manufacturers*
Diphenadione—*Dipaxin*
Levothyroxine sodium—*Letter, Synthroid*
Liothyronine sodium—*Cytomel*
Liotrix—*Euthroid, Thyrolar*

Phenindione—*Hedulin*
Phenprocoumon—*Liquamar*
Thyroglobulin—*Proloid*
Thyroid—*Thyrar*
Thyroxine fraction—*Various manufacturers*
Warfarin potassium—*Athrombin-K*
Warfarin sodium—*Coumadin Sodium, Panwarfin*

Prepared and evaluated by the Scientific Review Subpanel on Anticoagulants and reviewed by Practitioner Panel III.

Warfarin—Vitamin K

Summary—The interaction between warfarin and vitamin K is well documented. Warfarin inhibits the vitamin K-dependent synthesis of clotting factors II, VII, IX, and X and vitamin K antagonizes the inhibitory effect of warfarin. In cases of excessive hypoprothrombinemia due to administration of warfarin, phytonadione (vitamin K_1) is the vitamin K of choice. However, excessive intake of this vitamin, particularly from food (*e.g.,* green leafy vegetables), should be avoided in patients stabilized on oral anticoagulants.

Related Drugs—The coumarin (**acenocoumarol, dicumarol,** and **phenprocoumon**) and indandione (**anisindione, diphenadione,** and **phenindione**) anticoagulants all have essentially the same action within the body, their differences being mainly quantitative rather than qualitative (1).

Available drugs with vitamin K activity include **menadione** (and its water-soluble salts) and **phytonadione.** These compounds restore clotting factor synthesis in persons deficient in vitamin K.

Pharmacological Effect and Mechanism—Compounds with vitamin K activity are essential for hepatic synthesis and release of clotting factors II, VII, IX, and X, collectively called the vitamin K-dependent clotting factors. Their abnormally low plasma concentration is often described as hypoprothrombinemia (2). The mechanism by which vitamin K promotes the production of these factors has not been established (3, 4). All usual diets supply amounts of vitamin K that permit rates of synthesis of vitamin K-dependent clotting factors sufficient to replace any catabolic losses (2).

Coumarin anticoagulants inhibit the vitamin K-dependent synthesis of factors II, VII, IX, and X. The degree of suppression of clotting factor synthesis at any time depends on the serum anticoagulant levels (5, 6). The mechanism of interference by coumarins with the action of vitamin K remains unclear (3). Vitamin K antagonizes the inhibitory effect of coumarins on hepatic synthesis of vitamin K-dependent clotting proteins, and high doses reverse the effect of all coumarins. During coumarin therapy, therefore, the amount of vitamin K available at the site of synthesis always influences the rate of clotting factor synthesis (2).

Evaluation of Clinical Data—The effectiveness of vitamin K as an antidote for warfarin overdose is well documented (1, 2). Phytonadione has been shown to be more effective than menadione in this respect (7, 8).

There is little information on the effect of dietary intake of vitamin K on anticoagulant control. In one study (9), 10 healthy subjects were given a vitamin K-free diet for 3 weeks. There was a small but statistically significant increase in the average weekly prothrombin time in these subjects. One patient stabilized on a fixed dose of warfarin (5 mg/day po) experienced a sharp prothrombin time rise on three occasions in response to a vitamin K-free diet. On another three occasions, he showed a sharp fall in prothrombin time in response to a high vitamin K diet. None of the 10 subjects experienced any bleeding episodes.

There was an anecdotal report (10) of a patient who experienced a loss of anticoagulant (dicumarol) control after excessive ingestion of green leafy vegetables (which have relatively high levels of vitamin K) but specific details are lacking.

■ The concurrent administration of vitamin K significantly antagonizes the effects of warfarin and should be avoided except in cases where an antidote for warfarin overdose is desirable. The effect of dietary intake of vitamin K on warfarin control has not been determined.

Recommendations—Concurrent administration of vitamin K with anticoagulants should be avoided. A well-balanced diet and avoidance of significant changes in intake of vitamin K-containing foods (*e.g.*, green leafy vegetables) should be recommended to patients stabilized on anticoagulants.

If vitamin K is to be used as an antidote for warfarin overdose, phytonadione is more effective than menadione and would be the drug of choice (7, 8).

References

(1) R. A. O'Reilly and P. M. Aggeler, "Determinants of the Response to Oral Anticoagulant Drugs in Man," *Pharmacol. Rev.*, *22*, 35 (1970).

(2) J. Koch-Weser and E. M. Sellers, "Drug Interactions with Coumarin Anticoagulants," *N. Engl. J. Med.*, *285*, 487 (1971).

(3) D. Deykin, "Warfarin Therapy," *N. Engl. J. Med.*, *283*, 691, 801 (1970).

(4) I. L. Woolf and B. M. Babior, "Vitamin K and Warfarin. Metabolism, Function and Interaction," *Amer. J. Med.*, *53*, 261 (1972).

(5) R. Nagashima *et al.*, "Kinetics of Pharmacological Effects in Man: The Anticoagulant Action of Warfarin," *Clin. Pharmacol. Ther.*, *10*, 22 (1969).

(6) R. A. O'Reilly and G. Levy, "Kinetics of the Anticoagulant Effect of Bishydroxycoumarin in Man," *Clin. Pharmacol. Ther.*, *11*, 378 (1970).

(7) M. J. Finkel, "Vitamin K_1 and the Vitamin K Analogues," *Clin. Pharmacol. Ther.*, *2*, 794 (1961).

(8) P. Griminger, "Biological Activity of the Various Vitamin K Forms," *Vitam. Horm.*, *24*, 605 (1966).

(9) J. A. Udall, "Human Sources and Absorption of Vitamin K in Relation to Anticoagulation Stability," *J. Amer. Med. Ass.*, *194*, 127 (1965).

(10) "Leafy Vegetables in Diet Alter Prothrombin Time in Patients Taking Anticoagulant Drugs," *J. Amer. Med. Ass.*, *187* (11), 27 (1964).

[For additional information, see *Anticoagulant Therapy*, p. 358.]

Nonproprietary and Trade Names of Drugs

Acenocoumarol—*Sintrom*
Anisindione—*Miradon*
Dicumarol—*Various manufacturers*
Diphenadione—*Dipaxin*
Menadiol sodium phosphate—*Kappadione, Synkayvite*
Menadione—*Various manufacturers*

Menadione sodium bisulfite—*Hykinone*
Phenindione—*Hedulin*
Phenprocoumon—*Liquamar*
Phytonadione—*AquaMephyton, Konakion*
Warfarin potassium—*Athrombin-K*
Warfarin sodium—*Coumadin Sodium, Panwarfin*

Prepared and evaluated by the Scientific Review Subpanel on Anticoagulants and reviewed by Practitioner Panel IV.

Basic Principles of Drug Interactions:
An Overview

DRUG INTERACTIONS: GENERAL MECHANISMS

Drug Interactions: General Mechanisms

The great variation in the chemical structures, the physical properties, and the pharmacological effects of the numerous compounds used as therapeutic agents suggests that any two drugs, administered concurrently, might interact in virtually an endless number of ways. However, experimental findings and clinical experience have shown that the great majority of interactions occur by a small number of relatively specific basic mechanisms.

An understanding of the mechanism involved with a particular interaction is essential in interpreting, preventing, and treating specific interactions. It also provides a means of remembering and classifying the large number of individually reported interactions. An understanding of the mechanisms involved may be useful, to a limited degree, in predicting the possibility of previously unreported interactions by virtue of the drug's characteristics that are similar to other known interacting drugs. However, the present predictive capability is not sufficiently advanced to permit generalizations in most cases. Rather, the practitioner will be heavily dependent on future reports in the literature to extend his or her knowledge. As in all branches of science, progress is largely based on the current ability to quantitate certain events of interest.

To provide the practitioner with a background for entry into the original literature and to better understand some of the more technical aspects of the monographs, quantitative relationships and terms which are used frequently—half-life, volume of distribution, protein binding constant, rate constant for elimination, and renal clearance—are discussed. Future predictive ability will depend largely on the extent to which additional information is obtained and correctly applied to these quantitative concepts.

General Considerations

The increase in the potency and number of new drugs has contributed immeasurably to modern drug therapy, but like all progress it has also created new problems. A problem of increasing concern is the greater incidence of adverse effects when two or more drugs are given concurrently.

It is clear that either the therapeutic or toxic effects of a drug can be greatly modified by interactions with other drugs, foods, environmental substances (*e.g.,* aromatic hydrocarbons and insecticides), or endogenous substances (*e.g.,* hormones, neurohumoral transmitters, and vitamins). Deaths or serious hypertensive crises have been reported when monoamine oxidase inhibitors were administered with some prescription drugs such as amphetamines and tricyclic antidepressants, over-the-counter drugs such as phenylpropanolamine in cold preparations, and some foods containing tyramine (see *Imipramine–Tranylcypromine,* p. 103, and *Phenylpropanolamine–Tranylcypromine,* p. 188).

Many other less dramatic, but clinically significant drug interactions have been reported. It is difficult to estimate how often drug interactions have contributed to increased toxicity or decreased therapeutic efficacy. A possible correlation has been noted between the significant increase in adverse effects and the use of multiple drug therapy. Unfortunately, only very dramatic effects are usually perceived, and many clinically significant interactions no doubt have been overlooked.

Although information on the number of patients involved in drug interactions is limited, there are many reports on potential drug interactions. Long lists of such interactions have been compiled. Many of these reports are based on insufficient data, a limited number of patients, or animal data alone.

There are several basic problems in interpreting and using existing information to reduce the incidence and severity of adverse effects due to drug interactions including the following: (*a*) evaluation of the validity and clinical significance of reported drug interactions, (*b*) detection and prevention of drug interactions that are known to be potentially hazardous, (*c*) determination of the significance of a reported drug interaction for a specific patient, and (*d*) recognition of previously unreported interactions.

An understanding of the mechanisms involved in drug interactions is essential to provide a rational basis for classifying, interpreting, preventing, and treating adverse interactions.

Drugs can also interact outside the body. Chemical and physical interactions of drugs in intravenous fluids may negate pharmacological effects before the drug is ever given. Drugs and their metabolites in blood or urine samples may interfere with the clinical laboratory analysis of endogenous substances (*e.g.,* glucose or 17-ketosteroids) which may lead to serious misdiagnosis. A discussion of these *in vitro* interactions involves different principles than *in vivo* drug interactions. Therefore, they will not be considered here. The reader is directed to other reviews describing these important types of interactions (1–4).

Basically, the events that determine the onset, duration, and intensity of a drug effect and the sites involved in drug interactions can be divided into the following two categories:

(1) The transport processes that deliver and remove the drug molecules to and from the site of action including absorption, metabolism, excretion, and tissue distribution.

(2) The effect of the drug on the organism after the drug molecules reach the site of action or receptor site, *i.e.,* that component of the reactive biological system which interacts with the drug to initiate the biological response. The total biological response also may involve an additional sequence of biochemical events or homeostatic mechanisms which may or may not be dependent upon the initial drug effect at the receptor site. These factors and potential sites of interaction are shown in Fig. 1.

The effect of a drug or substance on the onset, duration, and intensity of the pharmacological effect of a second drug is usually through an increase or decrease of one of the events in these two categories. Viewed in this way, most drug actions and interactions can be seen as variations on a few basic themes, differing quantitatively but essentially following a few recurring patterns.

The basic factors affecting transit to and from the receptor site that can be altered by drug interactions can be summarized as follows:

Factors affecting transit of active drug to the site of action
- the rate and extent of absorption of the drug into the systemic circulation (plasma)
- distribution of active drug to the site of action
- metabolism of inactive drug to biologically active metabolite

Factors affecting removal of active drug from the site of action
- redistribution from site of action to other tissues
- metabolism of active drug to inactive metabolite
- excretion of active drug from the body (*e.g.,* urinary, biliary, or pulmonary excretion)

It is apparent that the small fraction of drug available to bind to the receptor site (usually <1% of total drug in the body) is determined by a tug of war between the

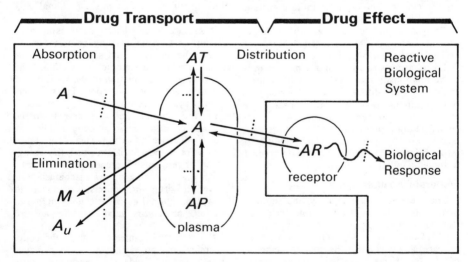

Figure 1—*Schematic diagram of some mechanisms involved in drug action and potential sites of drug interactions (designated by dotted lines). Key: A = free (unbound) active species, M = drug eliminated by drug-metabolizing enzymes, A$_u$ = drug elimination pathways of excretion of unchanged drug (e.g., urinary, biliary, or pulmonary excretion), AP = drug reversibly bound to plasma proteins, AT = drug reversibly localized in tissue (e.g., fat, muscle, and organs), and AR = drug reversibly bound to some part of the reactive biological system which initiates the biological effect, usually referred to as the "receptor site."*

dynamic rate processes: absorption, elimination (metabolism and excretion), and reversible plasma protein binding and tissue distribution. A few basic quantitative concepts are used to describe rate and equilibrium processes (pharmacokinetics).

Rate Constants and Biological Half-Life— A particularly useful concept to describe a rate process is the rate constant. The rate of transfer of an amount of drug from one location to another location (*e.g.*, drug in the body transferred to drug in the urine by renal excretion) or from one chemical form to another (*e.g.*, metabolism of active drug to inactive drug) is usually* simply proportional to the amount of drug available for transfer:

$$R = kA \qquad \text{(Eq. 1)}$$

where R is the rate of transfer, A is the amount of drug available for transfer, and k is simply a constant which describes the relationship between R and A. Thus, as A increases or decreases, the rate R will also increase or decrease by a proportional amount which is governed by the rate constant, k.

A simple but useful analogy in visualizing these relationships is to imagine a container of water with an opening in the bottom through which the water flows. The rate (R) that the water leaves the container is dependent on the amount (A) of water in the container which is changing and the size of the opening which is constant (k). The water represents the drug in the body, and the size of the opening represents the rate constant for the process (Fig. 2).

This rate constant is a valuable tool because it permits a transfer process to be characterized by a single number which gives the rate of transfer corresponding to any amount of drug present. Determination of a rate constant allows quantitative comparison of two different rate processes (*e.g.*, metabolism by two different pathways or comparison of the same pathway in two different groups of patients).

A single transfer process is usually represented as:

$$A_{body} \xrightarrow{\ k_u\ } A_{urine}$$

---

* The rate constant that is consistent with these conditions is termed the first-order rate constant. In some cases, the rate is independent of the amount of drug available for transfer (zero-order transfer) or may be a more complicated relationship such as is involved in the saturation of some metabolic processes.

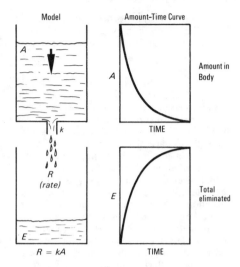

Figure 2—*Hydrodynamic model illustrating the relationships among the rate of transfer (R), the amount of drug available for transfer (A), the rate constant of transfer (k), and the amount of drug eliminated (E). Corresponding amount–time curves are shown at the right.*

where the rate constant (k_u) designates the specific process involved.

A series of consecutive rate processes such as the absorption of drug into the body (k_a) followed by elimination from the body by renal excretion (k_u) can be expressed as:

$$A_{gut} \xrightarrow{\ k_a\ } A_{body} \xrightarrow{\ k_u\ } A_{urine}$$

The rate constant k_a or k_u can be varied to determine the effect of changes in the relative rates of the processes of absorption and elimination on the amount of drug in the body. Examples of this approach are given in the subsequent discussion on the absorption mechanisms.

Often a drug is simultaneously removed from the body by more than one process (*e.g.*, by metabolism and renal excretion), each process being governed by its own rate constant:

$$A_b \overset{k_u}{\underset{k_m}{\rightrightarrows}} \begin{matrix} A_u \\ M \end{matrix}$$

When this occurs, the overall rate of removal is simply the sum of the individual rates of removal:

rate of total elimination	=	rate of metabolism	+	rate of excretion

(Eq. 2)

The rate constant to describe the rate of total elimination is the sum of all individual rate constants and will be represented here by the symbol K:

$$K = k_m + k_u \qquad \text{(Eq. 3)}$$

This relationship can again be visualized by the simple hydrodynamic analogy shown in Fig. 3. The rates of removal by each of the pathways are proportional to the amount of water in the container (analogous to the amount of drug in the body) and the individual sizes of the openings (analogous to the rate constants for metabolism, k_m, and excretion, k_u). The rate of removal of water would be the same if one larger opening was substituted for the two openings (analogous to K). The additive contribution of each individual process to the total elimination of drug is particularly important in understanding drug interactions. Many interactions affect only metabolism or only excretion. Thus, the contribution of the remaining pathways is important in determining the significance of the interaction.

The rate constant is expressed in units of reciprocal time and may be interpreted as the fraction of the amount of the unmetabolized drug in the body which will be eliminated in unit time. For example, a rate constant of 0.1 hr^{-1} means that one-tenth (or 10%) of the amount of drug present in the body at any given time will be eliminated per hour. More frequently, the rate of elimination is described by the biological half-life. The overall elimination rate constant (K) of a drug is related to the biological half-life ($t_{1/2}$) through the equation:

$$t_{1/2} = \frac{0.693}{K} \qquad \text{(Eq. 4)}$$

The biological half-life is the time for 50% of the drug to be eliminated (by all pathways) from the body. It is one of the most frequently altered parameters involved in drug interactions and is one of the most important quantitative parameters in relating serum drug levels to pharmacological effects. The clinical significance of changes in $t_{1/2}$ values caused by drug interactions will be discussed further in a later section on drug interactions affecting drug elimination.

Reversible and Irreversible Reactions— When the transfer of a drug by a particular process is essentially unidirectional, it can be considered to be an irreversible process. Absorption, metabolism, and excretion are essentially unidirectional and can often be conveniently considered as irreversible processes. Other transfer processes such as tissue distribution, protein binding, and binding at the receptor site are bidirectional reversible rate processes characterized by both the forward and reverse rates. For example, binding of drugs with plasma proteins can be expressed as:

$$A + P \underset{k_2}{\overset{k_1}{\rightleftharpoons}} AP$$

where A is the unbound drug in plasma water, P is the plasma proteins, and AP is the drug bound to plasma protein.

If the processes described by k_1 and k_2 are sufficiently rapid compared to other competing rate processes, apparent equilibrium may be reached which can be described by an equilibrium constant, K_p. In most cases, the ratio of A to AP (or the percent of drug that is bound) is constant over a range of plasma concentrations. Competing drugs which change this ratio may also affect the relative ratios of bound and unbound drug at the receptor site and reversible sites of distribution in the tissues. The degree to which each reversible process is affected depends on the relative values of the equilibrium and rate constants.

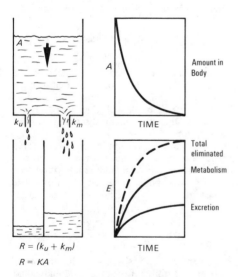

Figure 3—*Hydrodynamic model illustrating elimination by two pathways, metabolism and urinary excretion, and the relationship of the overall elimination rate constant (K) to the individual rates (k_m and k_u) (K = k_m + k_u).*

Quantitative Methods—Most drug interactions in humans are detected by qualitative observations during the clinical use of several drugs concurrently which result in either increased toxic effects or decreased therapeutic effects. To determine the mechanisms involved in the observed clinical effects, subsequent definitive studies usually involve quantitative measurements on: (*a*) some measurement of pharmacological response which can be easily quantitated such as prothrombin times, serum glucose levels, blood pressure, ECG's, and/or (*b*) the time course of serum levels of the active drug and metabolites.

Rationale of Serum Level Studies—The value of serum drug level studies in determining mechanisms of interactions is apparent from inspection of Fig. 1. The concentration of free drug in serum is central to all events and is the common denominator reflecting changes in the reversible processes of plasma protein binding, tissue distribution, and drug receptor binding. It also directly reflects the amount of drug entering the body by absorption and eliminated from the body through metabolism and excretion. This relationship should not be surprising since the systemic circulation evolved as the normal means of supplying all nutritive substances and endogenous hormones to all body cells, as well as the usual means of eliminating products of catabolism from all cells of the body.

A frequent criticism of serum level studies, usually from individuals unfamiliar with their interpretation, is that they are of limited value because tissue concentrations are more significant relative to pharmacological effects. Tissue levels are actually of very limited practical value in most studies in humans because it is usually impossible to sample the tissues containing the receptor site. Changes in tissue concentrations of other tissues are usually much less sensitive than serum level studies in predicting the combined effects of absorption, elimination, and distribution on the amount of drug at the site of action. Serum level curves alone, however, can sometimes be misinterpreted unless additional information is available such as the fraction of drug which is protein bound, the fraction of drug absorbed, and changes in metabolite levels. Ideally, both pharmacological effect and serum levels should be quantitated.

Volume of Distribution—Serum level studies also can provide a quantitative estimate of the extent of tissue distribution using a parameter termed the volume of distribution (V_d). When a drug is injected intravenously, there is a rapid decline of the serum level representing distribution of drug to the tissues (called the distributive phase) followed by a slower decline which represents the elimination of drug from the body. After the distributive phase, the ratio of drug in serum and tissue is often essentially constant and the total amount of drug in the body at a given time (Q_b) can be related to the serum concentration (C_p) by a capacity term (or proportionality constant) which is the volume of distribution (V_d):

$$Q_b = (V_d)(C_p) \qquad \text{(Eq. 5)}$$

This relationship is the basis for using serum levels to determine the elimination of total drug from the body. Drug interactions that change the ratio of drug in serum to drug in the tissues will be reflected by changes in the volume of distribution.

Analysis of serum levels yields the following parameters which can be used, together with measurements of pharmacological effects, to deduce mechanisms of interactions: (*a*) rate constant for absorption, (*b*) amount of drug absorbed, (*c*) rate constant for metabolism, (*d*) rate constant for renal excretion, (*e*) overall rate constant for total elimination and biological half-life, (*f*) extent of tissue distribution and volume of distribution, and (*g*) plasma protein binding affinity equilibrium constant and fraction bound.

These general principles now can be used to examine specific sites of interactions.

Interactions Affecting Drug Absorption

Clinical Considerations of Interactions Affecting the Rate and Amount of Drug Absorbed—Interactions during the absorptive phase result in either or both of the following potentially clinically significant effects (5):

(1) Increase or decrease in the relative rate of absorption (k_a).

(2) Increase or decrease in the amount of drug absorbed (F). Figure 4 shows the effect of these changes on serum levels.

A decrease in the fraction of drug absorbed is equivalent to a decrease in the dose given, with the obvious clinical implications. Although a drug may eventually be completely absorbed, it may be absorbed so slowly that: (*a*) it may never reach effective serum levels, (*b*) the rate of onset may be greatly delayed when prompt relief of acute symptoms, such as pain, is needed, or (*c*) the slow rate of absorption may act to sustain release and unduly prolong an effect.

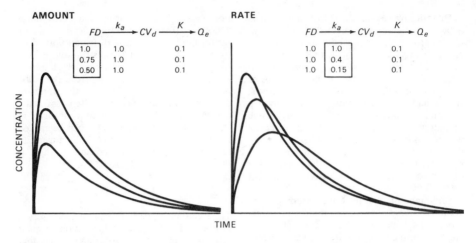

AMOUNT

RATE

CONCENTRATION

TIME

Figure 4—*Effects of changes in the rate constant of absorption* (k_a) *and fraction absorbed* (F) *on serum levels, following a single dose. In the left curve, only F is changed; in the right curve, only k_a is changed.* [*Adapted with permission from W. H. Barr, Drug Inform. Bull., 3, 27 (1969).*]

For example, the hypnotic effects of slowly absorbed barbiturates may lead to "hangover" effects in the morning.

It is important to distinguish between types of drugs and clinical situations where decreased rates of absorption are clinically significant and those where this type of interaction may occur but is not of concern. As a general rule, a decreased rate of absorption is most often important for drugs that are given as a single dose in clinical situations requiring a rapid onset of activity (*e.g.,* analgesics such as aspirin, antiasthmatics such as isoproterenol and theophylline, and hypnotics such as pentobarbital).

The rate of absorption is usually not important for compounds that are given in multiple-dose regimens to achieve a constant serum level such as antibiotics, sedatives, or tranquilizers. The reason for this is that the average steady-state serum level in a multiple-dose regimen is affected by the fraction of drug absorbed (*F*) but not usually by the relative rate of absorption (k_a).

The effects of changes in the rate and amount of drug absorbed on multiple-dose plasma levels are shown in Fig. 5. Illustration of these points is shown by the effect of food which frequently interferes with the absorption of drugs. Food affects the rate of absorption of aspirin but not the total amount absorbed. This effect might be clinically significant when treating a headache but probably is not significant in treating rheumatoid arthritis where multiple doses are given.

Food also affects the relative rate of absorption of sulfonamides but not the total amount absorbed. Since the average serum level during multiple dosing is the critical factor in sulfonamide therapy, the effect of food on the rate of absorption is not clinically significant. On the other hand, food may affect the amount of tetracycline absorbed but may not effect the relative rate of absorption (Fig. 6). This decrease will affect the plateau levels during multiple dosing and may be quite important clinically (see *Tetracycline–Aluminum, Calcium, and Magnesium Ions,* p. 227).

There are several ways in which the rate and amount of absorption of a drug can be modified. Like other types of drug interactions, most drug interactions during absorption are simple alterations of one of the steps involved in normal mechanisms of absorption. The events involved in absorption (6) and the potential sites of drug interactions are shown in Fig. 7.

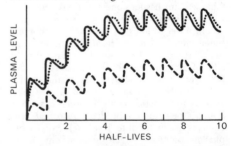

PLASMA LEVEL

HALF-LIVES

Figure 5—*Effects of changes in the relative rate of absorption (* k_a *) and fraction absorbed (F) on steady-state plateau plasma levels during multiple dosing. Key: ——, normal; ···, rate absorbed decreased; and - - -, amount absorbed decreased.*

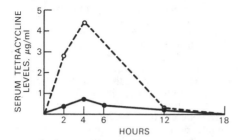

Figure 6—*Effect of food on the fraction of tetracycline absorbed after administration of 500 mg of tetracycline. Key:* ●, *30 min after a meal; and* ○. *fasting.* [Data from W. M. Kirby et al., Antimicrob. Ag. Chemother., 1, 286 (1961).]

Effect of Ionization on Drug Transport across Cell Membranes—A basic principle in pharmacology is that the rate of passive transport of a drug across cell membranes is proportional to the lipid solubility of the drug. For weak electrolytes (acids and bases), the unionized species has sufficient lipid solubility to pass rapidly through the membrane, while the polar ionized species does not. Thus, the ionization tendency of the drug (indicated by the pKa) and the pH of the aqueous environment affect the rate of transfer by changing the fraction unionized. Transfer of acids across biological membranes will be favored by low pH and transfer of bases will be favored by high pH (Fig. 8). The pH of the gastrointestinal (GI) lumen fluids can vary greatly, which may affect the transport of drugs in some

cases. The reabsorption of drugs from tubular urine can be affected by changes in urinary pH. Although the pH effect on renal reabsorption may result in clinically significant changes in drug elimination, which will be discussed later, the effect of pH changes on passage of drug across the GI membrane has been exaggerated in many reviews on drug interactions. Intestinal absorption of drug from commonly prescribed solid dosage forms involves other factors which are generally more important than the effect of pH on transport of drug across the mucosal cell.

Effect of pH Changes on Ionization and Dissolution of Drug during Absorption—Early classic studies on drug absorption from solutions perfused through rat intestine clearly showed that the rate of absorption was proportional to the fraction of unionized drug in solution (7). The frequent generalization that absorption of acidic drugs will be decreased by antacids which raise intragastric pH is not always warranted and is an example of the danger in extrapolating from animal studies, carried out under special experimental conditions, to clinical situations where additional factors may be involved.

Most drugs are administered orally as solid dosage forms (capsules, suspensions, or tablets) and the slowest (rate limiting) step is usually the rate at which the drug goes into solution (dissolution rate).

Although ionization decreases passage of drug across membranes, it increases the rate of dissolution. Even though a large amount of the drug in solution is ionized, the rate of

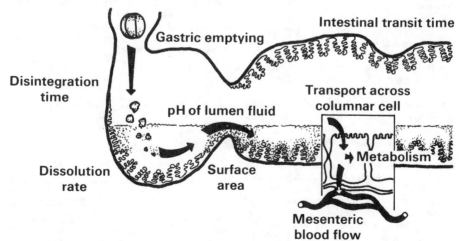

Figure 7—*Potential sites of drug interactions during drug absorption.* [Adapted with permission from *W. H. Barr*, Amer. J. Pharm. Ed., 32, 958 (1968).]

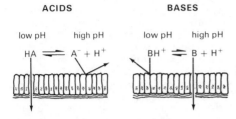

Figure 8—*Effect of pH on the fraction an acidic or basic drug which is unionized and able to pass across cell membranes.*

reversible proton transfer is so rapid that as soon as the unionized fraction in solution is absorbed it is almost immediately replenished. In the usual clinical situation, the drug is in contact with the absorbing site for a sufficient period of time (as opposed to a perfused animal intestine) that this reversible process continues until all drug is absorbed.

Antacids may tend to decrease absorption of basic drugs and increase absorption of acidic drugs because of effects on the dissolution rates. For example, administration of sodium bicarbonate will increase the rate of absorption of solid dosage forms of aspirin (8) but will greatly decrease the amount of tetracycline absorbed (9). Administration of antacids, food, or milk may reduce the absorption of bases, particularly poorly soluble drugs.

The rate of dissolution in gastric fluids and intestinal fluids is dependent on three principal (10) factors:

- the properties of the drug and dosage form [This is the subject of biopharmaceutics and is discussed in other reviews (11, 12).]
- the conditions at the site of dissolution, including pH, interfering substances, surfactants, and motility
- residence time at sites of dissolution which is dependent on gastric emptying and intestinal transit time

Gastric Emptying and Dissolution—Weak bases dissolve most rapidly in the acid pH of the stomach but are best absorbed in the more alkaline regions of the intestine. Foods (particularly fatty meals) or drugs such as atropine or other parasympatholytics will increase gastric pH and delay gastric emptying and may decrease the fraction dissolved and delay the absorption rate if dissolution is the rate-limiting step. Decreased gastric emptying may decrease absorption of drugs degraded in the acidic conditions

of the stomach such as erythromycin and penicillin G.

The rate of gastric emptying of particles is less than the rate of emptying of drug in solution when food is present. Food may, therefore, affect "spansule" type timed-release products or poorly dissolved drugs more than drugs administered in solution or rapidly dissolved drugs.

Dissolution in Intestinal Fluids—Poorly soluble drugs will pass into the intestine where they may slowly dissolve for several hours. Griseofulvin, a very insoluble drug, is absorbed over 20–30 hr. Absorption of griseofulvin is decreased by phenobarbital (see *Griseofulvin–Phenobarbital*, p. 77). The absorption of dicumarol, another poorly soluble drug, is decreased by heptabarbital (13). The mechanism involved in these reductions is not known but possibly involves effects of barbiturates on intestinal motility or transit time. The possible effect of barbiturates on other poorly soluble drugs, *e.g.*, digitalis and phenytoin (diphenylhydantoin), should be considered.

Methylphenidate, a sympathomimetic, has been reported to inhibit metabolism of the anticoagulant ethyl biscoumacetate (14). Inspection of the serum drug curve (Fig. 9) shows that the peak concentration is greatly delayed and the area under the curve is not appreciably altered, suggesting that the rate of absorption is also decreased. Amphetamine has been shown to decrease absorption of several anticonvulsants in rats (15). Unfortunately, there have been very few well-controlled studies on drug interactions in humans during the absorptive phase. The effect of laxatives and antidiarrheal agents on intestinal transit time and drug absorption is an obvious possibility but has not been studied sufficiently.

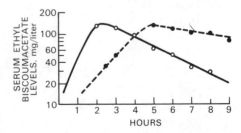

Figure 9—*Effect of methylphenidate on serum drug levels of ethyl biscoumacetate. Key:* o, *before methylphenidate administration; and* ●, *after methylphenidate administration. [Adapted with permission from L. K. Garrettson et al., J. Amer. Med. Ass., 207, 2053 (1969).]*

Physicochemical Interactions during Absorption—Several substances can bind or solubilize drugs which may alter absorption. Kaolin reduces the absorption of lincomycin (see *Lincomycin–Kaolin,* p. 135). Cholestyramine, a quaternary ion-exchange resin used to bind intestinal bile salts and reduce serum cholesterol levels, also binds with many drugs (10). Antacids containing polyvalent cations (aluminum, calcium, or magnesium) chelate with tetracycline; this mechanism is thought to be responsible for the decreased absorption of tetracycline. Actually, any antacid, regardless of the presence of polyvalent cations, may decrease dissolution and absorption of tetracycline (see *Tetracycline–Aluminum, Calcium, and Magnesium Ions,* p. 227). Chelation may be involved in the great reduction of serum levels of various tetracycline products when small doses (200 mg) of ferrous sulfate are given concurrently (see *Tetracycline–Ferrous Sulfate,* p. 231).

Surfactants used as stool softeners, such as dioctyl sodium sulfosuccinate, may increase solubilization of some poorly soluble drugs such as digitalis. Enhancement of digitalis toxicity by surfactants has been noted in animals but studies in humans are not available.

Physiological Factors—There are several possible physiological factors which may affect drug absorption and may be in turn influenced by other drugs. There is presently no documentation of these effects in humans, however. It has been suggested that amino acid derivatives such as methyldopa (16) are actively transported and amino acids in foods may compete for active transport. The intestinal mucosa contains enzymes capable of metabolizing many drugs. Inhibition or induction of metabolism at this site may affect the total amount of drug absorbed. Intestinal monoamine oxidase may be inhibited by monoamine oxidase inhibitors, increasing the amount of sympathomimetic amines, such as tyramine in foods, which reaches the systemic circulation (see *Phenylpropanolamine–Tranylcypromine,* p. 188).

Interactions Affecting Drug Elimination

Clinical Implications of Changes in Rate of Drug Elimination and Biological Half-Life—Elimination of drugs usually occurs by metabolism and excretion (*e.g.,* renal or biliary). Although the processes are quite dissimilar in the mechanisms involved and the factors affecting them, they both result in changes in the elimination rate constant

and the biological half-life. The biological half-life of a drug is one of the most important values in quantitative pharmacology since it provides the following information:

(1) The half-life determines the overall rate of elimination and the amount of drug remaining in the body at a given time. The half-life is the time for one-half of the drug to be eliminated from the body. For example, if 100 mg of drug is present at a given time and the half-life of the drug is 4 hr, 50 mg will be eliminated in the first 4 hr. In the second 4 hr, 50% of the remaining amount will be eliminated (25 mg); in the third half-life, 50% of the remaining drug will be eliminated (12.5 mg), and so on. After six half-lives, elimination of the drug is essentially complete (over 98%) (Fig. 10). It can be seen that the decline of drug in the body is exponential. If the amount in the body or corresponding serum levels are plotted on semilog paper, a straight line results from which the half-life can be determined easily. Half-lives of drugs vary from a few minutes to months. The long half-life of monoamine oxidase inhibitors is one reason that they can interact with a drug 2 weeks after the last dose.

(2) The half-life determines the average serum concentration after steady-state levels are reached during multiple dosing, as shown by (17):

$$\overline{C} = \frac{1.44\,(FD)\,(t_{1/2})}{V_d\,\tau} \qquad \text{(Eq. 6)}$$

where $\overline{C}$ is the average serum level at steady state, D is the dose given, F is the fraction of the dose absorbed, V_d is the volume of distribution, and τ is the time interval between doses. It can be seen that a drug interaction that doubles the half-life will double the average serum level (Fig. 11). Drug interactions that decrease the half-life by 50% will reduce the steady-state serum levels to one-half of their original value.

(3) The time to reach steady state during multiple dosing is about six half-lives if doses are given at intervals close to the half-life. For drugs with very long half-lives, it may take several weeks before steady-state levels are reached. Phenobarbital has a half-life of 2–3 days which may provide one reason for the several days required for enzyme induction by this drug.

With an understanding of the very great importance of changes in half-lives on single-dose and multiple-dose serum levels, drug interactions that influence the half-life through effects on drug metabolism and excretion will now be examined.

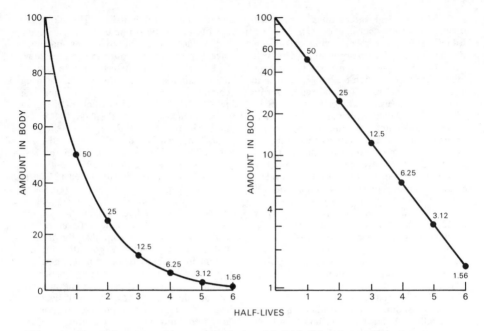

Figure 10—*Plots of the amount of drug in the body at each half-life. When the amount is plotted on a regular scale (left), an exponential decline is observed. When the amount is plotted on a logarithmic scale (right), a straight line is observed which is used to determine the half-life.*

Interactions Affecting Drug Metabolism

Clinical Significance of Changes in Drug Metabolism—The importance of drug metabolism in eliminating a drug from the body can be appreciated by the fact that the half-life of alcohol would be 30 days if the drug was not metabolized. The implication that the effects of a New Year's celebration would persist until February is indeed quite staggering.

A more serious example, which is not hypothetical, is the problem with some in-

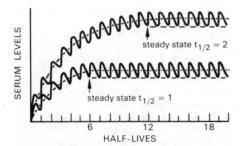

Figure 11—*Effect of a change in half-life on the steady-state serum levels and the time to reach steady-state serum levels.*

secticides. DDT is very slowly metabolized and has a half-life of several months. Accumulation of toxic effects of this substance occurs not only in one species but in a predator-chain, upsetting an entire ecosystem rather than just a single organism.

Drugs are transformed—by a variety of oxidative, reductive, and conjugating pathways including hydroxylation, dealkylation, deacetylation, and glucuronide conjugation—to more polar metabolites which are then more readily excreted. These biotransformations take place principally in the smooth endoplasmic reticulum (microsomal fraction) of the hepatic cell. These processes are poorly developed in the neonate. In past years, many infants died from overdoses of chloramphenicol because it was not realized that glucuronide conjugation of the drug proceeded at a slower rate, which increased the half-life to 25 hr compared to 4 hr in adults. Metabolizing capacity also seems to be reduced in the elderly.

Enzyme Induction—In recent years, it has been shown in animals that literally hundreds of drugs in virtually all pharmacological classes can induce an increase in the size and enzyme content of the endoplasmic reticulum and, therefore, increase the rate of metabolism of many drugs (18, 19).

Although there have been fewer documented reports in humans, there is no doubt that enzyme induction occurs and that it is quite important clinically. Butabarbital, phenobarbital, secobarbital, and other barbiturates induce the metabolism of dicumarol and warfarin, reducing the anticoagulant effect. An increase of the dose is then required to obtain the same clinical effect. A danger occurs when the inducer is withdrawn. Metabolism returns to normal and serum levels may reach toxic levels (see *Warfarin–Phenobarbital*, p. 291).

Barbiturates including heptabarbital, pentobarbital, phenobarbital, and secobarbital have been shown in humans to reduce serum levels or the pharmacological effect of phenytoin (diphenylhydantoin) and griseofulvin (see *Phenytoin–Phenobarbital*, p. 205, and *Griseofulvin–Phenobarbital*, p. 77). Enzyme induction has been stated to be the mechanism involved. In some cases, other mechanisms such as decreased absorption may be responsible.

The fact that other sedatives, such as glutethimide, also have been shown to induce metabolism in humans might lead to the speculation that a sedative effect is related to an inductive effect. Actually, the pharmacological effect is quite unrelated to the inductive effect. It just happens that sedatives are fairly lipid-soluble drugs and are continuously given over long periods. Most substances that fit these two criteria are probably capable of being enzyme-inducing agents.

DDT is a good inducer (20) even though it is not a drug *per se* and is itself very slowly metabolized. Alcohol is not appreciably lipid soluble but can apparently induce hepatic microsomal enzymes if large amounts are ingested over a long period. The half-lives of phenytoin (diphenylhydantoin), tolbutamide, and warfarin were significantly reduced in patients who had received alcohol (250 g/day for 3 months) (21) (see *Tolbutamide–Alcohol*, p. 240, and *Warfarin–Alcohol*, p. 265). Hydrocortisone is both an endogenously produced hormone and a therapeutic agent which is extensively metabolized and is apparently subject to increased metabolism which is induced by other corticosteroids.

Intravenous doses of hydrocortisone can be life saving in the treatment of acute asthma. It has been shown that asthmatic patients previously taking other corticosteroids did not respond to the usual intravenous dose of 100 mg (22). Much larger doses (300–1000 mg) were necessary to reach the minimum effective plasma level of 1.0 μg/ml which is necessary for effective treatment of acute life-threatening asthma attacks (Fig. 12). Another study (23) showed that the hydrocortisone half-life in chronically ill patients receiving steroids is significantly lower than the half-life in untreated patients.

Thus, these studies (22, 23) may provide one explanation for increasing mortality of steroid-treated (or undertreated) patients with status asthmaticus. More important, they suggest the basis for a more rational dosage regimen based on the patient's drug history. Phenobarbital and phenytoin (diphenylhydantoin) were shown to increase metabolism of corticosteroids in humans, and prior use of these drugs may also complicate emergency treatment of status asthmaticus requiring higher doses of hydrocortisone (see *Dexamethasone–Phenobarbital*, p. 42, and *Dexamethasone–Phenytoin*, p. 45). With the increasing quantities of foreign substances in the environment and the widespread drug use, many people may be in a chronic state of enzyme induction. One report (24) showed that the half-lives of antipyrine in normal (control) subjects averaged 13.1 hr with a large range (5.2–35 hr). Half-lives in subjects exposed to insecticides averaged 7.7 hr with a smaller range (2.7–11.7 hr) (Fig. 13). The great range in the normal population may be representative of varying degrees of enzyme induction. Smoking, for example, will increase drug metabolism by the human placenta (25).

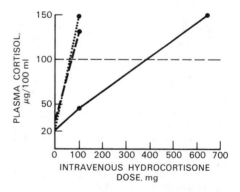

Figure 12—*Comparison of the dose necessary to raise plasma levels of hydrocortisone above 100 μg/100 ml 30 min after injection in nonsteroid-treated asthmatic subjects (---), steroid-treated asthmatic subjects (——), and control subjects (.........). [Adapted with permission from J. Dwyer et al., Australas. Ann. Med., 16, 297 (1967).]*

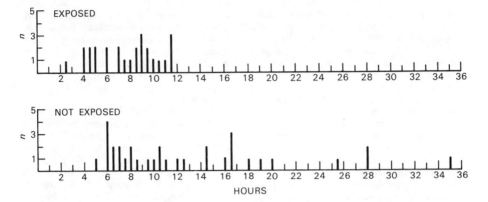

Figure 13—*Distribution of antipyrine half-lives in workers exposed to insecticides and unexposed subjects.* [*Adapted with permission from B. Kolmodin et al., Clin. Pharmacol. Ther., 10, 638 (1969).*]

Inhibition of Drug Metabolism—An early example of one drug decreasing the metabolism of another was the finding that proadifen (SK&F 525-A), a drug resembling the anticholinergic agent adiphenine, inhibited the metabolism of many drugs. Proadifen was never marketed but served to stimulate additional research in this area. There are now several clinically significant examples of inhibition of drug metabolism in humans by common therapeutic agents.

The metabolism of tolbutamide in humans is inhibited by a wide variety of compounds, with hypoglycemic episodes reported as a consequence in some cases (26). Phenytoin (diphenylhydantoin) metabolism is decreased by other drugs. An example of increases in half-lives of phenytoin and tolbutamide following administration of chloramphenicol is shown in Fig. 14 (27).

A dramatic increase in the half-life of phenytoin caused by pretreatment with dicumarol is shown in Fig. 15 (28). It is worthwhile to consider the clinical consequences of this reduction to one-fourth the expected rate of metabolism using the multiple-dose relationships described previously. It would be expected that average steady-state serum levels would increase fourfold but it would take six half-lives to reach the new level (9 days). Figure 16 shows that multiple-dose serum levels actually increased from 5 to about 15 μg/ml during the 7 days that dicumarol was administered (see *Phenytoin–Dicumarol*, p. 193).

The mechanism involved in these interactions is not known. It is significant that there appears to be considerable overlap in pairs of drugs involved in inhibition of metabolism (29–31). Some of these pairs are shown in Fig. 17. It appears that a common mechanism may be operative, possibly competitive inhibition of hydroxylation. Interaction between other pairs of these drugs should be considered even though they have not been specifically studied.

The therapeutic effect of monoamine oxidase inhibitors (*e.g.*, isocarboxazid, pargyline, phenelzine, and tranylcypromine) is due in part to their ability to inhibit the enzyme monoamine oxidase, which metabolizes sympathomimetic amines in the tissue. The ability of these drugs to inhibit enzymes does not appear to be limited to monoamine oxidase. Monoamine oxidase inhibitors were reported to inhibit metabolism of phenindione and possibly other drugs (32). Studies in animals indicate that several monoamine

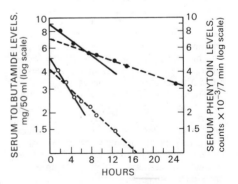

Figure 14—*Plots of the serum levels of tolbutamide (o) and phenytoin (diphenylhydantoin) (●) before (···) and after (___) chloramphenicol (3 g iv) administration. The tolbutamide half-life increased from 5 to 8.75 hr, and the phenytoin half-life increased from 10.5 to 22 hr. [Adapted with permission from L. K. Christensen and L. Skovsted, Lancet, iii, 1397 (1969).]*

oxidase inhibitors inhibit liver microsomal enzymes.

Another drug that is used therapeutically for its ability to inhibit a specific enzyme is disulfiram. This drug inhibits aldehyde dehydrogenase, leading to accumulation of acetaldehyde and unpleasant symptoms when alcohol is ingested. It also inhibits the metabolism of phenytoin (diphenylhydantoin), leading to toxic symptoms (see *Phenytoin–Disulfiram*, p. 195), and has been reported to enhance the anticoagulant effects of warfarin in one patient (33).

Several other drugs are said to have disulfiram-like effects including the sulfonylureas and the anti-infective, furazolidone. Furazolidone also inhibits monoamine oxidase (34), which lends support to the possibility of a common mechanism.

The metabolic pathways including glycine, glucuronide, and sulfate conjugation also can be inhibited. Glycine conjugation of salicylic acid is decreased by aminobenzoic acid (35). Salicylamide appears to block glucuronide conjugation of acetaminophen and salicylic acid (36, 37).

It is reported that several drugs which normally induce metabolism have a biphasic effect. Large doses may initially inhibit metabolism followed by the slower process of induction. Large doses of phenobarbital were reported to inhibit the metabolism of phenytoin in some subjects (see *Phenytoin–Phenobarbital*, p. 205).

Interactions Affecting Renal Excretion

Clinical Significance—Interactions that affect renal excretion of drugs will be clinically significant only when the drug or its active metabolite is appreciably eliminated by the renal route. For example, the hypoglycemic agent, tolbutamide, is metabolized extensively and very little of the drug appears intact in the urine. Interactions at the renal level would have little or no effect on the half-life of tolbutamide. Dicumarol, however, increases the hypoglycemic effect of tolbutamide by inhibiting metabolism rather than excretion (see *Tolbutamide–Dicumarol*, p. 245). Phenylbutazone enhances the effects of acetohexamide by interfering with the tubular secretion of its active metabolite, hydroxyhexamide, but it has no effect on the parent compound (see *Tolbutamide–Phenylbutazone*, p. 247).

Mechanisms of Renal Excretion—Drugs are eliminated by urinary excretion through three mechanisms: glomerular filtration, tubular reabsorption, and active tubular secretion (Fig. 18).

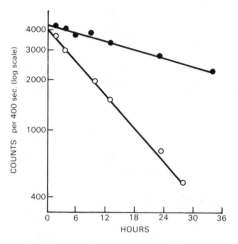

Figure 15—*Increase in half-life of phenytoin (diphenylhydantoin) by dicumarol due to inhibition of metabolism. Key: ○, before dicumarol administration (half-life = 9 hr); and ●, after dicumarol administration (half-life = 36 hr). [Adapted with permission from J. M. Hansen et al., Lancet, ii, 265 (1966).]*

Glomerular filtration is a simple filtration process of drug which is not bound to plasma proteins and is not greatly affected by other drugs, except in a few cases where highly protein-bound drugs are displaced by a second drug. Disease states do affect glomerular filtration, however, and may greatly increase the half-life of some drugs by decreasing the glomerular filtration rate.

Active Secretion—Many acidic drugs are transported from the blood across the proximal tubular cell into the tubular urine against a concentration gradient by an active (energy requiring) process. There are apparently two systems which actively transport drugs across the tubular epithelium, one for acidic drugs and one for basic drugs. Very little is known about interactions at the latter site. Acidic drugs that are transported include the penicillins; most anti-inflammatory agents including indomethacin, oxyphenbutazone, phenylbutazone, and salicylic acid; uricosurics such as probenecid and sulfinpyrazone; the thiazide diuretics; and some hypoglycemics such as chlorpropamide (38).

Interactions can occur by competition of these agents for tubular transport (38). The effect of probenecid on increasing serum levels of penicillin is well known (see *Penicillin–Probenecid*, p. 175). Probenecid is said to decrease the renal clearance of indomethacin (see *Indomethacin–Probenecid*,

p. 108). Salicylates interfere with uric acid clearance of the more potent uricosurics, phenylbutazone, probenecid, and sulfinpyrazone (see *Sulfinpyrazone–Aspirin,* p. 226). Salicylates do not block the effect of probenecid on penicillin excretion at the same serum levels (about 10 mg%) that block the uricosuric effect of probenecid (39). Concurrent use of probenecid and sulfinpyrazone does not alter the individual uric acid clearance obtained with each drug alone (40). Probenecid inhibits urinary secretion of the *p*-hydroxy metabolite of sulfinpyrazone. The mechanisms involved in tubular secretion are rather complex and are not completely understood.

Reabsorption—Drug delivered to tubular urine by glomerular filtration and tubular secretion is concentrated as water is reabsorbed; the reabsorption of water increases the concentration gradient between drug in urine and blood. If the drug possesses sufficient lipid solubility, it may passively diffuse into the blood. Very lipid-soluble drugs may be completely reabsorbed. The reabsorption of weak electrolytes can be influenced greatly by the pH of the tubular urine which determines the fraction unionized and transferred. Half-lives of some drugs can be greatly changed by changes in urinary pH induced by alkalizers such as sodium bicarbonate or urinary acidifiers such as ammonium chloride. These drugs generally have the following properties (41). They are weak acids (pKa 3–7) or weak bases (pKa 7–11). The unionized form is lipid soluble (high oil–water partition coefficient). They are eliminated appreciably (>20%) by urinary excretion.

An increase in urinary pH increases the tubular reabsorption of weak bases, therefore decreasing the elimination and increasing the half-life. Acidification of urine increases urinary excretion of bases and decreases their half-lives (41). The magnitude of these effects can be quite significant. The half-life of amphetamine, a weak base, is doubled when urinary pH is increased from 5 to 8, which may lead to sleepless nights for a person taking the drug during the day (42, 43).

Clearances of quinidine and its optical isomer quinine are greatly affected by urinary pH, resulting in changes in ECG recordings and potential toxicities. Quinidine renal clearance is reduced to one-tenth the expected level when urine pH below 6.0 is increased to 7.5 (44). Other bases which may show pH dependence are amitriptyline, ephedrine, imipramine, meperidine, and methamphetamine (41).

Acidification of urine increases and alkalinization decreases the half-life of some weak acids. The half-life of sulfaethidole, a weakly acidic sulfonamide, is decreased from 11.4 hr at a urinary pH of 5 to a half-life

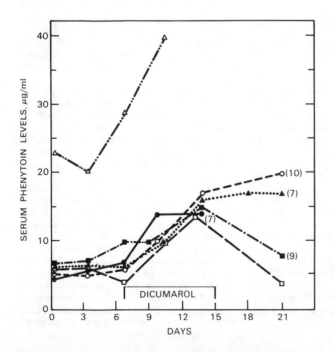

Figure 16—*Effect of dicumarol on steady-state serum levels of phenytoin (diphenylhydantoin) in six subjects. The numbers in parentheses indicate the peak serum level of dicumarol. [Adapted with permission from J. M. Hansen et al., Lancet, ii, 265 (1966).]*

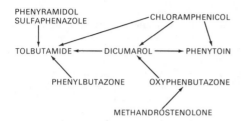

Figure 17—*Pairs of drugs which have been reported to result in decreased metabolism. Drug at arrow tail will inhibit metabolism of drug at arrow head.*

of only 4.2 hr at pH 8 (45). Other weak acids which show pH-dependent urinary excretion include nalidixic acid, nitrofurantoin, phenobarbital, and salicylic acid (41).

Interactions Affecting Drug Distribution

As shown in Fig. 1, drugs are reversibly bound to tissue, plasma proteins, and the receptor. The ratio of free drug to bound drug at each of these sites depends on the properties of the drug, the patient, and the presence of other substances.

Distribution to Tissues—Drug distribution to various tissues is governed by three major factors: the blood flow to tissues, the mass of the tissue, and the affinity of the tissue for the drug. A drug is initially transferred rapidly from blood to tissues with high blood flow (*e.g.,* brain, liver, and kidney) and is then redistributed to tissues with lower blood flow but higher affinity for the drug (*e.g.,* muscle or fat). For example, the hypnotic effect of thiopental is terminated by the lipid-soluble drug being drawn away from the initial site of distribution in the brain to tissues of greater mass and affinity such as muscle and fat (46).

Many drugs are highly localized in specific tissues. The concentration of the antimalarial drug quinacrine is 22,000 times greater in the liver than in the serum after 14 days of treatment. When a second antimalarial drug, pamaquine, is administered even months after quinacrine was given, toxic effects of pamaquine may occur because of decreased tissue binding sites available to it (47).

The increased activity of the neuromuscular blocker, hexafluorenium bromide, in the presence of cyclopropane and other "inert" lipid-soluble compounds has been attributed to their abilities to displace the drug from nonspecific tissue storage sites (48).

Pharmacokinetic evidence indicates that probenecid increases serum levels of penicillins by decreasing the volume of distribution as well as inhibiting renal secretion (see *Penicillin–Probenecid,* p. 175) (49).

Plasma Protein Binding—Most drugs and endogenous compounds (*e.g.,* bilirubin and hormones) are reversibly bound to a varying extent to proteins (principally albumin)

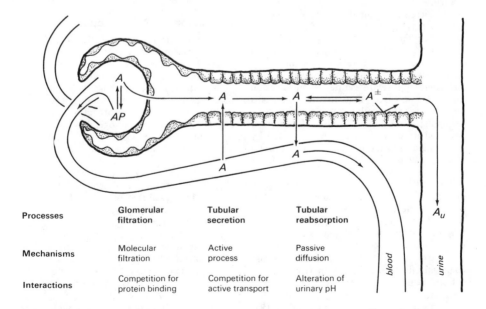

Figure 18—*Mechanisms of renal elimination and potential sites of drug interactions.*

circulating in the plasma. Plasma protein binding is a very important factor in determining the intensity and duration of drug effect. Plasma proteins are frequently the site of drug interactions.

The fraction of total drug bound to protein is a function of the concentration of drug in the plasma, the concentration of the plasma protein, the number of binding sites on the protein, and the equilibrium affinity constant.

The fraction of bound drug decreases as the total serum concentration of drug increases or the concentration of protein decreases. Binding may be decreased by a second drug which also binds at the same site, depending on the relative concentrations and affinity constants of the two drugs. Displacement might increase, decrease, or have no effect on the amount of drug at the receptor site, depending on the relative rates of tissue distribution and elimination of the drug. Decreased plasma protein will generally be significant only for drugs which are highly protein bound ($>90\%$ bound). This effect is easily appreciated by considering two examples, a drug that is 95% bound and one that is 50% bound. If 5% of the highly bound drug is displaced, the concentration of free drug available to diffuse to the site of action is increased twofold, from 5 to 10%. If 5% of the poorly bound drug is displaced, the increase of free drug is only 10% (from 50 to 55%), which is inconsequential.

An increase in the fraction of unbound drug in plasma available to diffuse to tissue may alter the rates of all irreversible and reversible processes. Generally, the fraction of drug at the tissue receptor is increased, leading to increased pharmacological effects. However, the relative rate of elimination may be increased due to the increased amount of drug available in the liver to be metabolized and the increased fraction of unbound drug in plasma to be extracted by glomerular filtration. Decreased protein binding usually does not affect the rate of active tubular secretion.

The ratio of drug in tissue to drug in plasma will be increased, resulting in an increase in the apparent volume of distribution. The net result of all of these effects is that the biological effect may be increased but the plasma concentration is decreased.

An example of both increased pharmacological effects and slightly increased elimination occurs when phenylbutazone is given with warfarin (97% bound). The half-life of warfarin is slightly decreased (Fig. 19). In this example, phenylbutazone interferes with the assay of warfarin and, unless a correction is made, the half-life would appear to increase, leading to erroneous conclusions on the mechanism involved (50). Displacement of anticoagulants from protein binding sites by phenylbutazone analogs has led to serious bleeding episodes (see *Warfarin–Phenylbutazone*, p. 295). Tolbutamide is a highly protein-bound drug which reportedly may be displaced from protein binding sites, leading to severe hypoglycemic crises (51). Moreover, it has been speculated that several drugs including phenylbutazone, salicylates, and sulfonamides may also be displaced. Methotrexate, a potentially toxic antineoplastic drug which is sometimes used for treatment of less severe diseases such as psoriasis, has been reported to be displaced from plasma protein sites by salicylates and sulfonamides. Although the clinical significance of these drug interactions has not been established, the potential hazards of increased methotrexate toxicity require that concurrent use of these drugs be avoided (see *Methotrexate–Aspirin*, p. 150, and *Methotrexate–Sulfisoxazole*, p. 156).

Several pairs of drugs compete for plasma protein binding sites, leading to increased biological effects (Fig. 20). Although all possible combinations have not been tested, it appears that there is very little specificity among these drugs, and the possibility of competition among these highly bound drugs should be considered.

Interactions at Site of Action

Once a drug reaches the site of action, a second drug may modify the ultimate pharmacological effect by altering the site of action in several ways including: (*a*) competition for the receptor site, (*b*) alteration of the receptor, (*c*) alteration of the other components at the site of action, and (*d*) effects on a different biological system which has similar or opposite effects and may augment or diminish the total biological response.

Understanding these types of interactions usually depends on a thorough knowledge of each biological system involved.

Competition of one agent for another at the receptor site is a well-known phenomenon in pharmacology. Many therapeutic agents such as atropine, propranolol, and tubocurarine have little or no intrinsic activity but can occupy a receptor and block the effects of an active substance such as acetylcholine or epinephrine (16).

Receptor site competition provides one explanation for the increased mortality in

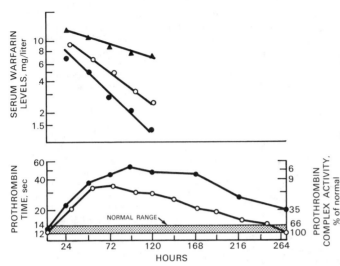

Figure 19—*Serum levels of warfarin (dose of 1.5 mg/kg) and anticoagulant effect when given alone and with phenylbutazone. Key:* ▲, *after phenylbutazone administration (uncorrected values);* ○, *before phenylbutazone administration;* and ●, *after phenylbutazone administration (corrected values).* [*Adapted with permission from P. M. Aggeler et al., N. Engl. J. Med., 276, 496 (1967).*]

patients taking isoproterenol by inhalation. Isoproterenol is metabolized to 3-methyliso-proterenol, a weak blocker of the β-adrenergic receptor site, which blocks the effects of the parent compound and also increases airway obstruction. Increased use of isoproterenol leads to greater accumulation of 3-methylisoproterenol, leading to progressive deterioration of the asthmatic condition (52). An even more serious consequence of the β-adrenergic blockade may occur if epinephrine is given parenterally for an acute asthmatic attack. Since epinephrine can stimulate both the α- and β-adrenergic receptors, an exaggerated effect may occur leading to death (53, 54).

Other agents may interact with the active site to modify the intensity of the response through noncompetitive processes. Thyroxine is said to increase the anticoagulant effect of warfarin in this manner (see *Warfarin–Thyroid,* p. 301). Potassium depletion (*e.g.,* by diuretics) sensitizes the heart to the pharmacological effects of the digitalis glycosides (see *Digitalis–Chlorothiazide,* p. 52).

Modification of other components involved at the site of action can occur by blocking specific metabolizing enzymes at the site of action (*e.g.,* acetylcholinesterase and monoamine oxidase) or by blocking uptake or facilitating release of norepinephrine from storage sites.

Enhancement of effects, elicited by drugs which act at different sites of the same system or different systems with similar biological response, is well known. Sedation may

be increased by any combination of alcohol, some antihistamines, barbiturates, narcotic analgesics, and phenothiazines, all of which probably have different sites of action. The small amount of blood loss caused by the direct effect of aspirin on gastric mucosa is usually benign but may be quite hazardous when anticoagulants are administered (see *Warfarin–Aspirin,* p. 270).

Clinical Factors

Not all drug interactions are hazardous. In fact, many types of interactions have been used to therapeutic advantage. Enzyme induction by phenobarbital or DDT has been used to reduce bilirubin levels in neonatal hyperbilirubinemia or excessive cortisol levels in patients with increased adrenocortical activity (Cushing's syndrome). Displacement of penicillin from plasma proteins by salicylates or inhibition of renal secretion by probenecid may increase serum and tissue antibacterial levels. Alteration of urinary pH to increase urinary drug excretion is frequently useful in the treatment of drug overdose.

The potentially deleterious interactions may be classified by the severity and the frequency of occurrence. A few interactions are quite severe and occur almost always when the two drugs are given concurrently. Interactions between monoamine oxidase inhibitors and sympathomimetic amines or between warfarin and phenylbutazone are obvious examples of therapeutic incompatibilities. In these cases, the course of action

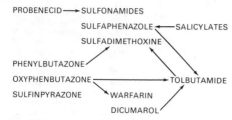

PROBENECID ⟶ SULFONAMIDES

Figure 20—*Some pairs of drugs that are reported to compete for plasma protein binding sites. Drug at arrow tail will displace drug at arrow head.*

is clear. Surveillance systems must be established to prevent their concurrent use.

Interactions between drugs such as phenobarbital and phenytoin (diphenylhydantoin) that are neither frequent nor severe are also rather simple to handle. The two drugs are usually used with the knowledge that dosage adjustments may be necessary. Unfortunately, many interactions fall in the less predictable class that may be severe but occur only in a few patients depending on the dosage regimen of each drug, the age, physiological, and pathological conditions of the patient, and a host of other unknown variables. In these cases, value judgments must usually be made on the total information available (which is often incomplete) and the course of therapy must be monitored closely.

A rather good example of the variation that occurs between different individuals can be obtained from the data given in Fig. 16. Five of the subjects receiving phenytoin (300 mg/day) averaged serum levels of 5 μg/ml which is below the levels usually associated with toxicity (about 20 μg/ml). The sixth subject attained serum levels of 23 μg/ml. When dicumarol was given, this subject's serum level reached the toxic level of 40 μg/ml, whereas the serum levels of the other five individuals increased to only 15 μg/ml. Unless prior knowledge of the serum levels of each subject was available, one would be hard pressed to explain why a toxic effect might occur in only one subject. If the initial maintenance dose was doubled in the other five subjects, the steady-state serum levels would still be below usual toxic levels. Addition of dicumarol at this dosage level might increase the serum levels sufficiently to result in toxic effects in all five patients. Thus, dose and individual variation can be extremely important factors.

Duration of therapy also is a critical factor. Enzyme induction requires several days to take effect and may not occur unless a drug is taken chronically. Inhibition of metabolism usually occurs rapidly. An increase in the half-life may not be immediately apparent, however, until a new steady-state plateau is reached which requires six half-lives. Likewise, an interaction which involves competition for protein binding occurs immediately and is a transient effect, disappearing when the second drug is removed (55).

There are some general guidelines that indicate the types of patients and drugs most likely to be involved in drug interactions. The age of the patient is apparently one of the most critical factors in determining the potential severity of an interaction. Examination of a large number of interactions which were fatal or nearly fatal shows that in the majority of the cases the age of the subject was more than 50 years. Infants, because of decreased metabolic and renal excretory functions, are also particularly susceptible to drug interactions.

Several disease states such as glaucoma, hypertension, ulcer, and diabetes predispose a patient to adverse reactions in general. Patients taking chronic medication including corticosteroids, oral contraceptives, sedatives, and tranquilizers or alcoholics are more susceptible as are patients taking doses at the upper limit of the dosage range of inherently toxic agents such as methotrexate. Drugs that must be titrated to the individual such as anticoagulants, anticonvulsants, digitalis, hypoglycemics, and quinidine are involved frequently in drug interactions.

From previous discussion, other types of drugs that present potential problems are poorly absorbed drugs (griseofulvin), highly protein-bound drugs (anti-inflammatory drugs, oral anticoagulants, and some sulfonamides), drugs that are appreciably eliminated by active tubular excretion (uricosurics), weak electrolytes that are tubularly reabsorbed (many narcotic analgesics and sympathomimetics), and drugs metabolized by aromatic hydroxylation.

References

(1) N. A. Pelissier and S. L. Burgee, "Guide to Incompatibilities," *Hosp. Pharm., 3,* 15 (1968).
(2) F. C. Cross *et al.,* "The Effect of Certain Drugs on the Results of Some Common Laboratory Diagnostic Procedures," *Amer. J. Hosp. Pharm., 23,* 235 (1966).
(3) M. P. Elking, Sr., and H. F. Karat, "Drug Induced Modifications of Laboratory Test Values," *Amer. J. Hosp. Pharm., 25,* 484 (1968).
(4) J. T. Hicks, "Drugs Affecting Laboratory Values," *Hosp. Form. Manage., 2,* 19 (1967).

(5) W. H. Barr, "Factors Involved in the Assessment of Systemic or Biological Availability," *Drug Inform. Bull., 3,* 27 (1969).

(6) W. H. Barr, "Principles of Biopharmaceutics," *Amer. J. Pharm. Ed., 32,* 958 (1968).

(7) L. W. Schanker, in "Physiological Transport of Drugs," N. J. Harper and A. B. Simmonds, Eds., Advances in Drug Research Series, vol. 1, Academic, London, England, 1964, pp. 72–106.

(8) "Handbook of Non-Prescription Drugs," G. B. Griffenhagen and L. L. Hawkins, Eds., American Pharmaceutical Association, Washington, DC 20037, 1971, p. 33.

(9) W. H. Barr *et al.,* "Decrease of Tetracycline Absorption in Man by Sodium Bicarbonate," *Clin. Pharmacol. Ther., 12,* 779 (1971).

(10) D. G. Gallo *et al.,* "The Interaction between Cholestyramine and Drugs," *Proc. Soc. Exp. Biol. Med., 120,* 60 (1965).

(11) J. G. Wagner, "Biopharmaceutics: Absorption Aspects," *J. Pharm. Sci., 50,* 359 (1961).

(12) G. Levy, in "Prescription Pharmacy," J. B. Sprowls, Ed., Lippincott, Philadelphia, Pa., 1963, pp. 31–94.

(13) P. M. Aggeler and R. A. O'Reilly, "Effect of Heptabarbital on the Response to Bishydroxycoumarin in Man," *J. Lab. Clin. Med., 74,* 229 (1969).

(14) L. K. Garrettson *et al.,* "Methylphenidate Interaction with Both Anticonvulsants and Ethyl Biscoumacetate," *J. Amer. Med. Ass., 207,* 2053 (1969).

(15) H. H. Frey and E. Kampmann, "Interaction of Amphetamine with Anticonvulsant Drugs. II. Effect of Amphetamine on the Absorption of Anticonvulsant Drugs," *Acta Pharmacol. Toxicol., 24,* 310 (1966).

(16) H. F. Morrelli and K. L. Melmon, "The Clinician's Approach to Drug Interactions," *Calif. Med., 109,* 380 (1968).

(17) J. G. Wagner *et al.,* "Blood Levels of Drug at the Equilibrium State after Multiple Dosing," *Nature, 207,* 1301 (1965).

(18) A. H. Conney, "Pharmacological Implications of Microsomal Enzyme Induction," *Pharmacol. Rev., 19,* 317 (1967).

(19) J. R. Gillette, in "Animal and Clinical Pharmacological Techniques in Drug Evaluation," P. E. Siegler and J. H. Moyer, III, Eds., Year Book, Chicago, Ill., 1967, pp. 48–66.

(20) R. Kuntzman, "Drugs and Enzyme Induction," *Ann. Rev. Pharmacol., 9,* 21 (1969).

(21) R. M. H. Kater *et al.,* "Increased Rate of Clearance of Drugs from the Circulation of Alcoholics," *Amer. J. Med. Sci., 258,* 35 (1969).

(22) J. Dwyer *et al.,* "A Study of Cortisol Metabolism in Patients with Chronic Asthma," *Australas. Ann. Med., 16,* 297 (1967).

(23) H. J. Schwartz *et al.,* "Steroid Resistance in Bronchial Asthma," *Ann. Intern. Med., 69,* 493 (1968).

(24) B. Kolmodin *et al.,* "Effect of Environmental Factors on Drug Metabolism: Decreased Plasma Half-Life of Antipyrine in Workers Exposed to Chlorinated Hydrocarbon Insecticides," *Clin. Pharmacol. Ther., 10,* 638 (1969).

(25) R. M. Welch *et al.,* "Stimulatory Effect of Cigarette Smoking on the Hydroxylation of 3,4-Benzpyrine and the N-Demethylation of 3-Methyl-4-monomethylaminoazobenzene by Enzymes in Human Placenta," *Clin. Pharmacol. Ther., 10,* 100 (1969).

(26) O. M. Spurny *et al.,* "Protracted Tolbutamide-Induced Hypoglycemia," *Arch. Intern. Med., 11,* 53 (1965).

(27) L. K. Christensen and L. Skovsted, "Inhibition of Drug Metabolism by Chloramphenicol," *Lancet, ii,* 1397 (1969).

(28) J. M. Hansen *et al.,* "Dicoumarol-Induced Diphenylhydantoin Intoxication," *Lancet, ii,* 265 (1966).

(29) S. I. Cullen and P. M. Catalano, "Griseofulvin-Warfarin Antagonism," *J. Amer. Med. Ass., 199,* 582 (1967).

(30) H. M. Solomon and J. J. Schrogie, "Effect of Phenyramidol and Bishydroxycoumarin on Metabolism of Tolbutamide in Human Subjects," *Metabolism, 16,* 1029 (1967).

(31) H. Kutt *et al.,* "Depression of Parahydroxylation of Diphenylhydantoin by Antituberculosis Chemotherapy," *Neurology, 16,* 594 (1966).

(32) K. Reber and A. Studer, "Beeinflussung der Wirkung Einiger Indirekter Antikoaguantien Durch Monaminoooxydase—Hemmer," *Thromb. Diath. Haemorrh., 14,* 83 (1965).

(33) E. Rothstein, "Warfarin Effect Enhanced by Disulfiram," letter to the editor, *J. Amer. Med. Ass., 206,* 1574 (1968).

(34) W. A. Pettinger *et al.,* "Inhibition of Monoamine Oxidase in Man by Furazolidone," *Clin. Pharmacol. Ther., 9,* 442 (1968).

(35) G. Levy and L. P. Amsel, "Kinetics of Competitive Inhibition of Salicylic Acid Conjugation with Glycine in Man," *Biochem. Pharmacol., 15,* 1033 (1966).

(36) G. Levy and J. Procknal, "Drug Biotransformation Interactions in Man I. Mutual Inhibition in Glucuronide Formation of Salicylic Acid and Salicylamide in Man," *J. Pharm. Sci., 57,* 1330 (1968).

(37) G. Levy and H. Yamada, "Drug Biotransformation Interactions in Man III: Acetaminophen and Salicylamide," *J. Pharm. Sci., 60,* 215 (1971).

(38) I. M. Weiner and G. H. Mudge, "Renal Tubular Mechanisms for Excretion of Organic Acids and Bases," *Amer. J. Med., 36,* 743 (1964).

(39) W. P. Boger *et al.,* "Probenecid and Salicylates: The Question of Interaction in Terms of Penicillin Excretion," *J. Lab. Clin. Med., 45,* 478 (1955).

(40) J. M. Perel *et al.,* "Studies of Interactions among Drugs in Man at the Renal Level: Probenecid and Sulfinpyrazone," *Clin. Pharmacol. Ther., 10,* 834 (1969).

(41) M. D. Milne, "Influence of Acid-Base Balance on Efficiency and Toxicity of Drugs," in Symposium on Interaction between Drugs, *Proc. Roy. Soc. Med., 58,* 961 (1965).

(42) A. H. Beckett and M. Rowland, "Urinary Excretion Kinetics of Amphetamine in Man," *J. Pharm. Pharmacol., 17,* 628 (1965).

(43) A. M. Asatoor *et al.,* "The Excretion of Dextroamphetamine and Its Derivatives," *Brit. J. Pharmacol. Chemother., 24,* 293 (1965).

(44) H. B. Kostenbauder *et al.,* "Quinidine Excretion in Aciduria and Alkaluria," *Ann. Intern. Med., 71,* 927 (1969).

(45) H. B. Kostenbauder *et al.,* "Control of Urine pH and Its Effect on Sulfaethidole Excretion in Humans," *J. Pharm. Sci., 51,* 1084 (1962).

(46) B. B. Brodie, "Displacement of One Drug by Another from Carrier or Receptor Sites," in Symposium on Interaction between Drugs, *Proc. Roy. Soc. Med., 58,* 946 (1965).

(47) B. B. Brodie, in "Absorption and Distribution of Drugs," T. Binns, Ed., Livingstone, Edinburgh, Scotland, 1964, p. 16.

(48) C. J. Cavallito *et al.,* "Influence of Anesthesia on the Neuromuscular Blocking Activity of Mylaxen," *Anesthesiology, 17,* 547 (1956).

(49) M. Gibaldi and M. A. Schwartz, "Apparent Effect of Probenecid on the Distribution of Penicillins in Man," *Clin. Pharmacol. Ther.,* 9, 345 (1968).

(50) P. M. Aggeler *et al.,* "Potentiation of Anticoagulant Effect of Warfarin by Phenylbutazone," *N. Engl. J. Med., 276,* 496 (1967).

(51) L. K. Christensen *et al.,* "Sulphaphenazole-Induced Hypoglycaemic Attacks in Tolbutamide-Treated Diabetics," *Lancet, ii,* 1298 (1963).

(52) J. W. Paterson *et al.,* "Isoprenaline Resistance and the Use of Pressurised Aerosols in Asthma," *Lancet, ii,* 426 (1968).

(53) A. G. McManis, "Deaths following IV. Epinephrine in Patients Using Isoproterenol," *Med. J. Aust., 2,* 76 (1964).

(54) W. D. Refshauge, "Deaths due to Epinephrine and Self Administered Isoproterenol," *Med. J. Aust., 1,* 93 (1965).

(55) J. Koch-Weser and E. M. Sellers, "Drug Interactions with Coumarin Anticoagulants," *N. Engl. J. Med., 285,* 487, 547 (1971).

Pharmacological Aspects of Drug Interactions: Therapeutic Classes

Acid–Base Balance Therapy

Total body fluids are composed of intracellular (65%) and extracellular (35%) fluids. There are major differences in the composition of these two fluids. The extracellular fluid is more accessible, more precisely defined, and better understood. Thus, the acid–base status of an individual is usually reported in terms of the pH of arterial blood. The actual hydrogen-ion concentration of arterial blood is 4×10^{-8} Eq/liter, and the pH is 7.4. An arterial pH below 7.4 is considered abnormal and constitutes acidosis or acidemia, while a pH above 7.4 constitutes alkalosis or alkalemia; pH values below 7.0 or above 7.8 usually are fatal—acidosis causing coma and alkalosis causing convulsions.

Acid–base regulation is necessary to protect the body from the effects of acid metabolic end products which are continually formed. For example, enzymatically catalyzed metabolic reactions are pH dependent. An increase in pH beyond the optimal value may produce hyperexcitability and tetany, while a decrease in pH may cause coma. The pH of the extracellular fluids is represented by the relationship between sodium bicarbonate and carbonic acid or by the tension of càrbon dioxide, expressed as the partial pressure of carbon dioxide (pCO_2) in the blood:

$$pH = 6.09 + \log \frac{[HCO_3^-]}{0.0307\, pCO_2} \qquad (Eq.\ 1)$$

The quantity of carbon dioxide dissolved in the fluid is proportional to the pCO_2. It is expressed in millimoles per liter and is equal to $0.0307\, pCO_2$. If the bicarbonate concentration and pH are known, pCO_2 can be calculated from Eq. 1. If pCO_2 and pH are known, the bicarbonate concentration can be calculated.

Control of Acid–Base Balance

Normally, the acid–base balance is controlled by physiological buffers, by the respiratory system, and by the kidneys. The bicarbonate–carbonic acid system is one of the two major buffer systems and is, in fact, the only buffer system subject to rapid compensatory regulation. The phosphate buffer represents the other major buffer system, although buffer activity is also provided by the proteins of the plasma, hemoglobin, and intracellular proteins.

An increase in extracellular fluid pH tends to inhibit ventilation, while a depression in pH or an increase in pCO_2 tends to increase ventilatory exchange. Thus, the respiratory system regulates the acid–base balance by varying the rate of carbon dioxide removal. Increased alveolar ventilation increases removal of the gas and lowers the hydrogen-ion concentration. When the cellular metabolic rate increases, the pCO_2 in venous blood rises, causing a decrease in pH. The lower pH stimulates the respiratory center to increase the depth and the rate of respiration, which lowers carbon dioxide pressure and increases the removal of carbon dioxide. As the process continues, the pH of body fluids again approaches normal values, normalizing respiratory depth and rate.

The kidneys, providing the slowest method of regulation, act by varying the rate of removal of hydrogen ions from body fluids. The kidneys counteract respiratory acidosis by increased secretion of hydrogen ions, retention of bicarbonate, and synthesis of ammonia. This process results in decreased urinary pH.

Therapeutic Indications

Alkalizers—There are a number of major disturbances of the acid–base balance which may require alkalizer therapy. Respiratory acidosis occurs whenever there is inadequate alveolar ventilation. The primary disorder involves retention of carbon dioxide. Any condition that decreases pulmonary ventilation can thus lead to respiratory acidosis. If the pH defines acidosis and there is no discernible base excess or deficit, the disturbance would be judged respiratory in nature. Conditions that may lead to respiratory acidosis include damage to the respiratory center, obstruction of airways, pneumonia, pulmonary edema and fibrosis, emphysema (due to decreased alveolar surface), and cardiopulmonary disease.

Metabolic acidosis is a loss of acid–base regulation due to any cause other than respiratory. It may result from an accumulation of metabolic acids or from a loss of alkali. Accumulation of organic acids occurs in uncontrolled diabetes mellitus, where excessive fat metabolism increases the quantity of ketone bodies. Organic acids that have been identified in such a process include lactic acid, β-hydroxybutyric acid, and acetoacetic acid. Prolonged and severe diarrhea and severe vomiting may cause excessive loss of alkali. Kidney disorders also may cause metabolic acidosis. Disease of the kidney tissue may cause uremic acidosis; renal failure may cause accumulation of phosphates and sulfates, resulting in mineral acidosis; and renal tubular disease may cause impaired ammonia synthesis and impaired tubular reabsorption of sodium chloride, leading to hyperchloremic acidosis.

The normal compensatory response to acidosis, hyperventilation, may occur in extreme acidosis or when the muscles of respiration are weakened. Acidosis is best evaluated by calculation of the base deficit or negative base excess. The normal value for bicarbonate averages from 21 to 25 mEq/liter (1); if the base deficit is more than 5 mEq/liter or if the plasma bicarbonate level is less than 20 mEq/liter, then alkalizer therapy is indicated (2). The need for therapy can also be established by estimating the difference between normal and current total carbon dioxide content and multiplying this by 50% of the body weight in kilograms (1).

Administration of sodium bicarbonate is the treatment of choice when alkali reserves require replenishment in severe metabolic acidosis (3). Other alkalinizing agents such as sodium lactate offer no advantage over sodium bicarbonate and have the additional disadvantage of requiring metabolic breakdown before liberating bicarbonate. For example, lactate is converted to glycogen and bicarbonate. It also can be oxidized to bicarbonate, water, and carbon dioxide. Of course, either of the two processes delays the desired therapeutic effect (1, 4, 5). In selecting a therapeutic agent, it must be kept in mind that the tricarboxylic acid cycle may not function efficiently, since severe metabolic acidosis tends to depress enzymatic activity. Thus, the conversion of lactate to bicarbonate may be further delayed, and, in fact, fractions of lactate may be excreted unchanged (4).

In respiratory acidosis, the administration of sodium bicarbonate alone is not recommended, as it would restore the pH to normal levels but would not correct the carbon dioxide excess (4). Additionally, correction of the pH alone may depress the respiratory stimulus and cause further retention of carbon dioxide. Treatment of respiratory acidosis with sodium bicarbonate alone presents the distinct danger of mental confusion and coma, due to a fall in pH of the cerebrospinal fluid to 7.25, as carbon dioxide readily penetrates into the cerebrospinal fluid and bicarbonate does not (4).

Alkalizers are also frequently used in hyperacidity of the gastrointestinal (GI) tract. They raise gastric pH, alleviating hyperchlorhydria and decreasing proteolytic enzyme activity. Nonabsorbable antacids generally have relatively little effect on systemic acid–base balance and have only a limited effect —compared to absorbable antacids such as sodium bicarbonate—on gastric pH. However, they absorb onto or coat sensitive areas of the gastroduodenal epithelium.

Another use of alkalizers is in urological disorders, where they may be employed to reduce the irritating quality of urine during bladder inflammation, to prevent calculus formation, to increase the effectiveness of certain drugs (whose urinary excretion is pH dependent), and to combat acidosis associated with renal failure (6). Urinary alkalinization (to pH 7.5–8.0) has proven useful in the management of porphyria by increasing the degree of ionization and, therefore, the rate of excretion of coproporphyrin and urobilinogen (7). Urinary alkalinization with sodium bicarbonate (4–8 g/day) (8) may initially benefit gouty patients with very high serum uric acid levels by markedly enhancing uric acid excretion.

Most commonly, sodium bicarbonate is used in urology. Potassium acetate and potassium citrate also are used, sometimes advantageously, as they do not neutralize gastric juice or disturb digestion. Sodium citrate, given orally, is claimed to be most palatable if administration of an alkalizer over a prolonged period is desired; but, of course, the citrates cannot be administered intravenously as they would interfere with the blood-clotting mechanism (6).

Acidifiers—The major acid–base disturbance requiring acidifier therapy is alkalosis. Respiratory alkalosis is only rarely encountered clinically. It may occur physiologically as a result of hyperventilation due to low atmospheric levels of oxygen. Nonetheless, it is a rare clinical entity. Metabolic alkalosis is an infrequent occurrence compared to metabolic acidosis. The ingestion of large amounts of sodium bicarbonate or other alkaline material is most often responsible for its onset. Less frequently, it may be the result of the vomiting of the gastric contents with a concomitant loss of gastric acid. Metabolic alkalosis can also arise from a loss of potassium induced by drug administration (*e.g.*, corticosteroids or diuretics) and diarrhea. Enhanced excretion of potassium results in an increase in hydrogen-ion secretion in the urine which enhances the tubular reabsorption of bicarbonate. Cellular ion exchange can be affected to the extent that hydrogen ions may be transported into cells in exchange for potassium ions. This process only serves to increase the degree of alkalosis.

Ammonium chloride has been used occasionally in the treatment of metabolic alkalosis in the absence of hepatic dysfunction. Hepatic transformation of ammonium chloride to urea and chloride ions results in a decrease in extracellular fluid pH and a correction of the alkalosis. However, it may result in an increased loss of potassium and sodium ions which would only aggravate the condition.

Arginine hydrochloride has been suggested (9) as an acidifying agent in place of ammonium chloride. While no more efficient in providing chloride ion, it does provide chloride without the danger of ammonia intoxication. This factor would be of obvious importance in treating those patients with underlying hepatic disease. Suggested treatment of metabolic alkalosis was based upon the correction of dehydration (by administration of salt and water), the correction of any potassium deficit (by the oral or parenteral administration of potassium salts), and the supply of adequate amounts of carbohydrate to minimize protein catabolism and ketonemia (10).

Two relatively minor indications for acidifier therapy involve deficient gastric secretion of hydrochloric acid (hypochlorhydria and achlorhydria) and urinary acidification. Hypochlorhydria and achlorhydria generally have been treated by the administration of an acidulant such as diluted hydrochloric acid or glutamic acid hydrochloride. Urine acidification often has been a requisite for treatment of urinary tract infections with some anti-infective agents (e.g., methenamine mandelate). A decreased urine pH, per se, may be effective in controlling or eliminating urinary tract infections. To this end, acidifiers such as ammonium chloride (6–8 g/day) and ascorbic acid (4–12 g/day) have been used effectively.

Contraindications, Side Effects, and Interactions

Alkalizers—The administration of systemic alkalizers such as sodium bicarbonate induces metabolic alkalosis, although in most instances the drug is eliminated so rapidly that a serious degree of alkalosis does not occur. However, administration of sodium bicarbonate also augments potassium excretion which could lead to an intensification of the alkalosis. Additionally, the development of hypokalemia could pose a serious problem for the patient maintained on cardiac glycosides, as cardiotoxicity is enhanced in the presence of hypokalemia (see Digitalis–Chlorothiazide, p. 52).

In some conditions, such as chronic renal failure, acidosis may be accompanied by hypocalcemia. When this occurs, treatment of the acidosis without attention to the calcium imbalance may precipitate an episode of hypocalcemic tetany (10). Therefore, hypocalcemic, acidotic patients should be treated initially by the infusion of calcium gluconate prior to the correction of the acidosis (1).

The route and rate of administration of alkalizers are also important. Thus, hemorrhagic liver necrosis was observed in newborn infants with respiratory acidosis who were treated with sodium bicarbonate and tromethamine via the umbilical vein, but this condition did not occur when the drugs were administered via the umbilical artery (11). Intravenous administration of sodium bicarbonate has become a standard practice in the treatment of metabolic and respiratory acidosis in premature infants (12–14). Sodium bicarbonate should be administered slowly because of the danger of respiratory depression or the possibility of seizures due to low total calcium or low ionized calcium. Calcium levels should be assessed periodically.

Finally, caution must be exercised with patients for whom sodium intake is restricted (1, 4). Thus, the use of sodium bicarbonate in patients with cardiovascular disease may not be prudent.

Gastric alkalizers have posed problems for the clinician, particularly when other drugs have been administered concurrently (15). The absorption and excretion of other drugs often can be affected. Thus, the amount of drug available for absorption from the GI tract can be reduced by adsorption of the drug onto the surface of finely divided solids, as found in suspensions of aluminum hydroxide or milk of magnesia. Complexation of drugs with metal ions, present in nonabsorbable gastric alkalizers, also can render a drug unavailable for absorption. A rise in intragastric pH, alone or coupled with changes in the gastric emptying time following alkalizer administration, may be sufficient to alter drug absorption significantly by affecting drug dissolution. This effect was demonstrated for tetracycline (see Tetracycline–Aluminum, Calcium, and Magnesium Ions, p. 227) (16). Finally, the prolonged ingestion of large amounts of absorbable gastric alkalizers could affect urinary pH and alter the urinary excretion of drugs whose dissociation is pH dependent.

The pH of the tubular fluid, the pKa, and the partition coefficient of a drug can influence renal tubular transport of many drugs. Changes in urinary pH also can alter the rate of urinary excretion. Most drugs are weak organic acids or bases. It is usually the ionized portion of the drug molecule that is water soluble and can thus be excreted by the kidney. In an alkaline urine, weak bases will be more unionized and less water soluble and will thus be reabsorbed, while acidic drugs will be more ionized and thus be more prone to excretion.

If the urine is at a pH at which the drug is present primarily in the ionized form, the possibility of passive reabsorption of the drug may be considerably reduced. Systemic drug levels may thus be diminished. If the urine is at a pH at which the drug is unionized, the possibility of passive reabsorption is enhanced, resulting in higher systemic levels (17–19). The following drugs could be affected by changes in urinary pH (19), i.e., they could be excreted more rapidly at different urinary pH values.

Acid Urine: amitriptyline, amphetamine, chloroquine, desipramine, imipramine, mecamylamine, meperidine, methamphetamine, nortriptyline, quinacrine, quinidine, and quinine.

Alkaline Urine: acetazolamide, phenobarbital, phenylbutazone, salicylic acid, sulfaethidole, and sulfathiazole.

Sodium citrate, the preferred urinary alkalinizer when prolonged alkalinization is needed, should only be employed along with a low calcium diet. Alkaline urine will precipitate calcium; thus, milk and milk products must be avoided by the patient (6).

Acidifiers—The problems inherent in the use of a systemic acidifier such as ammonium chloride have been noted previously. The gradual onset of hypokalemia could present a grave problem for patients maintained on cardiac glycosides.

The administration of acetazolamide or ammonium chloride occasionally has led to the development of a painful crisis in patients with sickle cell disease (20, 21). Patients in such a crisis have low levels of sodium bicarbonate and have been treated successfully with 0.17 M (1/6 M) sodium lactate intravenously and sodium citrate orally. Relief of symptoms, with either treatment, was obtained within 48 hr. The use of sodium citrate orally was recommended as it is economical, more readily available, and easily administered (21).

The use of acidifiers to decrease urine pH may involve additional difficulties. The ingestion of large doses of ascorbic acid in humans can lead to a significant increase in urinary oxalate excretion (22). Hyperoxa-

luria could favor renal damage due to the formation of oxalate stones. Urate or cystine stone formation may be induced by the ingestion of large doses of ascorbic acid in patients with gout or cystinuria (23). The effect of a decrease in urine pH on the excretion of other drugs has been discussed previously.

References

(1) "The Pharmacological Basis of Therapeutics," 5th ed., L. S. Goodman and A. Gilman, Eds., Macmillan, New York, NY 10022, 1975, pp. 769–780.

(2) "Current Therapy 1974," H. F. Conn, Ed., Saunders, Philadelphia, Pa., 1974, pp. 452–455.

(3) "Current Therapy 1972," H. F. Conn, Ed., Saunders, Philadelphia, Pa., 1972, p. 426.

(4) B. W. Gunner, "Intravenously Administered Sodium Bicarbonate," Med. J. Aust., 1, 275 (1967).

(5) H. E. Eliahou et al., "Acetate and Bicarbonate in the Correction of Uraemic Acidosis," Brit. Med. J., 4, 399 (1970).

(6) "Drugs of Choice, 1975," W. Modell, Ed., Mosby, St. Louis, Mo., 1975, p. 563.

(7) P. W. M. Copeman, "Porphyria. Successful Treatment by Alkalinization of Urine with Sodium Bicarbonate Assessed by Experimental Suction Blister Apparatus," Brit. J. Dermatol., 82, 385 (1970).

(8) "Drugs of Choice, 1974," W. Modell, Ed., Mosby, St. Louis, Mo., 1974, p. 482.

(9) "Cecil–Loeb Textbook of Medicine," P. B. Beeson and W. McDermott, Eds., Saunders, Philadelphia, Pa., 1975, p. 839.

(10) "Harrison's Principles of Internal Medicine," 6th ed., vol. 2, M. Wintrobe et al., Eds., McGraw-Hill, New York, N.Y., 1970, pp. 1371–1385.

(11) V. E. Goldenberg et al., "Hepatic Injury Associated with Tromethamine," J. Amer. Med. Ass., 205, 81 (1968).

(12) R. Usher, "Reduction of Mortality from Respiratory Distress Syndrome of Prematurity with Early Administration of Intravenous Glucose and Sodium Bicarbonate," Pediatrics, 32, 966 (1963).

(13) M. E. R. Stoneman and R. M. Owens, "Effects of Intragastric Sodium Bicarbonate in Infants with Respiratory Distress," Arch. Dis. Childhood, 43, 155 (1968).

(14) W. Feldman et al., "Severe Metabolic Acidemia in Infants: Clinical and Therapeutic Aspects," J. Can. Med. Ass., 94, 328 (1966).

(15) P. P. Lamy and M. E. Kitler, "Untoward Effects on Drugs. I. (Including Non-Prescription Drugs)," Dis. Nerv. Syst., 32, 17 (1971).

(16) W. H. Barr et al., "Decrease of Tetracycline Absorption in Man by Sodium Bicarbonate," Clin. Pharmacol. Ther., 12, 779 (1971).

(17) L. H. Block and P. P. Lamy, "Drug Interactions," J. Amer. Pharm. Ass., NS9, 202 (1969).

(18) P. P. Lamy and M. E. Kitler, "The Actions and Interactions of OTC Drugs," Hosp. Form. Manage., 5 (1), 19 (1970).

(19) M. M. Reidenberg, "Renal Function and Drug Action," Saunders, Philadelphia, Pa., 1971, pp. 9–11.

(20) J. P. Knochel, "Hematuria in Sickle Cell Trait: The Effect of Intravenous Administration of Distilled Water, Urinary Alkalinization, and Diuresis," *Arch. Intern. Med., 123,* 160 (1969).

(21) L. Barreras and L. W. Diggs, "Sodium Citrate Orally for Painful Sickle Cell Crisis," *J. Amer. Med. Ass., 215,* 762 (1971).

(22) M. P. Lamden and G. A. Chrystowski, "Urinary Oxalate Excretion by Man following Ascorbic Acid Ingestion," *Proc. Soc. Exp. Biol. Med., 85,* 190 (1954).

(23) "Vitamin C—Were the Trials Well-Controlled and Are Large Doses Safe?" *Med. Lett., 13,* 46 (1971).

Adrenergic Therapy

Drugs that stimulate structures innervated by adrenergic (sympathetic) nerves are referred to as adrenergic or sympathomimetic agents. Because of the various effects produced, these drugs are widely used in clinical medicine, have a large number of physiological effects, and are often used in conjunction with other therapeutic agents. The occurrence of unfavorable interactions is therefore common. Interactions primarily occur with three broad classes of drugs—anesthetic agents, antihypertensive drugs, and monoamine oxidase inhibitors—and several miscellaneous agents.

Therapeutic Indications

Adrenergic drugs have five broad actions. The first involves a peripheral effect on smooth muscle, producing an excitatory effect (vasoconstriction) on blood vessels supplying the skin, mucous membranes, abdominal viscera, and salivary and sweat glands. The second is an inhibitory or relaxing action on smooth muscles in several areas including the bronchi, gut wall, and blood vessels supplying skeletal muscles. A cardiac-stimulating effect is responsible for increased heart rate and force of contraction of cardiac muscle. Central nervous system (CNS) effects include increased excitability and some degree of respiratory stimulation. Finally, increased metabolic activity is manifested by enhanced glycogenolysis in muscle and liver and by enhanced lipolysis with liberation of free fatty acids. A particular drug is chosen for use by virtue of its specific action(s).

Sympathomimetic agents are effective temporarily in the acute management of hypotension and shock. Levarterenol and metaraminol are used to raise blood pressure to improve blood flow to vital organs. However, vasoconstriction is a feature of shock and may be aggravated by these drugs which can seriously impair blood flow to the kidneys and liver. Dopamine, an endogenous catecholamine, is also useful in shock and has the advantage of increasing renal blood flow (1).

There is greater rationale for the use of adrenergic agents in shock associated with myocardial infarction where vasopressors may enhance venous return and improve coronary blood flow and myocardial function. Some sympathomimetic agents increase myocardial work and predispose the patient to arrhythmias. Therefore, in some circumstances, drugs such as isoproterenol or mephentermine may be used to stimulate myocardial function while avoiding peripheral vasoconstriction. However, levarterenol or metaraminol may be indicated when both increased cardiac function and peripheral vasoconstriction are desired.

Sympathomimetic drugs including ephedrine, epinephrine, and isoproterenol are used in the treatment of Stokes–Adams attacks due to complete heart block. Several adrenergic drugs also have been used to treat peripheral vascular insufficiency, especially intermittent claudication, and to increase cerebral blood flow. These agents act primarily at β-receptor sites, are long acting, and can be given by mouth. The value of such drugs as isoxsuprine and nylidrin is not well established. Pressor drugs such as methoxamine and phenylephrine are of value in the treatment of paroxysmal atrial tachycardia.

Epinephrine and isoproterenol are important agents in the treatment of acute asthma; epinephrine is specifically indicated in the management of anaphylaxis and hypersensitivity seen with acute drug reactions or insect stings. Other uses, related to specific α- or β-receptor activity, include control of topical bleeding, decongestion of mucous membranes in allergic rhinitis, dilation of the pupils for ophthalmic examination, and prevention of posterior synechiae in uveitis.

The CNS effects of sympathomimetic drugs also can be utilized therapeutically. Unfortunately, they may produce side effects that limit their effectiveness. Noncatecholamine drugs such as amphetamine, diethylpropion, and phenmetrazine are used, with questionable effectiveness, as anorexic drugs. Amphetamines and ephedrine are used to treat narcolepsy, postencephalitic parkinsonism, hyperkinetic states in children, and some forms of epilepsy (2).

Pharmacological Mechanisms

The basic structure of all sympathomimetic drugs consists of an aromatic nucleus (the benzene ring) and an aliphatic portion (ethylamine). Substitutions can be made on either or both portions, yielding a large number of sympathomimetic agents with varying activity. The presence of hydroxyl groups at the 3- and 4-positions of the benzene ring gives rise to the catecholamines, including dopamine, epinephrine, isoproterenol, and norepinephrine. The noncatechol group of sympathomimetic amines includes amphetamine, ephedrine, mephentermine, metaraminol, methamphetamine, methoxamine, and phenylephrine. Other related amines which are used clinically include levodopa and methyldopa.

Sympathomimetic drugs may be broadly classified in two other ways. The first depends on their action on adrenergic receptor sites, classified as either α- or β-sites. Their effect is usually excitatory on α-receptors and inhibitory on β-sites. An important exception to this general rule is that sympathomimetic amines produce excitatory action on the heart where receptors are predominantly of the β-type. The clinical response to these drugs can, therefore, often be predicted by knowledge of their selectivity in reacting with each type of receptor. For example, isoproterenol, a β-adrenergic stimulator, produces both cardiac excitatory effects and the relaxation of bronchial musculature. Phenylephrine, on the other hand, is an α-adrenergic stimulator and causes neither of these effects but produces a vasopressor effect by constricting peripheral vascular beds. Most sympathomimetic drugs, however, affect both α- and β-receptors, although the ratio of such stimulation varies greatly.

The other classification is determined by whether a drug directly stimulates adrenergic receptor sites or acts indirectly *via* release of norepinephrine from adrenergic neurons (3). Epinephrine, isoproterenol, levarterenol, and methoxamine have a direct effect. Mephentermine is a compound with an indirect-release mechanism. The amphetamines, ephedrine, metaraminol, phenylephrine, and phenylpropanolamine occupy an intermediate position since they possess both direct and indirect activity (4). A knowledge of this action is especially important in terms of interactions between such sympathomimetic drugs and compounds used in the treatment of hypertension which deplete neuronal stores of norepinephrine.

Contraindications

In general, contraindications to the use of sympathomimetic amines are relative and relate to the fact that most agents have multiple effects, one of which may be desirable therapeutically while the other(s) may be deleterious. Epinephrine, for example, is the drug of choice in acute asthma, but in a patient with asthma and severe hypertension, the disadvantage of the pressor effect may outweigh the therapeutic benefit of bronchodilation.

Interactions

Anesthetic Agents—There are reports of adrenergic drug-induced arrhythmias occurring whenever adrenergic drugs are used concurrently with almost all general anesthetics (ether and nitrous oxide may not interact with adrenergic agents).

In terms of this adrenergic–anesthetic reaction, the adrenergic agents appear to act through β-adrenergic stimulation.

Anesthetic agents in order of decreasing sensitization potential in dogs are as follows: trichloroethylene, ethyl chloride, cyclopropane, halothane, chloroform, methoxyflurane, and fluroxene. Regardless of whether a similar ranking is applicable to humans, it is clear that anesthetic agents, especially halogenated compounds, and sympathomimetic drugs may interact and produce serious cardiac arrhythmias. This complication may occur with intramuscular as well as subcutaneous injections of sympathomimetic drugs, although the margin of safety is much greater than with intravenous use. Usually, untoward reactions of this type result from the injection of too high a concentration of the drug into a highly vascular area. Adrenergic drugs can be administered subcutaneously with relative safety if minimal doses are used and hypoxia, hypercapnia, and acidosis are avoided (see *Halothane–Epinephrine,* p. 90).

Antihypertensive Drugs—One group of drugs used to treat hypertension acts by blocking postganglionic sympathetic nerve activity. Agents of this type used clinically include guanethidine, methyldopa, and reserpine. Several mechanisms of action have been proposed for these drugs, including depletion of neurotransmitter (norepinephrine) stores, direct prevention of neurotransmitter release, and decreased neurotransmitter formation either by early blockade of synthesis or synthesis of a similar but less active "false" neurotransmitter. These drugs may act by more than one mechanism and the contribution of each to a given effect is difficult to assess.

Following synthesis within adrenergic nerve terminals, norepinephrine exists in equilibrium between small amounts free in the cytoplasm and concentrated amounts within storage granules. Nerve stimulation causes a release of the neurotransmitter from these granules and discharge from the neuron to the extracellular regions where it may react with adrenergic receptor sites of effector cells. Excess norepinephrine is then removed from the extracellular site by an active transport mechanism and returned to the nerve cell. This so-called "norepinephrine pump" mechanism represents the second source of norepinephrine found in adrenergic nerve sites. Small amounts not removed from the extracellular site are enzymatically metabolized by catechol-*O*-methyltransferase while excess amounts in the cytoplasm, if not stored in granules, are metabolized by monoamine oxidase. The entire process of synthesis, storage, and release of norepinephrine is nonspecific, and compounds not ordinarily present may accumulate within the neuron and replace the physiological neurotransmitter (5).

Guanethidine is the prototype of drugs that interfere with postganglionic sympathetic nerve activity. The antihypertensive effect is apparently related to both blockade of release of norepinephrine from adrenergic nerve cells (as shown by the hypotensive effect before depletion of catecholamines) and progressive depletion of tissue stores with chronic administration (6). Because it depletes norepinephrine stores within the neuron, guanethidine also diminishes the subsequent pressor response to indirect-acting sympathomimetic amines. In addition, a supersensitive response by effector cells may be seen with long-term therapy, probably explained by chronic absence of mediator stimulation of such receptors (7). Guanethidine blocks adrenergic neurons selectively, is concentrated in cells *via* the norepinephrine pump, and displaces norepinephrine (8). The uptake of guanethidine, in turn, is prevented by drugs that interfere with the membrane transport system. Guanethidine thus reduces sympathetic tone of the peripheral vasculature, resulting in a decrease in blood pressure, most pronounced in the upright position and greater in hypertensive than in normotensive subjects. It has little effect on catecholamine levels in either the adrenal medulla or the CNS.

Laboratory and clinical data indicate that the antihypertensive effect of guanethidine can be antagonized by the concurrent administration of sympathomimetic drugs (see *Guanethidine–Dextroamphetamine*, p. 86, and *Phenylephrine–Guanethidine*, p. 186). Amphetamines and ephedrine act in large part as indirect sympathomimetic agents *via* release of norepinephrine. They, as well as guanethidine, compete with norepinephrine for active transport into and storage within the neuron. When guanethidine is given and bound within neurons, subsequent administration of these sympathomimetic agents results in displacement of guanethidine, reversing the antihypertensive effect of the drug.

There are a few clinical reports describing untoward side effects from the interaction of sympathomimetic agents given to individuals receiving guanethidine. However, there are good experimental data in humans to show that adrenergic drugs, especially dextroamphetamine and methamphetamine, can displace guanethidine and reverse its antihypertensive effect.

Reserpine and other rauwolfia compounds have also been widely used in the treatment of hypertension. The effect of these drugs is similar to that of guanethidine in causing depletion of catecholamine stores. In contrast to guanethidine, reserpine also produces depletion of catecholamines in the CNS and produces tissue depletion of 5-hydroxytryptamine as well (9). However, neither of these effects appears to play a significant role in the action of reserpine on adrenergic blockade.

The action of reserpine on adrenergic neurons probably occurs by two mechanisms of action. It depletes catecholamine stores, an action which is antagonized by monoamine oxidase inhibitors. In addition, reserpine decreases norepinephrine synthesis by blocking uptake of dopamine by storage granules within neurons which have the ability to synthesize this catecholamine (10). The reduction of tissue catecholamines can be demonstrated almost immediately and is maximal by 24 hr. Furthermore, once established, the impairment of amine storage persists for long periods (11). For this reason, repeated doses may have a cumulative effect even when administered at weekly intervals.

As a consequence of tissue catecholamine depletion by reserpine, the effect of indirect- and mixed-acting sympathomimetic amines may be altered (see *Ephedrine–Reserpine*, p. 67). Early reports (12, 13) described either potential or real hazards of circulatory depression in individuals during general anesthesia who had received prior reserpine therapy. A 40% incidence of severe circulatory depression was reported in 40 cases (14).

Five cases were reported indicating a lack of response to indirect-acting sympathomimetic agents, and the use of norepinephrine was recommended if a pressor agent was required (15). It was suggested that treatment with reserpine should be discontinued for 2 weeks prior to elective surgery. Other studies in animals and humans showed that reserpine therapy did not necessarily predispose subjects to circulatory instability; another report (16) concluded that withdrawal of reserpine therapy prior to surgery was not warranted. Another study (4) provided reasonable guidance by pointing out that the response to indirect-acting sympathomimetic drugs may be diminished by tissue depletion of catecholamines following reserpine therapy, but it can easily be dealt with by the use of direct-acting adrenergic drugs (see *Reserpine–Halothane*, p. 220).

Methyldopa is included as an adrenergic blocking agent even though the relationship between tissue catecholamine depletion and the antihypertensive effect is unclear. Furthermore, it is considered as a sympathomimetic amine, although it is actually an amino acid. Pharmacologically, the drug acts by inhibiting the enzyme dopa decarboxylase and preventing conversion of dopa to dopamine and the subsequent formation of norepinephrine. Methyldopa is converted to α-methylnorepinephrine which can displace and replace norepinephrine in adrenergic neurons. Release of this "false transmitter," which is less active than norepinephrine, may be responsible for the hypotensive effect (17).

In common with guanethidine and reserpine, methyldopa is capable of antagonizing the cardiovascular actions of indirect-acting sympathomimetics such as amphetamine but not norepinephrine (18). This information is derived from animal studies, and there are no clinical reports of this interaction. The possibility is a real one, however, and the same precautions should be observed when using adrenergic pressor agents in patients receiving methyldopa (4).

Monoamine Oxidase Inhibitors—Monoamine oxidase inhibitors are used for the treatment of psychiatric illness, especially depression, and hypertension (19). There has been a decrease in their use recently because of serious hepatic toxicity. There are two broad classes of these drugs (see *Antidepressant Therapy*, p. 373). The first group consists of hydrazine derivatives; these drugs are used primarily for the treatment of depression. Currently used agents of this group include isocarboxazid and phenelzine.

The other group contains nonhydrazine drugs which are structurally related to amphetamine and includes pargyline and tranylcypromine. Pargyline is used primarily in the treatment of hypertension. Although monoamine oxidase inhibitors block oxidative deamination of sympathomimetic amines, there is no clear relationship between this pharmacological action and their therapeutic effectivenesss. They act by forming stable, irreversible complexes with monoamine oxidase. Since there is no impairment of catecholamine synthesis and since monoamine oxidase regulates intracellular amine levels, administration of monoamine oxidase inhibitors results in an excessive accumulation of norepinephrine within cells, including adrenergic neurons, although synthesis is decreased. In addition, monoamine oxidase inhibitors prevent destruction of other amines, (*e.g.*, tyramine) which are hydroxylated to amine products such as octopamine. They, like norepinephrine, are stored in granules and released by nerve stimulation but have a blunted pharmacological effect (false transmitters) (20). This partial adrenergic blockade may account for the hypertensive effect of such compounds.

A sudden pharmacological stimulus of adrenergic neurons can release large amounts of norepinephrine, leading to a hypertensive crisis in patients receiving monoamine oxidise inhibitors (see *Phenylpropanolamine–Tranylcypromine*, p. 188). Such release may be caused by large amounts of tyramine (present in certain foods, especially cheese and wine), by the concurrent administration of a sympathomimetic amine precursor such as levodopa (see *Levodopa–Phenelzine*, p. 128), or by drugs that mimic sympathomimetic actions (see *Imipramine–Tranylcypromine*, p. 103). All sympathomimetics which are indirect or mixed acting pose the same potential hazard.

Miscellaneous Agents—Various other drugs produce an effect on adrenergic neurons and may have clinical significance if they are being used at a time when sympathomimetic agents are also required.

Phenothiazine derivatives, of which chlorpromazine is the prototype, have significant effects on the autonomic nervous system. They may cause strong adrenergic blockade, possibly by impairment of uptake of norepinephrine and dopamine by storage granules (21). Chlorpromazine causes a complex series of effects on the cardiovascular system, only some of which relate to adrenergic blockade and result in decreased standing or sitting blood pressure, but not orthostatic hypertension (22). Tolerance develops within several weeks, however, and blood pressure returns to normal levels. There are also experimental data showing that chlorpromazine can interfere with the pressor effect of indirect-acting adrenergic drugs but not that of epinephrine (see *Chlorpromazine–Amphetamine*, p. 27).

In humans, chlorothiazide administration blunts the pressor response to sympathomimetic amines, including norepinephrine (23). The mechanism here is not due to adrenergic blockade but possibly relates to a change in contractility of arteriolar smooth muscle fibers. This diminished response to sympathomimetic amines, both direct and indirect acting, may be a significant clinical problem in patients receiving thiazide diuretic drugs who require pressor agents.

Tricyclic antidepressants have also been reported to antagonize the antihypertensive effect of guanethidine (see *Guanethidine–Desipramine*, p. 83). Concurrent administration of narcotic analgesics (with the possible exception of morphine) and monoamine oxidase inhibitors has resulted in serious CNS excitation and depression (see *Meperidine–Phenelzine*, p. 142).

References

(1) L. I. Goldberg, "Dopamine—Clinical Uses of an Endogenous Catecholamine," *N. Engl. J. Med., 291*, 707 (1974).

(2) "The Pharmacological Basis of Therapeutics," 5th ed., L. S. Goodman and A. Gilman, Eds., Macmillan, New York, NY 10022, 1975, pp. 477–513.

(3) E. Muscholl, "Indirectly Acting Sympathomimetic Amines," *Pharmacol. Rev., 18*, 551 (1966).

(4) M. H. Alper et al., "Pharmacology of Reserpine and Its Implications for Anesthesia," *Anesthesiology, 24*, 524 (1963).

(5) I. J. Kopin, "False Adrenergic Transmitters," *Ann. Rev. Pharmacol., 8*, 377 (1968).

(6) A. L. Boura and A. F. Green, "Adrenergic Neurone Blocking Agents," *Ann. Rev. Pharmacol., 5*, 183 (1965).

(7) N. Emmelin and J. Engstrom, "Supersensitivity of Salivary Glands following Treatment with Bretylium and Guanethidine," *Brit. J. Pharmacol., 16*, 315 (1961).

(8) J. R. Mitchell and J. A. Oates, "Guanethidine and Related Agents I. Mechanism of Selective Blockade of Adrenergic Neurons and Its Antagonism by Drugs," *J. Pharmacol. Exp. Ther., 172*, 100 (1970).

(9) M. Holzbauer and M. Vogt, "Depression by Reserpine of the Noradrenaline Concentration in the Hypothalamus of the Cat," *J. Neurochem., 1*, 8 (1956).

(10) C. O. Rutledge and N. Weiner, "The Effect of Reserpine upon the Synthesis of Norepinephrine in the Isolated Rabbit Heart," *J. Pharmacol. Exp. Ther., 157*, 290 (1967).

(11) P. W. Taylor, Jr., et al., "A New Effect of Reserpine: Accumulation of Glycoprotein in the Submaxillary Gland," *J. Pharmacol. Exp. Ther., 156*, 483 (1967).

(12) D. L. Crandell, "The Anesthetic Hazards in Patients on Antihypertensive Therapy," *J. Amer. Med. Ass., 179*, 495 (1962).

(13) M. Minuck, "Reaction to Drugs during Surgery and Anaesthesia," *Can. Med. Ass. J., 82*, 1008 (1960).

(14) C. S. Coakley et al., "Circulatory Response during Anesthesia of Patients on Rauwolfia Therapy," *J. Amer. Med. Ass., 161*, 1143 (1956).

(15) C. H. Ziegler and J. B. Lovette, "Operative Complications after Therapy with Reserpine and Reserpine Compounds," *J. Amer. Med. Ass., 176*, 916 (1961).

(16) W. M. Munson and J. A. Jenicek, "Effect of Anesthetic Agents on Patients Receiving Reserpine Therapy," *Anesthesiology, 23*, 741 (1962).

(17) M. D. Day and M. J. Rand, "A Hypothesis for the Mode of Action of α-Methyldopa in Relieving Hypertension," *J. Pharm. Pharmacol., 15*, 221 (1963).

(18) C. A. Stone et al., "Effect of α-Methyl-3,4-dihydroxyphenylalanine (Methyldopa), Reserpine, and Related Agents on Some Vascular Responses in the Dog," *J. Pharmacol. Exp. Ther., 136*, 80 (1962).

(19) I. J. Kopin et al., " 'False Neurochemical Transmitters' and the Mechanism of Sympathetic Blockade by Monoamine Oxidase Inhibitors," *J. Pharmacol. Exp. Ther., 147*, 186 (1965).

(20) R. A. Cohen et al., "False Neurochemical Transmitters," *Ann. Intern. Med., 65*, 347 (1966).

(21) K. F. Gey and A. Pletscher, "Influence of Chlorpromazine and Chlorprothixene on the Cerebral Metabolism of 5-Hydroxytryptamine, Norepinephrine and Dopamine," *J. Pharmacol. Exp. Ther., 133*, 18 (1961).

(22) B. Koral et al., "Effects of Chronic Chlorpromazine Administration on Systemic Arterial Blood Pressure in Schizophrenic Patients: Relationship of Body Position to Blood Pressure," *Clin. Pharmacol. Ther., 6*, 587 (1965).

(23) D. Aleksandrow et al., "Influence of Chlorothiazide upon Arterial Responsiveness to Norepinephrine in Hypertensive Subjects," *N. Engl. J. Med., 261*, 1052 (1959).

Analgesic Therapy (Narcotic)

Within the realm of rational therapeutics, the potent analgesics include the opiates and their synthetic derivatives and certain opiate congeners (such as ethoheptazine, pentazocine, and propoxyphene).

Therapeutic Indications

Morphine-like analgesics relieve severe, acute, and chronically recurring pain. Their central action also alleviates the apprehension associated with painful experiences. They should be reserved for the pain associated with renal, ureteral, or biliary colic; acute myocardial infarction; vascular occlusion; extensive surgical procedures; fractures; burns; and unusual cases where other alternatives are not available (1–9).

Because of their history and the high risk of drug dependence, the morphine-type analgesics are seldom indicated for long-term use. Tolerance to some initial pharmacodynamic effects eventually develops with prolonged and repeated administration. Development of tolerance may be minimized by using the smallest effective dose of the narcotic as infrequently as possible. When nonopioid analgesics have failed, as in terminal or incurable disorders with pain, the morphine-type analgesics usually are employed to ameliorate the discomfort.

In addition to their analgesic value, the opiates offer a selective spectrum of therapeutic application. They are known to produce sedation and sleep if insomnia is due to pain or cough. The opiates listed for moderate to severe pain (Table I) are generally considered to produce equianalgesia, arising from analgesic drug doses comparable to 10 mg iv of morphine in a 70-kg male, the optimal dose of morphine. For example, camphorated tincture of opium and diphenoxylate are used specifically to control diarrhea. Apomorphine stimulates emesis and is useful in the removal of orally ingested poisons. The narcotic antagonists, levallorphan, nalorphine, and naloxone, are employed to reverse narcotic-induced depression of respiration. Codeine suppresses cough and exhibits antitussive effects with a favorable balance between analgesia and side effects. Frequently, better analgesia is obtained from the use of codeine and aspirin or propoxyphene and aspirin than from the single drug entity alone for mild pain.

Morphine improves cardiovascular and respiratory function in patients who have acute pulmonary edema. The traditional use of narcotics and anticholinergics for preoperative sedation is diminishing since more specific anxiolytic drugs have been effectively and safely administered (4). Methadone is an acceptable agent for detoxification of patients dependent on narcotics (1, 10, 11). It prevents abrupt withdrawal symptoms and the euphoric effects of heroin and other narcotics.

Pharmacological Mechanisms

The narcotic analgesics exert their major pharmacological action on the central nervous system (CNS) (5–7). They act on the smooth muscles and exocrine glands of the respiratory and gastrointestinal (GI) tracts. All are characterized by quantitative differences in analgesic, antitussive, and antidiarrheal effects. They tend to dull the sensitivity of the reflex mechanisms; the involuntary reflexes may fail to respond to respiratory irritants for cough, to increases in carbon dioxide tension for respiration, to bulk content in the intestines for defecation, and to distention of the urinary bladder for urination.

The opiates elicit both stimulant and depressant effects on the CNS. They alter the perception of the pain stimulus, the propagation of pain impulses at selective points along the cerebrospinal chord, and the responses to the pain experience (6). They may elevate the pain threshold, an action that is more readily shown in animals than in humans. Their influence on the psychic reactions to pain is a salient feature of narcotic analgesia. In addition to relieving clinical pain, they increase the ability to tolerate pain.

Drowsiness or mental clouding and certain behavioral changes are clinical manifestations of opiate usage. Disturbances in mood often cause euphoria or dysphoria. In the presence of fear or pain, any alleviation of uneasiness and feelings of aggressiveness may produce pleasure (5). This effect can provoke a compulsion to repeat the drug-taking experience. Contrary to the unrealistic sense of well-being or euphoria, some patients receiving morphine-type drugs experience dysphoria, restlessness, and malaise.

In general, the degree of respiratory depression of opiates parallels their analgesic potency and increases progressively with increments in dosages. The opiates reduce the sensitivity of the respiratory center in the medulla to carbon dioxide tension. This reduction results in a slowed rate of breathing and a diminished respiratory minute volume. Irregular or periodic breathing may occur with high concentration of opiates in the body.

Most opiates suppress the cough reflex, but this effect is not directly related to analgesic potency. The antitussive action appears to be a separate pharmacological effect and is not common to all narcotic analgesics. Dextromethorphan, a nonanalgesic narcotic derivative, also possesses antitussive properties (5). Codeine is effective for suppressing involuntary cough (15 mg po) and pathological cough (30 mg po) (5). Ethylmorphine and oxycodone show comparable

effectiveness while the other effects of hydromorphone, levorphanol, methadone, and morphine do not allow for their routine use in cough suppression. In contrast to the previously cited analgesics, alphaprodine, meperidine, and pentazocine lack adequate antitussive activity for clinical use.

Large doses of morphine (0.5–3.0 mg/kg iv) induce anesthesia. Preliminary studies (12) suggest that patients undergoing cardiac surgery with minimal circulatory reserve can safely receive high doses of morphine when ventilation is controlled.

Movement and changes of body position of patients augment the adverse reactions to

Table I—MAJOR THERAPEUTIC INDICATIONS OF OPIATES AND SYNTHETIC OPIOIDS

Phenanthrene Alkaloids:	
Camphorated Tincture of Opium	Antidiarrheal
Codeine	Analgesic for mild to moderate pain
	Antitussive for cough
Morphine	Analgesic for moderate to severe pain
	Management of acute pulmonary edema
Congeners of Phenanthrene:	
Apomorphine	Emetic for poisonings
Ethylmorphine	Antitussive for cough
Heroin[a]	Nontherapeutic agent for the support of drug dependence or "addiction" of the morphine type
Nalorphine	Narcotic antagonist
Naloxone	Narcotic antagonist
Others: Hydromorphone	Analgesics for moderate to severe pain
Oxycodone	
Oxymorphone	
Phenylpiperidine Series and Related Piperidine Moieties:	
Diphenoxylate	Antidiarrheal
Ethoheptazine[b]	Analgesic for slight pain
Fentanyl	Analgesic for operative pain
Meperidine	Analgesic for moderate to severe pain
Others: Alphaprodine	Analgesics for moderate to severe pain
Anileridine	
Piminodine	
Diphenylheptane Derivatives:	
Methadone	Analgesic for moderate to severe pain
	Management of drug dependence of the morphine type
Propoxyphene[b]	Analgesic for mild to moderate pain
Morphinan Analogs:	
Levallorphan	Narcotic antagonist
Levorphanol	Analgesic for moderate to severe pain
Benzomorphan Series:	
Pentazocine[b]	Analgesic for moderate pain

[a] Heroin is used therapeutically in Europe, but it is illegal in the United States.
[b] Synthetic derivatives described as nonnarcotics.

injectable opiates (5). The incidence of nausea and vomiting is highly dependent on a vestibular component which becomes more sensitive to movement during the induction phase of narcotic analgesia. The opiates act in the area postrema of the medulla to produce nausea and vomiting (6). They stimulate the chemoreceptor trigger zone which activates the vomiting center. They also depress the vomiting center; after the initial therapeutic dose, subsequent challenges with opiates are less likely to induce emesis. Morphine (15 mg sc) caused nausea in about 40% of ambulatory patients and vomiting in about 16%. These effects are uncommon in recumbent patients (5).

Opiates given to patients in the supine position for analgesia exert only slight cardiac and vascular effects. However, rapid intravenous administration and sudden alterations in gravitational stress may lead to orthostatic hypotension and syncope. Large doses depress the vasomotor center, promote peripheral vasodilatation, and slow the heart rate. The sharp transient fall in blood pressure may be due in part to the peripheral dilatation of arterioles and veins secondary to histamine release.

Opiate-induced histamine release may likewise be responsible for cutaneous vasodilation, producing the flushing, warmth, pruritus, and sweating that sometimes accompany the use of a narcotic drug. The retention of carbon dioxide and lowered oxygen tension from respiratory depression may cause cerebral vasodilation and increased intracranial pressure. Postural hypotension occurs infrequently with intramuscular, oral, or subcutaneous administration of opiates.

Opiates decrease GI motility and reduce biliary, gastric, and pancreatic secretions into the lumen of the gut (5–7). The stomach emptying time may be delayed for as long as 12 hr. The rate and digestive content of GI secretion may diminish, which may retard the digestion of food. The opiates increase the tone of intestinal smooth muscle, slow peristalsis, and invoke a loss of central perception to sensory stimuli for the defecation reflex. The delayed passage of bowel content allows for more complete absorption of water from the intestinal lumen. These actions have been utilized to treat diarrhea. However, constipation may ensue during opiate use, although some sources (2, 4, 5) claim that meperidine and its congeners are less constipating than most narcotics.

The elevation of biliary pressure from therapeutic doses of opiates is caused by biliary tract spasms or constriction of the sphincter of Oddi. The spasmogenic effect prevents the emptying of the biliary tree and obstructs biliary flow. The obstruction can produce abnormally high serum amylase and lipase levels; a rise in biliary tract pressure may accompany the use of any opiate and appears to be inconsistent and variable. The biliary effects from meperidine and pentazocine are less predictable, more variable, and not as great as those associated with morphine.

Opiates stimulate the release of antidiuretic hormone, increase the tone and contraction of the ureter, and constrict the sphincter of the urinary bladder. The central action of opiates also may contribute to urinary retention by reducing urinary urgency.

Changes in pupil size characterize the action of opiates. Miosis arises from the stimulation of the pupilloconstrictor centers of the oculomotor nerve and the inhibition of the pupillodilator centers of the hypothalamus (6). However, the anticholinergic activity of meperidine appears to dominate over miosis and results in mydriasis.

Contraindications

Most texts (2, 5, 13, 14) agree on the general contraindications to the morphine-type drugs. Patients with myxedema, Addison's disease, and hepatic cirrhosis are highly sensitive to the drugs and have suffered respiratory depression, stupor, and even coma from relatively small doses of narcotics.

Since opiates diminish ventilation and cause hypercapnia which may progress to cerebrovasodilatation and elevated intracranial pressure, they should not be administered in conditions where such actions are hazardous (*e.g.,* certain types of head injuries, cerebral edema, and delirium tremens). Of course, patient allergic sensitivity to an individual drug precludes the use and challenge of that particular agent.

Interactions

The morphine-type analgesics interact with drugs that affect the central and autonomic nervous systems (15–18). The interactions are based on their pharmacological and pharmacokinetic mechanisms. Any use of antihistamines, muscle relaxants, psychotropic drugs, or sedative–hypnotics with opiates may intensify their overlapping actions and may manifest toxicities, namely exaggerated effects on smooth muscle and respiratory depression. Doses of analgesics may need to be adjusted to avoid these enhanced reactions.

The antiemetic effects of phenothiazines are often used to prevent or control episodes of opiate-invoked vomiting. However, orthostatic hypotension and respiratory depression restrict the value of such drugs. It is unclear if the use of opiates and phenothiazines allows for a reasonable reduction in narcotic dosages and justifies the exposure to a phenothiazine. Any major advantage of such therapy over equianalgesic doses of an opiate alone is questionable (2).

Anticholinergics, such as atropine, can partially reverse the biliary tract spasms produced by the opiates (5). The GI and urinary tract effects are additive to those of the opiates. Adynamic ileus or severe constipation and urinary retention can occur during vigorous anticholinergic–analgesic therapy.

The concurrent use of propoxyphene (a methadone congener) and orphenadrine has been reported to cause mental confusion, anxiety, and tremors. Although clinical impressions differ, the resultant effects may be no more than the additive side effects of the two agents (see *Orphenadrine–Propoxyphene*, p. 163).

Monoamine Oxidase Inhibitors—Dangerous and even fatal reactions have been associated with the concurrent ingestion of drugs or foods and monoamine oxidase inhibitors. The signs and symptoms of such an interaction include excitation, convulsions, hallucinations, hypertension or hypotension, hyperpyrexia, sweating, muscle rigidity, and impaired ventilation. Most monoamine oxidase inhibitor–narcotic interactions have been associated with meperidine administration and resemble meperidine or anticholinergic intoxication. However, other narcotic analgesics have occasionally been implicated in producing exaggerated responses during concurrent monoamine oxidase inhibitor use. Morphine may be a useful alternative since evidence indicates that morphine can be used safely under these circumstances (see *Meperidine–Phenelzine*, p. 142).

Narcotic Antagonists—The clinically useful narcotic antagonists levallorphan, nalorphine, and naloxone are *N*-allyl analogs of levorphanol, morphine, and oxymorphone, respectively (15, 16, 19). All antagonize the respiratory depression of narcotics and analogs except that induced by pentazocine. Only naloxone is capable of counteracting the pentazocine-induced ventilatory depression.

The narcotic antagonists reverse the respiratory depression, the miosis, and the biliary

tract spasms produced by the morphine-type analgesics. Unlike levallorphan and nalorphine, however, naloxone does not seem to produce psychotomimetic effects, respiratory depression, or miosis. In opiate-dependent individuals, they may precipitate an acute abstinence syndrome which may be dangerous in the presence of other disorders or pathologies.

References

(1) Council on Mental Health, American Medical Association, "Narcotics and Medical Practice," *J. Amer. Med. Ass., 218,* 578 (1971).

(2) "AMA Drug Evaluations," 2nd ed., American Medical Association, Chicago, Ill., 1973, pp. 249–260.

(3) W. T. Beaver, "The Pharmacologic Basis for the Choice of an Analgesic. I. Potent Analgesics," *Pharmacol. Physicians, 4,* 1 (1970).

(4) L. E. Hollister, in "Clinical Pharmacology," K. L. Melmon and H. F. Morrelli, Eds., Macmillan, New York, NY 10022, 1972, pp. 490–499, 506–510.

(5) "The Pharmacological Basis of Therapeutics," 5th ed., L. S. Goodman and A. Gilman, Eds., Macmillan, New York, NY 10022, 1975, pp. 245–283.

(6) V. C. Sutherland, "A Synopsis of Pharmacology," Saunders, Philadelphia, Pa., 1970, pp. 240–269.

(7) A. Goth, "Medical Pharmacology," 7th ed., Mosby, St. Louis, Mo., 1974, pp. 283–298.

(8) "Manual of Medical Therapeutics," 21st ed., E. C. Boedeker and H. H. Dauber, Little, Brown, Boston, Mass., 1974, pp. 10–12.

(9) L. D. Vandam, "Drug Therapy: Analgetic Drugs—The Potent Analgetics," *N. Engl. J. Med., 286,* 249 (1972).

(10) "Methadone Maintenance," *Med. World News, 13,* 53 (March 17, 1972).

(11) "Methadone in the Management of Heroin Addiction," *Med. Lett., 14,* 13 (1972).

(12) E. Lowenstein *et al.,* "Cardiovascular Response to Large Doses of Intravenous Morphine in Man," *N. Engl. J. Med., 281,* 1389 (1969).

(13) "Drill's Pharmacology in Medicine," 4th ed., J. R. DiPalma, Ed., McGraw-Hill, New York, N.Y., 1971, pp. 324–361.

(14) M. Victor and R. D. Adams, in "Harrison's Principles of Internal Medicine," M. M. Wintrobe *et al.,* Eds., McGraw-Hill, New York, N.Y., 1974, pp. 681–685.

(15) J. H. Jaffe, "Narcotics in the Treatment of Pain," *Med. Clin. N. Amer., 52,* 33 (1968).

(16) L. Lasagna, "Drug Interaction in the Field of Analgesic Drugs," *Proc. Roy. Soc. Med., 58,* suppl., 978 (1965).

(17) H. B. Murphree, "Clinical Pharmacology of Potent Analgesics," *Clin. Pharmacol. Ther., 3,* 473 (1962).

(18) L. Lasagna, "The Clinical Evaluation of Morphine and Its Substitutes as Analgesics," *Pharmacol. Rev., 16,* 47 (1964).

(19) J. W. Lewis *et al.,* "Narcotic Analgesics and Antagonists," *Ann. Rev. Pharmacol., 11,* 241 (1971).

Analgesic Therapy (Nonnarcotic)

Nonnarcotic analgesics are exemplified by aspirin and also include *p*-aminophenols, ethoheptazine, ibuprofen, indomethacin, mefenamic acid, propoxyphene, and pyrazolones. All drugs in this series are analgesic and antipyretic and, with the exception of the *p*-aminophenols, mefenamic acid, and propoxyphene, are anti-inflammatory and antirheumatic as well (1). These agents relieve pain of diverse causes, including some of the most common complaints—tension headache, joint and muscle pain, and the malaise of viral infections. They lower elevated body temperature and reduce the inflammation of rheumatoid arthritis and rheumatic fever (2). Aspirin is by far the most important and most commonly used drug in this particular group. In a few cases, other nonnarcotic analgesics will offer an advantage over aspirin but most of them also are more toxic.

Salicylates

Therapeutic Indications—Salicylates have many systemic and a few local uses. Several uses are based upon tradition and empirical results rather than on a clear understanding of the mechanism of therapeutic benefit (2).

Therapeutic indications of salicylates include fever, somatic pain of mild to moderate intensity, gout, rheumatic fever, and rheumatoid arthritis. Salicylic acid is utilized primarily as a keratolytic while methyl salicylate is utilized as a counterirritant. Neither of these agents is used systemically; therefore, interactions are not of major importance.

Pharmacological Mechanisms—The temperature-lowering effect is usually rapid and effective in febrile patients, but it is seen infrequently when the temperature is normal. In toxic doses, aspirin may produce fever. Body temperature regulation requires a very fine balance between heat production and heat dissipation. The central nervous system (CNS), especially nuclei located in the hypothalamus, plays a major role in the regulation of peripheral mechanisms concerned with body heat production and loss. With salicylates, heat production is not inhibited, but heat loss is increased by increased peripheral blood flow and perspiration (2).

The analgesic effect of the salicylates also is due to an action on the CNS, the exact mechanism of which has not been elucidated clearly. The site of action is presumably subcortical since analgesic doses do not cause hypnosis, mental disturbances, or alterations in modalities of sensation other than pain. It is now felt that peripheral factors play only a minor role in the relief of pain afforded by the salicylates (2).

Salicylates increase the excretion of urates and, for this reason, they have been used in the treatment of gout. The uricosuric action of the salicylates, however, is dose dependent. Only large doses (5 g/day po) induce uricosuria and lower serum urate levels. This effect of salicylates is enhanced if an alkalinizing agent is given concurrently. Alkalinization of the urine increases the uricosuric effect of the salicylates by increasing the solubility of uric acid. Therefore, deposition of uric acid crystals in the renal tubules is prevented (3).

The basic mechanism of action of salicylates in rheumatic fever remains unknown. Although salicylates suppress the clinical signs and even improve the histological picture, subsequent tissue damage such as cardiac lesions and other visceral involvement are unaffected (2).

Various experimentally induced inflammatory and "arthritis-like" syndromes in animals are suppressed by salicylates, but the relevance to rheumatic diseases in humans is not clear. When salicylates are used for arthritis, there is significant analgesia that allows for more effective therapy. Additionally, there is an improvement in appetite and a sense of well-being. Salicylates also reduce the inflammation in joint tissues and surrounding structures by an unknown mechanism, possibly through inhibition of prostaglandin synthesis (2).

Contraindications—Contraindications for the use of salicylates include hypersensitivity and gastrointestinal (GI) disturbances, particularly hemorrhaging ulcers. Salicylates should be used with care in patients receiving anticoagulant therapy. They should be discontinued or at least the dosage should be reduced if any signs of toxicity appear (*i.e.*, ototoxicity or ulceration). Salicylates should be avoided in patients receiving uricosurics.

Interactions—*Alcohol*—Although controversial, concurrent ingestion of alcohol and large doses of salicylates (2–3 g) appears to increase the GI bleeding produced by the salicylates (see *Aspirin–Alcohol*, p. 16).

Aminosalicylic Acid—The mechanism of this interaction is not firmly established. Using aspirin to treat patients with apparent aminosalicylic acid toxicity resulted in a further increase of toxic symptoms (4).

Aminosalicylic acid may interfere with the conversion of salicylate to salicyluric acid, resulting in elevated serum salicylate levels. Further study is needed to assess the clinical significance of this interaction.

Anticoagulants—The possible interaction between salicylates and heparin is based largely on theoretical considerations. Drugs including aspirin in small daily doses inhibit platelet adhesiveness (5). In addition, salicylates may displace oral anticoagulants from plasma protein binding sites, thereby increasing the anticoagulant effect of the latter. Salicylates in large doses also reduce plasma prothrombin levels (2). The mechanism of salicylate-induced hypoprothrombinemia is not completely understood. Large doses of salicylates (> 3 g/day po) should be avoided in patients receiving oral anticoagulants (see *Warfarin–Aspirin*, p. 270).

Corticosteroids—Corticosteroids may decrease serum salicylate levels by increasing the glomerular filtration rate and decreasing tubular reabsorption of water. Decreasing the corticosteroid dosage in patients also receiving salicylates may result in an increasing serum salicylate level with the possibility of developing salicylism. Another factor to consider is that both corticosteroids and salicylates may be ulcerogenic, so caution should be exercised when they are administered concurrently (see *Aspirin–Hydrocortisone*, p. 18).

Hypoglycemic Agents—Salicylates may have an intrinsic effect on carbohydrate metabolism which tends to decrease hyperglycemia in diabetic patients. The hypoglycemic action may be seen in diabetic patients and also in nondiabetic subjects ingesting large doses of salicylates. Therefore, it is possible that sulfonylurea-induced hypoglycemia may be increased by salicylates. Salicylates should be given cautiously to patients receiving sulfonylurea hypoglycemics. It is not known whether insulin or phenformin would be similarly affected by salicylate administration (see *Chlorpropamide–Aspirin*, p. 36).

Uricosurics—Salicylates inhibit the uricosuric effect of phenylbutazone, probenecid, and sulfinpyrazone. Aspirin antagonizes sulfinpyrazone's ability to increase the renal excretion of uric acid and to reduce serum uric acid levels. Therefore, salicylates should be avoided in patients receiving these uricosurics (see *Sulfinpyrazone–Aspirin*, p. 226).

Miscellaneous—Aminobenzoic Acid: Aminobenzoic acid appears to block the conversion of salicylate to salicyluric acid, resulting in an increased serum salicylate level. This increase is apparently not too serious a problem clinically, but it should be kept in mind when these drugs are administered concurrently (2).

Methotrexate: Salicylates displace methotrexate from plasma protein binding sites, resulting in an increase in free methotrexate. Salicylates also retard the renal elimination of methotrexate, resulting in accumulation of the antineoplastic drug (see *Methotrexate–Aspirin*, p. 150).

Sulfonamides: Salicylates reportedly increase serum sulfonamide levels, presumably by displacement from plasma protein binding sites (6).

Aspirin may also interact with ascorbic acid, indomethacin, penicillin, and spironolactone, but the clinical significance of these drug interactions has not been established (see *Ascorbic Acid–Aspirin*, p. 12; *Indomethacin–Aspirin*, p. 105; *Penicillin–Aspirin*, p. 166; and *Spironolactone–Aspirin*, p. 223).

p-Aminophenols

Therapeutic Indications—Acetaminophen and phenacetin are useful for their analgesic and antipyretic effects in much the same manner as the salicylates.

Pharmacological Mechanisms—The analgesic and antipyretic effects of phenacetin have been postulated to be exerted mainly through its conversion to acetaminophen. However, evidence suggests that phenacetin *per se* is also active (2). The mechanisms of action of the analgesia and antipyresis of the *p*-aminophenols, although poorly understood, are presumably similar to those of the salicylates. Unlike the salicylates, these agents (particularly phenacetin) can cause methemoglobinemia which becomes significant when phenacetin is ingested in large quantities (about 2 g) (2). Methemoglobinemia can result in a decreased oxygen-carrying capacity of hemoglobin. These agents do not reduce swelling or edema since clinical anti-inflammatory action is not characteristic of *p*-aminophenols.

Contraindications—If a patient has a sensivity to this series of drugs, the agents should not be administered.

Interactions—From available evidence, there are few interactions with these agents. Therapeutic doses of acetaminophen, however, do appear to produce a slight, but not clinically significant, increase in the hypoprothrombinemic response when used in conjunction with oral anticoagulants (see *Warfarin–Acetaminophen*, p. 263).

Pyrazolone Derivatives

Therapeutic Indications and Pharmacological Mechanisms—The two main systemic effects of aminopyrine and antipyrine are analgesia and antipyresis. In this respect, they closely resemble acetaminophen, phenacetin, and the salicylates. Neither aminopyrine nor antipyrine exhibits the uricosuric effect of the salicylates, but both produce anti-inflammatory effects. Aminopyrine has been used in rheumatic fever. The mechanisms of antipyresis and analgesia are similar to those of the salicylates (2).

Phenylbutazone, a congener of aminopyrine and antipyrine, was introduced for the treatment of rheumatoid arthritis and related disorders. It is effective for such disorders, but its toxicity precludes long-term use. The mechanism of the anti-inflammatory effects of phenylbutazone is not known. The analgesic efficacy of phenylbutazone for pain of nonrheumatic origin in humans is less than that of aminopyrine and is inferior to that of the salicylates (2). The mechanisms of the antipyretic and analgesic effects are similar to the p-aminophenols and the salicylates. Phenylbutazone has a mild uricosuric effect which is probably attributable to one of its metabolites, sulfinpyrazone. Oxyphenbutazone is a hydroxyl analog of phenylbutazone and one of the major metabolic conversion products of the parent drug. It has the same spectrum of activity, therapeutic uses, and toxicity as the parent compound, and it shares the same indications, hazards, and contraindications for clinical use.

Contraindications and Side Effects—The pyrazolones are contraindicated for any patient with a history of hypersensitivity to these drugs. Aminopyrine can cause agranulocytosis so it is contraindicated for patients with this and similar blood dyscrasias (2). In addition, phenylbutazone is contraindicated for patients with hypertension and cardiac, renal, or hepatic dysfunction (2).

Interactions—Reports of interactions of aminopyrine and antipyrine with other drugs are quite rare. However, there are many reports of oxyphenbutazone and phenylbutazone interacting with other drugs.

Anabolic Steroids—The mechanism of this interaction is not established. Considerable increases in serum oxyphenbutazone levels have been reported in several patients who also received methandrostenolone. However, clinical reports of toxicity from their interaction are lacking (see *Oxyphenbutazone–Methandrostenolone*, p. 165).

Anticoagulants—The interaction between phenylbutazone and oral anticoagulants is one of the most important and critical interactions of coumarin anticoagulants. Phenylbutazone displaces coumarin anticoagulants from plasma protein binding sites and initially enhances the anticoagulant effect and the rate of metabolism. Phenylbutazone may also induce GI ulceration which could be quite hazardous in a patient receiving anticoagulants (see *Warfarin–Phenylbutazone*, p. 295).

Cholestyramine—Simultaneous administration of cholestyramine has delayed the absorption of phenylbutazone in rats. However, this drug interaction has not been studied in humans (see *Phenylbutazone–Cholestyramine*, p. 185).

Hypoglycemic Agents—Phenylbutazone administration has been shown to enhance the hypoglycemic activity of the sulfonylureas. The mechanism of this drug interaction is unclear, but it may be phenylbutazone-induced inhibition of sulfonylurea metabolism or excretion. Clinically significant symptoms of hypoglycemia may occur, and concurrent use of these drugs should be avoided (see *Tolbutamide–Phenylbutazone*, p. 247).

Salicylates—The uricosuric effects of salicylates were inhibited by phenylbutazone in four nongouty subjects (7). However, the long-term effects of the drug interaction were not studied and the clinical outcome was not determined.

Other Analgesics

Ethoheptazine—Ethoheptazine is structurally related to meperidine and produces its analgesic effect through CNS activity. It has a very low abuse potential and has low analgesic efficacy (2).

Ibuprofen—Ibuprofen is a phenylpropionic acid derivative used in the treatment of rheumatoid arthritis. In recommended doses (900–1600 mg/day po), its anti-inflammatory activity is inferior to that produced by therapeutic doses of aspirin. Ibuprofen has been reported to cause less GI bleeding than aspirin, although exacerbation of peptic ulcer by ibuprofen has been reported (8).

Animal studies showed that aspirin may decrease ibuprofen activity and serum levels, but this drug interaction has not been studied in humans (8). Ibuprofen has been shown not to enhance the hypoprothrombinemic effects of the oral anticoagulants (9–11) but may enhance platelet aggregation and should still be used cautiously if used concurrently with the oral anticoagulants.

Indomethacin—The main effects of indomethacin are antipyresis, analgesia, and anti-inflammation. The mechanism of the anti-pyresis is not known, but presumably it is similar to that of the salicylates (2). The analgesic effect is evident only in those conditions where pain accompanies an inflammatory response. Indomethacin uncouples oxidative phosphorylation in mitochondria isolated from cartilage and liver. The mechanism of action may be related to this effect (12). The anti-inflammatory effect in humans is evident when the drug is used for rheumatoid arthritis, other types of arthritis, and acute gout.

Indomethacin should not be used by pregnant women, children, persons operating machinery, or patients with psychiatric disorders, epilepsy, or parkinsonism. It is also contraindicated in individuals with renal disease or ulcerative lesions of the stomach or intestines (2).

Indomethacin may displace coumarin anticoagulants from plasma protein binding sites, thus enhancing the latter's effect. Although this drug interaction is not clinically significant, indomethacin is an ulcerogenic drug and may be harmful to patients receiving anticoagulants (see *Warfarin–Indomethacin*, p. 286).

Indomethacin appears to undergo renal tubular secretion which may be blocked by probenecid. This drug interaction is clinically significant. A reduction in indomethacin dosage would be necessary since accumulation of the drug occurs if probenecid is given concurrently (see *Indomethacin–Probenecid*, p. 108).

Aspirin may also interact with indomethacin, but the clinical significance of this interaction has not been established (see *Indomethacin–Aspirin*, p. 105).

Mefenamic Acid—This compound is indicated for short-term administration for relief of pain in conditions ordinarily not requiring the use of narcotics. It is contraindicated in patients with intestinal ulceration and in women of child-bearing potential.

Mefenamic acid has been shown to displace warfarin from human protein binding sites (13). Although evidence is limited, it is likely that mefenamic acid is capable of enhancing the effects of oral anticoagulants.

Propoxyphene—This agent is chemically and pharmacologically related to methadone.

It is used orally for the relief of mild to moderate pain. Propoxyphene is devoid of any anti-inflammatory and antipyretic activity.

There are reports that propoxyphene administered concurrently with orphenadrine can lead to an adverse reaction consisting of mental confusion, anxiety, and tremors. Current information indicates that this may represent the cumulative side effects of the two drugs rather than a true drug interaction. Therefore, concurrent use of these drugs need not be avoided (see *Orphenadrine–Propoxyphene*, p. 163).

References

(1) A. Goth, "Medical Pharmacology," 7th ed., Mosby, St. Louis, Mo., 1974, p. 416.

(2) "The Pharmacological Basis of Therapeutics," 5th ed., L. S. Goodman and A. Gilman, Eds., Macmillan, New York, NY 10022, 1975, pp. 325–358.

(3) T.-F. Yu and A. B. Gutman, "Study of the Paradoxical Effects of Salicylate in Low, Intermediate and High Dosage on the Renal Mechanisms for Excretion of Urate in Man," *J. Clin. Invest.*, 38, 1298 (1959).

(4) K. L. Melmon *et al.*, "Drug Interactions that Can Affect Your Patients," *Patient Care*, 1, 33 (1967).

(5) D. Deykin, "Current Concepts: The Use of Heparin," *N. Engl. J. Med.*, 280, 937 (1969).

(6) A. H. Anton, "The Effect of Disease, Drugs, and Dilution on the Binding of Sulfonamides in Human Plasma," *Clin. Pharmacol. Ther.*, 9, 561 (1968).

(7) J. H. Oyer *et al.*, "Suppression of Salicylate-Induced Uricosuria by Phenylbutazone," *Amer. J. Med. Sci.*, 251, 1 (1966).

(8) L. J. Davis, "Ibuprofen," *Drug Intel.*, 9, 501 (1975).

(9) D. Thilo *et al.*, "A Study of the Effects of the Anti-Rheumatic Drug Ibuprofen on Patients Being Treated with the Oral Anticoagulant Phenprocoumon," *J. Intern. Med. Res.*, 2, 276 (1974).

(10) M. J. Boekhout-Mussert and E. A. Loeliger, "Influence of Ibuprofen on Oral Anticoagulation with Phenprocoumon," *J. Intern. Med. Res.*, 2, 279 (1974).

(11) L. Goncalves, "Influence of Ibuprofen on Homeostasis in Patients on Anticoagulant Therapy," *J. Intern. Med. Res.*, 1, 180 (1973).

(12) M. W. Whitehouse, "Some Biochemical and Pharmacological Properties of Anti-Inflammatory Drugs," *Fortschr. Arzneim.*, 8, 321 (1965).

(13) E. M. Sellers and J. Koch-Weser, "Displacement of Warfarin from Human Albumin by Diazoxide and Ethacrynic, Mefenamic and Nalidixic Acids," *Clin. Pharmacol. Ther.*, 11, 524 (1970).

Anesthetic Therapy

General anesthesia is accomplished by the administration of several types of drugs. Preanesthetic medications are prescribed to allay anxiety, alleviate pain, smooth the induction of general anesthesia, and minimize some side effects of anesthetic drugs. Intraoperatively, one or more general anesthetic agents are used with other drugs to achieve the primary objectives of abolition of pain and awareness (*i.e.*, unconsciousness), suppression of autonomic and somatic reflexes, and provision of adequate skeletal muscle relaxation. Particular surgical procedures may require additional adjustments (*e.g.*, hypotension or hypothermia) for which still other drugs may be administered. Finally, drugs may be used to reduce the incidence and severity of postoperative delirium, nausea and vomiting, and other unpleasant effects associated with emergence from certain types of general anesthesia.

As such, general anesthesia invariably involves drug interactions, some of which may be purposefully intended since they are designed to ensure maximum comfort and safety for the patient. Of course, the inappropriate use of these numerous agents may contribute to the complications of anesthesia, which are frequently the result of drug interactions. Undesirable drug interactions can also develop between anesthetic agents and other drugs administered preoperatively and intraoperatively. In this setting, an awareness of drug interactions related to general anesthetics is essential.

In practice, the anesthesiologist considers the potential for detrimental drug interactions as well as the patient's physical status, the type of surgical procedure, and other factors in the preanesthetic evaluation of anesthetic risks and in the choice of anesthetic agents. Unsuspected interactions occurring intraoperatively usually develop rapidly, since drugs are administered either intravenously or by inhalation. With the customary close monitoring of the patient's condition, the effects of the interaction will usually become apparent quickly and permit adjustments (*e.g.*, alteration of the inspired concentration of the anesthetic) to be made promptly. However, there are also subtle interactions which produce effects that become apparent only later in the postoperative period (*e.g.*, kidney failure).

Although the anesthesiologist may have means readily available to treat the effects of some undesirable interactions (*e.g.*, mechanical support of depressed ventilation and vasopressor drugs for hypotension), there are sequelae of interactions for which the treatment is of uncertain and limited success (*e.g.*, a cerebrovascular accident or myocardial infarction). Obviously, avoidance is the best remedy for interactions that increase the risks of morbidity and mortality.

The general anesthetics include inhalational and intravenously administered agents. Inhalational anesthetics offer a distinct advantage over intravenous agents in that the depth of anesthesia can be regulated easily by varying the anesthetic concentration inhaled and by assisting or controlling the subject's ventilation. Yet, side effects from general anesthetics and from their interactions with other drugs can be troublesome to control while maintaining a level of anesthesia suitable for the operative procedure.

Individual anesthetic agents differ markedly in their anesthetic potency and side effects; for this reason, one or more drugs are used to achieve anesthesia.

Pharmacological Mechanisms

The depth of general anesthesia is usually proportional to the concentration (or partial pressure) of the anesthetic agents in the central nervous system (CNS). In the case of inhalational agents, the major determinant of depth of anesthesia at the steady state is the inhaled concentration of the anesthetic. The rate of change in anesthetic depth (*i.e.*, induction and emergence) is determined by the physicochemical properties of the anesthetic agent, by its concentration gradients between pulmonary alveoli and blood and between blood and CNS tissue, and by the physiological factors of ventilation and perfusion of the alveoli and perfusion of the CNS. Factors such as metabolism and nonpulmonary excretion of the anesthetic agent are of little practical significance in the control of anesthetic depth (although they may be important in the toxic effects of anesthetics on hepatic and renal functions).

The site of action and mechanisms of general anesthetic action in the CNS remain largely speculative. Consequently, little more than descriptive information is available regarding the interactions of general anesthetics with other drugs. In most instances, the basis of interactions of general anesthetics with other drugs outside the CNS also remains obscure.

Inhalational Anesthetics

Anesthetic gases include cyclopropane, ethylene, and nitrous oxide. Volatile liquids used for general anesthesia include enflurane, ether (diethyl ether), fluroxene, halothane, methoxyflurane, and trichloroethylene. Chloroform is a volatile liquid anesthetic but its toxicity precludes its use except when no other agent is available. Many of these agents are explosive and must be used with great caution.

The most important anesthetic complications arising during a surgical procedure are related to the effects of these agents on the CNS, reflex mechanisms, ventilation, and cardiovascular–renal systems. In addition, complications that become apparent postoperatively include prolonged muscle paralysis and delayed toxicity in vital organs (*e.g.,* the kidneys).

CNS—The inhalational type of general anesthetic depresses all CNS functions (apparent stimulation in light levels of anesthesia has been attributed to depression of inhibitory mechanisms); this depression is enhanced by other depressant drugs such as the narcotic analgesics, sedative–hypnotics, and tranquilizers. Early clinical reports indicated that enflurane could produce tonic–clonic seizures and involuntary motor activity. However, recent clinical observations suggest that seizures are rare and occur only with hyperventilation during anesthesia. Involuntary movements seldom occur (1).

Patients premedicated with morphine require lower concentrations of inhalational anesthetics to suppress reflex movements to painful stimuli (2). Such interactions may be useful in limiting the dose, thereby minimizing the toxicity of the inhalational agent on certain functions (*e.g.,* lower concentrations of halothane produce less depression of cardiac output). Additive toxicity may occur in other functions (*e.g.,* respiratory depression by morphine and halothane), but there is no clinical documentation that this toxicity occurs.

Reflex Mechanisms—Although the direct actions of general anesthetics are generally depressant on all organ systems, certain anesthetics elicit reflex activity which may be of a stimulant nature and obscure the depressant actions. As a result, physiological processes may remain at, or be increased above, their preanesthetic levels. Obviously, drugs that interfere with such reflex activity may alter rather drastically the responses of patients to these anesthetics. For example, blood pressure and cardiac output are maintained near preanesthetic levels at moderate levels of surgical anesthesia with cyclopropane or ether by reflex activation of the sympathetic nervous system (1, 3, 4). Anything interfering with these reflex mechanisms or with the cardiovascular actions of the catecholamines (*e.g.,* adrenergic receptor blocking drugs) will unmask the direct depressant effects of these anesthetics on the heart and lead to marked hypotension.

Ventilation—The control of ventilation is localized in the brain stem respiratory centers. These centers normally respond to an elevation in the partial pressure of carbon dioxide in the blood (pCO_2) by increasing the rate and depth of ventilation. General anesthetics and other CNS depressants, especially the narcotic analgesics, depress both the spontaneous rhythmic activity of the respiratory centers as well as their response to an elevated pCO_2. Concurrent use of general anesthetics with other depressant drugs produces at least some enhancement of depression of the respiratory centers.

Ventilation also can be affected by drugs that alter the function of skeletal muscle (intercostal and diaphragmatic), bronchial smooth muscle, and tracheo-bronchial secretory cells. Concurrent use of general anesthetics and skeletal muscle relaxants depresses ventilation to a greater extent than either agent alone, but the quantitative nature of the interaction is unknown. Cholinergic blocking drugs such as atropine reduce salivary and tracheo-bronchial secretions (and possibly bronchoconstriction) elicited by irritating anesthetic vapors (*e.g.,* ether). As a result, the cholinergic blocking drugs may improve the ventilatory exchange of oxygen, carbon dioxide, and anesthetic gases. On the other hand, in the absence of irritating vapors, atropine and scopolamine increase ventilatory dead space by producing bronchodilatation; this increase results in a lowered arterial pO_2 (5).

The use of intravenous anesthetics such as the barbiturates and ketamine is associated with hyperactivity of the airway reflexes which produce laryngospasm. The reflexes are stimulated by the accumulation of secretions. Anticholinergic drugs may reduce the incidence of laryngospasm by decreasing the activity of secretory cells lining the airway; they have no direct effect on laryngeal striated muscle.

Halothane relaxes bronchial smooth muscle and is the agent of choice for general anesthesia in asthmatic patients. The mechanism of bronchodilatation by halothane is unknown. Studies of the action of halothane on isolated cardiac tissue have suggested that low concentrations of halothane stimulate β-type adrenergic receptors (6, 7). Bronchial smooth muscle is relaxed by β-receptor stimulants. The interactions of halothane with other bronchodilators have not been studied, but the potential for significant interactions on both the pulmonary and cardiovascular systems is recognized.

Circulation—Blood pressure, pulse rate, central venous pressure, and ECG readings are the most frequently used means of monitoring cardiovascular function during the intraoperative period. Blood pressure is dependent primarily on cardiac output (cardiac rate times stroke volume), total peripheral resistance, and the volume of circulating blood. Drugs including the general anesthetics can alter blood pressure by acting directly on the heart and vascular smooth muscle and by influencing the cardiovascular regulatory functions of the autonomic nervous system. These actions suggest that the influence of the general anesthetics on the cardiovascular system can be varied and complex, and indeed they are. For example, general anesthetics depress isolated cardiac muscle. Yet cardiac output is maintained at preanesthetic levels and can be increased by the administration of atropine to the intact subject. These observations suggest that there is activation of both sympathetic and parasympathetic (cholinergic) nerves to the heart by general anesthetics. It is conceivable that general anesthetics will interact with any drug that affects autonomic nervous system function.

Since all general anesthetics have been shown to depress isolated cardiac muscle, maintenance of sympathetic tone is essential if profound decreases in cardiac output are to be avoided. For this reason, many authorities recommend that propranolol (a β-adrenergic receptor blocking agent which in adequate therapeutic doses eliminates the effects of catecholamines on the heart) should be withdrawn at least 24 hr before elective surgery is scheduled. Conversely, other authorities believe that for certain indications (*e.g.*, angina pectoris, thyrotoxicosis, and subvalvular aortic stenosis) propranolol therapy should be continued up to the time of anesthesia and surgery and administered intraperitoneally if necessary. However, if emergency surgery is necessary in a patient receiving propranolol, general anesthetics that are more potent cardiac depressants should be avoided (*e.g.*, halothane) (8). Furthermore, if it is necessary to augment cardiac function under such circumstances, the usual cardiac stimulants (*e.g.*, direct- and indirect-acting sympathomimetics) will be less effective than usual, larger doses may be required, and an alternative drug (*e.g.*, rapid-acting digitalis derivatives such as acetylstrophanthidin or ouabain) may have to be chosen.

In addition to propranolol, reserpine may interfere with the actions of cardiac stimulants and vasopressor drugs, but this interference has not been documented clinically (see *Ephedrine–Reserpine*, p. 67).

One serious drug interaction involves sensitization of the myocardium to catecholamines by cyclopropane and some of the halogenated hydrocarbon anesthetics (*e.g.*, chloroform, ethyl chloride, halothane, and trichloroethylene). In the presence of these anesthetics, the administration of epinephrine, isoproterenol, or levarterenol markedly increases the incidence of cardiac arrhythmias (see *Halothane–Epinephrine*, p. 90).

Neuromuscular Function—Some general anesthetics augment the muscle relaxant effects of the competitive neuromuscular blocking agents (*e.g.*, gallamine triethiodide, pancuronium, and tubocurarine). The dose of the competitive-type muscle relaxants should be reduced when cyclopropane, ether, halothane, or methoxyflurane is used (9). The consequences of not reducing the dosage of muscle relaxants are limited in the operative period to paralysis of respiration requiring controlled respiration (*i.e.*, maintained by mechanical assistance). Postoperatively, a prolongation of the neuromuscular blockade may occur, even if the effects of neuromuscular relaxants are adequately reversed by anticholinesterases (*e.g.*, neostigmine).

Aminoglycoside antibiotics (*e.g.*, neomycin) produce neuromuscular blockade and may cause additive effects on the neuromuscular blockade produced by other general anesthetics. This drug interaction would result in prolonged neuromuscular blockade or enhanced CNS depression (see *Ether–Neomycin*, p. 70).

Delayed Impairment of Vital Organ Functions—The two organs most frequently involved in the delayed onset of functional impairment following general anesthesia are the liver and kidneys. In the case of the liver, reversible depression of function is associated with the use of many different anesthetic agents and also may be the result of factors other than the anesthetic agent (*e.g.*, hypoxia or hypotension) (10). Hepatic necrosis and other liver abnormalities, sometimes irreversible, have been related to excessive dosage and prolonged or repeated use of certain anesthetic agents, hypoxia, or the presence of previously established liver disease (11, 12). The particular anesthetics include vinyl ether and theoretically all halogenated agents (chloroform, ethyl chloride, fluroxene, halothane, and methoxyflurane), although the incidence varies considerably among the individual agents. The mechanisms whereby anesthetic agents induce liver abnormalities are unknown, but current speculation centers on two possibilities: (a) the anesthetics or their metabolites act as haptens in the development of an immune response, and (b) the anesthetics are metabolized to hepatotoxic products (13). Under the latter circumstance, the toxicity of the anesthetics may be altered when the subject is receiving other drugs that induce or inhibit hepatic metabolism of the anesthetics.

In terms of postanesthetic renal disease, the role of the anesthetic agent, in most cases, has not been clearly defined. Chloroform, methoxyflurane, and vinyl ether are contraindicated with evidence of decreased renal function. Instances of renal tubular dysfunction, especially high output renal failure, have been reported in patients who have received methoxyflurane (14). This nephrotoxicity has been correlated with increases in the blood inorganic fluoride level which is released by the biotransformation of methoxyflurane (15). Furthermore, an increased incidence and severity of renal failure, sometimes with a fatal outcome, have been attributed to the concurrent use of methoxyflurane and tetracycline antibiotics (see *Tetracycline–Methoxyflurane*, p. 234) or aminoglycoside antibiotics (16).

Liver damage induced by anesthetics may impair the metabolism of other drugs such as phenytoin that are metabolized by the liver (see *Phenytoin–Halothane*, p. 200).

Although nearly all anesthetic drugs promote the release of antidiuretic hormone, clinically significant oliguria during general anesthesia usually is the result of inadequate renal perfusion. Many anesthetic agents produce cardiovascular changes that lead to reduced blood flow through the kidneys. Other drugs affecting the cardiovascular system may exaggerate the effects of anesthetic agents on renal function.

Intravenously Administered Anesthetics

Intravenously administered anesthetics include the ultra-short-acting barbiturates (*e.g.*, methohexital thiamylal, and thiopental) and nonbarbiturate compounds such as ketamine (a phencyclidine derivative). They provide a rapid, pleasant anesthetic induction but do not produce muscle relaxation. Frequently, they are used as a single dose for induction of anesthesia; for maintenance of anesthesia, they often are used with other agents. Diazepam (a benzodiazepine) has been used intravenously to produce sedation and amnesia for electric cardioversion (17) and as an adjunct for induction of anesthesia.

Except for a single intravenous dose (*i.e.*, induction), the effects of which are terminated primarily by redistribution of the drug from the CNS to other tissues (*e.g.*, muscle and fat), these agents depend on hepatic metabolism and renal excretion for termination of their action. Consequently, significant drug interactions may arise when these anesthetic agents are used in patients who are receiving drugs that modify the elimination processes.

The general pharmacology of all barbiturates is similar. Because the barbiturates do not provide analgesia or skeletal muscle relaxation except at very deep anesthetic levels, they are frequently administered with narcotic analgesics and muscle relaxants. Inappropriate dosages when such drugs are used concurrently can lead to a marked depression of vital functions, especially ventilation.

Ketamine provides relief of somatic but apparently not of visceral pain. Skeletal muscle relaxation does not occur and, in fact, muscle rigidity is often observed. Other side effects include hypertension, hyperactive pharyngeal and laryngeal reflexes, and postoperative dreaming and psychic changes which some patients find unpleasant (14). Major and minor tranquilizers may reduce ketamine-induced postoperative delirium, but their effectiveness is still controversial. The use of other drugs to overcome the shortcomings of ketamine obviously has the potential for both desirable and toxic drug interactions, but thus far few have been described.

A 50:1 combination of droperidol (a tranquilizer) and fentanyl (a narcotic analgesic) produces a general quiescence with psychic indifference to environmental stimuli (including painful stimuli) without loss of consciousness or muscle relaxation. The principal side effects and drug interactions are those of the antipsychotics (*e.g.*, chlorpromazine) and narcotic analgesics (*e.g.*, morphine).

Narcotic analgesics (*e.g.*, fentanyl, meperidine, and morphine) have been administered intravenously in conjunction with muscle relaxants (*e.g.*, tubocurarine) and nitrous oxide to provide analgesia, muscle relaxation, amnesia, and obtundation of undesirable reflexes. Very large intravenous doses of morphine (1–3 mg/kg) have been used for various types of cardiovascular surgery because of the minimal effects of morphine on cardiovascular function when ventilation is adequately supported (18). The effects of such large doses of morphine last long into the postoperative period. Often such an action is desirable since it provides for continuous postoperative analgesia and facilitates the patient's tolerance of mechanical ventilatory assistance and the endotracheal tube. However, attempts to reverse the respiratory depressant effects with narcotic analgesic antagonists (e.g., levallorphan, nalorphine, and naloxone) are often accompanied by elimination of analgesia and sedation as well.

References

(1) "The Pharmacological Basis of Therapeutics," 5th ed., L. S. Goodman and A. Gilman, Eds., Macmillan, New York, NY 10022, 1975, p. 95.

(2) L. J. Saidman and E. I. Eger, II, "Effect of Nitrous Oxide and of Narcotic Premedication on the Alveolar Concentration of Halothane Required for Anesthesia," Anesthesiology, 25, 302 (1964).

(3) "Drill's Pharmacology in Medicine," 4th ed., J. R. DiPalma, Ed., McGraw-Hill, New York, N.Y., 1971, p. 155.

(4) "The Pharmacological Basis of Therapeutics," 5th ed., L. S. Goodman and A. Gilman, Eds., Macmillan, New York, NY 10022, 1975, pp. 85, 90.

(5) Ibid., p. 69.

(6) A. M. Klide et al., "Stimulation of Adrenergic Beta Receptors by Halothane and Its Antagonism by Two New Drugs," Anesth. Analg., 48, 58 (1969).

(7) H. L. Price et al., "Evidence for Beta-Receptor Activation Produced by Halothane in Normal Man," Anesthesiology, 32, 389 (1970).

(8) "A Practice of Anaesthesia," 3rd ed., W. D. Wylie and H. C. Churchill-Davidson, Eds., Year Book, Chicago, Ill., 1972, pp. 325, 559, 665–666.

(9) "The Pharmacological Basis of Therapeutics," 5th ed., L. S. Goodman and A. Gilman, Eds., Macmillan, New York, NY 10022, 1975, p. 583.

(10) M. H. Dykes, "Anesthesia and the Liver. The Early Years: 1846–1912," Int. Anesthesiol. Clin., 8, 175 (1970).

(11) "Summary of the National Halothane Study. Possible Association between Halothane Anesthesia and Postoperative Hepatic Necrosis," J. Amer. Med. Ass., 197, 775 (1966).

(12) "A Practice of Anaesthesia," 3rd ed., W. D. Wylie and H. C. Churchill-Davidson, Eds., Year Book, Chicago, Ill., 1972, pp. 332–335, 1319, 1325–1327.

(13) M. H. Dykes and J. P. Bunker, "Hepatotoxicity and Anesthetics," Pharmacol. Physicians, 4, 1 (1970).

(14) "AMA Drug Evaluations," 2nd ed., American Medical Association, Chicago, Ill., 1973, pp. 223–238.

(15) R. I. Mazze et al., "Methoxyflurane Metabolism and Renal Dysfunction: Clinical Correlation in Man," Anesthesiology, 35, 247 (1971).

(16) M. J. Cousins and R. I. Mazze, "Tetracycline, Methoxyflurane Anaesthesia, and Renal Dysfunction," Lancet, i, 751 (1972).

(17) R. L. Kahler et al., "Diazepam-Induced Amnesia for Cardioversion," J. Amer. Med. Ass., 200, 997 (1967).

(18) E. Lowenstein, "Morphine 'Anesthesia'—A Perspective," Anesthesiology, 35, 563 (1971).

Antiarrhythmia Therapy

Cardiac arrhythmias are among the most complex clinical conditions to manage; they may vary from insignificant palpitations to serious medical emergencies that can terminate in death if not properly treated. Although dissimilar chemically and pharmacologically, the agents generally used to treat cardiac arrhythmias, lidocaine, phenytoin (diphenylhydantoin), procainamide, propranolol, and quinidine, possess certain common properties.

To understand the rationale behind the use of the antiarrhythmic agents, it is important to be aware of the electrophysiological changes that occur in myocardial tissue. (For a complete discussion of these events, see Reference 1.)

From an electrophysiological standpoint, arrhythmias may result from a disturbance in impulse formation or automaticity or from a disturbance in conduction or both (2). Arrhythmias arising from a disturbance in automaticity may be induced by such factors as changes in body pH, electrolyte imbalance, hormonal alterations, myocardial fiber stretch, or certain drugs (3). These arrhythmias are reflected in the action potential by changes in the rate of diastolic depolarization (phase 4 depolarization), with or without changes in the resting and threshold potential. Any drug that can act to depress spontaneous diastolic depolarization of ectopic pacemakers or that can decrease the rate of discharge from the sinoatrial (S-A) node can reverse arrhythmias of this type.

Cardiac arrhythmias arising from disorders of impulse conduction may occur when the normal time course of depolarization and repolarization is disturbed or when normal pathways of conduction are distorted, causing an acceleration or delay in the propagation of a given impulse (4). The propagation of impulses is dependent on the conduction velocity and the duration of the refractory period (4, 5). From the end of the refractory period to the completion of repolarization, a premature stimulus will elicit an abnormal response having a lower than normal velocity during upstroke of the action potential. The response also will have a reduced amplitude and, therefore, a decreased conduction velocity. As full repolarization is approached, upstroke velocity, action potential amplitude, and conduction improve.

Unfortunately, there are many confusing statements in the literature with respect to the effects of antiarrhythmic agents on the duration of the refractory period. Whether the effective refractory period and total action potential are increased, are decreased, or remain unchanged depends on interrelated factors including the concentration of the drug, the net effect of simultaneous changes in phases 2 and 3 of ventricular repolarization, and the membrane potential during repolarization at which the earliest premature response can be elicited (6). In the Purkinje and ventricular fibers, the shift of the membrane potential during diastole, from which the earliest premature response arises, results in a prolongation in the effective refractory period relative to the total duration of action potential.

A premature impulse propagating before full electrical recovery has occurred may undergo decrement block with the production of an arrhythmia (7). Therefore, agents that affect conduction velocity or the refractory period are capable of reversing disorders of impulse conduction. Lengthening or shortening the refractory period and decreasing or increasing the conduction velocity will lead to the arrest of ectopic circus movements, with the impulse being fired into surrounding tissue that is refractory to depolarization.

Therapeutic Indications

The treatment of cardiac arrhythmias is highly complex and will vary according to the clinical condition of the patient. The therapeutic indications are only a guide and the drugs discussed may not necessarily represent the only acceptable methods of treatment.

Drugs that alter the electrophysiological properties of the heart may be divided into two general groups: (*a*) those drugs that decrease the conduction velocity and automaticity (*e.g.,* lidocaine, procainamide, propranolol, and quinidine); and (*b*) those agents that enhance conduction velocity (*e.g.,* phenytoin). Bretylium tosylate, not yet commercially available in the United States, also enhances conduction velocity and may be classified in this latter group.

Clinically, procainamide and quinidine are indicated for treating various ventricular and supraventricular arrhythmias, including the conversion of atrial fibrillation and flutter to normal sinus rhythm (8, 9). Procainamide may be preferable to quinidine in patients who do not respond adequately to maximal doses of quinidine or in patients who experience undesirable side effects such as excessive bowel motility.

In some situations, it may be desirable to administer other drugs with either procainamide or quinidine. For example, if excessive widening of the QRS interval becomes evident in the treatment of ventricular tachycardia with either drug, it may be possible to continue suppression of the arrhythmia by the addition of a drug such as phenytoin which reverses the conduction delay in addition to reducing ectopic automaticity (10). Procainamide and quinidine should not be used in treating digitalis-induced tachyarrhythmias, because of a high incidence of atrioventricular (A-V) block (11). Oral procainamide and quinidine have been used prophylactically to reduce the incidence of the development of ventricular and supraventricular premature contractions and "premonitory" ventricular ectopic beats in patients with uncomplicated myocardial infarction (12, 13), but this treatment has not been generally recommended. In the treatment of atrial fibrillation, digitalis should be used prior to procainamide or quinidine to decrease the ventricular rate (14).

The most specific applications for the use of propranolol are in the treatment of ventricular tachyarrhythmias induced by digitalis and in the treatment of cardiac arrhythmias arising from increased sympathetic stimulation (15). The drug is also useful in the treatment of both supraventricular and ventricular arrhythmias due to the anesthetic agents and in the termination of premature ventricular contractions (16). In patients with digitalis-induced atrial tachycardia with A-V block, it is recommended that digitalis be discontinued and that phenytoin be used to initiate therapy (10).

The effectiveness of propranolol in the treatment of arrhythmias depends not only on the type of arrhythmia present but also on the clinical condition of the patient. For instance, only about 50% of the patients with atrial tachycardia and normal A-V conduction or only about 10% of cases with atrial tachycardia with A-V block reverts to normal sinus rhythm when treated with propranolol if these arrhythmias are not induced by digitalis excess or are found concurrent with the Wolff–Parkinson–White syndrome (17). However, in patients with this syndrome, recurrent paroxysmal supraventricu-

lar tachycardia may be suppressed by propranolol in more than 90% of such cases. Additionally, more than 90% of patients with paroxysmal supraventricular tachycardia caused by either digitalis or exercise responds favorably to treatment with propranolol (18).

Propranolol is not as effective as the other antiarrhythmic agents in treating ventricular arrhythmias which occur unrelated to an acute myocardial infarction, exercise, or digitalis excess; it is effective in abolishing ventricular premature depolarizations or ventricular tachycardia in about 40% of the cases (16). In an acute myocardial infarction, propranolol will abolish frequent ventricular premature depolarizations and ventricular tachycardia in only about 60–70% of the cases and may be more effective when used with small doses of quinidine (19). Propranolol is considered to be effective in more than 90% of the cases with frequent ventricular premature depolarizations or ventricular tachycardia associated with digitalis toxicity; it is nearly 100% effective in exercise-induced or paroxysmal ventricular tachycardias (16). This drug has also been useful with procainamide or quinidine in controlling ventricular tachycardia, as well as in converting chronic atrial fibrillation and flutter to normal sinus rhythm (20).

Lidocaine is indicated primarily for the rapid control of ventricular tachyarrhythmias occurring during cardiac surgery, cardiac catheterization, or the acute phase of a myocardial infarction (5). A continuous infusion of lidocaine has also been used prophylactically by a few investigators to decrease the likelihood of developing premature ventricular contractions and ventricular tachycardia in patients who are in the early stages of an acute uncomplicated myocardial infarction (21). The drug is most specific in circumstances where ventricular arrhythmias arise from disorders of automaticity and reentry mechanisms (5). However, it is considered to be relatively ineffective in the treatment of supraventricular arrhythmias.

Phenytoin has been used to treat cardiac arrhythmias arising from alterations in the mechanisms of reentry and ectopic pacemaker activity (5). Like lidocaine, phenytoin is considered to be more effective in treating ventricular rather than supraventricular arrhythmias and has been most effective in treating arrhythmias associated with digitalis toxicity, acute myocardial infarction, and open-heart surgery (6, 10). It appears to be ineffective in conversion of atrial flutter and fibrillation to sinus rhythm, although it may have some use in slowing the ventricular rate in these circumstances (22). Intravenous phenytoin in divided doses at approximately 10-min intervals, although more hazardous, is considered superior in effectiveness to oral therapy.

Pharmacological Mechanisms

Unfortunately, no systematic approach has been developed to group the antiarrhythmic agents according to their known mechanisms of action and to apply this approach to the treatment of specific cardiac arrhythmias. However, antiarrhythmic agents may be classified (6) generally into three distinct groups: (a) those agents that remove or prevent the factors responsible for the electrophysiological abnormality underlying the arrhythmia, (b) those agents that produce their effects by increasing vagal tone or decreasing sympathetic tone, and (c) those agents that exert their effects by directly altering the electrophysiological characteristics of the single myocardial fiber and the heart. The agents commonly referred to as antiarrhythmic agents fall primarily into the third category which includes such agents as lidocaine, phenytoin, procainamide, propranolol, and quinidine. The potassium salts, although not considered to be antiarrhythmic agents in themselves, can also be classified in this latter group since they have the capability of altering the electrophysiological characteristics of the myocardium.

Lidocaine—Although the mechanism of action of lidocaine at the cellular level has not been elucidated, the drug appears to act in many ways like procainamide or quinidine in myocardial tissue. There are, however, certain distinct differences seen with lidocaine that make it unique with respect to other antiarrhythmic agents.

Although the rate of diastolic depolarization and automaticity are usually decreased in ventricular tissue, there is no change in the sinus rate (23, 24). Likewise, S-A node action potential and atrial, A-V, and ventricular conduction are not appreciably affected (25, 26). Lidocaine also shortens the total action potential duration and the duration of the effective refractory period in the Purkinje fibers, while these durations in the ventricular fibers remain either unchanged or shortened (5). Thus, the duration of the effective refractory period relative to the duration of the action potential is lengthened in the ventricular fibers (8, 23).

Phenytoin—Although the effects of phenytoin on single Purkinje fibers are similar to those produced by lidocaine, this agent produces other electrophysiological effects dissimilar in many respects to other antiarrhythmic agents. It may produce an antiarrhythmic effect in one or more of the following ways (27): (a) by a direct effect on the myocardium, (b) by an anticholinergic effect, (c) by a direct central nervous system effect, and (d) by an effect on the coronary circulation. The most prominent effects, however, are thought to arise from a direct effect on the myocardial tissue.

Like procainamide and quinidine, phenytoin decreases the excitability and automaticity of the heart and appears to have a variable effect on the rate of rise of the action potential and conduction velocity by depressing diastolic depolarization. However, the duration of the action potential and the effective refractory period are shortened in the Purkinje fibers, and the membrane potential at the onset of the earliest premature response is shifted to a more negative value (6). Consequently, the duration of the effective refractory period is prolonged relative to the duration of action potential (4).

The drug has no significant effects on the sinus rate or conduction within the atria (28, 29). Although it has no consistent effect on A-V conduction in nonpathological conditions, if the A-V or intraventricular conduction has been prolonged by digitalis or other cardiac depressants, phenytoin may increase the conduction velocity in these areas (29).

Procainamide and Quinidine—Although procainamide and quinidine are dissimilar chemically, they produce similar clinical, electrocardiographical, and electrophysiological effects on the heart (30–32). Their beneficial effects are thought to be related to an alteration in the cell membrane permeability to sodium, but the exact nature of this effect is still uncertain (4). Quinidine is concentrated primarily in the cell membrane and exerts its fundamental antiarrhythmic effect at that location. Autoradiographic studies showed that the unchanged drug attaches to the lipoprotein of the cell membrane and this attachment apparently leads to alteration of cation transfer and depressed transmembrane activity (33).

The chemical structures of procainamide and quinidine may also give a clue to their beneficial antiarrhythmic effects. It has been suggested that the positive charge of the free tertiary nitrogen repels cations such as potassium or sodium which would otherwise cross the cell membrane (34). The facts that sodium influx during depolarization and potassium efflux during repolarization are decreased when the cells are exposed to excessive amounts of procainamide or quinidine lend support to this hypothesis. It may also be that the positively charged procainamide or quinidine molecule attracts the negatively charged dipole of water, thereby increasing the hydration of the membrane and slowing ionic diffusion (4). Additionally, these agents may chelate the calcium ion and effectively block the passage of this ion through the membrane, thus decreasing contractility (34).

Procainamide and quinidine also possess anticholinergic activity which may contribute to their antiarrhythmic effects (14). It is not clear, however, to what degree this action contributes to the effective control of cardiac arrhythmias.

In therapeutic doses, procainamide and quinidine depress conduction velocity throughout the heart (2, 8, 28, 29, 35), without significantly altering the sinus rate (30). Additionally, the slope of diastolic depolarization is decreased in the pacemaker sites in the atria and the ventricles (5). These effects have a net result of reducing the rate of impulse formation in the S-A node and producing an overall effect of suppressing arrhythmias secondary to enhanced automaticity.

The threshold and resting potential duration are usually unchanged or slightly increased in the Purkinje fibers and the effective refractory period is prolonged (2, 8, 34). When the effective refractory period is prolonged, the heart can be prevented from responding to rapid or premature stimulation. Reentry movement also may be interrupted since the reentrant impulses may find the originally depolarized tissue excitable. It has been suggested that the lengthening of the effective refractory period alone may adequately explain the therapeutic activity of these agents (5).

Propranolol—Propranolol is a potent β-adrenergic blocking agent that is available commercially as the racemic *dl*-mixture. The antiarrhythmic effects of this drug appear to be the result of two effects (5): (*a*) the inhibition of β-adrenergic stimulation in the heart, and (*b*) a direct action on the electrophysiological properties of the myocardium. Propranolol also produces some local anesthetic effect, but this is not sufficient to cause an antiarrhythmic response. The drug is thought to bind at the sacroplasmic reticulum where it may depress calcium transport by blocking the enzyme, adenyl cyclase, thereby reducing cyclic adenosine monophosphate formation (36, 37). It is uncertain, however, what relationship this effect may have on the overall antiarrhythmic effect.

The A-V nodal refractory time is prolonged relative to the duration of the action potential. Additionally, the ventricular rate is slowed because of the β-adrenergic blocking effect within the myocardium. This blocking effect also indirectly enhances the vagal effects within the heart which can result in a depressed conduction velocity (38). This indirect effect successfully contributes to the control of ventricular arrhythmias if propranolol is used with digitalis in the treatment of atrial fibrillation.

As with procainamide or quinidine, propranolol decreases the rate of phase 4 (diastolic) depolarization, thereby decreasing automaticity (39). The conduction velocity is also depressed in all parts of the myocardium (2). Propranolol also decreases the rate of firing of the normal sinus and other atrial pacemakers and is the only drug to do so at normal therapeutic dose levels (40). Thus, it is effective in the tachycardia produced by anxiety.

Contraindications

As with any therapeutic agent, known hypersensitivity to an antiarrhythmic agent precludes the use of that agent.

Both procainamide and quinidine are contraindicated in the presence of complete A-V block and should be used cautiously when an incomplete heart block exists (14). These agents also are contraindicated in digitalis toxicity in which there is a disorder of A-V conduction.

However, the use of procainamide or quinidine may be of value in patients who develop tachyarrhythmias as a direct result of digitalis therapy, and where no other effective treatment is available. These drugs also should be used cautiously in the presence of congestive heart failure, in hypotensive states, or in cases where a low cardiac output may exist, such as in an acute myocardial infarction. Procainamide or quinidine also should be used with caution in patients who have myasthenia gravis since it may antagonize the depolarizing effects of acetylcholine. Quinidine is contraindicated specifically in patients with a known history of thrombocytopenic purpura that resulted from prior quinidine administration.

Propranolol is contraindicated in patients with sinus bradycardia, a heart block of second degree or greater, cardiogenic shock, or right ventricular failure secondary to pulmonary hypertension. The drug also is contraindicated in patients who have congestive heart failure except in those cases where the failure is secondary to a tachyarrhythmia that is refractory to the cardiac glycosides or the diuretics. Propranolol is contraindicated in patients receiving cardiac depressant anesthetics such as chloroform or ether. Additionally, the drug is not to be used in patients who have bronchial asthma or during the pollen season in patients who have seasonal allergic rhinitis. The β-adrenergic blocking effects of propranolol in the bronchioles may contribute to an increased bronchoconstriction, thereby aggravating these conditions (41).

Propranolol should be used cautiously in patients with severe cardiovascular disease and in patients who have undergone electrical cardioversion. Additionally, the drug should be used carefully when administered with antidepressant drugs having adrenergic properties as well as with the monoamine oxidase inhibitors. In high sustained doses, propranolol may actually increase myocardial tension, thereby increasing one of the three major determinants of myocardial oxygen utilization (42).

Lastly, propranolol should be used with caution in those patients who are known or suspected diabetics. In diabetic subjects, propranolol may prolong insulin hypoglycemia and, more importantly, may prevent the recognition of an acute hypoglycemic reaction by masking such prominent premonitory signs as tachycardia, nervousness, or increased sweating (43–45).

Phenytoin is contraindicated in conditions where there is a high degree of heart block or marked bradycardia (46). It should be used cautiously in elderly patients and in patients who have impaired myocardial contractility or peripheral vasodilation and in severe congestive heart failure (47). As most serious adverse reactions to phenytoin occurred after intravenous administration, particular caution should be used whenever it is administered parenterally.

Very few specific contraindications are reported for lidocaine and, in general, the drug is considered to be relatively safe when used as directed. However, lidocaine is contraindicated in patients with marked hypoxia, severe respiratory depression, hypovolemia, shock, or marked bradycardia. In addition, the drug is not to be used in patients with severe liver or renal disease since the impaired metabolism or excretion associated with these conditions may markedly increase the serum levels of this agent and produce serious toxic reactions (15). The drug is also contraindicated in patients with a known hypersensitivity to other local anesthetic agents, as well as in patients exhibiting the Adams–Stokes syndrome or in patients with severe degrees of S-A, A-V, or intraventricular heart block (48).

Interactions

In general, few specific drug interactions of documented clinical significance have been reported for the commonly used antiarrhythmic agents. However, because of the potential toxicity of these agents as well as the instability of the condition that may be present, a great deal of caution should be used whenever other drugs, particularly those that affect the cardiovascular system, are administered with the antiarrhythmic agents.

Lidocaine—There are very few reported drug interactions regarding lidocaine. Since it produces some electrophysiological changes in the myocardium like those seen with procainamide, propranolol, or quinidine, an additive cardiac depressant effect may occur when lidocaine is given concurrently with these agents. Although it has been reported that lidocaine may enhance the muscle relaxant effects of succinylcholine, the dosage range of lidocaine reported for this interaction is much higher than that normally used in antiarrhythmic therapy (49).

Phenytoin—Phenytoin is responsible for a number of clinically significant interactions with drugs such as antitubercular agents (isoniazid), anticoagulants (dicumarol), and anticonvulsants [phenobarbital (see *Anticonvulsant Therapy,* p. 369, for a detailed discussion)].

Procainamide—Since procainamide is quite similar pharmacologically to quinidine, most of the drug interactions reported for quinidine may be applied to this drug, even though there is a lack of documentation regarding procainamide interactions. Therefore, those interactions with quinidine involving the enhanced neuromuscular blockade, the anticholinergic effects, the possible antihypertensive effects, and the additive cardiac depressant effects may be expected to involve procainamide as well. However, procainamide has not been reported to interact with the oral anticoagulants to enhance the hypoprothrombinemic effects of these agents and, therefore, may be an effective antiarrhythmic substitute for quinidine in patients receiving large doses of anticoagulants concurrently.

Propranolol—Propranolol, a potent β-adrenergic blocking agent, may antagonize the β-stimulating effects of drugs such as isoproterenol (50). This reaction may be significant, particularly in the severe asthmatic patient who must rely on these agents for clinical relief. Additionally, propranolol may aggravate preexisting bronchial asthma as well as chronic obstructive lung disease by initiating bronchoconstriction (14). The stimulatory effect of epinephrine on the heart is blocked by propranolol. If epinephrine is administered to a patient receiving propranolol, a reflex tachycardia may result (51).

Propranolol also has been involved in affecting the serum glucose response to hypoglycemia or exercise, presumably by inhibiting or interfering with the glycogenolytic action of the catecholamines (52, 53). This interaction is compounded by the fact that propranolol also may mask some of the more common warning signs for hypoglycemia such as excessive sweating, nervousness, and tachycardia which are adrenergic in origin. It is recommended that patients maintained on hypoglycemic agents who require propranolol be watched closely for these adverse effects (see *Insulin–Propranolol,* p. 114).

Although there are some reports that the anticholinergic activity of desipramine may antagonize the myocardial effects of propranolol, no valid clinical studies have been found to substantiate this claim (see *Propranolol–Desipramine,* p. 214).

Propranolol may have its myocardial effects enhanced by the concurrent administration of other antiarrhythmic agents (see *Propranolol–Quinidine,* p. 216). Additionally, it has been reported that propranolol enhances the effect of digitalis glycosides in patients receiving these drugs concurrently (54). However, the clinical significance of this drug interaction is doubtful.

Although propranolol is not considered to be an antihypertensive agent *per se,* a blood pressure-lowering effect may occur in hypertensive patients, particularly at high doses. Therefore, additive antihypertensive effects may be predicted with concurrent use of propranolol and the antihypertensive agents

(55–57). Likewise, the phenothiazines possess some α-blocking activity and may produce additive hypotensive effects with propranolol (58). Although this interaction is largely theoretical in nature, caution should be used when propranolol is administered concurrently with large doses of the phenothiazines. Propranolol also has been reported to enhance the neuromuscular blockade produced by the neuromuscular blockers (see *Tubocurarine–Propranolol,* p. 257).

Chlorpheniramine theoretically could antagonize the β-adrenergic blocking effect of propranolol and enhance its quinidine-like effect. However, no experimental or clinical data are available to support this possibility (see *Propranolol–Chlorpheniramine,* p. 213).

Quinidine—Quinidine is a weak base excreted primarily by the kidneys and its biological half-life may be prolonged considerably if the pH of the urine is increased (59–61). Therefore, drugs such as the carbonic anhydrase inhibitors, sodium bicarbonate, and the thiazide diuretics, all of which increase urinary pH, may serve to increase the lipid solubility and the tubular reabsorption of quinidine and thus prolong its therapeutic effects.

It is recommended that quinidine be used cautiously in patients who also are taking drugs that can alkalinize the urine. These individuals should be monitored closely for any signs of impending quinidine toxicity. If feasible, another diuretic that does not alkalinize the urine may be considered to replace the thiazide diuretics. Ethacrynic acid and furosemide can produce the same qualitative effects on electrolyte concentrations as the thiazide diuretics but will not alkalinize the urine and may be considered to be potentially effective substitutes. Likewise, procainamide may be given in place of quinidine in these patients since this drug apparently is not as greatly affected by changes in urinary pH as is quinidine. Obviously, a careful study of the patient's overall condition should be carried out before any substitute is recommended.

To a lesser extent, the nonabsorbable antacids have been involved in delaying the rate of absorption of quinidine in the gastrointestinal tract. This interaction is considered to be of minor clinical significance since the overall amount of absorption is not affected in these circumstances and the amount of physical adsorption is considered to be insignificant (see *Quinidine–Aluminum Hydroxide,* p. 218).

Since quinidine possesses a distinct anticholinergic activity in the myocardial tissues, other drugs having cholinergic blocking activity may produce additive vagolytic effects when used concurrently. On the other hand, drugs having cholinergic activity may be antagonized by quinidine.

Quinidine also may produce an additive hypoprothrombinemic effect in patients who have had their procoagulant factors depressed by oral anticoagulant administration. The mechanism for this interaction is thought to be due to the fact that quinidine, like the oral anticoagulants, decreases the synthesis of procoagulant factors. Although this interaction has not been well documented in human subjects, it may be considered clinically significant (see *Warfarin–Quinidine*, p. 297).

Because parenteral quinidine has the potential property of causing a reduction in blood pressure through peripheral dilation, it should be used cautiously in patients who have been stabilized on antihypertensive therapy (14).

The administration of quinidine parenterally may enhance the neuromuscular blocking effects and respiratory depression of certain surgical muscle relaxants such as decamethonium, succinylcholine, tubocurarine, or the magnesium salts (see *Tubocurarine–Quinidine*, p. 259). Administration of certain antibiotics such as kanamycin, neomycin, or streptomycin may result in enhanced muscle relaxation and, therefore, should carry the same general warning.

Quinidine also has been reported to enhance the effects of reserpine and the other rauwolfia derivatives and to increase myocardial depressant activity. Although the clinical data about this drug interaction are limited, the potential adverse effects due to the concurrent use of these drugs require that these drugs be used together cautiously (see *Quinidine–Reserpine*, p. 219).

Lastly, quinidine may be expected to produce additive cardiac depressant effects when used with other antiarrhythmic agents. Concurrent use of two cardiac depressants may be indicated and may result in an overall greater antiarrhythmic effect with less danger of drug toxicity, since smaller doses of each agent may be used. For example, concurrent administration of propranolol and quinidine in the treatment of chronic atrial fibrillation has resulted in a greater conversion to normal sinus rhythm in smaller doses than when either drug was used alone in greater therapeutic doses. These drugs also are effective in the reduction of ventricular premature beats complicating myocardial infarction (see *Propranolol–Quinidine*, p. 216).

References

(1) A. C. Guyton, "Textbook of Medical Physiology," 4th ed., Saunders, Philadelphia, Pa., 1971, pp. 162–172.

(2) J. C. Pamintuan *et al.*, "Comparative Mechanisms of Antiarrhythmic Agents," *Amer. J. Cardiol.*, 26, 512 (1970).

(3) B. F. Hoffman and P. F. Cranefield, "The Physiological Basis of Cardiac Arrhythmias," *Amer. J. Med.*, 37, 670 (1964).

(4) M. R. Rosen and H. Geiband, "Appraisal and Reappraisal of Cardiac Therapy," *Amer. Heart J.*, 81, 428 (1971).

(5) D. T. Mason *et al.*, "The Clinical Pharmacology and Therapeutic Applications of the Antiarrhythmic Drugs," *Clin. Pharmacol. Ther.*, 11, 460 (1970).

(6) L. S. Gettes, "The Electrophysiologic Effects of Antiarrhythmic Drugs," *Amer. J. Cardiol.*, 28, 526 (1971).

(7) B. F. Hoffman, in "The Myocardial Cell," S. A. Briller and H. L. Conn, Jr., Eds., University of Pennsylvania Press, Philadelphia, Pa., 1966, p. 251.

(8) J. R. Bigger and R. H. Heissenbuttel, "The Use of Procainamide and Lidocaine in the Treatment of Cardiac Arrhythmias," *Progr. Cardiov. Dis.*, 11, 515 (1967).

(9) M. Skolow, "The Present Status of Therapy of Cardiac Arrhythmias with Quinidine," *Amer. Heart J.*, 42, 771 (1951).

(10) A. N. Damato, "Diphenylhydantoin: Pharmacological and Clinical Use," *Progr. Cardiov. Dis.*, 12, 1 (1969).

(11) R. H. Helfant *et al.*, "The Electrophysiological Properties of Diphenylhydantoin Sodium as Compared to Procaine Amide in the Normal and Digitalis-Intoxicated Heart," *Circulation*, 36, 108 (1967).

(12) N. Anderssen *et al.*, "The Prophylactic Antiarrhythmic Effect of Quinidine in Myocardial Infarction. A Controlled Clinical Trial," *Acta Med. Scand.*, 184, 171 (1968).

(13) S. S. Bloomfield *et al.*, "Quinidine for Prophylaxis of Arrhythmias in Acute Myocardial Infarction," *N. Engl. J. Med.*, 285, 979 (1971).

(14) "The Pharmacological Basis of Therapeutics," 5th ed., L. S. Goodman and A. Gilman, Eds., Macmillan, New York, NY 10022, 1975, pp. 552, 676–678.

(15) R. E. Gianelly and D. C. Harrison, "The Antiarrhythmic Properties of Lidocaine and Propranolol: A Review," *Geriatrics*, 25, 120 (1970).

(16) D. Gibson and E. Sowton, "The Use of Beta-Adrenergic Receptor Blocking Drugs in Dysrhythmias," *Progr. Cardiov. Dis.*, 12, 16 (1969).

(17) G. Sloman and M. Stannard, "Beta-Adrenergic Blockade and Cardiac Arrhythmias," *Brit. Med. J.*, 4, 508 (1967).

(18) R. Gianelly *et al.*, "Propranolol in the Treatment and Prevention of Cardiac Arrhythmias," *Ann. Intern. Med.*, 66, 667 (1967).

(19) S. Stern, "Synergistic Action of Propranolol with Quinidine," *Amer. Heart J.*, 72, 569 (1966).

(20) L. S. Dreifus *et al.*, "Propranolol and Quinidine in the Management of Ventricular Tachycardia," *J. Amer. Med. Ass.*, 203, 736 (1968).

(21) V. Berstein *et al.*, "Lidocaine Intramuscularly in Acute Myocardial Infarction," *J. Amer. Med. Ass.*, 219, 1027 (1972).

(22) E. Flensted-Jensen and E. Sandoe, "Lidocaine as an Antiarrhythmic Experience in 68 Patients," *Acta Med. Scand.*, 185, 297 (1969).

(23) L. D. Davis and J. V. Temte, "Electrophysiological Actions of Lidocaine on Canine Ventricular Muscle and Purkinje Fibers," *Circ. Res.*, 24, 639 (1969).

(24) J. T. Bigger, Jr., and W. J. Mandel, "Effect of Lidocaine on the Electrophysiological Properties of Ventricular Muscle and Purkinje Fibers," *J. Clin. Invest.*, 49, 63 (1970).

(25) T. Sugimoto *et al.*, "Electrophysiologic Effects of Lidocaine in Awake Dogs," *J. Pharmacol. Exp. Ther.*, 166, 146 (1969).

(26) A. Morales-Aguilera and E. M. Vaughan Williams, "The Effects on Cardiac Muscle of Beta-Receptor Antagonists in Relation to Their Activity as Local Anaesthetics," *Brit. J. Pharmacol.*, 24, 332 (1965).

(27) E. N. Mercer and J. A. Osborne, "The Current Status of Diphenylhydantoin in Heart Disease," *Ann. Intern. Med.*, 67, 1084 (1967).

(28) B. J. Scherlag *et al.*, "The Contrasting Effects of Diphenylhydantoin and Procaine Amide on AV Conduction in the Digitalis-Intoxicated and the Normal Heart," *Amer. Heart J.*, 75, 200 (1968).

(29) B. I. Sassynik and P. E. Dresel, "The Effect of Diphenylhydantoin on Conduction in Isolated Blood-Perfused Dog Heart," *J. Pharmacol. Exp. Ther.*, 161, 191 (1968).

(30) B. F. Hoffman and P. F. Cranefield, "Pharmacology of Cardiac Arrhythmias," McGraw-Hill, New York, N.Y., 1960, p. 197.

(31) D. H. Singer and R. E. Ten Eick, "Pharmacology of Cardiac Arrhythmias," *Progr. Cardiov. Dis.*, 11, 488 (1969).

(32) B. Surawicz and K. C. Laseter, "Effects of Drugs on the Electrocardiogram," *Progr. Cardiov. Dis.*, 13, 26 (1970).

(33) H. L. Conn, Jr., and R. J. Luchi, "Some Cellular and Metabolic Considerations Relating to the Action of Quinidine as a Prototype Antiarrhythmic Agent," *Amer. J. Med.*, 37, 685 (1964).

(34) H. L. Conn, Jr., in "The Myocardial Cell," S. A. Briller and H. L. Conn, Jr., Eds., University of Pennsylvania Press, Philadelphia, Pa., 1966, p. 269.

(35) E. M. Vaughan Williams, "The Mode of Action of Quinidine on Isolated Rabbit Atria Interpreted from Intracellular Potential Records," *Brit. J. Pharmacol.*, 13, 276 (1958).

(36) R. A. Levine and J. A. Vogel, "Cardiovascular and Metabolic Effects of Adenosine 3',5'-Monophosphate *in vivo*," *Nature*, 207, 987 (1965).

(37) W. G. Nayler, "Calcium Exchange in Cardiac Muscle: A Basic Mechanism of Drug Action," *Amer. Heart J.*, 73, 379 (1967).

(38) A. G. Wallace *et al.*, "The Electrophysiologic Effect of Beta-Adrenergic Blockade and Cardiac Observation," *Bull. N.Y. Acad. Med.*, 43, 1119 (1967).

(39) K. Shigenobu *et al.*, "Membrane Effects of Pronethalol on the Mammalian Heart Muscle Fiber," *Jap. Heart J.*, 7, 494 (1966).

(40) R. H. Helfant *et al.*, "Effects of Diphenylhydantoin on Atrioventricular Conduction in Man," *Circulation*, 36, 686 (1967).

(41) G. Zaid and G. N. Beall, "Bronchial Response to Beta-Adrenergic Blockade," *N. Engl. J. Med.*, 275, 580 (1966).

(42) E. H. Sonnenblick and C. L. Skelton, "Myocardial Energetics: Basic Principles and Clinical Implications," *N. Engl. J. Med.*, 285, 668 (1971).

(43) H. F. Morrelli and K. L. Melmon, "The Clinician's Approach to Drug Interactions," *Calif. Med.*, 109, 380 (1968).

(44) P. D. Bewsher, "Propranolol, Blood-Sugar, and Exercise," *Lancet, i*, 104 (1967).

(45) M. N. Kotler *et al.*, "Hypoglycaemia Precipitated by Propranolol," *Lancet, ii*, 1389 (1966).

(46) M. Rosen *et al.*, "Diphenylhydantoin in Cardiac Arrhythmias," *Amer. J. Cardiol.*, 20, 674 (1967).

(47) G. C. Voight, "Death following Intravenous Sodium Diphenylhydantoin (Dilantin)," *Bull. Johns Hopkins Hosp.*, 123, 153 (1968).

(48) "American Hospital Formulary Service," American Society of Hospital Pharmacists, Washington, D. C., Section 24:04.

(49) J. E. Usubiaga *et al.*, "Interaction of Intravenously Administered Procaine, Lidocaine, and Succinylcholine in Anesthetized Subjects," *Anesth. Analg.*, 46, 39 (1967).

(50) W. L. Way *et al.*, "Recurarization with Quinidine," *J. Amer. Med. Ass.*, 200, 153 (1967).

(51) J. Kram *et al.*, "Propranolol," letter to the editor, *Ann. Intern. Med.*, 80, 282 (1974).

(52) R. D. Miller *et al.*, "The Potentiation of Neuromuscular Blocking Agents by Quinidine," *Anesthesiology*, 28, 1036 (1967).

(53) G. Lorentz *et al.*, "Influenza del Trattamento Reserpinico a Dosi 'Depletive' delle Catecholamine Tessutali sulla Sensibilità Miocardica alla Chinidina," *Folia Cardiol.*, 26, 316 (1967).

(54) R. Greene and C. C. Oliver, "Sensitivity to Propranolol after Digoxin Intoxication," *Brit. Med. J.*, 3, 413 (1968).

(55) H. J. Waal, "Hypotensive Action of Propranolol," *Clin. Pharmacol. Ther.*, 7, 588 (1966).

(56) M. Stannard and G. Sloman, "Haemodynamic Effects of Propranolol," letter to the editor, *Brit. Med. J.*, 1, 700 (1967).

(57) B. N. C. Prichard *et al.*, "Haemodynamic Studies in Hypertensive Patients Treated by Oral Propranolol," *Brit. Heart J.*, 32, 236 (1970).

(58) L. Baker *et al.*, "Beta Adrenergic Blockade and Juvenile Diabetes: Acute Studies and Long-Term Therapeutic Trial. Evidence for the Role of Catecholamines in Mediating Diabetic Decompensation following Emotional Arousal," *J. Pediat.*, 75, 19 (1969).

(59) R. F. Knows *et al.*, "Variation in Quinidine Excretion with Changing Urinary pH," abstract, *Ann. Intern. Med.*, 68, 1957 (1968).

(60) R. E. Gerhardt *et al.*, "Quinidine Excretion in Aciduria and Alkaluria," *Ann. Intern. Med.*, 71, 927 (1969).

(61) M. D. Milne, "Influence of Acid-Base Balance in the Efficacy and Toxicity of Drugs," *Proc. Roy. Soc. Med.*, 58, 961 (1965).

Anticoagulant Therapy

It has been more than 30 years since anticoagulant drugs were first used in medical practice. In the late 1930's, heparin was first utilized in clinical trials; the first clinical trials with oral anticoagulants began in the early 1940's. More than a million patients each year receive anticoagulant therapy, acute or long term, for the management of thromboembolic states (1).

The intended purpose of heparin or oral anticoagulant therapy is to prevent thrombus formation in conditions that might predispose the patient to their development or to prevent the growth of an existing thrombus or thrombi. Neither heparin nor oral anticoagulants will lyse existing thrombi. Experimental drugs such as urokinase and streptokinase are showing promise as thrombolytic agents (especially for pulmonary emboli), but further study is necessary before such drugs can be made available for general use.

Because of the numerous pathological states in which anticoagulant therapy has proven of potential usefulness, the difficulties of establishing suitably controlled studies, and a lack of standardization of laboratory control of anticoagulation, the therapeutic indications, dosage, and duration of use of these drugs are subject to considerable controversy.

Some studies indicate that drug interactions may occur more frequently with oral anticoagulants than with any other pharmacological class. Data from the Boston Collaborative Drug Surveillance Program indicated that oral anticoagulants accounted for about 5% of adverse drug reactions in a large number of hospitalized patients (260 out of 7017 monitored patients) (2). This frequency is undoubtedly because of their narrow therapeutic ratio, high protein binding properties, easily measured indexes of desired action (prothrombin time change and signs of hemorrhage), and extensive prescribing for patients often receiving several other drugs. There are few known *in vivo* drug interactions with heparin therapy, but there are numerous intravenous admixture (*in vitro*) incompatibilities.

Heparin is the anticoagulant of choice when rapid anticoagulation and antithrombotic activity are desirable (*e.g.*, in acute pulmonary embolus or deep vein thrombosis). Warfarin, if administered in a loading dose (40–60 mg), will exert measurable anticoagulant activity due to a reduction in factors VII, IX, and X in about 24 hr with maximal effect in 36–48 hr. However, antithrombotic activity will not be evident for at least 3–5 days since factor II (prothrombin) has a long biological half-life (3).

A preferable anticoagulant technique with warfarin is to initiate therapy with a moderate dose of warfarin (10–15 mg/day) until the prothrombin time begins to lengthen. The patient should then be titrated to a maintenance dose to stabilize the prothrombin time from 2 to 2.5 times control (20–30% prothrombin activity). This method is preferable to the traditional loading dose techniques as a precipitous fall in factor VII is avoided (3, 4).

Heparin has an advantage over coumarin or indandione anticoagulants for initial anticoagulation because of its immediate antithrombotic effects. Warfarin generally is preferred as the oral anticoagulant of choice because of more complete absorption (dicumarol is incompletely and erratically absorbed) and because the serum half-life is independent of dose (the dicumarol half-life decreases as dosage increases); dicumarol, however, is less expensive.

Indandione compounds are seldom used because they are more toxic than coumarin compounds.

Vitamin K deficiency, which could be due to various pathological conditions (*e.g.,* starvation or biliary insufficiency states) may increase the risk of bleeding or sensitivity to anticoagulants (1). Age and sex also appear to affect bleeding. There is evidence that the risk of hemorrhage is greater in elderly (over 60 years of age) females than in younger men or women treated with heparin (5). Any condition that might predispose the patient to the depletion of blood factors would be expected to be a risk factor.

Factors that may decrease the responsiveness of anticoagulants include pregnancy (a "hypercoagulable" state may occur) (6) and hereditary factors that cause more rapid metabolism of oral anticoagulants (demonstrated in animals only) or consist of a genetic mutation of the vitamin K–anticoagulant receptor site (6). Other case reports of genetic resistance have been cited (7, 8).

Therapeutic Indications

Anticoagulant therapy has been advocated for at least 35 different disease states (1), although there are only a small number for which sufficient documentation supports the use of such drugs.

Treatment and Prophylaxis of Deep Vein Thrombosis and Pulmonary Embolism— There is convincing evidence that anticoagulants reduce the incidence of thromboembolism in high-risk patients with obstetrical and surgical complications (9). In patients with massive deep vein thrombophlebitis of the lower extremities, anticoagulant therapy is continued until edema subsides. If refractory edema occurs, long-term anticoagulant therapy should be instituted (10). Low-dose heparin reduces the incidence of deep vein thrombosis after most major operations (11, 12) and after myocardial infarction (12, 13). Low-dose heparin is also effective in reducing the frequency of thromboembolism after elective surgery (12, 14). Heparin has not been shown to be effective in fracture of the hips or hip surgery (15).

Heparin is usually given in a dose of 5000 units about 2 hr before surgery and then 5000 units every 12 hr for 7–10 days. For myocardial infarction, heparin is begun within 12 hr of infarction and continued for 10 days (11–14). Preliminary results with heparin given every 8 hr suggest this may be a more effective regimen but also that it may be associated with a higher incidence of hemorrhage (15).

Pulmonary embolism most commonly arises from thrombosis of the veins of the lower extremities. Anticoagulant therapy for at least 6 weeks (16) to 6 months (17) has been advocated if pulmonary embolism occurs in response to a discrete event (*e.g.,* surgical procedure or obstetrical complication). Therapy for an indefinite period (17) has been suggested if the cause is unknown; recurrent emboli suggest that consideration be given to surgery or longer (possibly lifetime) therapy. The duration of treatment is highly individualized and controversial. In certain patients, the benefit-to-risk ratio for use of anticoagulants may be low due to other factors that might predispose the individual to hemorrhage (*e.g.,* ulcer or interacting drugs).

Acute Myocardial Infarction—Anticoagulant therapy is controversial in this disease state since results of some well-controlled studies do not demonstrate any clear advantages. A reduction in mortality of patients adequately anticoagulated has been noted (18). Although use of anticoagulants in hospitalized patients with myocardial infarction is frequent, the decision as to their use is largely subjective and should depend upon patient history and the quality of the supporting laboratory (19). It has been suggested (20) that oral anticoagulant therapy has not been shown to cause a statistically significant decrease in deaths or in residential strokes among patients with acute myocardial infarction. It was recommended that patients should receive anticoagulant therapy after acute myocardial infarction during hospitalization unless there are relative or absolute contraindications or deficiencies in laboratory monitoring facilities. This recommendation is based upon strong clinical impressions of efficacy, the mortality rate from acute myocardial infarctions, and the suggestion in some studies that anticoagulants may decrease thromboembolic episodes and diminish pulmonary and systemic emboli (20).

It is questionable whether anticoagulants influence the course of mural thrombosis and there is no evidence to suggest that the course of infarction is influenced (19). It has been proposed that pathological data (at necropsy), but not clinical data, suggest a favorable effect of anticoagulants on mural thrombi (20). More recent data (21), however, indicate that anticoagulant therapy is of little or no value once the patient with myocardial infarction is discharged from the hospital.

Recurrent Myocardial Infarction—The use of anticoagulants to prevent reoccurrence of myocardial infarction is even more controversial; most well-controlled studies have not demonstrated justification for long-term anticoagulant therapy (22, 23). It is possible, however, that improper anticoagulant control (usually inadequate dosage) may be responsible for the poor results (1, 9).

Prophylaxis of Transient Ischemic Attacks or for Recurrent Cerebral Emboli—The evidence is favorable but not conclusive for use of anticoagulants in the first condition (4, 24). However, the evidence is somewhat more favorable for use in the latter condition (4, 24).

Peripheral Arterial Embolism—Acute and long-term therapy has resulted in improvement in patients with peripheral arterial embolism (9, 25). However, there are no controlled trials that support the efficacy of anticoagulants in arterial thrombi (20). Since such thrombi are largely composed of platelets which are unaffected by anticoagulants, a beneficial response would not be anticipated.

Other conditions in which anticoagulants are used include excessive traumatic injury, gangrene, frostbite of extremities, and prevention of systemic embolization in patients with artificial heart valve implants.

Rheumatic Mitral Stenosis and Atrial Fibrillation—There is evidence that anticoagulants reduce the incidence of peripheral thromboembolic events when mitral valvular disease is present, especially if atrial fibrillation coexists (26). Since patients with atrial fibrillation are at greater risk of incurring peripheral emboli at the time of cardioversion, full anticoagulation 1 week prior to electrical or drug- (usually quinidine) induced cardioversion is recommended with maintenance therapy for about 3 months afterward (27).

Disseminated Intravascular Coagulation—Heparin therapy is effective in stopping the progressive consumption of intrinsic coagulation factors (which results in coagulation in small blood vessels). It is adjunctive therapy in addition to other therapeutic means that are directed at the underlying cause. Heparin therapy, however, is not indicated in all patients with disseminated intravascular coagulation (28).

Pharmacological Mechanisms

Mechanism of Physiological Coagulation—To understand the pharmacological mechanism of anticoagulants, it is necessary to understand the normal physiological coagulative process. Figure 1 indicates the process of coagulation (simplified) and clot lysis with notation of where oral anticoagulants and heparin act.

Mechanism of Pharmacological Action of Anticoagulants—Heparin inhibits the formation of thrombin and blocks the enzymatic action of activated thrombin in the conversion of fibrinogen to fibrin. Once thrombin is formed, it acts as a catalyst for the cascade phenomenon. While large doses of heparin prevent the formation of thrombin, small ("mini-doses") of heparin enhance antithrombin activity. Antithrombin prevents the activation of factor X, common to the extrinsic and intrinsic systems. This effect indirectly results in blocking formation of large quantities of thrombin, thus preventing fibrin clot formation (29).

The highly acidic nature of heparin seems to be necessary for its activity since agents that neutralize its acidity block its pharmacological activity. Heparin does not interfere with prothrombin production.

Oral anticoagulants are thought to antagonize the action of vitamin K, which is a necessary cofactor for the synthesis of coagulation factors II, VII, IX, and X by the liver. Oral anticoagulants also may cause irreversible inhibition of transport of vitamin K_1 to its intracellular site of action in the liver (based on rat experimentation and use of vitamin K_1) (9). It is apparent, however, that such inhibition is not absolutely irreversible, since large doses of vitamin K may enter the cell by other mechanisms that are not inhibited by oral anticoagulants. Thus, vitamin K may be useful in oral anticoagulant overdosage (9). Abnormal prothrombin has been detected in patients treated with anticoagulants. The appearance of this abnormal prothrombin is attributed to an anticoagulant-induced release of imperfect or precursor molecules into the circulation (30).

Laboratory Parameters for Measurement of Oral Anticoagulant Activity—Oral anticoagulants effect their pharmacological action by reducing blood stores of the four factors (II, VII, IX, and X) that require vitamin K for their synthesis. Measurement of prothrombin time is the most useful laboratory test for clinical monitoring of patients. The prothrombin time is sensitive to factors II, VII, and X. It is possible, therefore, for bleeding to occur secondary to factor IX deficiency even in the presence of a normal prothrombin time. Other tests that have been used infrequently include the prothrombin and proconvertin (P and P), the thrombotest, and the partial thromboplastin time (PTT) (4).

Prothrombin time is an indirect test of the clotting ability of blood (Fig. 1). The one-stage method of Quick (most common test method) is performed by collecting a small sample (4–5 ml) of venous blood, adding the blood to a sodium citrate or oxalate mixture, and then adding thromboplastin and calcium. The time required for formation of fibrin threads is measured electronically, and results are compared to normal blood (control). Usually two samples of control blood and test blood are averaged to arrive at the reported value.

The normal range for prothrombin time is 11–13 sec. Each laboratory computes its own control value daily and this value is used as a comparison to the prothrombin time of the anticoagulated blood of the patient. Therapeutic levels are generally considered to be from 2 to 2.5 times that of the control plasma (31). Unfortunately, commercial thromboplastin is obtained from animal sources and there is considerable variability from one reagent to another.

Studies now suggest that a good therapeutic level when using commercial reagents is from 1.25 to 1.75 times the normal value or 15–30% of normal prothrombin activity. The optimum level of prothrombin concentration is 20–25% for prolonged therapy. Use of the conventional 2–2.5 times normal prothrombin time may lead to overanticoagulation with increased incidence of hémorrhage (31).

Prothrombin activity may be plotted against prothrombin time, although each laboratory must determine its own plot. A prothrombin activity of 20–30% is the usual range to which the patient receiving an anticoagulant is titrated. Clinicians are not in

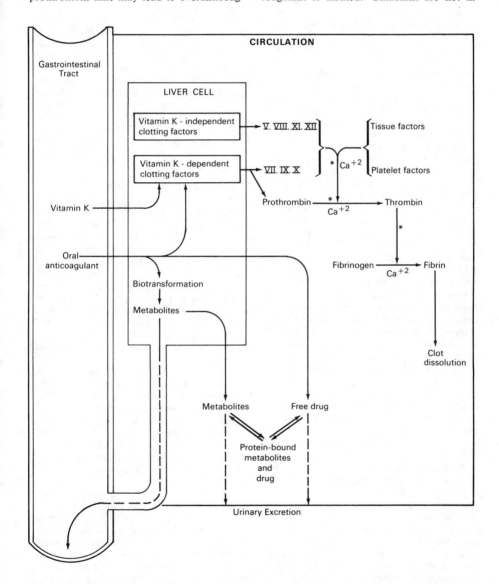

Figure 1—*Schematic representation of blood coagulation mechanisms and points of anticoagulant effects. [Adapted with permission from "The Pharmacological Basis of Therapeutics," L. S. Goodman and A. Gilman, Eds., (5th Ed.); Macmillan, New York, NY 10022, 1975, p. 1351.]*

agreement, however, as to the optimum prothrombin concentration.

Numerous drugs interfere with prothrombin determinations, resulting in increased or decreased test values (32).

Laboratory Parameters for Measurement of Heparin Activity—Heparin is the drug of choice for acute situations requiring anticoagulants because of its rapid action. The dosage of heparin is still sometimes monitored by Lee–White clotting time, despite its long end-point, poor reproducibility, and necessity for bedside determination (31). The Lee–White time should be kept at 2–2.5 times the control value (normal control is between 5 and 10 min). Clotting time should be measured just prior to initiating therapy and once daily before heparin is administered.

The activated partial prothrombin time (APTT) is now most commonly used to measure heparin activity. This test is more accurate and reproducible than the Lee–White test and it is considerably less time consuming. A level of 2–3 times the control is considered therapeutic for the activated partial prothrombin time, although the upper limit clinically is frequently 2.5 times the control. Other tests advocated for monitoring heparin therapy are the Celite and BaSon activated whole blood coagulation time (33).

Route for Administration of Heparin—Heparin should be administered only intravenously. Some authorities consider the continuous infusion method to be preferred over intermittent therapy since it avoids the "peaks and valleys" of the latter form of therapy and less heparin is required (34). Data from a controlled trial indicate that intermittent heparin is associated with a significantly higher incidence (seven times greater) of hemorrhage than constant infusion (35). Fluid overload and the necessity of constant supervision are disadvantages of this method of administration (36). Unfortunately, carefully controlled studies have not yet clearly supported either method as being more effective.

Intramuscular administration should be avoided because it results in variable absorption, more pain, and hematoma formation. Subcutaneous administration is not as acceptable as intermittent intravenous administration, but it is the next best choice if intravenous therapy is not possible. The subcutaneous route of administration of heparin has been associated with a considerable incidence of serious hemorrhagic complications (36). Absorption by this route is variable and, in case of toxicity, neutralization is more difficult (37).

Contraindications

Various specific conditions may exist in the case of a particular patient that contraindicate anticoagulant therapy. These include: (*a*) acute completed stroke (anticoagulants may be harmful by increasing the incidence of hemorrhage) (10); (*b*) active ulcerative disease of the gastrointestinal (GI) tract (38); (*c*) recent hemorrhage (38); (*d*) severe hypertension and renal or liver disease (38); (*e*) subacute bacterial endocarditis (26); (*f*) traumatic surgery (38); (*g*) recent cerebral hemorrhage and recent operation on the central nervous system (CNS) or eye (38); (*h*) pregnancy during first trimester or after 37 weeks of gestation (39); and (*i*) during breast feeding [heparin (39) should be used since oral anticoagulants are excreted in the breast milk].

Heparin Drug Interactions

Heparin interacts with aspirin and ethacrynic acid. Although antihistamines, dextran (see *Heparin–Dextran*, p. 94), digitalis, nicotine, quinine, and tetracycline have been stated to interfere with the anticoagulant activity of heparin, there is no substantial literature support for such "interactions." The chemical interaction occurring between heparin and protamine is well known. This interaction is used clinically to antagonize the anticoagulant effect of heparin. Additionally, chemical (*in vitro*) interactions can be expected to occur due to the acidity of the drug.

Aspirin—In a review of heparin therapy (37), it was advocated that concurrent aspirin administration be "scrupulously avoided." While documentation to support this interaction is incomplete, it would be prudent to avoid concurrent therapy whenever possible. Inhibition of platelet adhesiveness by aspirin impairs operation of an effective defense mechanism in the patient receiving heparin.

Ethacrynic Acid—Intravenously administered ethacrynic acid can cause GI bleeding. A significantly higher incidence of GI bleeding has been attributed to the concurrent use of intravenous ethacrynic acid and heparin (40). Furosemide may be a safer agent when diuretic therapy is indicated in the patient receiving heparin.

Oral Anticoagulants—Because oral anticoagulant drugs require 5 or more days to depress all four clotting factors effectively (4), therapy with these drugs should be initiated at about the same time as heparin. Such therapy is only necessary when oral anticoagulant therapy is indicated following a course of heparin. High serum levels of heparin prolong the prothrombin time and prevent proper interpretation of the test as a guide to oral anticoagulant dosage. This problem can be minimized by drawing blood for the prothrombin test just prior to a dose of heparin (9, 37). It has been advocated that 1 day of heparin therapy be omitted so that a prothrombin time totally uninfluenced by heparin may be obtained (3). Since difficulty is encountered when heparin is given subcutaneously, the most practical method is to give heparin by intermittent intravenous injection.

Probenecid—A single case report suggests that probenecid may increase the anticoagulant effect of heparin by increasing its reabsorption (41). Further study is needed to establish whether this drug interaction is clinically significant.

Oral Anticoagulant Drug Interactions

All oral anticoagulants marketed in the United States are coumarin or indandione derivatives. Of the coumarin derivatives, warfarin is the most widely prescribed. The indandione compounds are seldom used because of greater toxicity.

Numerous drug interactions of oral anticoagulants have been documented. Most commonly, warfarin has been implicated in clinical reports, dicumarol less commonly, and acenocoumarol, ethyl biscoumacetate, and phenindione rarely. It may be assumed that most reported interactions apply to all coumarin drugs, even though clinical documentation may be lacking.

Alcohol—Moderate, occasional ingestion of alcoholic beverages appears to have little effect on oral anticoagulant control. However, patients ingesting large amounts of alcohol, patients with a long history of alcohol consumption, or patients with liver dysfunction may sustain significant effects from alcohol on their anticoagulant therapy. The serum half-life of oral anticoagulants may be shortened with resultant antagonism of activity, presumably due to microsomal enzyme induction. Preferably, patients should avoid moderate to heavy alcohol consumption, especially over long periods. Sudden changes in alcohol consumption require corresponding alterations in oral anticoagulant dosage (see *Warfarin–Alcohol,* p. 265).

Analgesics—*Acetaminophen*—Any interference that may exist when acetaminophen is administered to oral anticoagulant-treated patients appears minor. Acetaminophen is an acceptable substitute for salicylates as an antipyretic or analgesic in patients receiving oral anticoagulants, but it has no anti-inflammatory action (see *Warfarin–Acetaminophen,* p. 263).

Indomethacin—Indomethacin theoretically may displace oral anticoagulants from protein binding sites and enhance their activity (42), but other data indicate that this effect is not clinically significant. However, indomethacin causes gastric ulceration and hemorrhage and inhibits platelet aggregation. Thus, caution is necessary if indomethacin is used. Ibuprofen may be a preferable alternative, but it may inhibit platelet aggregation. Therefore, concurrent administration of ibuprofen and warfarin still requires close monitoring (see *Warfarin–Indomethacin,* p. 286).

Mefenamic Acid—Highly protein-bound mefenamic acid displaces warfarin *in vitro* and significantly prolongs prothrombin time *in vivo* in patients receiving warfarin (43). The drug interaction may be clinically significant and alternative analgesics that do not interact would be preferable.

Pyrazolones—The pyrazolones (oxyphenbutazone, phenylbutazone, and sulfinpyrazone) enhance the hypoprothrombinemic action of oral anticoagulants in all patients by displacing the latter drugs from plasma protein binding sites. Additionally, pyrazolones inhibit platelet aggregation and have an ulcerogenic effect which may predispose the patient to GI hemorrhage. Such drugs should be avoided; alternative therapy is dependent upon the condition being treated (see *Warfarin–Phenylbutazone,* p. 295).

Salicylates—The salicylates (principally aspirin) enhance the action of oral anticoagulants. The salicylates interact principally by causing direct mucosal blood loss and inhibiting platelet aggregation. Aspirin causes hypoprothrombinemia, but it is usually only significant with doses of aspirin greater than 3 g/day. The salicylates should be avoided, but acetaminophen or ibuprofen may be a suitable alternative (see *Warfarin–Aspirin,* p. 270).

Aminosalicylic acid has been implicated in dogs (44) and in humans (single case report) (45) as a drug that enhances the effects of oral anticoagulants. More clinical data are needed before the clinical significance of this interaction can be established.

Antacids—It has been widely suggested that antacids interact with oral anticoagulants by alkalinizing the gut to promote ionization and prevent absorption. In clinical doses, antacids do not cause such an effect and the interaction is not clinically significant (see *Warfarin–Aluminum and Magnesium Ions*, p. 266).

Antibiotics—Although numerous interactions have been purported to occur with various antibiotic drugs, few have a sound basis. Broad spectrum antibiotics (*e.g.,* chloramphenicol and tetracycline, in particular) have been cited as causing hypoprothrombinemia by suppressing intestinal flora necessary for synthesis of vitamin K. Bacterial synthesis of vitamin K is important only when dietary intake of vitamin K is markedly decreased (46) (see *Warfarin–Tetracycline*, p. 299). Several antibiotics, however, do interact, apparently by other mechanisms.

Chloramphenicol—Chloramphenicol has been shown to inhibit the metabolism (probably by microsomal enzyme inhibition) of dicumarol (47). Presumably this may apply to other oral anticoagulants. Since chloramphenicol is rarely a drug of choice, alternative therapy should often be possible. When chloramphenicol therapy is necessary in patients receiving oral anticoagulants, the prothrombin time should be monitored closely.

Griseofulvin—Griseofulvin's antagonism of oral anticoagulant activity has been documented clinically, and there is sufficient evidence to suggest that this interaction is significant in some patients, possibly in a dose-dependent manner. Frequent prothrombin time monitoring of patients receiving these drugs concurrently is recommended (see *Warfarin–Griseofulvin*, p. 285).

Nalidixic Acid—Nalidixic acid displaces warfarin from protein binding sites *in vitro*. No data are available with respect to its effects in humans. Because of the lack of convincing evidence, the decision as to whether to use an alternative antimicrobial agent must depend upon individual patient circumstances. The same drug interaction may occur with oxolinic acid, but supporting clinical data are lacking.

Neomycin—Oral neomycin may enhance the effects of oral anticoagulants occasionally, possibly due to neomycin-induced steatorrhea or direct action on intestinal mucosa (46).

Rifampin—Rifampin has been documented (48, 49) as causing an enhancement of the effects of oral anticoagulants (acenocoumarol and warfarin). Effects occur in 5–8 days after rifampin therapy is initiated

and persist for 5–7 days after rifampin is discontinued. Rifampin may interfere with liver metabolism by increasing coagulation factor synthesis or causing anticoagulant degradation.

Sulfonamides—Sulfonamides have been reported to enhance the effects of oral anticoagulants by decreasing vitamin K production in the gut (unlikely) and, on long-term administration or in large doses, by causing anticoagulant displacement from protein binding sites (46). The latter explanation seems more reasonable and the long-acting sulfonamides, which are more highly protein bound than shorter acting derivatives, would seem more likely to interact. There is a lack of convincing evidence, however, and the degree of enhancement may not be significant.

Anticonvulsants—Dicumarol may increase the serum levels and half-life of phenytoin (diphenylhydantoin). In addition, the concurrent administration of phenytoin and dicumarol decreases the serum levels and anticoagulant effect of dicumarol. Patients receiving these drugs concurrently should be monitored closely for signs of toxicity from phenytoin or for a decrease in the anticoagulant effect of dicumarol (see *Phenytoin–Dicumarol*, p. 193).

Antidepressants—Tricyclic antidepressants may enhance the effects of oral anticoagulants. Nortriptyline caused an increase in the biological half-life of dicumarol, probably by inhibition of hepatic microsomal enzymes (46). However, there have been no published reports of enhanced anticoagulant effects due to tricyclic antidepressants. Monoamine oxidase inhibitors have not been shown to enhance the effects of oral anticoagulants in humans (46).

Antihistamines—In animals, some antihistamines cause hepatic microsomal enzyme induction and impair platelet function *in vitro*. Clinical significance has not been demonstrated in humans (see *Warfarin–Diphenhydramine*, p. 282).

Diuretics—Although high doses (125–500 mg/kg) of hydrochlorothiazide enhanced the anticoagulant effect by protein binding displacement of ethyl biscoumacetate in rats (46), no significant effect occurs in humans. Theoretically, diuretics may increase the concentration of clotting factors by loss of plasma volume and increase clotting factor synthesis by reducing hepatic congestion, thereby antagonizing the effect of oral anticoagulants (46). In one published study (50), no significant effects of thiazides on warfarin were observed. Ethacrynic acid displaces oral anticoagulants *in vitro* from human albumin (43, 51) and may have enhanced warfarin's hypoprothrombinemic effect in one patient (52). The data, although limited, indicate that this drug interaction may be clinically significant.

Hypoglycemics—Dicumarol increases the serum half-life of tolbutamide and may cause symptoms of hypoglycemia. This effect usually occurs 3–4 days after initiating dicumarol therapy. If dicumarol and a hypoglycemic drug must be given concurrently, insulin, which has not been reported to interact with dicumarol, may be substituted for tolbutamide. Otherwise, the tolbutamide dose should be adjusted accordingly whenever dicumarol is added to or withdrawn from the drug regimen (see *Tolbutamide–Dicumarol*, p. 245).

Phenformin has been reported (single case) to enhance the activity of warfarin. The proposed mechanism is an increased fibrinolytic effect caused by phenformin seen during the first few months of treatment (53). Controlled studies are required to determine the significance of this interaction in humans.

Hypolipidemics—The three major drugs used in hyperlipoproteinemias represent many different mechanisms of drug interactions.

Cholestyramine—Cholestyramine binds oral anticoagulants and may decrease absorption and oral anticoagulant effects. Cholestyramine also binds bile acids and may decrease the absorption of dietary vitamin K, possibly enhancing oral anticoagulant effects. Individual patient monitoring and titration are necessary to achieve proper control (see *Warfarin–Cholestyramine*, p. 278).

Clofibrate—Clofibrate is strongly protein bound and enhances the effects of oral anticoagulants by displacing them from protein binding sites. Other mechanisms, not yet clearly defined, may also be important. Enhanced oral anticoagulant activity occurs in many, but not all, patients (see *Warfarin–Clofibrate*, p. 280).

Dextrothyroxine—Dextrothyroxine enhances the effect of oral anticoagulants in most patients and a reduction in the dosage may be necessary. The exact mechanism of this interaction is unknown (see *Warfarin–Thyroid*, p. 301).

Sedative–Hypnotics—Most sedative–hypnotics that significantly affect oral anticoagulant activity cause a decreased hypoprothrombinemic effect. In most instances, the major mechanism responsible is hepatic microsomal enzyme induction, causing a decreased serum anticoagulant half-life.

Barbiturates—There is little reason to doubt that all barbiturates induce microsomal enzymes. All classes of barbiturates have been demonstrated to antagonize oral anticoagulants clinically except the thio (ultra short) derivatives. Time and dosage parameters have not been clearly identified (see *Warfarin–Phenobarbital*, p. 291).

Benzodiazepines—Chlordiazepoxide, clonazepam, clorazepate, diazepam, flurazepam, nitrazepam, and oxazepam do not have any significant effect on oral anticoagulant therapy (see *Warfarin–Chlordiazepoxide*, p. 276).

Chloral Hydrate—Although transient minor enhancement of the oral anticoagulant effect occurs when chloral hydrate is given concurrently, more recent evidence indicates that this enhancement is not clinically significant (see *Warfarin–Chloral Hydrate*, p. 273).

Ethchlorvynol—Ethchlorvynol may antagonize oral anticoagulant activity by hepatic microsomal enzyme induction (54), but the clinical significance of this interaction is not well established.

Glutethimide—Glutethimide also antagonizes the action of oral anticoagulants by causing hepatic microsomal enzyme induction. A chemically related drug, methyprylon, has not been implicated as interacting with oral anticoagulants (see *Warfarin–Glutethimide*, p. 284).

Meprobamate—Although meprobamate has been reported to antagonize oral anticoagulant activity by hepatic microsomal enzyme induction, the interaction has not been shown to be significant in humans (see *Warfarin–Meprobamate*, p. 288).

Steroids—Anabolic C-17-alkylated steroids (methandrostenolone and others) enhance the effects of oral anticoagulants. The mechanism is not known, although many have been suggested (see *Warfarin–Methandrostenolone*, p. 289).

Glucocorticoids have been implicated in enhancing oral anticoagulant effects (46, 55), but clinical evidence of any well-defined effects is lacking (46). Oral contraceptives (estrogen component) have been suggested, although not clinically documented, as inhibitors of oral anticoagulant activity (56). It is probable that the mechanism involves the ability of estrogens to increase serum levels of vitamin K-dependent clotting factors (46).

Thyroid and Antithyroid Drugs—Significant enhancement of oral anticoagulant activity has been demonstrated for dextrothyroxine (see *Warfarin–Thyroid*, p. 301). Hyperthyroidism (hypertensive disease or exogenous hormone administration) may accelerate catabolism and further deplete the concentration and activity of the factors (57–59). Published documentation of this interaction (except for dextrothyroxine) is lacking, however.

Antithyroid drugs (*e.g.*, propylthiouracil) or hypothyroidism may antagonize the action of oral anticoagulants by causing a slow rate of metabolism of vitamin K-dependent clotting factors (57), but published documentation is lacking.

Vitamin K and Analogs—Vitamin K antagonizes the inhibitory effects of oral anticoagulants on hepatic synthesis of vitamin K-dependent clotting factors. This effect is useful in reversing the toxic effects of oral anticoagulant overdosage. Patients with improper dietary habits could conceivably ingest enough foods to antagonize (*e.g.*, green leafy vegetables) or to enhance (*e.g.*, onions) the normal therapeutic response to oral anticoagulants. Such an effect would be exceedingly rare (see *Warfarin–Vitamin K*, p. 303).

Miscellaneous—*Allopurinol*—Allopurinol was shown to cause microsomal enzyme inhibition and to enhance the effect of dicumarol in one study (60). One patient in a subsequent study showed a 30% reduction in the elimination rate constant of warfarin (61). No change in prothrombin ratios occurred in any of the volunteers, however. Enhanced warfarin activity occurred in a patient previously stabilized on the anticoagulant who also received both allopurinol and indomethacin (62). Since indomethacin has been shown not to affect the hypoprothrombinemic effect of warfarin (see *Warfarin–Indomethacin*, p. 286), the enhanced hypoprothrombinemia may have been due to the concurrent administration of allopurinol. Generally, allopurinol would appear not to be contraindicated in patients receiving oral anticoagulants, but more frequent monitoring may be advisable.

Ascorbic Acid—Isolated case reports suggest that ascorbic acid (vitamin C) in large doses may antagonize the hypoprothrombinemic effect of oral anticoagulants, but no clinical studies support these observations. However, the practitioner should be aware of the potential drug interaction and should inquire about ascorbic acid intake in anti-coagulant-treated patients who respond erratically (see *Warfarin–Ascorbic Acid*, p. 268).

Carbamazepine—Antagonism of oral anticoagulants (warfarin) by carbamazepine has been noted in two of three patients studied (63). The proposed mechanism is that carbamazepine causes microsomal enzyme induction and decreases the oral anticoagulant half-life and activity. The antagonistic effect developed slowly over 2 weeks after initiation of carbamazepine and returned to baseline levels about 2 weeks after therapy was discontinued. Controlled studies are required to determine the significance of this interaction.

Diazoxide—Diazoxide displaces warfarin from protein binding sites *in vitro* (46, 51). This effect has not been confirmed in humans.

Disulfiram—It has been clearly shown that disulfiram enhances the hypoprothrombinemic effect of oral anticoagulants in most, but not all, patients (64–66). It is thought that disulfiram inhibits the enzymes in the liver responsible for hydroxylation of oral anticoagulants, thus increasing the serum level and half-life of unchanged anticoagulant (66).

Glucagon—High doses (25 mg or more for 2 days) of glucagon (as used investigationally to treat congestive heart failure) enhanced warfarin activity in most patients (67). This interaction may also occur with other oral anticoagulants. The mechanism of the interaction is not known.

Mercaptopurine—In a single case report, mercaptopurine has been noted to decrease the anticoagulant effect of warfarin. Hepatic enzyme induction was suggested as the likely mechanism of action (68).

Methylphenidate—One study (69) suggested that methylphenidate prolonged the half-life of ethyl biscoumacetate (no longer marketed) by hepatic enzyme inhibition. However, a more recent, better controlled study (70) demonstrated that methylphenidate did not affect the activity of ethyl biscoumacetate.

Quinidine and Quinine—Cinchona alkaloids (cinchophen, quinidine, and quinine) may enhance the effect of oral anticoagulants in some patients. The incidence of this interaction does not appear to be great, but the severity of the clinical outcome of this drug interaction is sufficient to recommend that concurrent administration of the drugs be avoided whenever possible (see *Warfarin–Quinidine*, p. 297).

Smoking—Cigarette smoking has been reported to increase the metabolism and decrease the therapeutic response to chlordiazepoxide, diazepam, pentazocine, and propoxyphene. A collaborative study, however, found no evidence for different maintenance doses of warfarin in smokers and nonsmokers (71).

Vitamin E—A recent case report suggests that vitamin E may enhance oral anticoagulant activity and cause hemorrhage in vitamin K-deficient patients (72).

Numerous other drugs or classes of drugs have been reported to interact with oral anticoagulants (46, 73). Such reports are based upon observations, animal experiments, or *in vitro* data; there is no evidence that the interactions are important in humans when therapeutic doses are used. These drugs or classes include acetylcholine, activated charcoal, aminosalicylate salts, atropine, bile salts, bromelains, chlorobutanol, digitalis glycosides, chloroquine, epinephrine, glyceryl guaiacolate, haloperidol, isoniazid, mineral oil, narcotics, niacin, paraldehyde, penicillin, phenothiazines, protamine sulfate, reserpine, riboflavin, theophylline, and vitamin D.

References

(1) I. Wright, "A Critical Evaluation of Anticoagulant Therapy," *Geriatrics*, 24, 96 (1969).
(2) H. A. Jick, "Drugs—Remarkably Nontoxic," *N. Engl. J. Med.*, 291, 824 (1974).
(3) R. O'Reilly and P. Aggeler, "Studies on Coumarin Anticoagulant Drugs: Initiation of Warfarin Therapy Without a Loading Dose," *Circulation*, 38, 169 (1968).
(4) D. Deykin, "Warfarin Therapy," *N. Engl. J. Med.*, 283, 691, 801 (1970).
(5) H. Jick *et al.*, "Efficacy and Toxicity of Heparin in Relation to Age and Sex," *N. Engl. J. Med.*, 279, 284 (1968).
(6) R. A. O'Reilly and P. M. Aggeler, "Determinants of the Response to Oral Anticoagulant Drugs in Man," *Pharmacol. Rev.*, 22, 35 (1970).
(7) J. Zager *et al.*, "Coumarin Resistance in a Negro Woman," *Ann. Intern. Med.*, 78, 775 (1973).
(8) D. B. Barnett and B. W. Hancok, "Anticoagulant Resistance: An Unusual Case," *Brit. Med. J.*, 1, 608 (1975).
(9) W. Coon and P. Willis, "Some Aspects of the Pharmacology of Oral Anticoagulants," *Clin. Pharmacol. Ther.*, 11, 312 (1970).
(10) "Current Therapy," H. Conn, Ed., Saunders, Philadelphia, Pa., 1969, p. 219.
(11) T. J. M. V. Vroonhoven *et al.*, "Low-Dose Subcutaneous Heparin *Versus* Oral Anticoagulants in the Prevention of Postoperative Deep-Venous Thrombosis. A Controlled Clinical Trial," *Lancet, i*, 375 (1974).
(12) "More Evidence on Prophylactic Low-Dose Heparin," *Drug Ther. Bull.*, 12, 57 (1974).
(13) C. Warlow *et al.*, "A Double-Blind Trial of Low Doses of Subcutaneous Heparin in the Prevention of Deep-Vein Thrombosis after Myocardial Infarction," *Lancet, ii*, 934 (1973).

(14) G. Lahnborg *et al.*, "Effect of Low-Dose Heparin on Incidence of Postoperative Pulmonary Embolism Detected by Photoscanning," *Lancet, i*, 329 (1974).
(15) A. N. Nicolaides *et al.*, "Small Doses of Subcutaneous Heparin in Preventing Postoperative Deep Venous Thrombosis," *Amer. Heart J.*, 87, 261 (1974).
(16) "Cecil–Loeb Textbook of Medicine," P. B. Beeson and W. McDermott, Eds., Saunders, Philadelphia, Pa., 1975, p. 919.
(17) "Current Therapy," H. Conn, Ed., Saunders, Philadelphia, Pa., 1975, p. 126.
(18) R. Ebert *et al.*, "Long-Term Anticoagulant Therapy after Myocardial Infarction. Final Report of the Veterans Administration Cooperative Study," *J. Amer. Med. Ass.*, 207, 2263 (1969).
(19) "Cecil–Loeb Textbook of Medicine," P. B. Beeson and W. McDermott, Eds., Saunders, Philadelphia, Pa., 1975, p. 1015.
(20) S. Wessler *et al.*, "Coumarin Therapy in Acute Myocardial Infarction," *Arch. Intern. Med.*, 134, 774 (1974).
(21) C. Merskey and A. Drapkin, "Long-Term Anticoagulant Therapy after Myocardial Infarction," *J. Amer. Med. Ass.*, 230, 208 (1974).
(22) A. Seaman *et al.*, "Long-Term Anticoagulant Prophylaxis after Myocardial Infarction," *N. Engl. J. Med.*, 281, 115 (1969).
(23) S. Ritland and T. Lygren, "Comparison of Efficacy of 3 and 12 Months' Anticoagulant Therapy after Myocardial Infarction. A Controlled Clinical Trial," *Lancet, i*, 122 (1969).
(24) "Duration of Anticoagulant Therapy for Thromboembolism," *Med. Lett.*, 13, 70 (1971).
(25) "Cecil–Loeb Textbook of Medicine," P. B. Beeson and W. McDermott, Eds., Saunders, Philadelphia, Pa., 1975, p. 920.
(26) "Coumarin and Indandione Derivatives," Section 20:12.04, Hospital Formulary Service, American Society of Hospital Pharmacists, Washington, D.C., July 1973.
(27) "Duration of Anticoagulant Therapy for Thromboembolism," *Med. Lett.*, 13, 71 (1971).
(28) J. Corrigan, "Disseminated Intravascular Coagulation," *S. Med. J.*, 67, 474 (1974).
(29) H. L. Bleich and E. S. Boro, "Actions and Interactions of Antithrombin and Heparin," *N. Engl. J. Med.*, 292, 146 (1975).
(30) M. Brozovic and L. Gurd, "Rate of Appearance of Abnormal Prothrombin following Initiation of Oral-Anticoagulant Treatment," *Lancet, ii*, 427 (1971).
(31) H. Latham, "Diagnosis and Treatment of Bleeding Disorders by the Primary Physician," *Va. Med. Mon.*, 99, 306 (1972).
(32) M. P. Elking and H. F. Karat, "Drug Induced Modifications of Laboratory Test Values," *Amer. J. Hosp. Pharm.*, 25, 484 (1968).
(33) J. E. Congdon, "Monitoring Heparin Therapy in Hemodialysis. A Report on the Activated Whole Blood Coagulation Time Tests," *J. Amer. Med. Ass.*, 226, 1529 (1973).
(34) M. Swanson and L. Cacace, "Heparin Therapy by Continuous Intravenous Infusion," *Amer. J. Hosp. Pharm.*, 28, 792 (1971).
(35) E. W. Salzman *et al.*, "Management of Heparin Therapy. Controlled Prospective Trial," *N. Engl. J. Med.*, 292, 1046 (1975).
(36) P. C. Raich *et al.*, "Heparin Therapy," *Amer. Family Physician*, 10, 163 (1974).
(37) D. Deykin, "The Use of Heparin," *N. Engl. J. Med.*, 280, 937 (1969).

(38) J. Holcenberg and J. Veltkamp, "Drug Therapy V. Oral Anticoagulant Therapy," *Northwest Med.*, *69*, 421 (1970).

(39) J. Hirsch *et al.*, "Clinical Experience with Anticoagulant Therapy during Pregnancy," *Brit. Med. J.*, *1*, 270 (1970).

(40) D. Slone *et al.*, "Intravenously Given Ethacrynic Acid and Gastrointestinal Bleeding— A Finding Resulting from Comprehensive Drug Surveillance," *J. Amer. Med. Ass.*, *209*, 1668 (1969).

(41) G. Sanchez, "Enhancement of Heparin Effect by Probenecid," *N. Engl. J. Med.*, *292*, 48 (1975).

(42) B. I. Hoffbrand and D. A. Kininmonth, "Potentiation of Anticoagulants," *Brit. Med. J.*, *2*, 838 (1967).

(43) E. M. Sellers and J. Koch-Weser, "Displacement of Warfarin from Human Albumin by Diazoxide and Ethacrynic, Mefenamic, and Nalidixic Acids," *Clin. Pharmacol. Ther.*, *11*, 524 (1970).

(44) N. R. Eade, "Potentiation of Bishydroxycoumarin in Dogs by Isoniazid and *p*-Aminosalicylic Acid," *Amer. Rev. Resp. Dis.*, *103*, 792 (1971).

(45) T. H. Self, "Interaction of Warfarin and Aminosalicylic Acid," *J. Amer. Med. Ass.*, *223*, 1285 (1973).

(46) J. Koch-Weser and E. M. Sellers, "Drug Interactions with Coumarin Anticoagulants," *N. Engl. J. Med.*, *285*, 487, 547 (1971).

(47) L. Christensen and L. Skovsted, "Inhibition of Drug Metabolism by Chloramphenicol," *Lancet*, *ii*, 1397 (1969).

(48) F. Michot *et al.*, "Rimactan (Rifampizin) und Antikoagulatientherapie," *Schweiz. Med. Wochenschr.*, *100*, 583 (1970).

(49) J. A. Romankiewicz and M. Ehrman, "Rifampin and Warfarin: A Drug Interaction," *Ann. Intern. Med.*, *82*, 224 (1975).

(50) D. S. Robinson and D. Sylwester, "Interaction of Commonly Prescribed Drugs and Warfarin," *Ann. Intern. Med.*, *72*, 853 (1970).

(51) E. M. Sellers and J. Koch-Weser, "Kinetics and Clinical Importance of Displacement of Warfarin from Albumin by Acidic Drugs," *Ann. N.Y. Acad. Sci.*, *179*, 213 (1971).

(52) R. J. Petrick *et al.*, "Interaction between Warfarin and Ethacrynic Acid," *J. Amer. Med. Ass.*, *231*, 843 (1975).

(53) T. J. Hamblin, "Interaction between Warfarin and Phenformin," *Lancet*, *ii*, 1323 (1971).

(54) S. I. Cullen and P. N. Catalano, "Griseofulvin-Warfarin Antagonism," *J. Amer. Med. Ass.*, *199*, 582 (1967).

(55) L. T. Sigell and H. C. Flessna, "Drug Interactions with Anticoagulants," *J. Amer. Med. Ass.*, *214*, 2035 (1970).

(56) J. J. Schrogie *et al.*, "Effect of Oral Contraceptives on Vitamin K-Dependent Clotting Activity," *Clin. Pharmacol. Ther.*, *8*, 670 (1967).

(57) M. B. Walters, "The Relationship between Thyroid Function and Anticoagulant Therapy," *Amer. J. Cardiol.*, *11*, 112 (1963).

(58) V. G. Apostolos, "Enhancement of Warfarin Induced Hypoprothrombinemia by Thyrotoxicosis," *Johns Hopkins Med. J.*, *131*, 69 (1973).

(59) T. H. Self *et al.*, "Warfarin Induced Hypoprothrombinemia, Potentiation by Hyperthyroidism," *J. Amer. Med. Ass.*, *231*, 1165 (1975).

(60) E. S. Vesell *et al.*, "Impairment of Drug Metabolism in Man by Allopurinol and Nortriptyline," *N. Engl. J. Med.*, *283*, 1484 (1970).

(61) M. D. Rawlins and S. E. Smith, "Influence of Allopurinol on Drug Metabolism in Man," *Brit. J. Pharmacol.*, *48*, 693 (1973).

(62) T. H. Self *et al.*, "Drug Enhancement of Warfarin Activity," *Lancet*, *ii*, 557 (1973).

(63) J. M. Hansen *et al.*, "Carbamazepine-Induced Acceleration of Diphenylhydantoin and Warfarin Metabolism in Man," *Clin. Pharmacol. Ther.*, *12*, 539 (1971).

(64) E. Rothstein, "Warfarin Effect Enhanced by Disulfiram," *J. Amer. Med. Ass.*, *206*, 1574 (1968).

(65) E. Rothstein, "Warfarin Effect Enhanced by Disulfiram (Antabuse)," *J. Amer. Med. Ass.*, *221*, 1052 (1972).

(66) R. A. O'Reilly, "Interaction of Sodium Warfarin and Disulfiram (Antabuse) in Man," *Ann. Intern. Med.*, *78*, 73 (1973).

(67) J. Koch-Weser, "Potentiation by Glucagon of the Hypoprothrombinemic Action of Warfarin," *Ann. Intern. Med.*, *72*, 331 (1970).

(68) A. S. D. Spiers and R. S. Mibashan, "Increased Warfarin Requirement during Mercaptopurine Therapy: A New Drug Interaction," *Lancet*, *ii*, 221 (1974).

(69) L. K. Garrettson *et al.*, "Methylphenidate Interaction with Both Anticonvulsants and Ethyl Biscoumacetate: A New Action of Methylphenidate," *J. Amer. Med. Ass.*, *207*, 2053 (1969).

(70) D. E. Hague *et al.*, "The Effect of Methylphenidate and Prolintane on the Metabolism of Ethyl Biscoumacetate," *Clin. Pharmacol. Ther.*, *12*, 259 (1971).

(71) A. A. Mitchell, "Smoking and Warfarin Dosage," *N. Engl. J. Med.*, *287*, 1153 (1972).

(72) J. L. Corrigan and F. I. Marcus, "Coagulopathy Associated with Vitamin E Ingestion," *J. Amer. Med. Ass.*, *230*, 1300 (1974).

(73) D. Bernstein, "Drugs Known to React with Coumarin-Type Anticoagulants—Revised," *Drug Intel.*, *8*, 172 (1974).

Anticonvulsant Therapy

Loccock first reported the usefulness of bromides in hysteroepilepsy in 1857. In 1912, an account of the beneficial effects of phenobarbital as an anticonvulsant opened the way for significant drug therapy in epilepsy. Since that time, many agents have been tested, some proving quite useful in the control of convulsive disorders. However, the ideal agent remains to be found; the utility of many available drugs is restricted by their sedative effect and/or varying degrees of toxicity and by varying degrees of effectiveness, particularly in certain types of epilepsy (*e.g.*, psychomotor epilepsy).

Epilepsy, a symptom and not a disease, is among the most common chronic neurological disorders. A definition of this symptom is difficult because of the widely varying clinical picture presented. Epilepsy has been defined (1) as a "symptom of paroxysmal and abnormal discharge in the brain that may be induced by a variety of pathological processes of genetic or acquired origin."

Drug therapy, although not curative, reportedly has resulted in either complete control or marked reduction of seizures in 85% of the patients treated (2). The control depends to some extent on the origin or type of seizure being treated. For example, seizures that arise from the temporal lobe generally are not as amenable to drug therapy as other seizures. In selecting an agent for therapy, several factors should be considered: (*a*) demonstrated effectiveness of the drug against the various types of epilepsy, (*b*) relative toxicity of the agents from which selection is to be made, (*c*) cost of the agent since therapy is generally chronic, and (*d*) ease of laboratory determination of serum levels. The mode and site of action of an agent also may be considered in certain situations.

Therapeutic Indications

The choice of the anticonvulsant agent(s) for a particular patient is dependent upon careful diagnosis of the seizure type. Some convulsive disorders may be mimicked by breath-holding spells with syncope or hysterical episodes. The history, not only as reported by the patient but also as described by a close relative or friend, can prove to be one of the most useful keys to accurate diagnosis (2). The therapeutic indications for the anticonvulsant drugs are listed in Table I.

A single drug at minimal dosage generally is selected to initiate anticonvulsant therapy. If seizure abatement is not accomplished initially, the dosage is increased until control is obtained or until toxic effects begin to appear. If the latter situation occurs, dosage of the initial drug is decreased and a second agent is added. Changes in therapy should be limited, as a rule, to one agent so that clinical results can be assessed with maximum confidence (3). Additionally, determination of serum anticonvulsant levels may be of assistance in achieving the desired effect more rapidly.

The anticonvulsant drugs are categorized according to the seizure pattern in which the agent is effective: (*a*) those effective against major and focal seizures, (*b*) those effective against petit mal, (*c*) those effective against psychomotor seizures, (*d*) those effective against infantile myoclonic seizures, and (*e*) those effective against status epilepticus.

The therapeutic approach to seizures that are focal at onset and those that are generalized at onset is somewhat similar. Either phenobarbital or phenytoin (diphenylhydantoin) is employed initially. Phenobarbital is chosen frequently because of a high therapeutic index and relative lack of serious toxicity (4). If the single drug is not successful, then several drugs may be used concurrently, *e.g.*, in order of choice, phenytoin–phenobarbital, phenytoin–primidone, mephenytoin–primidone, and phenytoin–mephenytoin (2, 5).

Generalized nonconvulsive seizures include petit mal; the occurrence of petit mal attacks usually begins in childhood and rarely persists after the age of 30 years. When properly diagnosed, true petit mal is less common than psychomotor seizures and myoclonic forms (6, 7). When true petit mal has been diagnosed, based on its characteristic EEG of 3 cps spike and wave discharge, ethosuximide is considered the drug of choice (2, 5, 8). The drug is effective, has a low incidence of hematological complications, and does not cause nephrotoxicity.

A complication frequently induced by the control of petit mal seizures is the appearance of grand mal attacks. Therefore, the administration of an anticonvulsant effective against grand mal seizures with an agent effective against petit mal is advisable (6). The various forms of petit mal seizures respond to ethosuximide or trimethadione,

Table I—ANTICONVULSANTS FREQUENTLY EMPLOYED IN TREATMENT OF VARIOUS EPILEPTIC SEIZURES

Seizure Type	Drug Therapy
Grand mal and focal motor	Barbiturates: phenobarbital, primidone Hydantoins: ethotoin, mephenytoin, phenytoin
Petit mal	Acetazolamide Oxazolidinediones: paramethadione, trimethadione Succinimides: ethosuximide, methsuximide
Psychomotor	Methsuximide Primidone Phenacemide (if no other agent successful)
Infantile myoclonic	Adrenocorticotropic hormone (ACTH) Diazepam
Status epilepticus	Diazepam (adults), intravenous Phenobarbital (children), intravenous Phenytoin

although the benzodiazepines may yield better results (9).

Common mistakes (4, 6) that result in treatment failures are: (a) improper classification of seizure type, possibly resulting in the use of ineffective drugs; (b) failure to obtain effective serum levels because of fear of toxicity; (c) an insufficient trial period and frequent shifting of drugs; (d) poor communication with the patient in understanding the importance of the drug regimen; and (e) sudden withdrawal of a drug, leading to severe exacerbation of seizures.

Withdrawal convulsions are most likely to occur when a new drug is added to the regimen or when the patient experiences a seizure-free period of several years and the decision is made to discontinue completely anticonvulsant therapy.

As anticonvulsant drugs are used for both acute (emergency) and chronic therapy, it is important to note that these drugs are not devoid of toxicity. (A table of the toxic effects of the anticonvulsant agents is presented in Reference 10.)

Pharmacological Mechanisms

The precise pharmacodynamic mechanisms of the anticonvulsant drugs have not been defined clearly. Generally, the drugs employed appear to act by suppressing the seizure focus and/or by preventing the spread of impulses through normal neuronal tissue. Most anticonvulsants are recognized as neuronal depressants with certain variations. Hydantoin drugs reduce posttetanic potentiation of synaptic transmission, while the oxazolidinediones decrease postsynaptic excitation following repetitive stimulation (10).

The stabilizing effect that the hydantoins and primidone exert upon excitable neuronal membranes is apparently through alteration of ion permeability and membrane polarization. For example, phenytoin has been shown to decrease the intracellular sodium level in brain cells and skeletal and cardiac muscle cells. Sodium efflux from the neuron is promoted probably through influences on the sodium pump, resulting in a tendency toward stabilization of the threshold against hyperexcitability (11).

Interactions

The interactions that occur with the anticonvulsant drugs primarily involve the hydantoin derivatives (e.g., phenytoin). The drugs that reportedly interact with phenytoin fall into a number of different pharmacological classes. However, the interactions for the most part involve an alteration of the metabolism of phenytoin. The interaction is thus dependent upon the route of metabolism of the offending drug or its ability to alter enzyme systems rather than the specific pharmacological actions.

The major site of metabolism for phenytoin is the liver, where it is converted primarily to 5-(p-hydroxyphenyl)-5-phenylhydantoin. This para-hydroxylation reaction apparently is carried out in the microsomal enzyme system.

Some agents may induce the enzyme system, thus speeding the metabolism of phenytoin so as to effect inadequate seizure control in some patients; other drugs inhibit the system either competitively or noncompetitively. The net result is a slowing of phenytoin metabolism, increased serum levels of free drug, and the potential for development of toxicity. Additionally, it is possible that both types of effects may occur simultaneously; in the case of phenobarbital, a variable outcome in net effect depends on such factors as the doses of the interacting drugs and the individual characteristics of metabolism.

Drugs for which there is at least minimal clinical evidence of interaction include alcohol, antitubercular agents (aminosalicylic acid and isoniazid), benzodiazepines, carbamazepine, chloramphenicol, dicumarol, disulfiram, methylphenidate, and phenobarbital. Other agents for which there is less substantial evidence for interaction with phenytoin are chlorpromazine, dimenhydrinate, estrogens, meprobamate, prochlorperazine, propoxyphene, and reserpine (12, 13).

The more clinically significant interactions appear to result from the inhibition of the metabolism of phenytoin. There is, for example, considerable clinical evidence of an isoniazid–phenytoin interaction. This particular phenomenon results in toxicity for approximately 10–20% of the patients receiving the two drugs. It is dependent upon the patient's ability to acetylate isoniazid; the genetically slow acetylators are the only persons who encounter problems. The mechanism by which isoniazid inhibits *para*-hydroxylation is unknown. Aminosalicylic acid and cycloserine also have shown inhibitory properties, but much higher (*in vitro*) concentrations are required to produce the same effect as isoniazid (13). It is conceivable that a patient receiving isoniazid–aminosalicylic acid or isoniazid–cycloserine may have more potential for toxicity if phenytoin is part of the therapy (see *Phenytoin–Isoniazid*, p. 202).

Other drugs that apparently inhibit the *para*-hydroxylation of phenytoin are dicumarol and, conceivably, other oral anticoagulants (see *Phenytoin–Dicumarol*, p. 193), the benzodiazepine drugs (chlordiazepoxide and diazepam) (14), disulfiram (see *Phenytoin–Disulfiram*, p. 195), and chloramphenicol (15). In the case of the latter two drugs, investigations showed that serum phenytoin levels are increased within a matter of hours after a dose of the suspect drugs. This fact suggests that the interaction is not due to alteration of the synthesis of metabolizing enzymes but to an inhibition of microsomal enzyme activity.

Animal studies indicated that methylphenidate is a weak competitive inhibitor of hepatic drug metabolism, and at least one case report is available that implicates initiation of methylphenidate therapy in phenytoin toxicity. More recent studies reveal little effect on the levels of anticonvulsants when methylphenidate is administered (see *Phenytoin–Methylphenidate*, p. 204). Phenylbutazone (16) and sulfonamides (17, 18) also have been reported to increase the half-life of phenytoin, but the clinical significance of this effect has not been established.

Drugs that alter the enzyme system in such a way as to increase the rate of metabolism of phenytoin include alcohol, carbamazepine, and folic acid. Alcohol and carbamazepine probably exert their effect by a nonspecific induction of the microsomal enzyme system (19, 20). In regard to folic acid, it is known that folate deficiency frequently accompanies long-term anticonvulsant therapy. Folic acid in an optimum amount is believed to accelerate the conversion of phenytoin to its inactive metabolite, but it appears that the magnitude of this effect is such that control is interrupted in only a few patients (see *Phenytoin–Folic Acid*, p. 197).

Phenytoin increases the metabolic inactivation of vitamin D, possibly by induction of hepatic microsomes. This effect is more prominent with concurrent phenobarbital or primidone (see *Vitamin D–Phenytoin*, p. 261).

Phenytoin invalidates the dexamethasone suppression test and the oral metapyrone test (see *Dexamethasone–Phenytoin*, p. 45).

Phenytoin also increases the metabolism of doxycycline, although the clinical significance of the drug interaction is not established (21).

The interaction of phenobarbital and phenytoin must be considered since these two drugs are frequently employed in concurrent anticonvulsant therapy. The effect of phenobarbital on phenytoin is probably the result of a combination of factors. Phenobarbital causes enzyme induction, which would result in decreased phenytoin levels, but at the same time, phenobarbital also may competitively inhibit the activity of the enzyme. With both actions apparent, the net result depends on time, individual variation, and the dose of phenobarbital. It was suggested that the stimulation of phenytoin metabolism may be of short duration. The phenomenon is further complicated by the fact that both drugs have anticonvulsant effects (see *Phenytoin–Phenobarbital*, p. 205).

Aspirin displaces phenytoin from plasma protein sites *in vitro*, but the clinical significance of this observation has not been determined.

Although it has been reported that phenytoin may enhance digitalis-induced bradycardia or decrease serum digitoxin levels, there is no evidence that these effects are clinically significant (see *Digitalis–Phenytoin*, p. 57).

The clinical significance of many of these interactions is not clearly established since, in most instances, there are only a few case reports available. It is probable that most of these interactions can occur clinically but on an infrequent basis and usually without a significant clinical effect. As noted earlier, the development of toxicity due to inhibition of the metabolism of phenytoin seems to be the most frequently encountered interaction. The potential for interaction may be managed by closely monitoring a patient when other medications are added to the anticonvulsant drug regimen.

Serum drug levels should be determined at the first sign of phenytoin toxicity (*e.g.*, constant lethargy, gait ataxia, and nystagmus). The recommended serum level for phenytoin is 10–20 µg/ml (13). Although considerable individual variation exists, nystagmus generally appears when the serum phenytoin level reaches 20 µg/ml or higher. Gait ataxia is observed at levels around 30 µg/ml with constant lethargy seen at levels approaching 40 µg/ml (13). If toxicity occurs, phenytoin should be discontinued or the dosage should be reduced until toxic signs and symptoms disappear. Then phenytoin can be reinstituted or the dosage can be adjusted until therapeutic levels are attained.

References

(1) R. P. Schmidt and B. J. Wilder, "Epilepsy," F. A. Davis Co., Philadelphia, Pa., 1968, pp. 2–4, 142, 170.
(2) W. L. Griggs, "Epilepsy—Practical Medical Treatment," *Mod. Treat., 8,* 258 (1971).
(3) H. J. Grossman, "Therapy of Childhood Seizures," *Curr. Psychiat. Ther.,* Grune and Stratton, New York, N.Y., 1970, pp. 11–13.
(4) J. G. Millichap, "Drug Treatment of Convulsive Disorders," *N. Engl. J. Med., 286,* 464 (1972).
(5) W. E. Karnes, "Medical Treatment for Convulsive Disorders," *Med. Clin. N. Amer., 52,* 959 (1968).
(6) "Current Therapy," H. Conn, Ed., Saunders, Philadelphia, Pa., 1972, p. 651.
(7) J. Holowach *et al.,* "Petit Mal Epilepsy," *Pediatrics, 30,* 893 (1962).
(8) J. F. Schwartz, "Recent Advances in Treating Epileptic Children," *Postgrad. Med., 44,* 107 (December 1968).
(9) "Anticonvulsant Drugs," vol. II, J. Mercier, Ed., Pergamon Press, Oxford, England, 1973, p. 585.
(10) "Cecil–Loeb Textbook of Medicine," P. B. Beeson and W. McDermott, Eds., Saunders, Philadelphia, Pa., 1971, p. 269.
(11) "The Pharmacological Basis of Therapeutics," 5th ed., L. S. Goodman and A. Gilman, Eds., Macmillan, New York, NY 10022, 1975, p. 206.
(12) H. Kutt and K. Verebely, "Metabolism of Diphenylhydantoin by Rat Liver Microsomes. I. Characteristics of the Reaction," *Biochem. Pharmacol., 19,* 675 (1970).
(13) H. Kutt and F. McDowell, "Management of Epilepsy with Diphenylhydantoin Sodium. Dosage Regulation for Problem Patients," *J. Amer. Med. Ass., 203,* 969 (1968).
(14) F. J. E. Vajda *et al.,* "Interaction between Phenytoin and the Benzodiazepines," letter to the editor, *Brit. Med. J., 1,* 346 (1971).
(15) L. K. Christensted and L. Skovsted, "Inhibition of Drug Metabolism by Chloramphenicol," *Lancet, ii,* 1379 (1969).
(16) P. B. Andreason *et al.,* "Diphenylhydantoin Half-Life in Man and Its Inhibition by Phenylbutazone: The Role of Genetic Factors," *Acta Med. Scand., 193,* 561 (1969).
(17) K. Siersbaek-Nielsen *et al.,* "Sulfamethizole-Induced Inhibition of Diphenylhydantoin and Tolbutamide Metabolism in Man," *Clin. Pharmacol. Ther., 14,* 148 (1973).
(18) J. M. Hansen *et al.,* "Sulthiame (Ospolot) as Inhibitor of Diphenylhydantoin Metabolism," *Epilepsia, 9,* 17 (1968).
(19) R. M. H. Kater *et al.,* "Increased Rate of Clearance of Drugs from the Circulation of Alcoholics," *Amer. J. Med. Sci., 258,* 35 (1969).
(20) J. M. Hansen *et al.,* "Carbamazepine-Induced Acceleration of Diphenylhydantoin and Warfarin Metabolism in Man," *Clin. Pharmacol. Ther., 12,* 539 (1971).
(21) O. Penttilä *et al.,* "Interaction between Doxycycline and Some Antiepileptic Drugs," *Brit. Med. J., 2,* 470 (1974).

Antidepressant Therapy *

Pharmacological agents for the treatment of depressive psychoses were not introduced until the late 1950's. The monoamine oxidase inhibitors were developed first and later the tricyclic antidepressants became available (1). In addition to these antidepressant drugs, psychomotor stimulants such as the amphetamines are still used. The newer drugs differ from the psychomotor stimulants in that they have a preferential effect on mood and behavior, and clinical studies indicate that they are effective in certain cases of the depressive syndrome (1).

Monoamine Oxidase Inhibitors

The first monoamine oxidase inhibitors were derivatives of hydrazine, a hepatotoxic substance. Hydrazine derivatives still commercially available include isocarboxazid and phenelzine. Modification of the phenylalkylamine side chain, as found in the chemical structure of amphetamine, resulted in the nonhydrazine monoamine oxidase inhibitors pargyline and tranylcypromine. Pargyline is used primarily for the treatment of hypertension. The other monoamine oxidase inhibitors have been used primarily in the treatment of mental depression and certain phobic-anxiety states. Because of their potential interaction with many foods and drugs, their use has diminished significantly.

Pharmacological Mechanisms—The mechanism of action of the monoamine oxidase inhibitors in producing an antidepressant effect or a hypotensive effect is unknown. The effects of monoamine oxidase inhibition are seen primarily in organ systems influenced by dopamine, epinephrine, 5-hydroxytryptamine, and norepinephrine.

Following drug administration, the concentrations of dopamine, 5-hydroxytryptamine, and norepinephrine increase in brain and other tissues, with the resultant effect that the amounts of certain metabolites of the monoamines in the urine are decreased. Specifically, the concentration of 5-hydroxyindoleacetic acid (the major metabolite of 5-hydroxytryptamine) is reduced, and there is a decreased excretion of 3-methoxy-4-hydroxymandelic acid with an increased excretion of normetanephrine and metanephrine. The latter two compounds result from the action of catechol-*O*-methyltransferase

on norepinephrine and epinephrine, respectively.

The monoamine oxidase inhibitors do not interfere with the enzymes that synthesize the biogenic amines nor do they interfere with the release of the amines by pharmacological agents such as amphetamine or tyramine. It would be speculative to causally relate the antidepressant or hypotensive effects of these compounds to monoamine oxidase inhibition because the clinically used monoamine oxidase inhibitors are not specific for inhibiting the degradation of the monoamines. They also inhibit the metabolic degradation of a number of drugs such as acetanilid, barbiturates, cocaine, and meperidine. This mechanism is believed to be related to their ability to inhibit the drug-metabolizing enzymes associated with the smooth endoplasmic reticulum located in the liver. Because of this property, they may prolong and intensify the action of many drugs.

Contraindications—Monoamine oxidase inhibitors are contraindicated in patients with a known hypersensitivity to such drugs, with conditions such as pheochromocytoma and congestive heart failure, or with a history of liver disease. They should not be given to patients receiving sympathomimetic drugs or to patients who consume foods high in tryptamine or tyramine. Also, they should not generally be used with central nervous system (CNS) depressants (narcotics) or with tricyclic derivatives. They should be discontinued at least 10 days before elective surgery requiring general anesthesia. In cases of emergency surgery, the anesthesiologist should be warned against using parenteral anesthetic preparations, whereas ether and other anesthetics may be used at lower doses. Such drugs should be used with great caution in elderly or debilitated patients because of their effects on blood pressure, and they should not be used in patients with a history of, or suspected, cerebrovascular disease. Their use during pregnancy has not been established, and they are not recommended for use in children. They have variable effects on convulsive thresholds and should be used with great caution in epileptic patients.

Interactions—*Analgesics*—Concurrent administration of meperidine and monoamine oxidase inhibitors has resulted in excitatory and/or depressant CNS effects leading to coma and death. Concurrent use of meperi-

---

* Monoamine oxidase inhibitors and tricyclic compounds are covered in this discussion.

dine, particularly in high doses, should be avoided in patients receiving monoamine oxidase inhibitors. The effects of concurrent administration of other narcotic analgesics and monoamine oxidase inhibitors have not been established (see *Meperidine–Phenelzine*, p. 142).

Antiarrhythmics—Concurrent use of propranolol and monoamine oxidase inhibitors is considered contraindicated by the manufacturer and one investigator (2), but no clinical data are available to support these precautions.

Antihypertensives—Monoamine oxidase inhibitors have been reported to antagonize the antihypertensive effects of guanethidine (3). The significance of this interaction has not been established, but patients receiving these drugs concurrently should be monitored for a possible reversal of guanethidine's antihypertensive effect.

Autonomics—Levodopa (50 mg or more) causes a significant rise in blood pressure and related symptoms when given to patients receiving a monoamine oxidase inhibitor. To avoid this reaction, a tricyclic antidepressant may be substituted for the monoamine oxidase inhibitor or a carbidopa–levodopa combination product may be used instead of levodopa (see *Levodopa–Phenelzine*, p. 128).

Unpublished animal data and one case report (4) suggest that the concurrent administration of methyldopa and monoamine oxidase inhibitors may result in hallucinations. Although evidence for an interaction is limited and unreliable, patients receiving such therapy should be monitored for possible excitatory CNS effects.

Phenylpropanolamine and other indirect- and mixed-acting sympathomimetic amines produce a hypertensive crisis and related symptoms in some individuals receiving monoamine oxidase inhibitors. This interaction is infrequent but is usually severe and can be fatal. Sympathomimetics and tyramine-containing foods should be avoided in patients taking monoamine oxidase inhibitors (see *Phenylpropanolamine–Tranylcypromine*, p. 188).

Diuretics—The concurrent administration of thiazide diuretics and monoamine oxidase inhibitors may result in hypotension. The significance of this interaction is not established since the only documentation for its occurrence is a single case report (5).

Hypoglycemics—Administration of monoamine oxidase inhibitors to diabetic patients receiving insulin may result in an increased hypoglycemic response. Reduction of the insulin dose may be necessary in patients receiving these drugs concurrently (see *Insulin–Phenelzine*, p. 110).

Monoamine oxidase inhibitors may increase or prolong the hypoglycemia produced by sulfonylureas and possibly phenformin (6). The clinical significance of these interactions has not been established, but patients receiving such drugs concurrently should be monitored for symptoms of hypoglycemia (see *Insulin–Phenelzine*, p. 110).

Psychotropics—Severe reactions have been reported when tricyclic antidepressant drugs have been given concurrently with a monoamine oxidase inhibitor. Symptoms of this interaction include hyperpyrexia, excitability, fluctuations in blood pressure, and coma which can progress to death. Concurrent use of these drugs should be attempted only in carefully selected, closely supervised patients (see *Imipramine–Tranylcypromine*, p. 103).

Tricyclic Antidepressants

The chemical structure of these drugs is similar to the phenothiazines. Imipramine and promazine have the same structure except for the replacement of the sulfur with an ethylene bridge between the two benzene rings. In addition to imipramine, the other tricyclic antidepressants include amitriptyline, desipramine, doxepin, nortriptyline, and protriptyline. These agents are used primarily for their action on the CNS and are most effective in endogenous depression (7).

Pharmacological Mechanisms—The mechanism by which these agents produce their antidepressant action is unknown. One major pharmacological property is to reduce the inactivation of released norepinephrine by inhibiting the membrane pump of the adrenergic nerve terminal responsible for the reuptake of norepinephrine. This action allows norepinephrine to remain in higher concentrations at the receptor site for a longer period, resulting in supersensitization to released or injected norepinephrine (levarterenol) (8). Antidepressants may increase the norepinephrine concentration at the adrenergic receptors in the brain and the increased levels may be responsible for elevating mood (9).

Contraindications—Since tricyclic antidepressants may evoke seizures, these agents are contraindicated in patients with a history of seizure disorders (10). Tricyclic antidepressants may produce tachycardia and orthostatic hypotension and should not be used in patients with cardiovascular disease

(1, 10). The most frequent adverse reactions to tricyclic antidepressants result from their anticholinergic effects. These agents should be used with great caution in patients with urinary retention or glaucoma (1, 10).

Interactions—*Antiarrhythmics*—The anticholinergic activity of tricyclic antidepressants theoretically antagonizes the myocardial effects of propranolol. However, clinical evidence for this interaction is lacking and no additional precautions are necessary when these drugs are used concurrently (see *Propranolol–Desipramine*, p. 214).

Anticoagulants—The hypoprothrombinemic effect of dicumarol may be enhanced by nortriptyline (11). The clinical significance of this drug interaction has not been established and the interaction has not been studied with other coumarin anticoagulants or tricyclic antidepressants. Nevertheless, patients receiving anticoagulants should be monitored closely whenever tricyclic antidepressants are added to or withdrawn from the drug regimen.

Antihypertensives—Tricyclic antidepressants have antagonized the antihypertensive effects of methyldopa in humans (12) and in animals (13, 14). However, other studies in humans (15) failed to confirm this effect. Although this interaction is controversial, patients receiving these drugs concurrently should be monitored for a possible decrease in the antihypertensive effect. The antihypertensive action of guanethidine also may be antagonized by tricyclic antidepressants (see *Guanethidine–Desipramine*, p. 83).

Autonomics—Although concurrent administration of tricyclic antidepressants and reserpine may be effective in treating some depressed patients refractory to other forms of treatment, the potential hazards associated with their concurrent use indicate that such therapy should be limited to selected patients under close supervision (see *Imipramine–Reserpine*, p. 99).

Concurrent administration of a tricyclic antidepressant and amphetamines or methylphenidate may result in increased serum levels of the tricyclic antidepressant, resulting in an enhanced clinical response. This effect has been attributed to an inhibition of drug-metabolizing enzymes by amphetamines and methylphenidate (16).

Tricyclic antidepressants may have additive anticholinergic effects when used with other anticholinergic agents (17). Concurrent use of these agents may result in acute glaucoma and urinary retention. Patients receiving anticholinergic agents concurrently with a tricyclic antidepressant should be monitored to avoid development of these complications.

Administration of intravenous infusions of epinephrine may result in an increased pressor response and arrhythmias in patients receiving tricyclic antidepressants (18). Patients receiving these antidepressants should be monitored closely for such reactions whenever epinephrine is used.

Hormones—Estrogens may increase the number of toxic reactions to tricyclic antidepressants but clinical evidence for this interaction is limited and unreliable. Patients receiving these drugs concurrently should be observed closely for tricyclic-induced adverse reactions. If a reaction occurs, the dose of either the estrogen or tricyclic antidepressant should be reduced or one drug should be discontinued (see *Imipramine–Ethinyl Estradiol*, p. 97).

Psychotropics—Several cases of impaired motor function have been attributed to the concurrent administration of tricyclic antidepressants and benzodiazepines. However, these observations have not been confirmed by controlled clinical trials and it appears unlikely that concurrent use of these drugs will result in serious depressant effects (see *Amitriptyline–Chlordiazepoxide*, p. 8).

Tricyclic antidepressants enhance the CNS effects of meprobamate in animals, but the significance of this effect has not been established in humans. Patients receiving these agents concurrently should be cautioned to avoid driving or operating hazardous machinery while taking these drugs (see *Meprobamate–Imipramine*, p. 147).

Severe reactions have been reported when tricyclic antidepressants have been given concurrently with monoamine oxidase inhibitors. Symptoms of this interaction include hyperpyrexia, excitability, muscular rigidity, fluctuations in blood pressure, and coma which may progress to death. Concurrent use of these drugs should be attempted only in carefully selected, closely supervised patients (see *Imipramine–Tranylcypromine*, p. 103).

Concurrent administration of phenothiazines and tricyclic antidepressants may result in increases in the serum level of either agent (19, 20). The clinical significance of this interaction is not established, but the interaction may be beneficial in some instances.

Concurrent use of thioxanthene tranquilizers and tricyclic antidepressants may result in an increased pharmacological effect of either agent. The result of this interaction may be CNS stimulation, tremors, or arrhythmias. Although there has been a report of a possible interaction (21), the clinical significance of this interaction has not been established.

Haloperidol has been reported to decrease the urinary excretion of tricyclic antidepressants (18), but the clinical outcome of this interaction is unknown.

Sedative–Hypnotics—Limited data indicate that barbiturates may decrease the serum level of tricyclic antidepressants. The barbiturates should be considered a causative factor in barbiturate-treated patients who are unresponsive to tricyclic antidepressants (see *Nortriptyline–Phenobarbital*, p. 161).

Concurrent ingestion of alcohol and tricyclic antidepressants may result in enhancement of the CNS depressant effect of alcohol. Patients receiving tricyclic antidepressants should be cautioned to avoid alcohol especially when driving or operating hazardous machinery (see *Alcohol–Amitriptyline*, p. 1).

References

(1) "The Pharmacological Basis of Therapeutics," 5th ed., L. S. Goodman and A. Gilman, Eds., Macmillan, New York, NY 10022, 1975, pp. 174–187.

(2) J. Frieden, "Propranolol as an Antiarrhythmic Agent," *Amer. Heart J.*, *74*, 283 (1967).

(3) O. D. Gulati *et al.*, "Antagonism of Adrenergic Neuron Blockade in Hypertensive Subjects," *Clin. Pharmacol. Ther.*, *7*, 510 (1966).

(4) J. M. van Rossum, "Potential Danger of Monoamine Oxidase Inhibitors and Alphamethyldopa," *Lancet*, *i*, 950 (1963).

(5) M. Moser *et al.*, "Experience with Isocarboxazid," *J. Amer. Med. Ass.*, *176*, 276 (1961).

(6) P. I. Adnitt, "Hypoglycemic Action of Monoamineoxidase Inhibitors (M.A.O.I.'s)," *Diabetes*, *17*, 628 (1968).

(7) "Harrison's Principles of Internal Medicine," 7th ed., McGraw-Hill, New York, N.Y., 1974, pp. 1893–1894.

(8) J. Axelrod *et al.*, "Effect of Psychotropic Drugs on the Uptake of H3-Norepinephrine by Tissues," *Science, 133*, 383 (1961).

(9) J. J. Schildkraut *et al.*, "Norepinephrine Metabolism and Drugs Used in the Affective Disorders: A Possible Mechanism of Action," *Amer. J. Psychiat.*, *124*, 600 (1967).

(10) "Drill's Pharmacology in Medicine," 4th ed., J. R. DiPalma, Ed., McGraw-Hill, New York, N.Y., 1971, pp. 503–505.

(11) E. S. Vesell *et al.*, "Impairment of Drug Metabolism in Man by Allopurinol and Nortriptyline," *N. Engl. J. Med.*, *283*, 1484 (1970).

(12) A. G. White, "Methyldopa and Amitriptyline," *Lancet, ii*, 441 (1965).

(13) H. W. Van Spanning and P. A. Van Zwieten, "The Interaction between Alpha Methyl Dopa and Tricyclic Antidepressants," *Int. J. Pharmacol. Biopharm.*, *11*, 65 (1975).

(14) P. A. Van Zwieten *et al.*, "Interaction between Centrally Acting Hypotensive Drugs and Tricyclic Antidepressants," *Arch. Int. Pharmacodyn. Ther.*, *214*, 12 (1975).

(15) J. R. Mitchell *et al.*, "Guanethidine and Related Agents III. Antagonism by Drugs which Inhibit the Norepinephrine Pump in Man," *J. Clin. Invest.*, *49*, 1596 (1970). [Preliminary communication: J. R. Mitchell *et al.*, "Antagonism of the Antihypertensive Action of Guanethidine Sulfate by Desipramine Hydrochloride," *J. Amer. Med. Ass.*, *202*, 973 (1967).]

(16) P. Zeidenberg *et al.*, "Clinical and Metabolic Studies with Imipramine in Man," *Amer. J. Psychiat.*, *127*, 1321 (1971).

(17) G. Milner, "Gastro-intestinal Side Effects and Psychotropic Drugs," *Med. J. Aust.*, *2*, 153 (1969).

(18) A. J. Boakes *et al.*, "Interactions between Sympathomimetic Amines and Antidepressant Agents in Man," *Brit. Med. J.*, *1*, 311 (1973).

(19) L. F. Gram *et al.*, "Influence of Neuroleptics and Benzodiazepines on Metabolism of Tricyclic Antidepressants in Man," *Amer. J. Psychiat.*, *131*, 863 (1974).

(20) M. R. El-Yousef and D. H. Manier, "Tricyclic Antidepressants and Phenothiazines," letter to the editor, *J. Amer. Med. Ass.*, *229*, 1419 (1974).

(21) L. F. Gram and K. F. Overo, "Drug Interaction: Inhibitory Effect of Neuroleptics on Metabolism of Tricyclic Antidepressants in Man," *Brit. Med. J.*, *1*, 463 (1972).

Antihistamine Therapy

Antihistamines are drugs capable of preventing or diminishing several pharmacological actions of histamine by competitive inhibition of histamine at receptor sites in tissue (1). In addition to blocking the activity of histamine, the antihistamines possess sedative, local anesthetic, antispasmodic, and analgesic properties, quinidine-like activity, and cholinergic blocking activity.

Most antihistamines are derivatives of ethanolamine, ethylenediamine, piperazine, or propylamine. Drugs that are phenothiazines or derivatives also exhibit potent antihistaminic activity and have widespread clinical use because of this activity. In addition, several drugs of varied chemical structure are effective antihistamines as shown by *in vitro* and *in vivo* studies.

Therapeutic Uses

The antihistaminic drugs have the greatest application in the treatment of those allergic disorders in which symptoms result from immunoglobulin E (IgE) antibody–antigen interaction causing histamine release from tissue mast cells.

Respiratory Conditions—Seasonal allergic rhinitis (prototype disorder is ragweed hay fever) is treated quite effectively with antihistamines. The profuse rhinorrhea, nasal itching, and repetitive sneezing of the disease are more responsive to treatment than is the symptom of nasal obstruction (2).

Perennial allergic rhinitis and vasomotor rhinitis (in the latter disorder the symptoms are similar to perennial allergic rhinitis but no allergic etiology can be demonstrated) are less effectively treated with antihistamines than is seasonal allergic rhinitis. In perennial allergic rhinitis and vasomotor rhinitis, nasal blockage may be the predominant symptom and is only minimally responsive to antihistaminic drugs.

The role of antihistaminic drugs in the treatment of asthma has not been conclusively delineated. Histamine may be only one mediator of asthma. Another agent, called slow-reacting substance, has potent bronchoconstricting activity on human bronchi which is not blocked by antihistaminic drugs. Most studies of the efficacy of antihistamines in asthma either have not been properly controlled or have not included objective evidence of efficacy such as pulmonary function data. However, in a well-designed, double-blind crossover study, some patients clearly had amelioration of asthma while receiving an antihistamine (3).

Ophthalmological Conditions—Allergic conjunctivitis occurs concomitantly with seasonal allergic rhinitis and frequently is more bothersome to the patient than the nasal symptoms. Itching, conjunctival edema, and chemosis are only moderately relieved by antihistaminic drugs.

Dermatological Conditions—The pruritus of atopic dermatitis (atopic eczema), the most distressing symptom of the disease, is lessened by systemic antihistaminic therapy. Whether this is due to the inhibition of histamine effect or to the sedative action of the antihistamine is unknown. Most practitioners favor the latter explanation.

Contact dermatitis (prototype disorder is poison ivy) is due to a cell-mediated (delayed hypersensitivity) immune reaction and is not effectively treated with antihistamines, although they may be useful for the pruritis caused by this dermatitis.

Many urticarias, especially the acute variety, appear to be mediated by histamine and are effectively treated with antihistamines. Indeed, antihistamines are the drugs of choice in these conditions. The chronic urticarias are much more difficult to treat with antihistamines alone. Certain antihistamines, such as hydroxyzine, have been reported to be of special value in chronic urticaria. Angioedema is variably affected by antihistaminic therapy. In the hereditary autosomal dominant form of the disease, due to C-1 esterase inhibitor deficiency, antihistamines have not been effective. The vasoactive substance responsible for the disease is not histamine but a product of the complement system (4). In urticaria appearing on exposure to cold and known as cold urticaria, cyproheptadine, which has antihistaminic, anti-5-hydroxytryptamine, and antikinin activities, was extraordinarily effective (5).

Miscellaneous Allergic Conditions—When there is reasonable evidence that a particular allergic reaction is mediated by the action of histamine, one would expect antihistamines to have a favorable effect in treating the disorder. For example, the urticaria of an adverse drug reaction is effectively treated with antihistaminic drugs; late occurring nonurticarial reactions that are not histamine mediated are little affected by this treatment. Similarly, the urticaria of serum sickness-like reactions is responsive to antihistamines, while the other symptoms of the disorder are ameliorated to a lesser degree. Even in the treatment of acute systemic anaphylaxis in which histamine may play a role, epinephrine, not antihistamines, is the drug of choice for the treatment of the immediate problem. In this circumstance, antihistamines may be of value in blocking the effect of subsequent histamine release and are frequently administered for this reason. In conditions such as migraine headaches, gastrointestinal symptoms, and reactions to intravenous administration of blood components, the role of histamine as a mediator of the allergic reaction (if an allergic reaction can be implicated at all) has not been established.

Antihistamine Use Other than for Histamine Inhibition—Antihistamines, particularly those belonging to the ethanolamine, phenothiazine, and piperazine groups, are used extensively in the prophylaxis of motion sickness associated with air and sea travel.

The pronounced hypnotic effects of certain antihistamines, which limit their use in allergic disorders, make them valuable for this reason in selected patients. Diphenhydramine, in particular, is a safe and effective hypnotic in elderly persons. Methapyrilene hydrochloride is found in many over-the-counter "sleep-aids." It has minor sedative activity and may be used with other drugs such as scopolamine.

The sedative effects of antihistamines may explain their efficacy in the treatment of pruritis quite apart from their antihistaminic activity. The local anesthetic activity of antihistamines is utilized in situations in which the patient cannot tolerate the conventional local anesthetic drugs. However, their irritant properties following injection limit their use by this route. Diphenhydramine and tripelennamine are used quite effectively on an acute basis to provide oral mucous membrane analgesia in young children suffering from herpetic gingivostomatitis.

The anticholinergic effects of antihistaminic drugs make them useful therapeutic agents in parkinsonism. Diphenhydramine and certain phenothiazines are prescribed most often.

Pharmacological Mechanisms

Antihistamines are competitive antagonists of histamine. They compete with histamine for receptor sites in effector tissues without initiating a pharmacological effect. The histamine-blocking effect of antihistamines is the activity most easily understood.

Two types of histamine receptors mediate different physiological effects and are blocked by different histamine antagonists. The H_1 receptors mediate the effects of histamine on capillary permeability and on vascular, bronchial, and many other types of smooth muscle. The H_2 receptors are responsible for the effect of histamine on gastric secretion and may also play a role in histamine's stimulation of the heart. Both receptors seem to be involved in a synergistic manner in vasodilation and edema formation (6).

The beneficial effects of antihistamines in allergic disorders are explicable in terms of competitive inhibition of released histamine, thereby preventing the pharmacological effect of the latter on smooth muscle and capillary permeability. The mechanisms of the other activities of antihistamines are less well understood. The atropine-like effect of most antihistaminic drugs more than likely results from a competitive inhibition of acetylcholine (7). The latter property has also been proposed to explain the favorable effect of these drugs in prophylaxis of motion sickness and treatment of parkinsonism.

Contraindications

The major contraindication to the use of antihistamines relates to their sedative properties. Individuals who work at jobs or perform activities requiring a high degree of mental alertness should use these drugs with caution. The atropine-like activity of antihistamines which results in the drying of respiratory secretions has led some practitioners to interdict their use in asthma because of fear of worsening the airway problem due to inspissation of mucus. However, despite this theoretical objection, many practitioners believe that the use of antihistamines in an individual who has both allergic rhinitis and asthma (as is frequently the case) does not have an adverse effect on the asthma.

Little is known about the potential teratogenic effects of antihistamines; however, certain piperazine compounds have produced teratogenic effects in experimental animals and thus should not be given to pregnant women. Since antihistamines occasionally have a paradoxical effect in children, especially with overdosage, causing central nervous system (CNS) stimulation instead of the usual sedation, caution is indicated when used in children with convulsive disorders. A similar admonition may be given for individuals with asthma treated with high doses of ephedrine and theophylline, both of which are CNS stimulants.

Acute antihistaminic poisoning as a result of accidental ingestion is common and represents a serious problem in small children.

The CNS activity of the antihistamines dominates the clinical picture. Marked excitation leading to convulsions and terminating in cardiorespiratory collapse and coma in the absence of a specific antidote makes the condition particularly serious. However, with the recent general availability of life support systems, the acute phase of the episode is more easily managed. The cholinergic blocking activity of antihistamines should also be kept in mind when these drugs are prescribed for individuals with glaucoma.

Interactions

Anticholinergics—The cholinergic blocking effect of many antihistamines has an additive effect with anticholinergic drugs. The effects of excessive cholinergic blockade are usually of minor clinical significance. Patients with glaucoma are susceptible to an adverse effect as a result of this interaction but clinical documentation is lacking. A widely quoted adverse effect, dental caries and loss of teeth, occurs secondary to xerostomia produced by the concurrent use of diphenhydramine, tricyclic antidepressants, and trihexyphenidyl. Urinary retention may be a problem in older men with prostatic hypertrophy, and constipation may be bothersome.

Anticholinesterases—The significant anticholinergic activity of certain antihistamines antagonizes the miotic effect of the anticholinesterase drugs. Anticholinesterase drugs may have diminished activity in glaucoma patients treated with antihistamines, but this effect has not been observed clinically.

Catecholamines—Some but not all antihistamines enhance the cardiovascular action of epinephrine and norepinephrine. Apparently, this activity is due to inhibition of neuronal uptake of catecholamine (cocaine-like effect), resulting in an increased amount of unbound drug which is then available to react with the receptor sites in cardiac and vascular tissues (8).

The potential for increased catecholamine toxicity should be recognized when antihistaminic drugs and catecholamines are used concurrently, as is frequently the case. Since catecholamines, especially epinephrine, are potent histamine antagonists, the need for antihistaminic therapy is minimal when the former drugs are administered.

CNS Depressants—These agents include alcohol, anesthetics, barbiturates, bromides, hypnotics, narcotics, reserpine, scopolamine, and tranquilizers (9). Antihistamines have an additive sedative effect when used concurrently with these compounds. CNS depression may result from the concurrent use of antihistamines and other classes of CNS depressants.

Halogenated Insecticides—These compounds diminish antihistaminic activity by hepatic enzyme induction (10). Decreased efficacy of antihistamines may be anticipated in individuals whose occupation exposes them to halogenated insecticides. This effect may be remedied, if it occurs, by increasing the antihistaminic dose.

Hormones—Antihistamines, if given repeatedly, can decrease the effect of corticosteroids, estradiol, progesterone, and testosterone by hepatic enzyme induction (11). Diminished effectiveness of various hormones may result from concurrent antihistaminic therapy. However, the clinical significance of this interaction is open to question.

Various classes of antihistamines differ in their capacity to induce hepatic microsomal enzymes. Alternatives within antihistamines may have to be sought empirically, since only a relatively few antihistamines have been studied for their enzyme induction activity.

Nylidrin—The effects of antihistamines with the phenothiazine structure (*e.g.,* promethazine) are enhanced by nylidrin by displacement of the phenothiazine from receptor sites and tissues (12) and by the cerebral vasodilator effect of nylidrin. Although clinical documentation is lacking, phenothiazine activity may be enhanced by the concurrent use of nylidrin.

Miscellaneous—Drugs whose metabolism may be affected by the enzyme induction activity of antihistamines include griseofulvin, phenylbutazone, phenytoin (diphenylhydantoin), various anticoagulants, and the antihistamine itself, especially diphenhydramine. The degree of clinical significance of these reported interactions remains to be established.

References

(1) "The Pharmacological Basis of Therapeutics," 5th ed., L. S. Goodman and A. Gilman, Eds., Macmillan, New York, NY 10022, 1975, p. 603.
(2) "Current Therapy 1974," H. F. Conn, Ed., Saunders, Philadelphia, Pa., 1974, p. 568.
(3) J. M. Karlin, "The Use of Antihistamines in Asthma," *Ann. Allergy, 30,* 342 (1972).
(4) M. M. Frank *et al.,* "Epsilon Aminocaproic Acid Therapy of Hereditary Angioneurotic Edema. A Double-Blind Study," *N. Engl. J. Med., 286,* 808 (1972).
(5) A. A. Wanderer and E. F. Ellis, "Treatment of Cold Urticaria with Cyproheptadine," *J. Allergy Clin. Immun., 48,* 366 (1971).

(6) "The Pharmacological Basis of Therapeutics," 5th ed., L. S. Goodman and A. Gilman, Eds., Macmillan, New York, NY 10022, 1975, p. 595.

(7) E. R. Loew, "Pharmacological Properties of Antihistamines in Relation to Allergic and Nonallergic Diseases," *Boston Med. Quart., 3,* 1 (1952).

(8) L. Isaac and A. Goth, "The Mechanism of the Potentiation of Norepinephrine by Antihistaminics," *J. Pharmacol. Exp. Ther., 156,* 463 (1967).

(9) L. Lasagna, "Drug Interaction in the Field of Analgesic Drugs," *Proc. Roy. Soc. Med., 58,* 978 (1965).

(10) A. H. Conney *et al.,* "Effects of Pesticides on Drug and Steroid Metabolism," *Clin. Pharmacol. Ther., 8,* 2 (1967).

(11) A. H. Conney *et al.,* "Drug-Induced Changes in Steroid Metabolism," *Ann. N.Y. Acad. Sci., 123,* 98 (1965).

(12) J. Chu *et al.,* "The Clinical Determination of Unique Effect of Potentiation of Phenothiazine Medication by Nylidrin Hydrochloride," *Int. J. Neuropsychiat., 2,* 53 (1966).

Antihypertensive Therapy

Hypertension is one of the most prevalent diseases affecting the cardiovascular system; it has been estimated that hypertension affects approximately 23 million persons in the United States. It is difficult to discuss the actions and therapeutic uses of drugs utilized in the treatment of the disease when the physiological disturbances producing the characteristics associated with that particular pathological disturbance are not fully understood.

Although the precise etiology of hypertensive cardiovascular disease has not been elucidated, data were presented suggesting that the labile hypertensive reactions appear to be due to the response of the organism to stressors occurring in its environment. Selye (1, 2) described the characteristic physiological and behavioral responses occurring in the mammalian organism subjected to intensive environmental stimuli which he called the "general adaptation syndrome."

Experimental animals subjected to environmental stressors consisting of noxious sounds, flashing lights, and motion develop systolic hypertension, left ventricular hypertrophy, and hypertrophy of the zona fasiculata and zona reticularis of the adrenal cortex (3). The elevation in blood pressure is sustained even after the exposure to stressors has been discontinued for as long as 6 months.

Concomitant with the increase in the blood pressure, serum corticosterone levels increased almost threefold during 4 weeks of stress exposure (3); however, the plasma steroid levels declined to below normal by the end of the fifth week. There was an increase in the synthesis rate of brain norepinephrine during the first 4 weeks of stress exposure; however, the turnover of brain norepinephrine returned to prestress levels between the fifth and sixth weeks. The development of hypertension due to exposure to stressors could be divided into two phases (3): (a) the acute phase which is manifested by stimulation of central sympathetic centers and liberation of adrenocorticotropic hormone (ACTH) from the anterior pituitary, resulting in elevation of adrenal steroid secretion, and (b) the chronic phase which is associated with a reduction of the elevated plasma glucocorticoid levels and central sympathetic nervous system activity to prestress levels.

Additional studies were undertaken to investigate the role of the peripheral sympathetic nervous system in hypertension induced in rats by chronic intermittent exposure to environmental stress (4). Repeated doses of 6-hydroxydopamine sufficient to maintain an effective chemical sympathectomy were utilized in these studies. The results indicated that, unlike certain other models of hypertension, normal peripheral sympathetic function is an absolute requirement for stress-induced hypertension. Furthermore, the hypertension is not associated with any observable malfunction in peripheral sympathetic activity, such as alterations in transmitter uptake, release, adrenal medullary function, or adrenergic effector–receptor sensitivity.

Although two major factors contribute to blood pressure *per se*, *i.e.*, cardiac output and peripheral resistance, the elevation in blood pressure in hypertensive cardiovascular disease appears mainly to be due to increased peripheral resistance. The increase in sympathetic activity and plasma glucocorticoid levels would definitely be expected to increase peripheral resistance.

The chronic phase may involve several factors including: (a) an upward resetting of the carotid sinus and aortic arch baroreceptors, (b) increased production of renin by the kidney leading to increased plasma levels of angiotensin I and angiotensin II, and (c) increased sodium content of the vascular wall. The resetting of the baroreceptors diminishes the normal effects of the reflexogenic mechanisms in maintaining homeostasis. Therefore, both the systolic and diastolic pressures will be maintained at higher levels.

If, in fact, the plasma angiotensin II concentration increases, this increase will further enhance the progression of hypertensive cardiovascular disease by: (a) inducing a direct constriction of vascular smooth muscle, (b) increasing the rate of synthesis and release of aldosterone from the adrenal cortex, (c) interacting to enhance the activity of the sympathetic division of the autonomic nervous system at peripheral sites, (d) stimulating the release of epinephrine from the adrenal medulla, (e) stimulating the release of antidiuretic hormone, and (f) stimulating one or more central sympathetic structures, thereby increasing the outflow of sympathetic impulses.

Pathological changes associated with the development of hypertension and used to diagnose the status of this condition include left ventricular hypertrophy, changes in the vasculature of the retina, kidney damage, and alterations in myocardial conduction (ECG changes). If the elevation in blood pressure is not controlled, this progressive disease can accelerate the development of arteriosclerosis, eventually leading to coronary occlusion and/or cerebral vascular accidents (5). The increased peripheral resistance will also increase the workload of the left ventricle and possibly lead to congestive heart failure. There are currently a number of compounds and concurrent therapy that can be used to control the elevated pressure, thereby markedly prolonging the life of the patient.

Therapeutic Indications

Hypertensive cardiovascular disease is a progressive disease in which there is an initial labile hypertensive state which may be associated with the response of the individual to environmental situations. Eventually, this labile hypertension develops into a sustained hypertensive state. The main objective of drug therapy is to control the hypertensive state with compounds which will minimize the possibility of adverse reactions and will permit the patient to lead a relatively normal life. It has been postulated that the progression of hypertensive cardiovascular disease can be halted and possibly even reversed through the lowering of both systolic and diastolic blood pressure.

Pharmacological Mechanisms

The mechanisms of action of the antihypertensive compounds are not only complex but in many instances unknown. The compounds may interfere with central adrenergic outflow, ganglionic transmission, and peripheral adrenergic transmission; directly relax vascular smooth muscle; affect reflexogenic mechanisms; and possibly alter electrolyte balance. Although the mechanisms of action are complex and may involve various sites of action, they will be discussed according to their primary site of action.

Centrally Acting Compounds—Mebutamate is structurally related to meprobamate and was reported to be a centrally acting hypotensive agent. The compound produces sedative effects similar to meprobamate; however, it is still questionable whether mebutamate produces a specific antihypertensive effect via central mechanisms. Investigators utilizing dog cross-circulation preparations recorded splanchnic nerve activity; they concluded that the initial tran-

sient hypotension was largely due to direct vasodilator action since the sustained effect was attributed to an inhibition of sympathetic vasomotor tone, essentially at the spinal ganglion levels. These data suggest that spinal and/or peripheral mechanisms in conjunction with the sedative action of the compound are responsible for the weak hypotensive effects induced.

Clonidine is an imidazoline derivative producing hypotension, bradycardia, and sedation in relatively low doses. Several investigators (6–9) showed that this compound produces its hypotensive effect via central mechanisms. Data from dog cross-circulation studies showed that the compound produces a central hypotensive effect by reducing sympathetic outflow (10). Clonidine was a potent inhibitor of the spontaneous sympathetic outflow from the brain stem but was less effective on reflexly or centrally evoked discharges (11). The hypotensive effect of clonidine is due mainly to a decrease in cardiac output and a reduction in peripheral resistance.

Ganglionic Blocking Agents—The bisquaternary ammonium compounds (chlorisondamine, pentolinium, and trimethidinium) and mecamylamine lower arterial blood pressure through a specific paralysis of transmission at ganglionic synapses. The mechanism of action appears to be that of competitive inhibition because they block impulses at autonomic ganglia by raising the threshold of the ganglion cells to acetylcholine released at the preganglionic nerve endings. Since the antagonism is competitive, the intensity of the blockade increases as the concentration of the compounds in the extracellular space of the ganglion increases in relation to the acetylcholine release. Unfortunately, there is an inhibition of all autonomic ganglia; that is, these compounds do not selectively block either the sympathetic or parasympathetic systems. Many side effects, therefore, are due to diminished cholinergic outflow including dryness of the nose, mouth, and throat; constipation; impaired visual accommodation; and urinary retention.

The bisquaternary ammonium compounds are, in general, poorly absorbed from the gastrointestinal (GI) tract and, therefore, there is difficulty in maintaining consistent serum levels. This problem results in either an increase in side effects or a decrease in efficacy of the compound.

Mecamylamine hydrochloride is a secondary amine and differs from the bisquaternary ammonium compounds in that it is almost completely absorbed from the GI tract.

Since it is almost 100% absorbed, the hypotensive effects are more predictable than those obtained with bisquaternary ammonium compounds. Mecamylamine also has a much longer duration of action and a decreased tendency for the production of severe postural hypotension.

Compounds Affecting Postganglionic Adrenergic Neuronal Activities—Adrenergic neurotransmitter depleters such as reserpine and other rauwolfia alkaloids deplete both peripheral and central stores of catecholamines, thus interfering with sympathetic neuronal transmission. Although reserpine releases large quantities of norepinephrine, the sympathetic activity is not enhanced since the neurotransmitter passively diffuses from its storage sites and is deaminated by monoamine oxidase (12).

The available data suggest that reserpine acts through three specific mechanisms: (*a*) depletion of norepinephrine from peripheral binding sites, producing sympathetic blockade with a possibility of an initial inhibition of norepinephrine release (12); (*b*) depression of central sympathetic outflow; and (*c*) central nervous system (CNS) depression producing a decrease in tension and aggressiveness as well as a decreased response in the sympathetic centers to external stimuli.

Guanethidine releases norepinephrine from peripheral sympathetic neurons with little or no effect on norepinephrine stores in the brain (13). A selective accumulation of guanethidine was demonstrated in adrenergic neurons associated with the same granular fraction which contains the norepinephrine stores (13). The compound also blocks the release of norepinephrine from sympathetic nerve endings and to some extent inhibits the reuptake of norepinephrine. High doses of guanethidine (25 or 30 mg/kg/day ip) administered for 6 weeks to rats produced a more complete and longer lasting peripheral chemical sympathectomy than was possible with 6-hydroxydopamine (14).

Guanethidine antagonizes the hypertension induced by large doses of amphetamine or bilateral carotid occlusion and produces a relaxation of the nictitating membrane in dogs and cats. The compound enhances the pressor response to angiotensin, epinephrine, phenylephrine, and vasopressin. The hypotensive effects of guanethidine appear to be mainly due to a decrease in cardiac output rather than a reduction in peripheral resistance, and this reduction in cardiac output is usually associated with a reduction in the renal blood flow and glomerular filtration rate (15).

Inhibitors of Norepinephrine Release—Bethanidine sulfate inhibits the release of norepinephrine at sympathetic postganglionic neuronal sites without inhibiting the effects of circulating norepinephrine (16). After prolonged administration of bethanidine, the tissue stores of catecholamines are reduced, but to a much lesser degree than that induced by guanethidine. Studies showed that bethanidine prevents the release of norepinephrine by guanethidine (17, 18), and it has been suggested that the hypotensive effects may be due to the failure of norepinephrine release from sympathetic nerve endings.

Bretylium tosylate is a benzyl quaternary ammonium compound which selectively blocks the sympathetic nervous system without affecting the parasympathetic division. The compound accumulates selectively in adrenergic neurons in sufficient concentrations to impair conduction. Bretylium inhibits the release of norepinephrine when certain sympathetic neurons are stimulated; however, the effects of circulating catecholamines are enhanced. Therefore, the mechanism of action does not appear to be due to a peripheral depletion of norepinephrine or inhibition of the synthesis of norepinephrine but possibly to the prevention of the release of the sympathetic neurotransmitter. High concentrations of bretylium induce a curare-like paralysis; muscle weakness or fatigue was reported in patients treated with this compound.

Derivatives of phenylalanine were reported to inhibit the decarboxylation of dopa (dihydroxyphenylalanine) which, in the presence of the enzyme dopa decarboxylase, forms dopamine. Methyldopa is a potent dopa decarboxylase inhibitor *in vitro*, preventing the decarboxylation of dopa to dopamine and thus inhibiting norepinephrine synthesis. Methyldopa has been reported to deplete tissue stores of norepinephrine but this does not appear to be due to inhibition of dopa decarboxylase (19). It was suggested that methyldopa is metabolized to α-methylnorepinephrine which is bound in the tissues and acts as a false transmitter (19).

Other investigators (20) showed that methyldopa produces central hypotensive effects since infusion of small doses into the vertebral artery of anesthetized cats produced hypotensive effects whereas intravenous administration of the same doses failed to affect blood pressure. The suspected mechanism of the central hypotensive effect is thought to be methyldopa-initiated stimulation of the α-adrenergic receptors in the brain resulting in decreased pressor effects (21). Further evidence for methyldopa's central hypotensive effect was provided by the observation that the dopamine and norepinephrine content of the brain was reduced significantly while brain 5-hydroxytryptamine and cardiac norepinephrine levels remained normal. Additionally, the central component of the antihypertensive effects of methyldopa is also suggested by the fact that the compound produces some degree of tranquillity and CNS depression. Although the compound appears to act by interfering with peripheral adrenergic function and possibly *via* a central mechanism, the precise mechanisms of action are still unclear.

Monoamine Oxidase Inhibitors—One major side effect reported with the monoamine oxidase inhibitors has been postural hypotension; pargyline is a nonhydrazine monoamine oxidase inhibitor which produces postural hypotension and decreases vascular resistance. Although the exact mechanism of action of pargyline is not understood, inhibition of monoamine oxidase enhances the formation and accumulation of octopamine (22). Octopamine is then believed to be released by sympathetic nerve stimulation; however, since this amine is relatively inactive, a partial inhibition of sympathetic activity may result. The concept of "false transmitters" has received wide attention specifically with regard to methyldopa and pargyline. The role of dopamine and octopamine (22) in the mechanism of the antihypertensive actions of pargyline is still unclear.

α-Adrenergic Blocking Agents—Compounds that block stimulation of the α-adrenergic receptors produce a decrease in peripheral resistance and therefore a decrease in arterial pressure. Phenoxybenzamine is a β-haloalkylamine which produces prolonged blockade of α-adrenergic receptors. Although the compound selectively blocks the sympathetic division as well as circulating norepinephrine and epinephrine, its usefulness in the treatment of hypertension has been limited because it so firmly binds with the receptor that it produces severe postural hypotension and tachycardia. Phenoxybenzamine appears to affect covalent bond formation at the receptor site (23), thereby preventing the α-adrenergic neurotransmitter from reacting with the receptor.

Phentolamine, like phenoxybenzamine, blocks α-adrenergic receptors by competing with the naturally occurring neurotransmitter and other α-adrenergic stimulants. Phentolamine is only moderately effective

in blocking the α-adrenergic receptors and the duration of action is much less than phenoxybenzamine.

β-Adrenergic Blocking Agents—Propranolol, a β-adrenergic blocking compound, has been reported to produce hypotensive effects and augment the depressor effects of vasodilator antihypertensive compounds (24–26). Propranolol and other β-adrenergic blocking compounds have also been reported to attenuate the increased plasma renin activity induced by certain vasodilator compounds, such as the diuretics, hydralazine, and minoxidil (27, 28). Propranolol also has been found to antagonize the increase in heart rate induced by minoxidil and markedly decrease plasma renin activity in patients treated with minoxidil (29). Both *d*-propranolol and racemic propranolol administered by intraventricular injection to α-chloralose-anesthetized cats produced a decrease in blood pressure (30). The hypotension associated with propranolol therapy may have a central component that is independent of its β-adrenergic blocking property.

Compounds Acting Directly on Vascular Smooth Muscle—Hydralazine is a potent hypotensive compound which simultaneously dilates peripheral blood vessels, increases cardiac output, and, to some extent, increases blood flow. The pharmacology of hydralazine is complex and the precise mechanism of the hypotensive activity is not understood clearly. Hydralazine appears to act through both peripheral and central mechanisms; however, the peripheral effects predominate and the hypotensive effects in humans are due to decreased peripheral resistance induced by arterial vasodilatation. The compound is a nonspecific inhibitor of a variety of vasoconstrictor substances including angiotensin II, barium chloride, epinephrine, norepinephrine, serotonin, tyramine, and vasopressin. Hydralazine also inhibits dopa decarboxylase and, therefore, inhibits norepinephrine biosynthesis and may interfere with normal adrenergic transmission through this mechanism.

Sodium nitroprusside produces peripheral vasodilatation *via* a direct action on vascular smooth muscle (31). The compound has an extremely short onset and duration of action and is administered intravenously in the treatment of hypertensive crises.

Diuretics—The importance of electrolyte levels and electrolyte balance in the production and control of hypertension is well documented and the use of the low salt diets or salt-free diets has been recommended for the treatment of arterial hypertension. Oral diuretics were shown to possess hypotensive activity and/or to enhance the depressor effects produced by other antihypertensive compounds.

The mechanism of action of chlorothiazide and other benzothiadiazines on the cardiovascular system is not clearly understood; however, the hypotensive properties of these compounds were reported to be selective to hypertensive patients. Hydrochlorothiazide inhibited the pressor response to stimulation of adrenergic vasomotor fibers without influencing the vascular response to catecholamines and angiotensin II in experimental animals (32). The mechanisms by which the thiazides produce a decrease in arterial pressure are still not understood. The antihypertensive action does not appear to be related to the diuretic effects or to a decrease in plasma volume. Ethacrynic acid and furosemide are also oral diuretics possessing antihypertensive properties.

Compounds that antagonize the renal tubular action of aldosterone and related mineralocorticoids by competitive inhibition produce hypotensive effects in hypertensive rats. Spironolactone, an aldosterone antagonist, lowers blood pressure when administered orally. The compound differs from other orally effective diuretics in that, although there is an increase in sodium excretion, there is usually no change or an actual decrease in potassium excretion.

Compounds Affecting Reflexogenic Mechanisms—The veratrum alkaloids appear to produce vasodepressor actions through reflexogenic mechanisms. The compounds stimulate afferent reflex pathways from the carotid sinus, the aortic arch, and pulmonary arteries as well as act through the Bezold-Jarisch reflex in which the afferent fibers arise from the walls of the coronary arteries in the left ventricle. The pure alkaloids, protoveratrine A and protoveratrine B, appear to act almost exclusively *via* reflexogenic mechanisms (33). Cryptenamine, an alkaloidal mixture prepared from *Veratrum viride* by a nonaqueous triethylamine extraction procedure, was reported to have a ratio of emetic to effective hypotensive dose superior to that of other veratrum preparations. Cryptenamine also stimulates receptors in the carotid sinus-body complex (34) and sensitizes certain β-adrenergic receptors (34, 35).

Contraindications

The major contraindications for certain of the antihypertensive compounds are impaired renal function, decreased cardiac efficiency (especially with reserpine), and severe depression or melancholia (especially with reserpine or other centrally acting compounds).

Since an excessively elevated blood pressure must be lowered, there are truly no absolute contraindications for the use of one or more antihypertensive compounds. In such instances, it is a matter of selecting a compound which would be least deleterious. For example, in cases where renal function is impaired, the hypotensive agent should not produce a further decrease in blood flow to the kidneys. If a person's mood is depressed, a compound which would not further increase the depression of the individual should be administered.

Interactions

Clonidine–Desipramine—Desipramine and other tricyclic antidepressants may block the antihypertensive effects of clonidine (36) and concurrent administration of these drugs should be avoided.

Guanethidine–Alcohol—Alcohol may enhance the antihypertensive effects of guanethidine. Patients treated with guanethidine should be cautioned that they may experience symptoms of postural hypotension and that these symptoms may worsen if alcoholic beverages are ingested concurrently (see *Guanethidine–Alcohol*, p. 79).

Guanethidine–Chlorpromazine, Guanethidine–Desipramine, Guanethidine–Dextroamphetamine, and Phenylephrine–Guanethidine—Chlorpromazine, desipramine, and dextroamphetamine can reverse the hypotensive activity of guanethidine. Conversely, guanethidine enhances the pressor effects of phenylephrine. These drug interactions may be clinically significant and concurrent administration should generally be avoided (see *Guanethidine–Chlorpromazine*, p. 81; *Guanethidine–Desipramine*, p. 83; *Guanethidine–Dextroamphetamine*, p. 86; and *Phenylephrine–Guanethidine*, p. 186).

Pargyline–Tyramine—Pargyline is an antihypertensive agent with monoamine oxidase inhibitory activity which permits the accumulation of norepinephrine in intraneuronal binding sites. Under certain conditions, the ingestion of foods containing tyramine (fermented cheeses, herring, broad beans, chicken livers, and certain fermented beverages) will produce a release of large quantities of stored catecholamines normally metabolized by monoamine oxidase, resulting in a hypertensive crisis (see *Phenylpropanolamine–Tranylcypromine*, p. 188).

Reserpine–Antidepressants—Monoamine oxidase inhibitors such as pargyline prevent the intraneuronal destruction of norepinephrine; the tricyclic antidepressants such as imipramine prevent the reuptake of norepinephrine into neuronal binding sites. The administration of reserpine which produces the intraneuronal release of norepinephrine from both central and peripheral sites produced marked stimulatory effects in animals pretreated with either type of antidepressant. Reserpine has been used with little success to enhance the therapeutic effects of tricyclic antidepressants (see *Imipramine–Reserpine*, p. 99).

Reserpine–Barbiturates and Anesthetics—Reserpine may enhance the CNS depressant action of most barbiturates; the required dose of barbiturate anesthetics may need to be lowered in patients treated with reserpine (see *Thiopental–Reserpine*, p. 236).

Reserpine–Halothane—Early reports indicated that patients receiving rauwolfia alkaloids had an increased risk of hypotension when general anesthetics (*e.g.,* halothane) were given concurrently. However, more current data do not substantiate the earlier reports and these drugs may be given together without interacting (see *Reserpine–Halothane*, p. 220).

Reserpine–Digitalis—Several clinical and experimental reports indicate that concurrent use of cardiac glycosides and rauwolfia alkaloids may increase the likelihood of cardiac arrhythmias. This drug interaction appears to occur in only select patients (*e.g.,* those with atrial fibrillation) (see *Digitalis–Reserpine*, p. 58).

Reserpine–Quinidine—Reserpine may enhance the antiarrhythmic and cardiodepressant effects of quinidine. However, the clinical significance of the drug interaction is not established. When these drugs are used concurrently, the dose of quinidine may need to be decreased or an alternative antiarrhythmic agent should be selected (see *Quinidine–Reserpine*, p. 219).

Alternative Therapy

Unfortunately, all therapeutic agents discussed have major side effects and certain interactions which may limit their usefulness. The orally effective diuretics appear to be the most desirable compounds; however, they also produce adverse reactions such as hypokalemia, skin rash, increased serum uric acid levels, hyperglycemia, and other toxic effects. Although one common interaction is that they enhance the action of other antihypertensive compounds, this interaction can be used to attenuate certain adverse reactions commonly seen with this group. Therefore, the concurrent use of two or more hypotensive agents appears to be justified; since the diuretics do enhance the hypotensive activity of reserpine, hydralazine, and ganglionic blockers, they may be administered concurrently with one or more of these hypotensive agents. The use of concurrent therapy may decrease the incidence of adverse effects; however, special care should be taken with patients receiving such compounds as guanethidine, methyldopa, pargyline, and reserpine to prevent interactions with other drugs, especially cocaine, epinephrine, levarterenol, and tyramine.

References

(1) H. Selye, "A Syndrome Produced by Diverse Nocuous Agents," *Nature, 138,* 32 (1936).
(2) H. Selye, "The General Adaptation Syndrome and the Diseases of Adaptation," *J. Clin. Endocrinol., 6,* 117 (1946).
(3) H. H. Smookler and J. P. Buckley, "Relationships between Brain Catecholamine Synthesis, Pituitary Adrenal Function and the Production of Hypertension during Prolonged Exposure to Environmental Stress," *Int. J. Neuropharmacol., 8,* 33 (1969).
(4) H. H. Smookler *et al.,* "Hypertensive Effects of Prolonged Auditory, Visual, and Motion Stimulation," *Fed. Proc., 32,* 2105 (1973).
(5) "Arteriosclerosis," vol. II, National Institutes of Health, Bethesda, MD 20014, June 1971, pp. 71–79.
(6) H. H. Wang *et al.,* "Mechanism of Hypertensive Action of Mebutamate," *J. Pharmacol. Exp. Ther., 151,* 285 (1966).
(7) K. D. Bock *et al.,* "Klinische und Klinisch-Experimentelle Untersuchungen mit einer neuen Blutdrucksendenden Substanz: Dichlorphenylaminoimidazolin," *Deut. Med. Wochenschr., 91,* 1761 (1966).
(8) W. Hoefke and W. Kobinger, "Pharmacologische Wirkungen des 2-(2,6-Dichlorphenylamino)-2-imidazoline Hydrochloride einer neuen, Antihypertensiven Substanz," *Arzneim.-Forsch., 16,* 1038 (1966).
(9) R. W. Sattler and P. A. Van Zwieten, "Acute Hypotensive Action of 2-(2,6-Dichlorphenylamino)-2-imidazoline Hydrochloride (St-155) after Infusion into the Cat's Vertebral Artery," *Eur. J. Pharmacol., 2,* 9 (1967).
(10) G. P. Sherman *et al.,* "Evidence for a Central Hypotensive Mechanism of 2-(2,6-Dichlorophenylamino)-2-imidazoline (Catapresan, St-155)," *Eur. J. Pharmacol., 2,* 326 (1968).
(11) H. Schmitt *et al.,* "Cardiovascular Effects of 2-(2,6-Dichlorophenylamino)-2-imidazoline Hydrochloride (St-155) II. Central Sympathetic Structures," *Eur. J. Pharmacol., 2,* 340 (1968).
(12) B. B. Brodie, "Recent Views on Mechanisms for Lowering Sympathetic Tone," *Circulation, 28,* 970 (1963).
(13) C. C. Chang *et al.,* "Interaction of Guanethidine with Adrenergic Neurons," *J. Pharmacol. Exp. Ther., 147,* 303 (1965).

(14) G. Burnstock *et al.*, "A New Method of Destroying Adrenergic Nerves in Adult Animals Using Guanethidine," *Brit. J. Pharmacol.*, *43*, 295 (1971).

(15) M. Moser, "Guanethidine and Bethanidine in the Management of Hypertension," *Amer. Heart J.*, *77*, 423 (1969).

(16) R. W. Gifford, Jr., "Bethanidine Sulfate—A New Antihypertensive Agent," *J. Amer. Med. Ass.*, *193*, 901 (1965).

(17) E. Costa *et al.*, "Structural Requirements for Bretylium and Guanethidine-Like Activity," *Life Sci.*, *3*, 75 (1962).

(18) R. Kuntzinall *et al.*, "Reserpine and Guanethidine, Action of Peripheral Stores of Catecholamines," *Life Sci.*, *1*, 65 (1962).

(19) M. D. Day and M. J. Rand, "Some Observations on the Pharmacology of α-Methyldopa," *Brit. J. Pharmacol.*, *22*, 72 (1964).

(20) M. Henning and P. A. Van Zwieten, "Central Hypotensive Effect of α-Methyldopa," *Acta Pharmacol.*, *25*, suppl. 4, 25 (1967).

(21) A. Heise and G. Kroneberg, "Central Nervous α-Adrenergic Receptors and the Mode of Action of α-Methyldopa," *Naunyn-Schmiedeberg's Arch. Pharmakol.*, *279*, 285 (1973).

(22) I. J. Kopin *et al.*, "'False Neurochemical Transmitters' and the Mechanism of Sympathetic Blockade by Monoamine Oxidase Inhibitors," *J. Pharmacol. Exp. Ther.*, *147*, 186 (1965).

(23) M. S. Ghouri and T. J. Haley, "Structure-Activity Relationships in the Adrenergic Blocking Agents," *J. Pharm. Sci.*, *58*, 511 (1969).

(24) E. Gilmore *et al.*, "Treatment of Essential Hypertension with a New Vasodilator in Combination with Beta-Adrenergic Blockade," *N. Engl. J. Med.*, *282*, 521 (1970).

(25) K. O'Malley *et al.*, "Adrenergic Mechanism of Minoxidil-Induced Increase in Plasma Renin Activity," *Clin. Res.*, *21*, 953 (1973).

(26) R. Zacest *et al.*, "Treatment of Essential Hypertension with Combined Vasodilation and Beta-Adrenergic Blockade," *N. Engl. J. Med.*, *286*, 617 (1972).

(27) T. B. Gottlieb *et al.*, "Combined Therapy with Vasodilator Drugs and Beta-Adrenergic Blockade in Hypertension. A Comparative Study of Minoxidil and Hydralazine," *Circulation*, *45*, 571 (1972).

(28) W. A. Pettinger and H. C. Mitchell, "Minoxidil—An Alternative to Nephrectomy for Refractory Hypertension," *N. Engl. J. Med.*, *289*, 167 (1973).

(29) M. Velasco *et al.*, "Differential Effects of Propranolol on Heart Rate and Plasma Renin Activity in Patients Treated with Minoxidil," *Clin. Pharmacol. Ther.*, *16*, 1031 (1974).

(30) G. J. Kelliher and J. P. Buckley, "Central Hypotensive Activity of *dl*- and *d*-Propranolol," *J. Pharm. Sci.*, *59*, 1276 (1970).

(31) R. W. Gifford, in "Hypertension: Mechanisms and Management," Grune and Stratton, New York, N.Y., 1973, p. 808.

(32) P. Preziosi *et al.*, "On the Mechanism of the Antihypertensive Effect of Hydrochlorothiazide," *Boll. Soc. Ital. Biol. Sper.*, *36*, 1581 (1960).

(33) B. E. Abreu *et al.*, "Cardiovascular, Emetic and Pharmacodynamic Properties of Certain Veratrum Alkaloids," *J. Pharmacol. Exp. Ther.*, *112*, 73 (1954).

(34) B. S. Jandhyala and J. P. Buckley, "Pharmacology and Mechanism of Action of Cryptenamine," *J. Pharm. Sci.*, *55*, 888 (1966).

(35) M. L. Jandhyala and J. P. Buckley, "Mechanisms of Action of Cryptenamine," *J. Pharm. Sci.*, *57*, 1576 (1968).

(36) R. H. Briant *et al.*, "Interaction between Clonidine and Desipramine in Man," *Brit. Med. J.*, *1*, 522 (1973).

Anti-Infective Therapy

Anti-infective agents are the most widely prescribed class of drugs in the medical armamentarium. These ubiquitous agents also comprise the most diverse class of drugs with respect to chemical structure, physicochemical properties, and mechanisms of actions.

Therapeutic Indications

Anti-infective agents are employed in the treatment of systemic, respiratory, gastrointestinal (GI), genitourinary, circulatory, ophthalmic, skeletal, soft tissue, and topical infections. These agents are also used in the prophylaxis of infection as follows (1): (a) to protect healthy individuals against invasion by specific organisms to which they have been exposed (e.g., gonococci or group-A streptococci), (b) to prevent secondary bacterial infections in acutely ill individuals (e.g., patients with upper respiratory tract viral infections), (c) to reduce the risk of infection in certain chronically ill individuals (e.g., patients with bronchial asthma, emphysema, or colitis), and (d) to inhibit the spread of an infection from a localized area or to prevent infection in patients subjected to accidental trauma (e.g., head injuries involving skull fracture, penetrating brain wounds, or lacerations) or surgical procedures (e.g., abdominal surgery or oral surgery).

Anti-infective agents have also been used in situations other than the treatment or prophylaxis of infections. Tetracycline, for example, has been used in the diagnosis of malignancies (2). Antimalarials, such as chloroquine and quinacrine, have been employed in the treatment of lupus erythematosus (3) and rheumatoid arthritis (4). Some antibiotics (e.g., bleomycin, dactinomycin, and mithramycin) have been used primarily as antineoplastic agents. Amantadine, an antiviral compound, has been suggested for use in parkinsonism (5), although its effectiveness relative to levodopa has been questioned (6).

Precautions

The following general factors must be considered when using anti-infective agents: (a) the susceptibility of the invading organism to the chemotherapeutic agent, (b) the extent of organ dysfunction or the pathological state of the patient, (c) the possibility of an allergic or hypersensitivity reaction to the drug, (d) the extent of physiological development of the patient (particularly in the case of neonates), and (e) the potential teratogenicity of the drug when administered to women of child-bearing age.

Response Variants

A given chemotherapeutic regimen may not yield the expected results even though the invading organism is susceptible to the drug because of (a) organ dysfunction and atypical pharmacokinetic parameters, and/or (b) inherited enzyme abnormalities.

Organ Dysfunction and Atypical Pharmacokinetic Parameters—If some degree of renal or hepatic dysfunction is already present, there may be a tendency toward drug accumulation if the drug is eliminated via the renal or hepatic pathway. If drug accumulation continues unabated, the incidence of adverse reactions can increase markedly. In addition, many chemotherapeutic agents are potentially nephrotic or hepatotoxic (7–10).

Nephrotoxic: Amphotericin B, bacitracin, carbarsone, cephaloridine, colistin, gentamicin, kanamycin, neomycin, nitrofurantoin, paromomycin, polymyxins, streptomycin, sulfonamides, tetracycline, vancomycin, and viomycin.

Hepatotoxic: Aminosalicylic acid, carbarsone, chloramphenicol, erythromycin esters, ethionamide, isoniazid, nitrofurantoin, novobiocin, oleandomycin esters, penicillin G, rifampin, sulfonamides, and tetracyclines.

Continued administration of such agents could lead to a further impairment of organ function.

Chemotherapeutic agents potentially capable of causing renal or hepatic dysfunction in asymptomatic individuals must be employed cautiously (7–10). Renal and hepatic function should be assessed at the outset and during therapy, using whatever tests are indicated by the circumstances. Suggested antibiotic dosage regimens for patients with varying degrees of renal function are available (9, 10).

The efficiency of drug absorption, distribution, biotransformation, and excretion in the patients also must be considered. Absorption and elimination efficiency may decline with increasing age (particularly with geriatric patients). Drug distribution depends, in part, upon the compartmentalization of the patient (degree of obesity and edematous state), vascularity, and cardiovascular function.

As no two patients are alike functionally, compartmentally, or otherwise, the ideal approach to anti-infective dosing would involve the monitoring of serum or tissue levels of the drug and altering the dosing regimen in accordance with the results. The more empirical approach would involve the adjustment of dosage in accordance with the clinical response of the patient: an increase in dosage when therapy seems ineffective and a decrease in dosage when symptoms or signs of possible toxicity are evoked.

The neonate presents a special problem in chemotherapy. Few chemotherapeutic agents have been evaluated effectively in newborn and premature infants. Summaries of pharmacokinetic studies on ampicillin, colistin, kanamycin, methicillin, neomycin, oxacillin, and streptomycin were reported (11). The administration of equivalent doses (on a body weight basis) generally yielded higher peak serum levels and markedly prolonged serum half-lives when compared with results in older children and adults. With the exception of colistin, the decline in serum half-life correlated best with maturation of renal function. The postnatal age of the premature and newborn infant becomes the most important determinant in drug dosage, since renal function appears to change to a great extent during the first 2 weeks of postnatal life (11).

Other problems encountered in neonatal drug therapy reflect deficiencies in microsomal enzymes (12). The use of chloramphenicol in infants has occasionally resulted in toxicity or death even though the doses employed were considered safe and were well tolerated by older patients. The half-life of chloramphenicol in neonates is 26 hr, whereas in children 4–5 years of age the half-life is only 4 hr (13). Elimination of chloramphenicol as the glucuronide is impaired by the low activity of the glucuronide-conjugating system in the neonate. Underdeveloped renal function and bilirubin displacement from protein binding sites may also account for the poor elimination of the antibiotic and its toxicity, respectively.

Inherited Enzyme Abnormalities—The presence or absence of specific enzymes may alter the sensitivity of the patient to a given chemotherapeutic agent. Heightened sensitivity to primaquine and other 8-aminoquinolines, nitrofurantoin, sulfonamides, and sulfoxones has been reported in individuals having a glucose-6-phosphate dehydrogenase defect (14, 15). Relatively high incidences of glucose-6-phosphate dehydrogenase deficiency or defects are found in individuals of Mediterranean or African descent (15) (*e.g.,* the reported incidence in American blacks is 13%). Glucose-6-phosphate dehydrogenase activity should be determined prior to the use of the previously mentioned chemotherapeutic agents.

Isoniazid biotransformation and inactivation, *via* acetylation, are known to be affected genetically (14). Although approximately 50% of Americans can be classified as "rapid" inactivators, 90% of persons of Japanese descent can be so classified (16). The degree and rapidity of acetylation are important because isoniazid-induced peripheral neuritis is more commonly encountered in patients who are slow acetylators than in those who are fast acetylators. Isoniazid also is more effective in slow acetylators than in rapid acetylators. Serum level monitoring of isoniazid, at least in the initial stage of drug administration, is recommended to avoid adverse effects or therapeutic failure.

Dapsone, a sulfoxone used in the treatment of leprosy, is also subject to polymorphic acetylation in humans (17). However, the genetic significance of this has yet to be firmly established.

Interactions

Anti-infective agents currently used often differ markedly from one another structurally, pharmacodynamically, and pharmacokinetically.

Alcohol—A mild "disulfiram-like" reaction has been reported in patients taking furazolidone (18) and possibly metronidazole (see *Metronidazole–Alcohol,* p. 158). Furazolidone may affect alcohol intolerance either by virtue of its monoamine oxidase inhibition or by inhibition of alcohol dehydrogenase. Metronidazole may produce its effects by inhibition of alcohol-metabolizing enzymes. However, the precise mechanism of these potential interactions is not clear. The practitioner should be aware of the possibility of alcohol intolerance and should advise the patient to be cautious with respect to alcohol intake (frequency and amount).

Analgesics—Aspirin and other salicylates may displace acidic anti-infective agents (*e.g.,* aminosalicylic acid, penicillins, and sulfonamides) from their protein binding sites. The salicylates may also compete with some antibiotics (*e.g.,* penicillin) for renal excretion pathways. The result of this interaction would be the enhancement of anti-infective agent activity due to the increased serum level of the unbound form of the drug. The clinical significance of this interaction has not been established (see *Penicillin–Aspirin*, p. 166).

Anesthetics—Methoxyflurane anesthesia is occasionally accompanied by renal abnormalities (19). Clinical reports (20, 21) clearly document the occurrence of prolonged, acute renal failure following methoxyflurane anesthesia. Tetracycline administration was correlated with renal dysfunction induced by methoxyflurane (22). However, the association between tetracyclines and renal dysfunction is unclear, although data are available that show progressive azotemia in patients given tetracycline (23, 24). The tetracycline effect in humans is essentially prerenal and other antibiotics with an antianabolic mechanism would produce the same effect (see *Tetracycline–Methoxyflurane*, p. 234).

Rifampin may augment the hepatotoxicity of halothane (25), but this drug interaction is not well documented.

Aminoglycoside antibiotics (*e.g.,* kanamycin, neomycin, and streptomycin) produce neuromuscular blockade that may enhance the same effect produced by general inhalation anesthetics. The result is additive respiratory arrest or prolonged neuromuscular blockade (see *Ether–Neomycin*, p. 70).

Anticholinergics—Patients to whom high doses of anticholinergic drugs such as benztropine or trihexyphenidyl are given may require a smaller dose of the anticholinergic if treatment with amantadine is begun. Concurrent administration of amantadine and anticholinergics has resulted in the occurrence of anticholinergic side effects (*e.g.,* mental confusion and hallucinations) (26).

Anticoagulants (Oral)—Nalidixic acid displaces warfarin from albumin *in vitro* (27); highly protein-bound sulfonamides also may displace coumarin anticoagulants from their binding sites (28). Anticoagulant intensification also results from an interference with vitamin K synthesis by gut flora. Chloramphenicol, kanamycin, neomycin, streptomycin, sulfonamides, and tetracyclines may prolong prothrombin time, in part, by this mechanism (29) (see *Warfarin–Tetracycline*, p. 299). It has not been established whether or not these anti-infectives significantly influence anticoagulant activity.

Anticoagulant enhancement also may result from an inhibition of the hepatic microsomal enzymes responsible for the biotransformation of the anticoagulant. A marked increase in the half-life of dicumarol was reported following chloramphenicol administration over approximately 5–8 days (half-life for dicumarol increased by about two-to fourfold) (30).

The possibility of enhanced anticoagulant effect should not be regarded lightly, although problems such as those arising from interference with gut flora vitamin K synthesis may only gain significance when the dietary intake of vitamin K is severely restricted and the patient is receiving high doses. Prothrombin times should be monitored closely and the anticoagulant dosage should be adjusted, if necessary, in accordance with test results.

A decrease in the hypoprothrombinemic effect of warfarin was reported (31) with the addition of griseofulvin to the drug regimen. Enzyme induction by griseofulvin has been suggested as the cause of the decreased anticoagulant effect. Again, the prudent approach to this problem would involve the close monitoring of prothrombin times and the adjustment of anticoagulant dosage in accordance with test results (see *Warfarin–Griseofulvin*, p. 285).

Rifampin may increase warfarin elimination and cause a decrease in warfarin's hypoprothrombinemic activity (32). Until more clinical data are available, caution should be exercised when these drugs are used concurrently.

Anticonvulsants—Chloramphenicol was shown to retard significantly the biotransformation of phenytoin (diphenylhydantoin) in humans (30). As much as a two- to threefold increase in half-life may be observed, thus necessitating a reduction in the anticonvulsant dosage. Similarly, the addition of isoniazid to the drug regimen of patients taking phenytoin has resulted in toxicity due to increased serum levels and retarded biotransformation of the anticonvulsant (see *Phenytoin–Isoniazid*, p. 202).

Several sulfonamides have been shown to inhibit hepatic metabolism of phenytoin (33). Phenytoin stimulated the metabolism of doxycycline and caused a significant decrease in the half-life (34). However, no clinical manifestations of either drug interaction have been reported.

Anti-Inflammatory Agents—Acidic, protein-bound anti-inflammatory agents (*e.g.,* indomethacin, phenylbutazone, and salicylates) may displace or be displaced by acidic, protein-bound anti-infective agents (*e.g.,* aminosalicylic acid, nalidixic acid, penicillins, and sulfonamides). The result of the displacement would be an enhancement of activity of the displaced drug. There is a potential for increased toxicity, although it would be difficult to predict which of two drugs would be more readily displaced from its protein binding sites without some knowledge of the relative affinity of the drugs for plasma protein and their relative concentrations.

Antineoplastics—Methotrexate toxicity may be increased by the concurrent administration of sulfonamides as a result of an increase in the fraction of unbound methotrexate in the serum. Sulfonamides should be used with caution in patients receiving methotrexate (see *Methotrexate–Sulfisoxizole*, p. 156).

Corticosteroids—Rifampin induced the metabolism of corticosteroids and necessitated an increase in dosage of the corticosteroids (35).

Diuretics—The effectiveness of the anti-infective agents such as methenamine in urinary tract infections is diminished when urine pH rises above 5.5 (36). Diuretics, such as acetazolamide and the thiazides, can alkalinize the urine and thus theoretically would limit the usefulness of methenamine as well as its mandelate and hippurate salts as urinary tract anti-infective agents. Anti-infectives whose activity in the urine is not as markedly pH dependent (*e.g.*, nalidixic acid or nitrofurantoin) may be more appropriate than methenamine or its salts in this instance.

Administration of diuretics (*e.g.*, ethacrynic acid or furosemide) occasionally is accompanied by ototoxicity, particularly when the parenteral route has been employed. Concurrent administration of agents such as the aminoglycoside antibiotics (*e.g.*, amikacin, gentamicin, kanamycin, neomycin, paromomycin, and streptomycin) that have been associated with cochlear damage should be used with caution (see *Kanamycin–Ethacrynic Acid*, p. 120).

Furosemide may enhance the nephrotoxicity of cephalosporins (37). Renal function should be monitored closely when these agents are used concurrently.

Hematinics and Vitamins—Simultaneous administration of iron preparations and tetracyclines may lead to subtherapeutic serum tetracycline levels and should, therefore, be avoided. Oral administration of iron preparations should preferably follow tetracycline administration by at least 2–3 hr to allow gastric emptying and maximum intestinal absorption of the tetracycline to occur unimpeded (see *Tetracycline–Ferrous Sulfate*, p. 231).

Chloramphenicol will impair the hematological response to vitamin B_{12}, folates, and iron (38, 39). Alternative antibiotics should be selected in anemic patients receiving any of these products.

Although there is some evidence that pyridoxine may interfere with the activity of isoniazid, concurrent administration of these drugs does not alter the clinical effect of isoniazid (see *Isoniazid–Pyridoxine*, p. 118).

Hypoglycemics—The addition of chloramphenicol to a tolbutamide regimen was reported to result in the doubling of serum tolbutamide levels and, ultimately, in the prolongation of the tolbutamide half-life. The case of a patient treated with chloramphenicol who subsequently received tolbutamide also was described. A hypoglycemic coma ensued within a few days. Measurement of serum tolbutamide levels yielded an apparent half-life of 10 hr compared with a value of 4 hr previously noted in the same patient in the absence of chloramphenicol. Concurrent use of oral hypoglycemics and chloramphenicol may necessitate the lowering of the hypoglycemic dosage (see *Tolbutamide–Chloramphenicol*, p. 243).

Hypoglycemia has also been induced following the addition of sulfaphenazole to a tolbutamide regimen. Other reports appeared in which hypoglycemia was apparently induced by sulfisoxazole. Whether hypoglycemia is the result of displacement of the sulfonylurea hypoglycemic agent from its protein binding site by the sulfonamide or the result of enzyme inhibition (*e.g.*, the inhibition of tolbutamide carboxylation) is not certain at this point. The concurrent administration of sulfonylurea hypoglycemics and sulfonamide anti-infectives may result in hypoglycemia. A reduction in hypoglycemic dosage should be considered just prior to sulfonamide administration (see *Tolbutamide–Sulfaphenazole*, p. 250).

Muscle Relaxants—The aminoglycoside antibiotics (*e.g.*, gentamicin, neomycin, and streptomycin) act on the neuromuscular junctions as weak nondepolarizing agents, *i.e.*, they have a curare-like effect (see *Tubocurarine–Neomycin*, p. 254). Neuromuscular blockade with respiratory depression has occurred in patients given aminoglycoside antibiotics who were anesthetized with ether (see *Ether–Neomycin*, p. 70). The polymyxin antibiotics (*e.g.*, colistin and polymyxin B), bacitracin, and amphotericin B also can produce a neuromuscular blockade, although not necessarily by the same mechanism. All of these antibiotics should be used with extreme caution during or after surgery as the possibility of respiratory depression or myasthenia is not remote.

Oral Contraceptives—Rifampin has been reported to decrease the effect of oral contraceptives by enzyme induction (40). However, no decreased effectiveness of oral contraceptives has been attributed to this drug interaction.

Sedative–Hypnotics—Concurrent or recent administration of phenobarbital may result in lower serum levels of orally administered griseofulvin and, consequently, in ineffectiveness of the antifungal agent. Although the lower serum griseofulvin levels were initially ascribed to enzyme induction by phenobarbital, other data indicate that the mechanism may be interference by phenobarbital with griseofulvin absorption. Clinically, the removal of phenobarbital from the patient's drug regimen or an increase in griseofulvin dosage may be necessary to achieve control of the fungal infection (see *Griseofulvin–Phenobarbital*, p. 77).

Enzyme induction by the barbiturates has enhanced the metabolism of chloramphenicol (41) and doxycycline (42). The clinical outcome of this inhibition has not been determined.

Uricosurics—Probenecid and sulfinpyrazone compete with uric acid at renal tubule transport sites (43). Urinary excretion of other weak acids also can be affected by these uricosuric agents. Thus, aminosalicylic acid, cephalosporins, dapsone, nitrofurantoin, penicillins, and sulfonamides may be affected by concurrent use of probenecid or sulfinpyrazone. Diminished tubular secretion of these weak acids could result in higher and more sustained serum levels and, hence, an intensification of drug activity. Anti-infectives employed for lower urinary tract infections (*e.g.*, nitrofurantoin) may be less effective due to diminished urinary excretion of the drug in the presence of a uricosuric agent (see *Penicillin–Probenecid*, p. 175, and *Nitrofurantoin–Probenecid*, p. 159).

Sulfinpyrazone may displace sulfonamides from plasma protein binding sites (44), resulting in higher serum levels of unbound sulfonamide. This effect may necessitate a reduction in sulfonamide dosage.

One study suggested that probenecid interferes with hepatic uptake of rifampin resulting in increased serum levels of the anti-infective (45). This drug interaction could be judiciously used to diminish the need for large doses of rifampin. Unrecognized, it could lead to an increased incidence of adverse reactions due to rifampin.

Ethambutol has been shown to elevate serum urate levels in humans (46). Ethambutol administration may exacerbate an already existing gouty condition or hasten its development. The uricosuric dosage may have to be increased to maintain control.

Induction of Malabsorption—A transitory and reversible state of malabsorption may result from the oral administration of the aminoglycoside antibiotics (*e.g.,* kanamycin and neomycin) (47). This effect could result in diminished GI absorption and compromised therapeutic efficacy of other drugs, as has been indicated in the case of penicillin when given concurrently with neomycin (48). The practitioner should be alert for any indication of therapeutic failure. It may be necessary to revert to a nonenteral route, although normal absorption is usually evident within a few days after aminoglycoside administration ends (48).

Aminosalicylic acid may cause a mild malabsorption syndrome in some patients. Aminosalicylic acid reportedly can impair the absorption of rifampin (49) and vitamin B_{12} (50).

The use of antidiarrheal mixtures or antacids containing finely divided solids (*e.g.,* aluminum hydroxide, attapulgite, kaolin, and magnesium hydroxide) can markedly affect the GI absorption of anti-infectives (*e.g.,* clindamycin, isoniazid, lincomycin, and tetracyclines). Antidiarrheal or antacid preparations with adsorbing or binding capacity should not be administered along with the chemotherapeutic agent but rather 2–3 hr before or after the anti-infective. If this is impractical, it may be necessary to employ a different chemotherapeutic agent—one less affected by concurrent administration with the antidiarrheal or antacid product (see *Isoniazid–Aluminum Hydroxide*, p. 116; *Lincomycin–Kaolin*, p. 135; and *Tetracycline–Aluminum, Calcium, and Magnesium Ions*, p. 227). Sodium bicarbonate administration decreases significantly the extent of absorption of tetracycline in human subjects (51). The results were indicative of decreased tetracycline dissolution and suggested the avoidance of concurrent administration of any preparation that could raise intragastric pH.

References

(1) "The Pharmacological Basis of Therapeutics," 5th ed., L. S. Goodman and A. Gilman, Eds., Macmillan, New York, NY 10022, 1975, pp. 1157–1158.

(2) L. J. Sandlow and H. T. Necheles, "Tetracycline Fluorescence and Cytological Procedures Compared for the Detection of Malignancy," *J. Brit. Soc. Gastroenterol., 7,* 640 (1966).

(3) "AMA Drug Evaluations," 2nd ed., American Medical Association, Chicago, Ill., 1973, pp. 581–589.

(4) "Principles of Internal Medicine," vol. 2, 5th ed., T. R. Harrison *et al.,* Eds., Blakiston, New York, N.Y., 1966, p. 1355.

(5) "Parkinson's Disease and Amantadine Hydrochloride," *J. Amer. Med. Ass., 208,* 1180 (1969).

(6) K. R. Hunter *et al.,* "Combined Treatment of Parkinsonism with L-Dopa and Amantadine," *Lancet, ii,* 566 (1970).

(7) L. P. Garrod and F. O'Grady, "Antibiotic and Chemotherapy," E. & S. Livingstone, Edinburgh, Scotland, 1971, pp. 276–279.

(8) H. Smith, "Antibiotics in Clinical Practice," Pitman, London, England, 1970, pp. 283–291.

(9) C. M. Kunin, "A Guide to Use of Antibiotics in Patients with Renal Disease. A Table of Recommended Doses and Factors Governing Serum Levels," *Ann. Intern. Med., 67,* 151 (1967).

(10) R. J. Bulger and R. G. Petersdorf, "Antimicrobial Therapy in Patients with Renal Insufficiency," *Postgrad. Med., 47,* 160 (1970).

(11) S. J. Yaffe and H. J. Simon, in "The Control of Chemotherapy," P. J. Watt, Ed., E. & S. Livingstone, Edinburgh, Scotland, 1970, pp. 37–48.

(12) A. H. Conney, "Drug Metabolism and Therapeutics," *N. Engl. J. Med., 280,* 653 (1969).

(13) C. F. Weiss *et al.,* "Chloramphenicol in the Newborn Infant: A Physiologic Explanation of Its Toxicity when Given in Excessive Doses," *N. Engl. J. Med., 262,* 787 (1960).

(14) I. H. Porter, "Genetic Basis of Drug Metabolism in Man," *Toxicol. Appl. Pharmacol., 6,* 499 (1964).

(15) P. A. Marks and J. Banks, "Drug-Induced Hemolytic Anemias Associated with Glucose-6-phosphate Dehydrogenase Deficiency: A Genetically Heterogeneous Trait," *Ann. N.Y. Acad. Sci., 123,* 198 (1965).

(16) H. W. Harris *et al.,* "Comparison of Isoniazid Concentrations in the Blood of People of Japanese and European Descent," *Amer. Rev. Tuberc., 78,* 944 (1958).

(17) R. Gelber *et al.,* "The Polymorphic Acetylation of Dapsone in Man," *Clin. Pharmacol. Ther., 12,* 225 (1971).

(18) W. J. Parker, "Clinically Significant Alcohol-Drug Interactions," *J. Amer. Pharm. Ass., NS10,* 664 (1970).

(19) Committee on Anesthesia, National Academy of Sciences–National Research Council, "Statement Regarding the Role of Methoxyflurane in the Production of Renal Dysfunction," *Anesthesiology, 34,* 505 (1971).

(20) J. A. Frascino *et al.,* "Renal Oxalosis and Azotemia after Methoxyflurane Anesthesia," *N. Engl. J. Med., 283,* 676 (1970).

(21) N. K. Hollenberg *et al.,* "Irreversible Acute Oliguric Renal Failure, A Complication of Methoxyflurane Anesthesia," *N. Engl. J. Med., 286,* 877 (1972).

(22) E. Y. Kuzucu, "Methoxyflurane, Tetracycline, and Renal Failure," *J. Amer. Med. Ass., 211,* 1162 (1970).

(23) J. C. Bateman *et al.,* "Fatal Complications of Intensive Antibiotic Therapy in Patients with Neoplastic Disease," *Arch. Intern. Med., 101,* 476 (1958).

(24) R. B. Stott *et al.,* "Tetracyclines and Impaired Renal Function," *Lancet, ii,* 1378 (1971).

(25) J. A. Most and G. B. Markle, "A Nearly Fatal Hepatotoxic Reaction to Rifampin after Halothane Anesthesia," *Amer. J. Surg., 127,* 593 (1974).

(26) R. S. Schwab *et al.,* "Amantadine in the Treatment of Parkinson's Disease," *J. Amer. Med. Ass., 208,* 1168 (1969).

(27) E. M. Sellers and J. Koch-Weser, "Displacement of Warfarin from Human Albumin by Diazoxide and Ethacrynic, Mefenamic, and Nalidixic Acids," *Clin. Pharmacol. Ther., 11,* 524 (1970).

(28) D. Deykin, "Warfarin Therapy. II," *N. Engl. J. Med., 283,* 801 (1970).

(29) D. Bernstein, "Drugs Known to Interact with Coumarin-Type Anticoagulants—Revised," *Drug Intel., 8,* 172 (1974).

(30) L. K. Christensen and L. Skovsted, "Inhibition of Drug Metabolism by Chloramphenicol," *Lancet, ii,* 1397 (1969).

(31) S. I. Cullen and P. M. Catalano, "Griseofulvin-Warfarin Antagonism," *J. Amer. Med. Ass., 199,* 582 (1967).

(32) R. A. O'Reilly, "Interaction of Sodium Warfarin and Rifampin. Studies in Man," *Ann. Intern. Med., 81,* 337 (1974).

(33) K. Siersbaek-Nielsen *et al.,* "Sulfamethizole-Induced Inhibition of Diphenylhydantoin and Tolbutamide Metabolism in Man," *Clin. Pharmacol. Ther., 14,* 148 (1973).

(34) O. Penttila *et al.,* "Interaction between Doxycycline and Some Antiepileptic Drugs," *Brit. Med. J., 2,* 470 (1974).

(35) O. M. Edwards *et al.,* "Changes in Cortisol Metabolism following Rifampicin Therapy," *Lancet, ii,* 549 (1974).

(36) V. Knight *et al.,* "Methenamine Mandelate: Antimicrobial Activity, Absorption, and Excretion," *Antibiot. Chemother., 2,* 615 (1952).

(37) M. G. Dodds and R. D. Foord, "Enhancement by Potent Diuretics of Renal Tubular Necrosis Induced by Cephaloridine," *Brit. J. Pharmacol., 40,* 227 (1970).

(38) P. Saidi *et al.,* "Effect of Chloramphenicol on Erythropoiesis," *J. Lab. Clin. Med., 57,* 247 (1961).

(39) R. M. JiJi *et al.,* "Chloramphenicol and Its Sulfamoyl Analogue. Report of Reversible Erythropoietic Toxicity in Healthy Volunteers," *Arch. Intern. Med., 111,* 70 (1963).

(40) H. M. Bolt *et al.,* "Rifampicin and Oral Contraception," *Lancet, i,* 1280 (1974).

(41) D. L. Palmer *et al.,* "Induction of Chloramphenicol Metabolism by Phenobarbital," *Antimicrob. Ag. Chemother., 1,* 112 (1972).

(42) P. J. Neuvonen and O. Penttila, "Interaction between Doxycycline and Barbiturates," *Brit. Med. J., 1,* 535 (1974).

(43) I. M. Weiner and G. H. Mudge, "Renal Tubular Mechanisms for Excretion of Organic Acids and Bases," *Amer. J. Med., 36,* 743 (1964).

(44) A. H. Anton, "The Effect of Disease, Drugs, and Dilution on the Binding of Sulfonamides in Human Plasma," *Clin. Pharmacol. Ther., 9,* 561 (1968).

(45) S. Kenwright and A. J. Levi, "Impairment of Hepatic Uptake of Rifamycin Antibiotics by Probenecid, and Its Therapeutic Implications," *Lancet, ii,* 1401 (1973).

(46) A. E. Postlethwaite *et al.,* "Hyperuricemia Due to Ethambutol," *N. Engl. J. Med., 286,* 761 (1972).

(47) W. W. Faloon *et al.,* "Effect of Neomycin and Kanamycin upon Intestinal Absorption," *Ann. N.Y. Acad. Sci., 132,* 879 (1966).

(48) S. H. Cheng and A. White, "Effect of Orally Administered Neomycin on the Absorption of Penicillin V," *N. Engl. J. Med., 267,* 1296 (1962).

(49) G. Boman *et al.,* "Drug Interaction: Decreased Serum Concentrations of Rifampicin when Given with P.A.S.," letter to the editor, *Lancet, i,* 800 (1971).

(50) O. Heinevaara and I. P. Palva, "Malabsorption of Vitamin B_{12} during Treatment with Para Aminosalicylic Acid: A Preliminary Report," *Acta Med. Scand., 175,* 469 (1964).

(51) W. H. Barr *et al.,* "Decrease of Tetracycline Absorption in Man by Sodium Bicarbonate," *Clin. Pharmacol. Ther., 12,* 779 (1971).

Antineoplastic Therapy *

The present armamentarium of chemotherapeutic agents includes diverse families of compounds, which are classified as follows: (*a*) antimetabolites, including folic acid antagonists, purine analogs, pyrimidine analogs, and glutamine antagonists; (*b*) polyfunctional alkylating agents; (*c*) antibiotics; (*d*) natural products; (*e*) hormones; (*f*) radioactive isotopes; and (*g*) miscellaneous compounds. It is well documented that concurrent therapy with these compounds yields a benefit greater than the single entity. The beneficial effect of concurrent therapy is no doubt the result of many factors. Most successful antineoplastic drug regimens have been discovered through clinical trials based on cytotoxic principles.

Methotrexate

Indications—Methotrexate is indicated for treating women with trophoblastic tumors (choriocarcinoma, chorioadenoma destruens, and hydatiform mole), acute and subacute leukemias and leukemic meningitis (especially in children), and acute lymphoblastic leukemia (1). It has been used for lymphosarcoma (1) and mycosis fungoides (2) and for carefully selected patients for the symptomatic control of severe, recalcitrant, disabling psoriasis which is not adequately responsive to other forms of therapy (3, 4). Methotrexate has also been used in the treatment of other nonmalignant diseases such as chronic refractory ocular disease (*i.e.*, cyclitis, refractory uveitis, sympathetic ophthalmia syndrome, and pseudotumor of the eye) (5), Wegener's granulomatosis (6), psoriatic arthritis (5), dermatomyositis (7), and Reiter's syndrome (8, 9).

Contraindications—Methotrexate is contraindicated (1) in the presence of existing liver, bone marrow, or renal damage, particularly the latter because methotrexate is excreted by the kidney. In patients with renal insufficiency, methotrexate may produce functional and morphological changes in the kidney. It has been reported to act as an abortifacient and should not be administered during the first trimester of pregnancy.

Mechanism of Action—The mechanism of action of methotrexate in causing cellular injury must be viewed in relation to the normal biological function of folic acid. Ingested folic acid, although it is an essential

vitamin, is an inactive compound in mammalian tissue. To exert its biological effect, it must be converted by enzymatic reduction to tetrahydrofolic acid. The enzyme dihydrofolate reductase acts as the catalyst for this reaction. Once folic acid is reduced to the active coenzyme tetrahydrofolic acid, it acts as an acceptor of various one-carbon units to form a series of folate coenzymes. These folate coenzymes are then active in the transfer of one-carbon units to the essential reactions in the synthesis of nucleic acids and other materials.

Methotrexate exerts its activity by binding to dihydrofolate reductase and inhibiting the formation of tetrahydrofolic acid. When methotrexate toxicity occurs, it may be reduced if leucovorin is administered within 6 hr after the administration of methotrexate (see *Methotrexate–Leucovorin*, p. 154).

Metabolism—Methotrexate is rapidly absorbed from the gastrointestinal tract when administered in small doses (0.1 mg/kg) but not when large doses (10 mg/kg) are administered. Stool excretion was 39% with the large oral dose *versus* 7–9% following the small oral dose. Intravenous administration of doses of 0.1, 0.3, 1, 5, and 10 mg/kg yielded total recoveries of 67–101%, with 2–5% of this being recovered in the stool (10). About 50% of the drug is bound to plasma proteins (1, 10), although there is a report of protein binding as high as 69% (11). It is not significantly degraded in the body and is excreted mainly by the kidney (12) *via* glomerular filtration and active transport (12). The rate of excretion varies, with 40–50% of a small dose (2.5–15 mg/kg) to about 90% of a large dose (150 mg/kg) excreted unchanged within 48 hr, mostly in the first 8 hr (2). The drug not excreted during this time may remain bound to protein or dihydrofolate reductase for months.

Interactions—Because methotrexate binds to plasma proteins, it can be displaced from its binding sites and made available to react with dihydrofolate reductase. Those compounds that have been reported to displace methotrexate include aminobenzoic acid (13), chloramphenicol (14), phenytoin (diphenylhydantoin) (14), salicylates (see *Methotrexate–Aspirin*, p. 150), sulfonamides (see *Methotrexate–Sulfisoxazole*, p. 156), and tetracyclines (14). The clinical significance of this displacement is not established. Caution is necessary when these agents are administered concurrently with methotrexate.

---

* This discussion covers methotrexate and mercaptopurine.

Administration of methotrexate also impairs the immunological response. Smallpox vaccinations can result in generalized vaccinia in patients receiving methotrexate (15).

Cytarabine enhances the cell-kill effects of methotrexate when administered 48 hr before the initiation of methotrexate therapy. Methotrexate enhances the cell-kill effects of cytarabine when administered at least 30 min before initiation of cytarabine therapy. However, the clinical data to support these observations are inconclusive (see *Methotrexate–Cytarabine*, p. 151).

Mercaptopurine

Indications—Mercaptopurine is useful in the treatment of acute leukemia and chronic myelocytic leukemia (16). The use of mercaptopurine was suggested (5) for the following nonmalignant diseases: rheumatoid arthritis, systemic lupus erythematosus, lupus nephritis, steroid-resistant nephrotic syndrome, dermatomyositis, uveitis, active chronic hepatitis, lupoid hepatitis, plasma cell hepatitis, psoriatic arthritis, polyradiculoneuropathy (Guillain–Barre syndrome), autoimmune hemolytic anemia, and idiopathic thrombocytopenic purpura.

Contraindications—Mercaptopurine is contraindicated in patients with evidence of toxic hepatitis or biliary stasis (6).

Mechanism of Action—Like methotrexate, the mechanism of action of mercaptopurine (a purine antagonist) must be viewed in light of the normal metabolic pathways of other purines. Purines (*e.g.*, hypoxanthine and adenine) or their derivatives formed during biotransformation to nucleotides are essential to the production of RNA, various coenzymes, and ultimately, DNA.

Mercaptopurine is a sulfur-containing analog of hypoxanthine and adenine. Mercaptopurine, after its conversion to the active compound mercaptopurine ribonucleotide by the reaction of mercaptopurine with 5-phosphoribosyl-1-pyrophosphate (17), is capable of inhibiting the utilization of hypoxanthine and adenine.

Metabolism—Mercaptopurine is readily absorbed after oral administration, and about half of the dose is excreted within 24 hr. The degradation of mercaptopurine is known to follow two pathways: (*a*) enzymatic oxidation, catalyzed by xanthine oxidase, to 6-thiouric acid, and (*b*) methylation of the sulfhydryl group, followed by oxidation of the methylated derivatives and desulfuration to remove the sulfur as inorganic sulfate.

Interactions—Animal and human studies have confirmed that allopurinol inhibits the enzymatic oxidation of mercaptopurine at normal doses of both drugs within 24 hr. The interaction is clinically significant and requires an immediate · reduction in the dosage of mercaptopurine (see *Mercaptopurine–Allopurinol*, p. 148).

References

(1) "The Pharmacological Basis of Therapeutics," 5th ed., L. S. Goodman and A. Gilman, Eds., Macmillan, New York, NY 10022, 1975, pp. 1268–1273.

(2) J. C. Wright *et al.*, "Observations on the Use of Cancer Chemotherapeutic Agents in Patients with Mycosis Fungoides," *Cancer, 17*, 1045 (1964).

(3) "Psoriasis, Methotrexate and Cirrhosis," editorial, *J. Amer. Med. Ass., 212*, 314 (1970).

(4) "Methotrexate in the Treatment of Psoriasis," *Med. Lett., 14*, 41 (1972).

(5) A. D. Steinberg *et al.*, "Cytotoxic Drugs in Treatment of Nonmalignant Disease," *Ann. Intern. Med., 76*, 619 (1972).

(6) R. L. Capizzi and J. R. Bertino, "Methotrexate Therapy of Wegener's Granulomatosis," *Ann. Intern. Med., 74*, 74 (1971).

(7) A. N. Malaviya *et al.*, "Treatment of Dermatomyositis with Methotrexate," *Lancet, ii*, 485 (1968).

(8) G. A. Farber *et al.*, "Reiter's Syndrome. Treatment with Methotrexate," *J. Amer. Med. Ass., 200*, 171 (1967).

(9) R. L. Jetton and W. C. Duncan, "Treatment of Reiter's Syndrome with Methotrexate," *Ann. Intern. Med., 70*, 349 (1969).

(10) E. S. Henderson *et al.*, "The Metabolic Fate of Tritiated Methotrexate II. Absorption and Excretion in Man," *Cancer Res., 25*, 1018 (1965).

(11) D. G. Liegler *et al.*, "Renal Clearance and *In Vivo* Protein Binding of Methotrexate in Man and Changes Associated with Salicylate Administration," *Proc. Amer. Ass. Cancer Res., 8*, 41 (1967).

(12) D. G. Liegler *et al.*, "The Effect of Organic Acids on Renal Clearance of Methotrexate in Man," *Clin. Pharmacol. Ther., 10*, 849 (1969).

(13) R. L. Dixon *et al.*, "Plasma Protein Binding of Methotrexate and Its Displacement by Various Drugs," *Fed. Proc., 24*, 454 (1965).

(14) "Methotrexate: Antimetabolic Agent for Cancer Chemotherapy," Lederle Laboratories, Pearl River, N.Y., February 1971.

(15) J. Allison, "Methotrexate and Smallpox Vaccination," letter to the editor, *Lancet, ii*, 1250 (1968).

(16) "The Pharmacological Basis of Therapeutics," 5th ed., L. S. Goodman and A. Gilman, Eds., Macmillan, New York, NY 10022, 1975, pp. 1279–1280.

(17) R. W. Rundles *et al.*, "Effects of a Xanthine Oxidase Inhibitor on Thiopurine Metabolism, Hyperuricemia and Gout," *Trans. Ass. Amer. Physicians, 76*, 126 (1963).

Antipsychotic Therapy

The almost simultaneous introduction of chlorpromazine in France and reserpine in the United States led to a complete remodeling of psychiatric treatment; however, reserpine is no longer used for such purposes. By conservative estimate, at least 50 million patients have been treated with phenothiazines, butyrophenones, and thioxanthenes. Concomitant with the introduction of antipsychotic drugs, the number of resident patients in mental hospitals has been reduced by almost 50% in the past 15 years, in spite of the doubling of admissions. Without question, the development of the psychotropic agents has contributed considerably to this dramatic decrease.

Because of the large number of patients treated, concurrent use of an antipsychotic agent with a large number of other pharmaceuticals has likely occurred. In a patient receiving a particular drug or several drugs concurrently when some new symptom or syndrome appears, it is only natural to question the contribution of such agents.

Drugs in the "antipsychotic" class can and should be used in two different ways. The drug treatment of schizophrenia is analogous to the drug treatment of cardiac failure, *i.e.,* when the decision to "digitalize" has been made, a full course of treatment should be followed even though symptoms remit early. Although opinions differ, a 3-month period of antipsychotic drug therapy should constitute the minimum time before reduced doses or the withdrawal of medication is attempted. There is a strong body of opinion that favors maintaining schizophrenic patients on this type of drug indefinitely, since it is known that the relapse percentage is only one-fourth that of patients who discontinue treatment.

A second use of these drugs is in the treatment of the manic patient and of the patient with anxiety, agitation, hyperirritability, and excitement. In these patients, the dose should be titrated against the degree of disturbance and discontinued when there is no longer symptomatic indication for such usage. Anxiolytic agents and sedatives are preferred for short-term use because they work more rapidly and have fewer side effects than the antipsychotic agents. However, these drugs (*e.g.,* chlordiazepoxide and meprobamate) possess the disadvantages that tolerance sometimes develops and a continually increasing dose may be required. Dependence also may develop.

Other uses for the antipsychotic agents related to the psychiatric field are for porphyria, anorexia nervosa, chorea, tetanus, and amphetamine and lysergide (LSD) intoxication (1). However, the potential for extrapyramidal side effects or possibly irreversible disorders of the basal ganglia such as tardive dyskinesia detracts from the usefulness of these agents in these disorders.

Extrapyramidal symptoms often occur, especially the akathisia manifested by restlessness and tension. Failure to recognize this side effect and other parkinsonian-like manifestations is probably the most common error associated with this treatment. These side effects often respond well to antiparkinsonian medication. However, a reduction of the antipsychotic dosage also may be necessary. Continued use of the neuroleptic can often be accompanied by cessation of the antiparkinsonian drug after 3–6 months (see *Chlorpromazine–Benztropine,* p. 30).

When an antipsychotic drug is used as a sedative or anxiolytic agent, the dosage should be titrated against the intensity of the symptoms. When used as an antipsychotic agent (at a dose level roughly 5–10 times as great as that for anxiety), a prescribed course of medication should be followed with little regard to severity of symptoms once the decision to treat has been made.

Butyrophenones and Thioxanthenes, Phenothiazines, and Rauwolfia Alkaloids

Therapeutic Indications—A comparison of studies indicates that, except for promazine and mepazine, all antipsychotic drugs commercially available have equal efficacy in the treatment of psychoses. One drug is not particularly advantageous over the others. Most studies on comparative antipsychotic drug efficacy used chlorpromazine as the standard rather than comparing the drugs with each other.

Butyrophenones and Thioxanthenes—The butyrophenones and the thioxanthenes are generally less sedative than the phenothiazines. Haloperidol is often advocated for agitated patients and those with paranoid ideation. Extrapyramidal symptoms are said to occur even more frequently than with the phenothiazines, but there is little substantial evidence to support this suggestion.

Phenothiazines—The phenothiazines are sometimes divided into three subgroups on the basis of their pharmacological action and side chains (aliphatic, piperazine, and piperidyl). The aliphatic group tends to be sedative, the piperazine group tends to stimulate patients, and the piperidyl group is less sedative and possibly antidepressant. Table I lists the phenothiazines, thioxanthenes, and butyrophenones in decreasing order of sedative effect. This order has not been confirmed in controlled studies and does not take into account differences between individual patients. It should be regarded as a rough guide rather than a precise statement.

There is still a dispute as to whether timed-release preparations are more effective than conventional preparations either in terms of therapy or a reduction of side effects; it is not even clear whether divided doses are more effective than once-a-day administration. The general dose range has, however, been fairly well established. The determination of dosage form and frequency of administration depend on the individual case. If drowsiness proves to be a problem, the total dose might be given at bedtime. However, tolerance usually develops to the sedative effects and continued nighttime medication may not be necessary. If the medication acts as a stimulant and the pa-

tient has difficulty sleeping, the drug may be given in the morning.

Fluphenazine decanoate and fluphenazine enanthate are available as long-acting phenothiazine dosage forms. A single injection (25 mg) will last from 2 to 3 weeks. Some patients may require 50–75 mg or more. For patients who tend to forget medication or those who are resistant and agree to use the drug but have no intention of doing so, this depot-type administration is practical. The occurrence of extrapyramidal symptoms is extremely high so that initially a single parenteral injection of an antiparkinsonian agent should be given; this injection may be followed by continued oral administration of an antiparkinsonian drug. After several weeks or months, the antiparkinsonian drug frequently can be discontinued. In France, injectable fluphenazine has been used in much higher doses (up to almost 1000 mg in a single injection), but such usage has not been approved in the United States.

Other available phenothiazines are used in small doses for other purposes but probably act similarly to fluphenazine when used in high doses. These agents include acetophenazine for anxiety, methotrimeprazine for pain, and trimeprazine for treatment of pruritus.

Table I—DRUGS FOR TREATMENT OF SCHIZOPHRENIA
(Listed in Descending Order of Sedation; Activating Properties are in the Reverse Order)

Drug	Tablet Dosage Size, mg	Intensive Treatment Dose (three times daily), mg	Maintenance Dose (two or three times daily), mg
Chlorpromazine	10, 25, 50, 100, 200 (30, 75, 150, 200, 300) [a]	150–500	50–100
Triflupromazine	10, 25, 50	50–150	25–50
Thioridazine	10, 25, 50, 100, 150, 200	200–300	20–60
Mesoridazine	10, 25, 50, 100	50–100	10–25
Chlorprothixene	10, 25, 50, 100	50–100	25–50
Promazine	10, 25, 50, 100, 200	200–600	50–100
Mepazine	25, 50	100–150	50–100
Carphenazine	25, 100	50–100	25–50
Butaperazine	5, 10, 25	25–50	5–10
Thiopropazate	5, 10	20–30	5–15
Fluphenazine	1, 2.5, 5	2–8	1–4
Perphenazine	2, 4, 8, 16	4–16	2–8
Prochlorperazine	5, 10, 25 (10, 15, 30, 75) [a]	50–150	25–50
Trifluoperazine	1, 2, 5, 10	10–20	1–10
Haloperidol	0.5, 1, 2, 5	2–5	1–2
Thiothixene	1, 2, 5, 10	10–20	5–10

[a] Timed-release form.

Rauwolfia Alkaloids—The rauwolfia alkaloids, especially reserpine, in low doses, were widely used previously in the treatment of hypertension, particularly with diuretics or sedatives. Their use in the treatment of schizophrenia has all but ended because of the frequency of side effects (particularly severe depression), and because their efficacy is significantly less than that of the other antipsychotic agents currently available. Additionally, they cannot be used concurrently with electroconvulsive therapy.

Side Effects—A number of side effects must be kept in mind with antipsychotic therapy.

CNS and Anticholinergic Action—Extrapyramidal symptoms are common side effects. In addition to the restlessness of akathisia, there are various dystonias and, in rare instances, there is some evidence of tardive dyskinesia occurring, especially among the elderly who have some evidence of brain damage and arteriosclerosis. Antiparkinsonian drugs are remarkably effective for the extrapyramidal symptoms but of no use in the treatment of tardive dyskinesia and may aggravate these symptoms. The added anticholinergic action of such supplementary drugs may produce some blurring of vision, especially in older patients where the muscles of accommodation do not function as well as in the young. Reduced gastric motility and dryness of the mouth are quite common.

Any antiparkinsonian agent can produce toxic states including visual hallucinations in sensitive individuals. A schizophrenic patient who has been doing well with disappearance of auditory hallucinations and delusions but a few weeks later develops visual hallucinations and other psychotic manifestations should be tested by withdrawal of the antiparkinsonian agent to see whether it is the cause of the new symptoms. Otherwise, there is danger that increased rather than decreased medication might be used. Such recurrences occasionally have been blamed incorrectly on the phenothiazines. Frequently, the dose of the antiparkinsonian medication can be reduced or eliminated after the patient has been receiving the antipsychotic drug for a few weeks (see *Chlorpromazine–Benztropine,* p. 30).

Another neurological side effect of the antipsychotic agents is a slight lowering of the seizure threshold in susceptible individuals.

Occasionally, patients may develop allergic reactions to the antipsychotic agents. Photosensitivity is especially marked with chlorpromazine and is occasionally seen with other phenothiazines. Sun lotions containing aminobenzoic acid sometimes help to prevent the reaction. Avoidance of, or at least gradual exposure to, strong sunlight is indicated for patients receiving phenothiazines.

Endocrine Effects—Many endocrine effects have been attributed to antipsychotic drug therapy, but there are insufficient clinical data to identify them clearly.

Autonomic Nervous System Reactions—Some degree of dryness of the mouth is common in antipsychotic drug therapy and may increase dental caries as a xerostomic side effect of reduced salivary flow (2). Increased salivation also has been reported and may be related to the parkinsonian effects of the various drugs. Slowed gastrointestinal (GI) function is quite common; in severe cases, this effect can lead to a marked stasis. Nasal congestion is a rare side effect as are miosis and mydriasis. Glycerin-based cough drops are helpful for the dry mouth. Stool softeners rather than strong laxatives are recommended for constipation. All adverse reactions tend to be self-correcting.

All antipsychotic drugs, especially thioridazine, will inhibit ejaculation. This side effect does not usually prevent occurrence of the sexual climax.

Metabolic Side Effects—Some patients gain weight during phenothiazine therapy. It is unclear whether this is due to the drug or to increased caloric intake of the patients (3).

Lethargy and Drowsiness—Some patients complain of lethargy and drowsiness even when drug doses have been lowered to the minimal therapeutic level. These effects are more frequent with aliphatic phenothiazines than with other types, so that either a change of antipsychotic medication is indicated or at times small amounts of a stimulant drug can be added. Frequently, tolerance to the sedative effects of the drugs develops.

Hematological Dyscrasias—A variety of blood dyscrasias has been reported. Except for agranulocytosis, it is not certain that they are truly drug related. If patients complain of the sudden appearance of sore throat or give other evidence of infection, a white blood count and differential should be performed immediately. It is always prudent to have a hematological baseline for comparison before starting treatment. Such cases almost always occur in the second or third month of the treatment. A slight depression of the white blood count, if it remains within the normal range, is not sufficient reason for discontinuing treatment, unless there are actual clinical symptoms.

Liver Effects—Hepatic effects are usually manifested by jaundice during the first month of treatment. Occasionally, this jaundice is only subclinical so that if a fever with virus-like symptoms persists more than a few days, tests for abnormal liver function should be undertaken promptly. Almost any type of jaundice can be mimicked by the antipsychotic drugs and extra care should be exercised before making a diagnosis that may lead to surgery.

Cardiovascular Responses—Postural hypotension and tachycardia can appear as well as syncope in the presence of normal blood pressure and pulse rate. These effects are more likely to occur among the elderly. Usually such occurrences are near the beginning of drug use, recovery is spontaneous, and there is little tendency to subsequent recurrence. In the occasional patient in whom the reaction is severe, epinephrine is contraindicated as a vasopressor. Since the phenothiazines are α-adrenergic blockers, epinephrine administration results in a further lowering of blood pressure. Therefore, agents such as levarterenol or phenylephrine are indicated if pharmacological management is necessary.

Nonspecific Q and T wave abnormalities are commonly seen in the ECG of patients receiving phenothiazines.

Skin Pigmentation—Pigmentary change in exposed areas of the body has occurred after long-term use, especially in females. These changes are characterized by a darkening of the skin sometimes to a slate gray or a purplish hue as a result of a melanin change in the dermis. The color change tends to fade after the drug is discontinued. Chlorpromazine has been implicated most frequently with this adverse effect.

Ocular Changes—In patients receiving long-term therapy, minute deposits develop in the lens and cornea, but it is highly questionable whether these are clinically significant. There is some evidence to indicate that they occur more frequently in patients exposed to bright light. Additionally, pigmentary retinopathy has developed in patients treated with thioridazine. This reaction has occurred primarily in patients receiving more than the recommended dose of the drug.

Antiemetic Action—Since phenothiazines tend to reduce nausea and vomiting for a brief period, they may mask evidence of intestinal obstruction, brain tumor, or overdose of toxic drugs. Although other evidence of these conditions usually makes diagnosis apparent, the altered clinical picture because of the absent symptoms of emesis should be kept in mind.

Overstimulation—Some antipsychotic drugs, especially those at the activating end of the phenothiazine spectrum, occasionally produce undesirable overstimulation including insomnia. Changing the time of administration or changing the drug may be indicated.

Pharmacological Mechanisms—Many of the pharmacological changes are well understood. However, uncertainty exists as to whether the psychological changes are directly related to the pharmacological causes. The effects of chlorpromazine are known in some detail. One theory of the mechanism of action is that a decrease in reticular activity is important. Chlorpromazine has only a slight depressant action on the reticular formation, but it does depress the afferent input to this region.

There is evidence that phenothiazines may interact with the structurally similar flavo enzymes and thus influence the production of adenosine triphosphate. A pathological gene may lead to a marked reduction in activity of dopamine β-hydroxylase (or in the capacity to induce the enzyme under stress), which in turn results in incomplete conversion of dopamine to norepinephrine (4). Dopamine is oxidatively or enzymatically converted to 6-hydroxydopamine which is then taken up by the noradrenergic terminals and destroyed. Chlorpromazine antagonizes the norepinephrine-depleting action of hydroxydopamine.

Another action of antipsychotic agents is to enhance the breakdown of catecholamines as evidenced by increased urinary excretion of metabolites of the catecholamines.

Haloperidol may act by mimicking γ-aminobutyric acid and blocking the action of glutamic acid (5). Dopamine, norepinephrine, and other catecholamines are also blocked. γ-Aminobutyric acid increases the permeability of membranes to chloride ions which inhibit depolarization.

Contraindications—Conditions requiring careful consideration before use of antipsychotics include low white count with a shift to the left, conditions in which the patient has already received large amounts of central nervous system (CNS) depressants (alcohol, barbiturates, and narcotics), and the situation in which the patient is comatose. Those patients who have demonstrated hypersensitivity to phenothiazines manifested by blood dyscrasias or jaundice obviously should be treated with caution and only if the potential benefits outweigh the potential hazards.

Some drowsiness or lethargy may be evident, particularly during the first few days of use. Patients with occupations or activities involving machinery or in circumstances requiring high psychomotor control should be evaluated as to whether the drugs may be contraindicated. In such patients, trying an initial low or test dose is the best course to follow.

Interactions—The following interactions should be considered.

Adrenergic Blocking Agents—Adrenergic blocking agents such as phentolamine and propranolol should be used in lower doses when used concurrently with antipsychotic agents. The same is true for drugs used in the production of spinal or epidural anesthesia.

Antacids—Clinical studies indicate that the concurrent administration of chlorpromazine and aluminum or magnesium gel-type antacids results in a significant reduction in serum levels of the antipsychotic agent. The clinical effects of this interaction have not been determined (see *Chlorpromazine–Aluminum and Magnesium Ions,* p. 25).

Anticoagulants—Haloperidol was found to reduce the prothrombin time normally produced by phenindione (6). Close monitoring of prothrombin time is needed since ordinary doses of the anticoagulant may no longer be sufficient. Antithrombotic coumarins also are antagonized by haloperidol. The action may be through increased liver microsomal enzyme activity. This action increases the metabolic degradation of the anticoagulants, thereby reducing the anticoagulant effect. When haloperidol is discontinued, the anticoagulant effect may become more pronounced. The resulting increase in prothrombin time may reach a dangerous level unless the anticoagulant dosage is reduced (7).

Haloperidol probably affects indandione derivatives in a similar manner. It has been pointed out that there is only one case report indicating an interaction between haloperidol and an oral anticoagulant, although a few more cases had previously been reported (6–8). It is unclear whether these are the same cases of interaction referred to in other reports (9–12). Hence, it is difficult to estimate the frequency of this interaction.

Anticonvulsant Drugs—Phenothiazines and thioxanthenes lower the convulsive threshold in susceptible individuals, so that an increase in the dose of the anticonvulsant may be necessary. The clinical significance of this effect has not been established.

Antihypertensive Agents—Phenothiazines may enhance the hypotensive action of antihypertensive drugs due to their ability to produce α-adrenergic blockade (13). When a phenothiazine and an antihypertensive agent are used concurrently, a reduction in dosage of one or both agents may be necessary. However, chlorpromazine may inhibit the hypotensive effect of guanethidine, and presumably other antipsychotic drugs would do the same. Concurrent administration of these drugs should be avoided whenever possible (see *Guanethidine–Chlorpromazine,* p. 81).

Antiparkinsonian Agents—Antipsychotic drugs induce some degree of extrapyramidal symptoms. In most cases, there is an excellent response to antiparkinsonian agents. At times, if the antiparkinsonian agent induces somnolence or other undesired side effects, a different one may prove useful. For patients in whom side effects might discourage use of a needed antipsychotic agent, it is often advisable to give an antiparkinsonian agent at the initiation of antipsychotic treatment. After 1 or 2 months of use, the antiparkinsonian drug may no longer be necessary, and an attempt should be made to reduce the dose and eventually eliminate this adjunctive medication. If the patient is receiving both an antipsychotic and an antiparkinsonian agent, it is important to remember that the effects of the antipsychotic agent last at least a few days longer than the antiparkinsonian agent. Therefore, the latter should be continued for 4 days after the antipsychotic drug is discontinued (14). Premature withdrawal of the antiparkinsonian agent may precipitate extrapyramidal symptoms.

Antiparkinsonian agents may exacerbate tardive dyskinesia or intensify the anticholinergic properties of chlorpromazine (see *Chlorpromazine–Benztropine,* p. 30, and *Levodopa–Chlorpromazine,* p. 122).

CNS Depressants—Antipsychotic agents and barbiturates cause additive CNS effects. Because of this mutual enhancement, smaller than customary doses of such drugs may be necessary. Prolonged phenobarbital administration may decrease serum chlorpromazine levels and increase the urinary excretion of chlorpromazine, resulting in a decrease in chlorpromazine's effect (see *Phenobarbital–Chlorpromazine*, p. 183).

Although there is much controversy concerning the concurrent ingestion of alcohol and phenothiazines, the present evidence seems to indicate that there is a slight but not dangerous enhancement if both are used at "normal" levels. In instances where alcohol is used to excess, the effects may then be more serious than if the patient were not taking an antipsychotic drug. Haloperidol (but not chlorpromazine) was found to increase blood alcohol levels (15).

Epinephrine—Epinephrine should not be given to a patient receiving phenothiazines since, instead of raising blood pressure, it may result in a further fall. This effect appears to result from the partial α-adrenergic block produced by antipsychotic agents. The result is a paradoxical response to epinephrine. Levarterenol or phenylephrine is a safe and adequate substitute. This antagonism can be exploited advantageously in the use of chlorpromazine as a treatment of poisonings which involve amphetamine-like drugs (see *Chlorpromazine–Amphetamine*, p. 27).

Lysergide and Psilocybin—Chlorpromazine and most other antipsychotics are quite effective in antagonizing various hallucinogenic agents and are the most effective means of terminating the hallucinogenic state. The butyrophenones may be particularly advantageous because they are the most potent antidopaminergic drugs commercially available.

Monoamine Oxidase Inhibitors—There is some evidence of an additive orthostatic hypotensive effect, so that doses of monoamine oxidase inhibitors should be increased gradually. This precaution is especially important for patients in whom sudden hypotension may be dangerous.

Piperazine—Some animal studies and one case report suggest that concurrent use of chlorpromazine and piperazine may result in convulsions. Subsequent studies failed to confirm these findings (see *Chlorpromazine–Piperazine*, p. 34).

Preanesthetics and Anesthetics—Moderate prolongation of thiopental narcosis has been induced by haloperidol (16). Haloperidol enhances the effects of analgesics (17). The introduction of chlorpromazine was for the purpose of intensifying anesthetic and preanesthetic agents (18).

In general, all phenothiazines partially block the α-receptors of the sympathetic nervous system. Inhibition of the sympathetic controls by phenothiazines may induce a significant risk of cardiovascular collapse. Epinephrine administration is contraindicated in this situation.

Promethazine Hydrochloride—This drug should not be used as an adjunct to anesthesia in patients who have received any other phenothiazine over a prolonged period.

Stimulants—Pentylenetetrazol, picrotoxin, and similar agents may cause convulsions and should not be used to treat phenothiazine overdoses and should not be administered at other times when a stimulant is needed. Amphetamines are suitable alternatives since they also have an antagonistic effect on the phenothiazines and related preparations (see *Chlorpromazine–Amphetamine*, p. 27).

Thiazide Diuretics—Although clinical documentation is lacking, the use of thiazide diuretics with antipsychotic agents may result in lower blood pressure than when these diuretics are used alone.

Tricyclic Antidepressants—Concurrent administration of phenothiazines and tricyclic antidepressants may increase the pharmacological effects of either drug (19–21). Lowered doses of either drug may be necessary if these drugs are administered concurrently.

Lithium Salts

Therapeutic Indications—Lithium was first introduced as an agent for the treatment of mania in 1949 but, due to the previously disastrous results of its use as a salt substitute in the 1940's, it did not become accepted until the 1960's. Lithium is a unique psychotropic agent in that it is devoid of sedative, stimulant, and other pharmacological effects (22).

The primary indication for lithium is the treatment of the manic phase of manic-depressive illness (23). Lithium is also effective in the prophylactic suppression or modification of cyclic manic-depressive attacks in bipolar patients (24). Although lithium is also beneficial in some types of schizo-affective disorders, other agents are and should be used more routinely (25).

Lithium is administered orally as the carbonate salt. Peak serum levels occur within 1–2 hr after oral administration. Lithium is excreted by the kidneys and has a half-life of approximately 24 hr (26). In the acute manic phase of manic-depressive illness, lithium should be increased to achieve the desired clinical response or until toxicity occurs (usually at serum lithium levels rang-ing between 1.6 and 2.0 mEq/liter). When used for maintenance treatment, lithium dosage should be adjusted to attain a serum level between 0.6 and 1.2 mEq/liter, which generally corresponds to a dosage of 600–1700 mg/day (27). For best results, serum lithium levels should be determined 8–12 hr after the last dose. Since the full effect is usually not seen for 5–10 days, lithium is often used with other psychotherapeutic agents during the initial treatment period (22). Patients in a manic phase tolerate higher concentrations of lithium but may require a decrease in dosage when the mania is resolved (28).

Side Effects—As noted previously, ad-verse effects to lithium are typically seen when serum levels exceed 1.6 mEq/liter (18). GI disturbances, muscle weakness, and lethargy appear to be associated with peaks in serum levels and may disappear with continued treatment (27), while poly-uria and tremor may persist. Other effects not related to dosage seen with acute or chronic treatment include diffuse thyroid enlargement, hypothyroidism, or both. Withdrawal of lithium or administration of thyroid hormone is effective treatment (29). Lithium also may cause a diabetes insipidus syndrome related to a decrease in renal-concentrating ability (30).

Poisoning with lithium is often seen when the serum level exceeds 2.0 mEq/liter. The effects are CNS in origin and include drowsiness, slurred speech, and muscle twitching which progress to increased muscle tone, coma, and death from pul-monary complications. There is no specific antidote for lithium poisoning. Osmotic diuresis, alkalinization of the urine, and restoration of serum electrolytes are some measures that have been used successfully (31–33). Factors that may predispose a patient to lithium toxicity include renal im-pairment, cardiovascular disease, low sodium intake, and advanced age (31).

Pharmacological Mechanisms—The phar-macological mechanisms responsible for the therapeutic action of lithium are not well understood. Studies involving lithium's mode of action indicated that it involves alteration in body electrolytes (especially calcium, potassium, and sodium) or possibly alterations in brain amine metabolism. Like other psychotherapeutic agents, lithium has an effect on the dopamine system (34, 35), but few studies have focused on this effect. The effects of lithium on biogenic amines

include an increased turnover of norepineph-rine and possibly serotonin (34) and inhibi-tion of the release of both norepinephrine and 5-hydroxytryptamine (34, 35). Lithium also inhibits the activation of adenyl cyclase and alters the concentration of γ-aminobuty-ric acid and glutamate within the CNS (35).

Contraindications—Lithium should not be used in patients with renal or cardiovascular disease or in patients on low sodium or sodium-free diets. The only criteria for lithi-um administration are adequate kidney func-tion and salt intake.

Interactions—*Diuretics*—Thiazide diuret-ics can enhance the cardiotoxic and neuro-toxic effects of lithium. Concurrent use of these drugs should be avoided. When these drugs must be used together, the patient should be observed closely for symptoms of lithium toxicity. Close monitoring of serum electrolyte levels and maintenance of ade-quate fluid, potassium, and sodium intake also are necessary (see *Lithium Carbonate–Chlorothiazide*, p. 137).

Iodine—The concurrent administration of lithium carbonate and potassium iodide may enhance the hypothyroid and goiterogenic effects of either drug. Thyroid status should be determined before initiation of therapy and at periodic intervals to detect changes in thyroid function. If hypothyroid-ism develops, treatment with thyroid prep-arations and discontinuation of iodine-con-taining drugs are appropriate actions (see *Lithium Carbonate–Potassium Iodide*, p. 140).

References

(1) N. S. Kline and T. G. Scott, "Unusual Therapeutic Uses of Phenothiazines as a Clue to Mode of Action," *Agressologie, 9*, 319 (1968).

(2) L. Bahn, "Drug-Related Dental Destruction," *Oral Surg. Oral Med. Oral Pathol., 33*, 49 (1972).

(3) M. M. Singh *et al.*, "Weight as a Correlate of Clinical Response to Psychotropic Drugs," *Psychosomatics, 11*, 562 (1970).

(4) L. Stein, "Neurochemistry of Reward and Punishment: Some Implications for the Eti-ology of Schizophrenia," *J. Psychiat. Res., 8*, 345 (1971).

(5) P. A. J. Janssen, "The Pharmacology of Halo-peridol," *Int. J. Neuropsychiat., 3*, suppl. 1, 10 (1967).

(6) S. Grosshandler *et al.*, "Toxic Reactions Due to Drug Synergism and Antagonism," *Anesth. Analg., 47*, 345 (1968).

(7) I. S. Wright, "Recent Developments in Anti-thrombotic Therapy," *Ann. Intern. Med., 71*, 823 (1969).

(8) L. T. Sigell and H. C. Flessa, "Drug Inter-actions with Anticoagulants," *J. Amer. Med. Ass., 214*, 2035 (1970).

(9) D. L. Bernstein et al., "Drug Altered Warfarin Anticoagulation," Drug Ther., 5, 95 (1975).

(10) A. I. Sandler, "Interactions of Oral Coumarin Anticoagulants with Other Drugs," Drug Intel., 4, 146 (1970).

(11) D. B. Hunninghake, "Drug Interactions," Postgrad. Med., 47, 71 (1970).

(12) M. J. Ellenhorn and F. A. Sternad, "Problems of Drug Interactions," J. Amer. Pharm. Ass., NS6, 62 (1966).

(13) W. R. Martin et al., "Chlorpromazine III: The Effects of Chlorpromazine and Chlorpromazine Sulfoxide on Vascular Response to L-Epinephrine and Levarterenol," J. Pharmacol. Exp. Ther., 130, 37 (1960).

(14) N. S. Kline and J. M. Davis, in "Comprehensive Group Psychotherapy," H. I. Kaplan and E. J. Sadock, Eds., Williams and Wilkins, Baltimore, Md., 1971, pp. 328–369.

(15) P. L. Morselli et al., "Further Observations on the Interaction between Ethanol and Psychotropic Drugs," Arzneim.-Forsch., 2, 20 (1971).

(16) A. B. Dobkin, "Potentiation of Thiopental Anaesthesia: With Tigan, Panectyl, Benadryl, Gravol, Marzine, Histadyl, Librium, and Haloperidol (R 1625)," Can. Anaesth. Soc. J., 8, 265 (1961).

(17) F. Le Goaziou, "Use of Haloperidol (R 1625) in Premedication," Presse Med., 70, 578 (1962).

(18) H. Laborit and P. Huguenard, "L'hibernation Artificielle par Moyens Pharmacodynamiques et Physiques," Presse Med., 59, 1329 (1951).

(19) L. F. Gram and K. F. Overo, "Drug Interaction: Inhibitory Effect of Neuroleptics on Metabolism of Tricyclic Antidepressants in Man," Brit. Med. J., 1, 463 (1972).

(20) F. J. Kane and T. W. Taylor, "An Unusual Reaction to Combined Imipramine-Thorazine Therapy," Amer. J. Psychiat., 120, 186 (1963).

(21) K. Whitton, "Severe Toxic Reaction to Combined Amitriptyline and Thioridazine," Amer. J. Psychiat., 121, 812 (1965).

(22) L. E. Hollister, "Clinical Use of Psychotherapeutic Drugs I: Antipsychotic and Antimanic Drugs," Drugs, 4, 321 (1972).

(23) P. E. Stokes et al., "Efficacy of Lithium as Acute Treatment of Manic-Depressive Illness," Lancet, i, 1319 (1971).

(24) P. C. Baastrup et al., "Prophylactic Lithium. Double Blind Discontinuation in Manic-Depressive and Recurrent-Depressive Disorders," Lancet, ii, 326 (1970).

(25) R. F. Prien et al., "Comparison of Lithium Carbonate and Chlorpromazine in the Treatment of Mania. Report of the Veterans Administration and National Institute of Mental Health Collaborative Study Group," Arch. Gen. Psychiat., 26, 146 (1972).

(26) H. C. Caldwell et al., "A Pharmacokinetic Analysis of Lithium Carbonate Absorption from Several Formulations in Man," J. Clin. Pharmacol., 11, 349 (1971).

(27) M. Shou et al., "Pharmacological and Clinical Problems of Lithium Prophylaxis," Brit. J. Psychiat., 116, 615 (1970).

(28) M. Shou, "Lithium in Psychiatric Therapy and Prophylaxis," J. Psychiat. Res., 6, 67 (1968).

(29) S. Gershon, "Lithium in Mania," Clin. Pharmacol. Ther., 11, 168 (1970).

(30) T. A. Ramsey et al., "Lithium Carbonate and Kidney Function. A Failure in Renal Concentrating Ability," J. Amer. Med. Ass., 219, 1446 (1972).

(31) "Lithium, Its Role in Psychiatric Research and Development," S. Gershon and B. Shopsin, Eds., Plenum, New York, NY 10011, 1973, pp. 107, 115.

(32) K. Thomsen and M. Schou, "Renal Lithium Excretion in Man," Amer. J. Physiol., 215, 823 (1968).

(33) H. I. Hurtig and W. L. Dyson, "Lithium Toxicity Enhanced by Diuresis," N. Engl. J. Med., 290, 748 (1974).

(34) "Lithium, Its Role in Psychiatric Research and Development," S. Gershon and B. Shopsin, Eds., Plenum, New York, NY 10011, 1973, pp. 178–183.

(35) "The Pharmacological Basis of Therapeutics," 5th ed., L. S. Goodman and A. Gilman, Eds., Macmillan, New York, NY 10022, 1975, pp. 184–185.

Antitussive Therapy

The human organism possesses different and varied warning systems to protect against possible damage; one is the process of coughing.

If a cough is persistent and lasts for days or weeks, it may serve to alert the individual to the early stages of conditions such as emphysema, tuberculosis, or lung cancer. In such cases, it would be unwise to self-medicate and suppress the cough; instead a thorough physical examination should be undertaken to determine the etiology of the cough.

The cough may also be useful in clearing the respiratory passages of excessive secretions or foreign materials. Again, it may be unwise to suppress coughing.

If it has been determined that the cough is not serving a useful purpose, then failure to suppress the cough can cause much unnecessary discomfort for the patient. For such patients, the use of an antitussive agent is valid and may not only relieve the cough but also allow the patient to rest more easily and thereby speed recovery.

Therapeutic Indications

Antitussive agents fall into two major categories: narcotic antitussive agents and nonnarcotic antitussive agents.

Narcotic antitussive agents include codeine, hydrocodone, hydromorphone, levorphanol, methadone, and morphine. These agents, especially codeine, are among the more effective antitussive agents available. At effective dose levels, they possess some undesirable side effects including a constipating action and a possible addiction potential on prolonged use.

Many new nonnarcotic agents are also effective cough suppressants and lack the addiction potential of the narcotic agents. Representative nonnarcotic antitussive agents include noscapine, an antitussive agent approximately equal to codeine in effectiveness while lacking the side effects usually associated with narcotic antitussives, and dextromethorphan, an agent lacking the analgesic, addictive, central depressant, and constipating properties of narcotic antitussives.

Other nonnarcotic antitussives include benzonatate (less effective than codeine but producing fewer side effects and having a low toxicity), carbetapentane (equivalent to codeine as an antitussive), levopropoxyphene, and pipazethate [less potent than codeine but having a reported low incidence of side effects (1)].

In addition to antitussive agents, most cough suppressant preparations contain various other ingredients. The more important adjuvants include antihistamines, useful when the cause of the cough is allergic in nature; sympathomimetics, employed for their bronchodilatory activity; parasympatholytics, which help to decrease secretions in the upper respiratory tract; and expectorants (2).

Pharmacological Mechanisms

Since narcotic agents (*e.g.,* codeine and morphine) have a central analgesic action, their antitussive effects may also be due to a central mechanism.

The nonnarcotic antitussives may also produce their effects through a central mechanism, although another theory has been proposed (3) for some of these agents. According to this theory, irritation of the mucosa initially causes bronchoconstriction which excites the cough receptors; therefore, agents that cause bronchodilation should offer some relief from coughing.

Contraindications

The contraindications usually identified with antitussive preparations are many times associated with other ingredients generally included in such formulations, as well as with the antitussive agent itself.

Sympathomimetic agents should be used with caution in individuals with hypertension, diabetes mellitus, urinary retention, and hyperthyroidism.

Antihistamines may cause drowsiness and should be used cautiously in patients who operate machinery or automobiles.

Parasympatholytic agents are contraindicated in cases of glaucoma, constipation, advanced hepatic or renal damage, obstructive disorders, and stenosis.

Various antitussive preparations contain agents that are not recommended for use during pregnancy.

Interactions

Many deaths have resulted from the concurrent use of various types of depressant agents. Therefore, antitussive agents that are depressant in nature or that contain central nervous system depressants should be used with extreme caution if the patient is also consuming other depressant drugs (such as barbiturates or tranquilizers), since such concurrent use produces at least additive effects. In this context, the simultaneous ingestion of alcohol is a serious hazard (see *Diazepam–Alcohol,* p. 47; *Meprobamate–Alcohol,* p. 145; and *Phenobarbital–Alcohol,* p. 180).

Caution should be observed in the use of narcotic agents with coumarin-type anticoagulants as the narcotic may enhance the anticoagulant response (4). Neither the mechanism involved in this interaction nor the clinical significance has been established.

Tricyclic antidepressants may enhance respiratory depression and display additive anticholinergic effects (5).

Narcotic antitussive agents and dextromethorphan should also be used with caution in patients treated with monoamine oxidase inhibitors. While the mechanisms involved in these interactions remain to be established, deaths have resulted from the concurrent use of such agents (see *Meperidine–Phenelzine,* p. 142).

The concurrent use of narcotic agents and neuromuscular blocking agents may lead to atelectasis and respiratory depression.

Methotrimeprazine and procarbazine also may increase the respiratory depression produced by narcotic agents (6).

There remains some doubt as to the possibility of a drug interaction between narcotic agents and dexpanthenol.

References

(1) A. B. Amier and C. B. Rothman, "Evaluation of Pipazethate as an Antitussive Agent in Pediatric Practice," *J. New Drugs, 3,* 362 (1963).

(2) "Textbook of Organic Medicinal and Pharmaceutical Chemistry," C. O. Wilson *et al.,* Eds., Lippincott, Philadelphia, Pa., 1969, p. 669.

(3) H. Salem and D. M. Aviado, "Antitussive Drugs, with Special Reference to a New Theory for the Initiation of the Cough Reflex and the Influence of Bronchodilators," *Amer. J. Med. Sci., 247,* 585 (1964).

(4) M. Weiner, "Effect of Centrally Active Drugs on the Action of Coumarin Anticoagulants," *Nature, 212,* 1599 (1966).

(5) K. Melmon *et al.,* "Drug Interactions that Can Affect Your Patients," *Patient Care, 1,* 32 (1967).

(6) "The Pharmacological Basis of Therapeutics," 5th ed., L. S. Goodman and A. Gilman, Eds., Macmillan, New York, NY 10022, 1975, p. 1295.

Cardiac Glycoside Therapy

The rational use of cardiac glycosides in the treatment of cardiac insufficiency goes back almost 200 years, when Withering (1) published his "Account of the Foxglove" in 1785. Withering wrote: "It has a power over the heart, to a degree yet unobserved in any other medicine, and . . . this power may be converted to salutary ends." Considering the long history of use, it is interesting that the value of cardiac glycosides is currently increasing rather than decreasing (2).

The term digitalis includes a number of cardiac glycosides obtained from various plants including digitalis, squill, and strophanthus and is often used to designate the entire class of cardiac glycosides, rather than just those from digitalis. All cardiac glycosides have the same basic structure. This structure includes a cyclopentanoperhydrophenanthrene nucleus characteristic of steroid compounds, an unsaturated lactone ring at C-17, a hydroxyl group at C-14, and some type of sugar residue attached at C-3. The various glycosides differ in the type of the lactone ring, the number and type of sugar residues, and the number of other hydroxyl groups attached to the steroid nucleus (3, 4). The different sugar residues and additional hydroxyl groups yield compounds that differ in their rates of absorption, metabolism, and excretion (5).

In the last 60 years, a great deal of information has been obtained on the therapeutic use of cardiac glycosides. It has been established that the major use of the glycosides is in the treatment of congestive heart failure. However, it has only been in the last 25 years that specific information has become available about the pharmacology of these extremely complex compounds (6).

The cardiac glycosides are very important from a therapeutic standpoint and also from a toxicity standpoint. These agents have one of the lowest therapeutic indexes of all drugs used; it has been estimated that approximately 20% of the patients taking cardiac glycosides exhibit some type of toxic reaction (7, 8). The dosage of the glycosides varies greatly with each individual, and a certain expertise is required to treat adequately the cardiac insufficiency and, at the same time, prevent digitalis intoxication. It has been estimated that the therapeutic dose is approximately 35% of the fatal dose and that serious cardiac arrhythmias can develop at 60% of the fatal dose (2).

Patients treated with digitalis usually take it for prolonged periods and often receive other drugs. The factors of prolonged use, low therapeutic index, and multiple-drug treatment make the cardiac glycosides ideal candidates for drug interactions.

Therapeutic Indications

Congestive Heart Failure—The major indication for the cardiac glycosides is in the treatment of congestive heart failure (2, 6, 9). Years ago, digitalis was thought to be useful in congestive heart failure only in the presence of atrial fibrillation; now it is agreed that digitalis is of value in the treatment of congestive heart failure regardlesss of the etiology (9). Best results are obtained when the congestive heart failure is induced by conditions such as hypertension or atherosclerotic heart disease which do not impair the supply of energy to the myocardium (6).

Congestive heart failure results from the inability of the heart to pump sufficient blood to meet the metabolic demands of the tissues (10). Compensatory mechanisms are activated in an attempt to maintain cardiac output and to satisfy the needs of the body. Sodium and water retention occurs and results in an expansion of blood volume. The size of the heart increases in the face of expanded blood volume. The sympathetic nervous system is stimulated to increase the heart rate in an attempt to increase cardiac output (10).

The effects of digitalis on congestive heart failure include correcting all of the altered cardiac physiology that accompanies this condition. The diastolic size of the heart approaches normal, the heart rate slowly returns to normal, and sodium and water retention is reduced. The main action of digitalis is to increase the force of myocardial contractility (11).

Once digitalis has returned the failing heart to a state of compensation, its continued use helps prevent a recurrence of heart failure. Thus, it may be considered appropriate to maintain patients on digitalis, even though they are subsequently free of symptoms (6). However, in the absence of a known primary cardiac lesion, an attempt to withdraw digitalis should be made (12).

Atrial Fibrillation and Flutter—Atrial fibrillation and flutter are other indications for digitalis even in the absence of congestive heart failure (6, 9). Digitalis rarely terminates the altered atrial rhythms or arrhythmias, and the glycosides are not used for that reason. However, digitalis does maintain the ventricular rate at approximately normal levels by blocking atrioventricular (A-V) conduction (6, 9, 10, 13).

Pharmacological Mechanisms

Digitalis Effects—The major demonstrable effects of the cardiac glycosides are on the cardiovascular system and specifically on the heart. The major effect on the heart is a marked increase in the contractile force (11). In patients with congestive heart failure, this increased inotropic effect leads to an increased cardiac output, decreased heart size, decreased blood volume, and a transient diuresis. The diuresis helps eliminate the edema that results from the cardiac insufficiency. All of these effects are readily explained on the basis of the increased force of contraction (13).

Digitalis also can slow the heart rate in normal animals and this cardiac slowing is apparently mediated by vagal and extravagal actions (14). The cardiac slowing is not a prerequisite for the activity of digitalis in congestive heart failure in humans (6). The positive inotropic response of digitalis is definitely a direct effect of the glycosides and is not dependent on any extracardiac factor (11). It is certainly not dependent on catecholamine liberation or enhancement, because positive inotropism can be demonstrated in animals administered reserpine and in the presence of β-adrenergic blocking agents (4, 6).

Digitalis also affects conduction of electrical impulses within the heart. It depresses conduction in the A-V node, which accounts for its usefulness in treating conditions resulting from increased atrial rates (11).

Digitalis increases the inotropic response in the cardiac myofibril. There is some evidence that this is mediated by an increase in calcium in the sarcoplasmic reticulum (2, 4). Calcium is thought to initiate contraction by activating myosin adenosine triphosphatase to provide the necessary energy. Digitalis increases the exchangeable calcium fraction in the heart muscle without a detectable increase in total calcium content (4, 15).

Digitalis inhibits the enzyme sodium–potassium adenosine triphosphatase which may indirectly influence calcium movement. There is a correlation between the toxicity of the cardiac glycosides and the inhibition of sodium–potassium adenosine triphosphatase (16). According to one of the current theories, inhibition of sodium–potassium adenosine triphosphatase would lead to increased intracellular sodium. This increased intracellular sodium would result in better mobilization of calcium (11, 15). This theory is currently surrounded with a great deal of controversy and cannot be proved or disproved with current evidence. There are some investigators who claim that sodium–potassium adenosine triphosphatase is actually stimulated at therapeutic levels of digitalis and inhibited only at toxic levels (16).

Absorption, Distribution, Metabolism, and Excretion—The majority of drug interactions occur by altering the amount of drug in the body and the length of time it is there. The various cardiac glycosides differ greatly in their absorption, distribution, metabolism, and excretion. Digitoxin is almost completely absorbed orally; it is metabolized and excreted very slowly and is highly protein bound (97%) (17). The biological half-life in humans is about 7 days (17, 18). Digitoxin is excreted into the bile and generally reabsorbed from the gastrointestinal (GI) tract. This enterohepatic circulation markedly prolongs its half-life. In humans, digitoxin is partially metabolized to digoxin (19); however, the extent of this conversion and the pharmacological effects are not thoroughly understood.

Digoxin is more polar than digitoxin, is protein bound to a much lesser extent (23%), and is only about 80% absorbed orally. Digoxin is excreted fairly rapidly in the urine with little or no metabolism preceding excretion. The biological half-life of digoxin is about 34 hr (20).

Ouabain is much more polar and is absorbed very poorly after oral administration. For this reason, ouabain is usually given intravenously. Ouabain is a rapid-acting cardiac glycoside and is excreted in unchanged form in the urine. The biological half-life is less than 8 hr (2, 17).

Contraindications

There are few absolute contraindications to the use of cardiac glycosides. If congestive heart failure is present, the cardiac glycosides are usually the drugs' of choice, regardless of the presence of other syndromes.

Care is necessary in treating patients with renal or liver dysfunction due to the altered metabolism and/or excretion of the glycosides. In these cases, the patient must be monitored closely and the dose should be adjusted to compensate for the altered biological half-life (21, 22).

Response Variants

There are important conditions that influence a patient's response to digitalis (23).

Age—Infants and elderly individuals appear to be more sensitive to the actions of digitalis. The incidence of intoxication is much higher in these groups (24, 25).

Renal and Liver Dysfunction—It has already been mentioned that care must be exercised in treating patients with possible altered metabolic or excretory functions.

Thyroid Disease—The incidence of digitalis toxicity is higher among patients with thyroid disease. Hyperthyroid individuals require greater amounts of digitalis, and myxedematous patients require a smaller amount of digitalis (26). Treatment of these conditions can create problems in patients also requiring digitalis therapy (27).

Interactions

Calcium—An increase in the serum calcium levels can markedly enhance the action of the cardiac glycosides and a decrease in the serum calcium level will have the opposite effect (2, 6). Parenteral calcium preparations and calcium chelators (edetate sodium) should probably be used carefully in patients receiving digitalis (see *Digitalis–Calcium*, p. 50).

Diuretics—Diuretics are used frequently with digitalis to remove the edema associated with congestive heart failure more rapidly. All potent diuretics increase potassium, sodium, and water excretion. The resulting loss of potassium can lead to hypokalemia, which enhances the activity and toxicity of the cardiac glycosides (6, 28). The potent diuretics include chlorthalidone, ethacrynic acid, furosemide, the mercurial diuretics, metolazone, quinethazone, and the thiazide diuretics. The increased sensitivity to digitalis produced by diuretic-induced hypokalemia is the most serious interaction.

Measures to prevent or reduce these adverse interactions would include monitoring plasma potassium levels and where necessary supplementation with liquid potassium chloride, a potassium-rich diet, or the addition of a potassium-sparing diuretic (*e.g.*, amiloride, spironolactone, or triamterene) (see *Digitalis–Chlorothiazide*, p. 52).

Miscellaneous—There are a number of other drugs that have been shown to interact with glycosides in animals and occasionally in humans. The clinical significance of all of these interactions is still questionable.

Amphotericin B—Amphotericin B is known to cause potassium loss (29). Patients receiving this drug with cardiac glycosides should have plasma potassium levels monitored closely to minimize the danger of hypokalemic-induced digitalis toxicity.

Barbiturates—The barbiturates increase the hydroxylation of digitoxin to digoxin. It is doubtful that this effect markedly alters the therapy with the glycosides, because the extent of digoxin formation appears extremely low (19).

Cholestyramine—Studies indicate that ion-exchange resins such as cholestyramine reduce the serum level of cardiac glycosides when used concurrently. Although there is little clinical documentation, it is prudent to administer the cardiac glycosides 1.5 hr before cholestyramine (see *Digoxin–Cholestyramine*, p. 62).

Heparin—It has been demonstrated in animals that digitalis can increase blood coagulation and that heparin reduces the toxicity of digitalis. However, clinical investigations indicate no changes in coagulation time or heparin tolerance (6).

Phenytoin—Although it has been reported that phenytoin (diphenylhydantoin) may enhance digitalis-induced bradycardia or decrease serum digitoxin levels, there is little indication that these effects are clinically significant (see *Digitalis–Phenytoin*, p. 57).

Propantheline—The concurrent use of digoxin and propantheline may result in increased absorption of digoxin. This interaction may be significant only in patients taking digoxin tablets that exhibit slow release rates (see *Digoxin–Propantheline*, p. 65).

Rauwolfia Alkaloids—Several clinical and experimental reports indicate that the concurrent use of cardiac glycosides and rauwolfia alkaloids may increase the likelihood of cardiac arrhythmias. In most cases, these agents could probably be administered concurrently without adverse effects, but the possibility of serious drug-induced arrhythmias should be considered, particularly in patients with atrial fibrillation (see *Digitalis–Reserpine*, p. 58).

Spironolactone—Another drug which, for the time being, must be placed in the miscellaneous class is spironolactone. This potassium-sparing diuretic has been shown to prevent the toxicity of digitoxin in animals. The mechanism of this protection is unknown, but it probably involves altered metabolism and/or excretion of digitoxin. The serum levels of digitoxin are reduced markedly in animals pretreated with spironolactone. The clinical significance of this interaction is unknown at this time (see *Digitoxin–Spironolactone*, p. 61).

References

(1) W. Withering, "An Account of the Foxglove and Some of Its Medical Uses, with Practical Remarks on Dropsy and Other Diseases," G. G. J. Robinson and J. Robinson, London, England, 1785 (Reprinted in "Cardiac Classics," Mosby, St. Louis, Mo., 1941, pp. 305–443).

(2) "Drill's Pharmacology in Medicine," 4th ed., J. R. DiPalma, Ed., McGraw-Hill, New York, N.Y., 1971, pp. 780–808.

(3) S. E. Wright, "The Metabolism of Cardiac Glycosides," Thomas, Springfield, Ill., 1960, pp. 3–10.

(4) T. W. Smith and E. Haber, "Digitalis I," *N. Engl. J. Med., 289,* 945 (1973).

(5) G. R. Okita, in "Digitalis," C. Fisch and B. Surawicz, Eds., Grune and Stratton, New York, N.Y., 1967, pp. 13–27.

(6) "The Pharmacological Basis of Therapeutics," 5th ed., L. S. Goodman and A. Gilman, Eds., Macmillan, New York, NY 10022, 1975, pp. 676–679.

(7) P. L. Rodensky and F. Wasserman, "Observations on Digitalis Intoxication," *Arch. Intern. Med., 108,* 171 (1961).

(8) T. W. Smith and E. Haber, "Digitalis," *N. Engl. J. Med., 289,* 1125 (1973).

(9) A. F. Lyon and A. C. DeGraff, "Digitalis Therapy," Mosby, St. Louis, Mo., 1967, pp. 23–27.

(10) K. L. Melmon and H. F. Morrelli, "Clinical Pharmacology, Basic Principles in Therapeutics," Macmillan, New York, NY 10022, 1972, pp. 180–193.

(11) D. T. Mason, "Digitalis Pharmacology and Therapeutics: Recent Advances," *Ann. Intern. Med., 80,* 520 (1974).

(12) J. L. C. Dall, "Maintenance Digoxin in Elderly Patients," *Brit. Med. J., 2,* 705 (1970).

(13) T. W. Smith and E. Haber, "Digitalis," *N. Engl. J. Med., 289,* 1010 (1973).

(14) P. L. McLain *et al.,* "The Effect of Atropine on Digitoxin Bradycardia in Cats," *J. Pharmacol. Exp. Ther., 126,* 76 (1959).

(15) K. S. Lee and W. Klaus, "The Subcellular Basis for the Mechanism of Inotropic Action of Cardiac Glycosides," *Pharmacol. Rev., 23,* 193 (1971).

(16) K. Repke, "Metabolism of Cardiac Glycosides," *Proc. Int. Pharmacol. Meetings 1st, 3,* 47 (1963).

(17) T. W. Smith and E. Haber, "Digitalis," *N. Engl. J. Med., 289,* 1063 (1973).

(18) G. Okita *et al.,* "Metabolic Fate of Radioactive Digitoxin in Human Subjects," *J. Pharmacol. Exp. Ther., 115,* 371 (1955).

(19) B. T. Brown *et al.,* "C-12 Hydroxylation of Digitoxin," *Nature, 180,* 607 (1957).

(20) J. E. Doherty *et al.,* "Tritiated Digoxin Studies in Human Subjects," *Arch. Intern. Med., 108,* 531 (1961).

(21) R. W. Jelliffe *et al.,* "An Improved Method of Digitoxin Therapy," *Ann. Intern. Med., 72,* 453 (1970).

(22) R. W. Jelliffe, "Administration of Digoxin," *Dis. Chest, 56,* 56 (1969).

(23) A. Selzer and K. E. Cohn, "Production, Recognition and Treatment of Digitalis Intoxication," *Calif. Med., 113,* 1 (October 1970).

(24) E. K. Chung, "Guide to Digitalis Therapy. I," *Postgrad. Med., 47,* 100 (1970).

(25) G. A. Ewy *et al.,* "Digoxin Metabolism in the Elderly," *Circulation, 39,* 449 (1969).

(26) E. K. Chung, "Guide to Digitalis Therapy. II," *Postgrad. Med., 48,* 132 (1970).

(27) J. E. Doherty and W. H. Perkins, "Digoxin Metabolism in Hypo- and Hyperthyroidism. Studies with Tritiated Digoxin in Thyroid Disease," *Ann. Intern. Med., 64,* 489 (1966).

(28) B. Lown *et al.,* "Interrelationship of Digitalis and Potassium in Auricular Tachycardia with Block," *Amer. Heart J., 45,* 589 (1953).

(29) R. P. Miller and J. H. Bates, "Amphotericin B Toxicity. A Follow-Up Report of 53 Patients," *Ann. Intern. Med., 71,* 1089 (1969).

Corticosteroid Therapy

The therapeutic use of corticosteroids has gone through two experimental phases: trials in new diseases and trials with new compounds. It is now in a third phase: trials with new (high) dose levels. As there is no way to predict in advance optimal therapeutic dosage, this phase is necessary to delineate the limits of effective therapy. The valid therapeutic indications and contraindications are known (1–4).

Therapeutic Indications

The major use of corticosteroids is in anti-inflammatory therapy. They are used when less potent and/or less toxic therapy has been inadequate. Included in this category are collagen diseases such as rheumatoid arthritis, rheumatic carditis, systemic lupus erythematosus, polymyositis, polyarteritis, and erythema nodosum. Other disease entities for which corticosteroids are used include osteoarthritis, nephrotic syndrome, blepharitis, uveitis, thyroiditis, saccoidosis, chronic ulcerative colitis, and various skin disorders. Ideal therapy for most, if not all, of these would range from a brief intensive course of treatment to chronic treatment with the lowest effective dose.

Other conditions in which corticosteroids are useful include the treatment of allergic disorders such as bronchial asthma, suppression of the immune response in transplantation procedures, and autoimmune disorders such as hemolytic anemia and thrombocytopenia.

A third therapeutic indication is in the treatment of malignant disease, especially in certain leukemias and lymphomas. A fourth therapeutic category includes such phenomena as increased intracranial pressure and shock. Finally, corticosteroids are useful as substitution therapy in anterior pituitary or adrenal insufficiency and in the adrenogenital syndrome and as diagnostic agents in various clinical disorders.

Pharmacological Mechanisms

An essential feature of corticosteroids is their potent anti-inflammatory effect. These agents relieve the heat, swelling, pain, and generalized morbidity of a host of disorders characterized by tissue damage, whether the damaging agent is a microorganism, a bacterial or chemical toxin, UV light, or hypoxia. This effect is apparently mediated by stabilization of the lysosomal membrane, thus preventing the spillage of cathepsins and other enzymes from the lysosomal sac (5).

The mechanism of action by which corticosteroids suppress allergic or autoimmune reactions is unknown. Corticosteroids do not inhibit the elaboration of antibody and do not interfere with the antigen–antibody reaction, with the release of histamine from sensitized cells, or with the characteristic response of skin and smooth muscle to histamine. But even after this chain of events has run its course, the inflammatory response to histamine is minimized because (presumably) of the stabilization of the lysosomal membrane (4).

Corticosteroids have a potent catabolic effect on all lymphoid tissue through mechanisms which are poorly understood. This action may also partly explain the success of such therapy in allergic disorders. Malignant processes such as leukemia and lymphomas also respond somewhat to corticosteroids. Such therapeutic use is enhanced by concurrent administration of other antitumor drugs.

Finally, corticosteroids markedly decrease capillary permeability, increase cardiac output, and enhance the normal vasomotor responses. The capillary effects may be mediated through the lysosomal mechanism, although details are poorly understood. Corticosteroids in massive doses are believed to block the effect of a myocardial depressant factor which has been identified in certain cases of septic shock (6). The effect of corticosteroids on maintaining vasomotor tone is still conjectural.

Corticosteroids represent the essential secretion of the adrenal cortex, and doses equivalent to 25–50 mg of cortisone/day constitute adequate replacement in most patients with pituitary or adrenal failure. The latter may also require salt-retaining hormones to replace the absent aldosterone. In adreno-genital syndrome, the dose of corticosteroids is empirically chosen to produce suppression of pituitary adrenocorticotropic hormone (ACTH) secretion and thus of adrenal androgen production.

Contraindications

The primary contraindication to the use of corticosteroids is the lack of a clearcut diagnosis and prognosis. Without these, it is impossible to foretell the patient's response. All steroid treatment, except predetermined brief courses of 2 weeks or less, is likely to produce interference with the normal hypo-thalamic–pituitary–adrenal regulatory system and a rebound worsening of the primary problem when steroids are stopped abruptly (7). Since most patients treated with steroids experience striking feelings of well-being ir-respective of the effect of steroids on the primary disease process, such therapy may be difficult to stop and, therefore, should not be started except for well-considered reasons, particularly in view of the inevitable long-term side effects.

Tuberculosis (whether active or arrested) is usually felt to be an absolute contraindica-tion to any except substitution therapy with corticosteroids. If tuberculosis is a potential complication, concurrent antituberculosis therapy should be employed. Disseminated tuberculous infections are sometimes treated with corticosteroids in addition to specific antituberculosis drugs to minimize the toxic-ity of the infectious process.

Ocular herpes simplex and acute psychoses also are usually considered to be absolute contraindications to the use of cortico-steroids.

Relative contraindications include diver-ticulitis, active or latent peptic ulcer, osteo-porosis, diabetes mellitus, psychotic tenden-cies, any serious acute or chronic infection (especially if antibiotics are unavailable or unsatisfactory), myasthenia gravis, severe hypertension, thromboembolic phenomena, recent extensive surgery or burns, and the first trimester of pregnancy.

Response Variants

It is the obligation of the practitioner who initiates corticosteroid therapy to maintain careful and prolonged surveillance of its im-pact on four parameters: (a) therapeutic effect on the disease process, (b) emergence of side effects, (c) impact on the pituitary–adrenal axis, and (d) nonspecific withdrawal effects. The occurrence of clinically signifi-cant drug interactions will naturally compli-cate each task and will require reconsidera-tion of the benefit-to-risk ratio.

The pattern of objective measurements that might signal improvement necessarily depends on which condition is being treated, but it is imperative to discount almost com-pletely the general feeling of well-being that results from high corticosteroid doses.

An index of the magnitude of the problem of side effects is found in the prospective study of 50 patients with active rheumatoid arthritis (8). Corticosteroid therapy was discontinued early in about one-third of the patients, because it either had no apparent

therapeutic effect or because of remission. In another third, the development of severe side effects necessitated stopping the drugs. Such side effects included depression (10%), peptic ulcer (4%), and fatal termination (18%). The deaths were due to pneumonia (10%), surgery for ulcer (2%), cerebrovascular acci-dent (2%), heart failure (2%), and myocar-dial infarction (2%). In the remaining 32%, corticosteroid therapy was continued with benefit for 9–12 years, after which time most patients in this group had demonstrable evi-dence of osteoporosis of the spine in addition to other complications such as ulcer, hyper-tension, or mental symptoms. Posterior cap-sular cataracts are another possible compli-cation of long-term therapy; the pathogenesis is not clear.

Any dose of corticosteroids in excess of the equivalent of 100 mg of cortisone/day for 2 weeks results in derangement of the normal hypothalamic–pituitary–adrenal axis. The pituitary gland contains reasonably nor-mal amounts of ACTH but fails to respond to the normal stimuli for its release. The adrenal glands become atrophic. Once exo-genous corticosteroid treatment is discontin-ued, plasma cortisol and ACTH values fall to very low levels (7). Over several months, the ACTH level gradually rises to normal values and above, followed (with a lag of several months) by a return of plasma corti-sol to normal levels, after which plasma ACTH also becomes normal. Thus, for sev-eral months after discontinuing corticoste-roids, the patient experiences what has been termed (9) "the steroid withdrawal syn-drome." Symptoms include anorexia, lassi-tude, irritability, malaise, hypercalcemia, and pruritus. These symptoms gradually disap-pear. For 6–9 months, such patients are in danger of an Addisonian crisis if stressed by trauma, surgery, or acute severe infection. There is reasonably good evidence that this problem is minimized in patients whose long-term therapy is given on alternate days or in similar intermittent fashion (10).

Finally, there have been scattered reports of a peculiar myositis or vasculitis in a few patients with rheumatoid arthritis whose long-term steroid therapy was abruptly stopped. The mechanisms of these effects are unknown (11).

Interactions

All corticosteroids interact with a variety of drugs through three principal mechanisms.

Enzyme Induction—Metabolism of ste-roids is accomplished *via* an enzymatic degradation occurring in the smooth endoplasmic reticulum of the hepatic cells. These enzymes are readily induced by many drugs, including the antihistamines, barbiturates, and phenytoin (diphenylhydantoin). Thus, concurrent administration of these agents diminishes steroidal, pharmacological, and physiological effects (12).

The practitioner faced with the problem of such interactions has two alternatives. The corticosteroid dosage can be increased to maintain effective tissue levels of active steroid, or other drugs that do not produce this interaction with corticosteroids may be selected. In the case of antihistamines or antiepileptic drugs, however, this latter approach is usually impractical (see *Dexamethasone–Phenobarbital*, p. 42, and *Dexamethasone–Phenytoin*, p. 45).

Displacement from Binding Sites—Methandrostenolone displaces oxyphenbutazone from plasma protein binding sites and increases the drug's serum levels. Although no clinical effects have been noted, patients treated with these drugs concurrently should be monitored for signs of oxyphenbutazone-induced adverse effects (see *Oxyphenbutazone–Methandrostenolone*, p. 165).

Aspirin, in large doses, has displaced endogenous corticosteroids from plasma proteins in animals. However, the displacement was not observed in humans and the clinical significance of this effect is not established (see *Aspirin–Hydrocortisone*, p. 18).

Opposing Physiological Actions—A third clinical interaction is the prevention by corticosteroids of the hypoglycemic actions of oral agents and insulin. This interaction occurs because corticosteroids promote intense gluconeogenesis and glycogenolysis activity in the liver, thus raising the serum glucose. In diabetes mellitus, treatment with corticosteroids may result in deterioration of diabetic control as measured by blood and urine glucose tests. Patients originally nondiabetic may develop hyperglycemia and glycosuria while receiving prolonged anti-inflammatory corticosteroid therapy. If the patient is already taking oral hypoglycemic

agents for diabetes, the dose can be increased accordingly. Often, this dose is still ineffective and insulin must be used at a dose adequate to control the diabetes (see *Chlorpropamide–Cortisone*, p. 38).

Miscellaneous—Methandrostenolone and other C-17-alkylated androgens in therapeutic doses increase the hypoprothrombinemic action of warfarin significantly. The mechanism of action is unclear, but methandrostenolone may increase the affinity of the receptor sites for warfarin (see *Warfarin–Methandrostenolone*, p. 289).

References

(1) G. W. Liddle, "Clinical Pharmacology of the Anti-Inflammatory Steroids," *Clin. Pharmacol. Ther.*, 2, 615 (1961).

(2) G. W. Thorn, "Clinical Considerations in the Use of Corticosteroids," *N. Engl. J. Med.*, 274, 775 (1966).

(3) F. H. Meyers *et al.*, "Review of Medical Pharmacology," 2nd ed., Lange Medical Publications, Los Altos, Calif., 1970, pp. 314–325.

(4) "The Pharmacological Basis of Therapeutics," 5th ed., L. S. Goodman and A. Gilman, Eds., Macmillan, New York, NY 10022, 1975, pp. 1477–1502.

(5) G. Weissman, "The Many-Faceted Lysosome," *Hosp. Practice*, February 1968, p. 30.

(6) A. M. Lefer and R. L. Verrier, "Role of Corticosteroids in the Treatment of Circulatory Collapse States," *Clin. Pharmacol. Ther.*, 11, 630 (1970).

(7) A. L. Graber *et al.*, "Natural History of Pituitary–Adrenal Recovery following Long-Term Suppression with Corticosteroids," *J. Clin. Endocrinol. Metab.*, 25, 11 (1965).

(8) J. B. Nielsen *et al.*, "Long Term Treatment with Corticosteroids in Rheumatoid Arthritis," *Acta Med. Scand.*, 173, 177 (1960).

(9) T. T. Amatruda *et al.*, "A Study of the Mechanism of the Steroid Withdrawal Syndrome. Evidence for Integrity of the Hypothalamic–Pituitary–Adrenal System," *J. Clin. Endocrinol. Metab.*, 20, 339 (1960).

(10) R. L. Ney, "Alternate-Day Steroid Therapy," *Hosp. Practice*, August 1968, p. 57.

(11) G. T. Perkoff *et al.*, "Studies in Disorders of Muscle, XII, Myopathy Due to the Administration of Therapeutic Amounts of 17-Hydroxycorticoids," *Amer. J. Med.*, 26, 891 (1959).

(12) A. H. Conney, "Pharmacological Implications of Microsomal Enzyme Induction," *Pharmacol. Rev.*, 19, 317 (1967).

Diuretic Therapy

To maintain homeostasis, a proper balance between the external and internal environments must be achieved. The kidneys, under neurological and endocrine control, are largely responsible for maintaining this balance by regulating the volume and composition of body fluids (1). In individuals with no underlying pathology, the volume and composition of body fluids are generally governed by the body's needs. To maintain the proper degree of hydration and electrolyte balance, the kidneys eliminate or retain variable amounts of water and selected ions including bicarbonate, chloride, hydrogen, phosphate, potassium, sodium, and sulfate.

Individuals with underlying pathology (*e.g.,* disturbances in cardiac, hepatic, or renal function) often retain large amounts of sodium and water, resulting in expansion of extracellular fluid volume and in accumulation of fluid in the extravascular space. The rate at which edema fluid accumulates is a reflection of the disparity between sodium intake and sodium excretion (2). Although some patients can tolerate slight fluid retention with little discomfort, reducing the amount of edema fluid generally results in improving the patient's sense of well-being and functional capacity. In addition, the elimination of edema fluid can facilitate treatment of the primary pathological condition.

Therapeutic Indications

A major indication for the use of diuretic agents is the mobilization of edema fluid. As diuretic therapy is an empirical approach to the management of patients with edema and does not correct the underlying pathology, the use of diuretics should be regarded as symptomatic rather than curative therapy (3).

Cardiac Failure—Diuretics may be used successfully to relieve the edema associated with either right-sided or left-sided cardiac failure.

Right-Sided Heart Failure—Oral diuretics of moderate potency, *e.g.,* chlorthalidone and the thiazides, are usually effective in relieving peripheral edema resulting from right-sided failure. If the edema is refractory to this type of management, more potent diuretics (*e.g.,* ethacrynic acid, furosemide, or the mercurial diuretics) are indicated (4). Although the mercurial diuretics may promote adequate diuresis, they must be given parenterally, may produce many untoward reactions (including severe renal damage), and are self-limiting because of the production of systemic alkalosis (4). Ethacrynic acid and furosemide are both effective when administered orally and are generally considered to be less toxic than the mercurial diuretics. Intermittent administration may be more effective than continuous daily therapy in promoting a negative sodium balance and loss of edema (5). Additionally, this approach may be employed to allow the kidneys to correct possible electrolyte imbalance caused by the diuretics.

Parenteral diuretic therapy (usually ethacrynic acid or furosemide) may be indicated in patients with right-sided heart failure if it is accompanied by intestinal blockade or if vomiting is present. However, caution must be used because the rapid, copious diuresis occurring after intravenous administration of diuretics may cause peripheral circulatory failure (4). High doses of ethacrynic acid or furosemide administered intravenously have been associated with both transient and permanent deafness (6, 7). This effect is more likely to occur if the patient's renal function is impaired (7).

Once the edema has been corrected, thiazide diuretics may be used to prevent edema from reoccurring. If these agents do not control or prevent recurrent edema, it may be necessary to use ethacrynic acid or furosemide. Although the latter drugs are more potent than the thiazides, they may also be used in ambulatory outpatients (8) as well as in hospitalized patients. The use of spironolactone or triamterene with either ethacrynic acid, furosemide, or the thiazides can enhance the natriuretic effect of the latter agents (9). Additionally, both spironolactone and triamterene conserve potassium, decreasing or eliminating the need for potassium supplements (10). These drugs should be used with caution, particularly in patients with impaired renal function, since they can produce hyperkalemia (3, 11).

Left-Sided Heart Failure—Mild left-sided heart failure may respond well to the administration of thiazide diuretics. In more severe cases characterized by pulmonary edema, administration of ethacrynic acid or furosemide intravenously may be necessary to promote a more rapid diuresis (12, 13). In some cases, however, clinical improvement precedes significant diuresis. This fact suggests that a brisk diuresis may not be a prerequisite to clinical improvement in acute pulmonary edema (14).

Generally, excessive salt and water intake should be restricted in patients with either peripheral or pulmonary edema. Daily weighing of the patient serves to monitor the patient's water balance and allows the practitioner to adjust diuretic therapy accordingly. Close attention should be paid to the patient's potassium balance, particularly if the patient is receiving cardiac glycosides. It must be emphasized that diuretic agents only provide symptomatic relief and do not constitute treatment of the primary disorder (the drug of choice is one of the cardiac glycosides).

Hepatic Disease—Decreased plasma osmotic pressure, resulting from the liver's inability to synthesize albumin, and portal hypertension are evident in patients with parenchymal liver disease and result in the formation of edema and ascites. A decrease in the circulating blood volume results in secondary hyperaldosteronism, a diminished glomerular filtration rate, excessive renal tubular reabsorption of sodium, and hypokalemia.

In mild cases, the replenishment of plasma albumin, by providing adequate protein, carbohydrate, and vitamin intake, may be sufficient to correct the edema (4). In more severe cases, diuretic therapy is indicated. Care must be taken not to disturb the precarious electrolyte balance of the cirrhotic patient by the overuse of diuretics. The dose of diuretic should be the smallest possible to achieve a gradual diuresis. Severe sodium restriction is often more effective and safer than diuretic therapy of any kind (15). The use of an aldosterone antagonist (e.g., spironolactone or triamterene) alone or with a thiazide diuretic also may be indicated.

The thiazides may aggravate borderline hepatic disease. Therefore, caution is essential if these agents must be employed in the treatment of cirrhotic edema and ascites (16, 17). Their usefulness depends in part on an adequate glomerular filtration rate (>20–25 ml/min) (18). The secondary hyperaldosteronism present in many cirrhotic patients contributes to salt and water retention.

Intractable ascites may require the use of ethacrynic acid or furosemide. These agents produce azotemia and hepatic encephalopathy more frequently than do the thiazides (16). Potassium-sparing diuretics or potassium supplements may be indicated to prevent hypokalemic alkalosis caused by hepatic disease.

Renal Disease–Nephrotic Syndrome—Edema in patients with the nephrotic syndrome is less responsive to thiazide diuretics than is cardiac or cirrhotic edema (4). Use of corticosteroids is the treatment of choice in this condition (19). Excessive aldosterone secreted by these patients contributes to the formation of edema, and aldosterone antagonists such as spironolactone have been suggested, but this type of therapy has proven unsuccessful. Patients with resistant edema usually respond to high doses of ethacrynic acid or furosemide. If these measures fail, an osmotic diuretic such as mannitol may be effective in inducing diuresis.

Chronic Renal Failure—Diuretics are often effective in the control of the hypertension, azotemia, and edema associated with renal failure.

Salt restriction and the diuretics are important in the control and sometimes in the reduction of azotemia. It has been shown that, as the glomerular filtration rate falls, the percentage of filtered sodium excreted increases. Patients with renal pathology can be separated into two groups: severe "salt wasters" and "non-salt wasters."

Salt wasters will develop severe azotemia if supplemental sodium chloride is not administered. These patients require sodium chloride doses of 10–20 g/day in addition to their normal dietary intake. Patients who are not salt wasters also should receive sodium chloride doses of 2–5 g/day in addition to a normal salt diet. These patients also must be adequately hydrated. Significant improvement in renal function and a decrease in uremia have been demonstrated in patients with chronic renal failure receiving adequate sodium and fluids (20).

It is in the adequately hydrated patient with excess sodium that a diuretic would be expected to induce a significant diuresis with excretion of urea and creatinine (4). Ethacrynic acid and furosemide are the diuretics of choice in renal failure because of their potency and tendency to increase renal blood flow. Large doses of ethacrynic acid or furosemide (800–1000 or 800–1500 mg/day, respectively) are often required to treat patients with edema and/or azotemia (4, 21, 22).

Acute Renal Failure—Metolazone may be useful in patients with a glomerular filtration rate less than 20 ml/min and in unresponsive patients, if treated concurrently with furosemide (23). Diuretics may be useful in the early stages of acute failure. They are efficacious in maintaining an adequate urine output in early renal failure secondary to circulatory dysfunction when decreased renal perfusion may progress to acute tubular necrosis (4).

There is good evidence to support the use of mannitol as a prophylactic agent in any situation likely to give rise to acute tubular necrosis (24–26). Ethacrynic acid or furosemide is sometimes administered concurrently with mannitol to manage oliguric patients. The success achieved with this regimen is attributed to the ability of the two former agents to reach the renal tubule without depending on glomerular filtration (27).

Diabetes Insipidus—Thiazide diuretics are used in the management of diabetes insipidus due to pituitary or renal tubular disease. These agents decrease urine output directly attributable to sodium depletion. Patients with primary polydipsia should not receive thiazides because dilutional hyponatremia can ensue (28). This condition results from the ability of the thiazide diuretics to inhibit the excretion of solute-free water.

Hypertension—Thiazide diuretics are accepted as the most useful diuretics in all types of systemic hypertension. In the treatment of mild hypertension, the thiazides may be effective when used alone. In more severe hypertension, however, they must be administered with other antihypertensive agents. When this is done, smaller doses of the antihypertensive agent may be used and side effects can be minimized (29). The antinatriuretic effects of drugs as guanethidine, hydralazine, mecamylamine, and reserpine can be reversed by the thiazides (30). Ethacrynic acid and furosemide are as effective as the thiazides in the treatment of hypertension (4). In view of their potency, greater risk of side effects, and short duration of action, they probably should not be used in place of the thiazides in the routine management of hypertension (4). Spironolactone can be used to control increased blood pressure when it is associated with elevated mineralocorticoid production (31, 32) and in low renin hypertension (33). Triamterene exhibits only a mild antihypertensive activity when used alone. However, when used with a thiazide diuretic, spironolactone and triamterene serve the additional purpose of suppressing potassium loss (34).

Pregnancy—Edema in pregnancy, except when secondary to renal disease, responds to thiazide diuretic therapy (35), although mild edema of pregnancy probably should not be treated with diuretics (36). The toxemias may require the use of more rapidly acting, potent diuretics such as ethacrynic acid or furosemide. The use of thiazides as prophylactic agents against toxemia of pregnancy must be approached with caution because of possible fetal and maternal morbidity, especially with regard to hematopoietic disorders (4, 37).

Drug Poisoning—The osmotic diuresis induced by mannitol is useful in hastening the excretion of barbiturates and salicylates. Alkalinization of the urine with acetazolamide or sodium bicarbonate may result in the enhanced excretion of weak organic acids. Acetazolamide should not be used in the treatment of salicylate poisoning because of potential enhancement of salicylate-induced latent acidosis. Acidification of urine with ammonium chloride may result in enhanced excretion of weak organic bases. Intravenous administration of ethacrynic acid or furosemide may further enhance the excretion of certain drugs (38). When diuretics are used in the treatment of drug overdosage, it is important to hydrate the patient adequately to maintain the diuresis.

Miscellaneous—Mannitol is useful in the acute reduction of cerebrospinal and intraocular fluid pressure and volume. It enhances the diffusion of water from these fluids into the plasma and the extracellular space by increasing the osmolarity of plasma and establishing an osmotic gradient between plasma and transepithelial fluids.

Acetazolamide also is used to decrease intraocular pressure. Unlike mannitol, however, it produces a fall in intraocular pressure by inhibiting aqueous humor formation (1). This action is independent of the systemic acid–base balance changes produced by acetazolamide. Because acetazolamide use results in systemic acidosis, it is used as an anticonvulsant in the treatment of some types of epilepsy. It also is effective in treating certain patients with periodic paralysis (39). Initially found effective in the hyperkalemic-type periodic paralysis, acetazolamide also is effective in the hypokalemic type as well, although the mechanism for this action is not well understood. The systemic acidosis produced by acetazolamide alters potassium movement across the cell membrane and may be partially responsible for the drug's effectiveness (40). Some investigators also recommend thiazides for the treatment of hypercalciuria and renal tubular acidosis (41).

Pharmacological Mechanisms

The diuretics' major pharmacological effect is to block sodium reabsorption in the renal tubules. The action subsequently results in natriuresis and diuresis. However, the mechanisms by which the diuretics accomplish this inhibition are largely unknown and the sites of action are varied.

Osmotic Diuretics—Mannitol is a hexahydroxy alcohol and exemplifies the osmotic diuretic. It is essentially not metabolized and is only minimally reabsorbed when presented to the renal tubules. The hyperosmolarity of the glomerular filtrate prevents water reabsorption from the proximal tubule, resulting in diuresis and natriuresis. A water diuresis can be produced by mannitol without significant loss of sodium if distal tubular reabsorption of sodium is active. This effect can lead to the production of hypernatremia because of the loss of water without the loss of sodium (1). Isosorbide and glycerol are osmotic diuretics used to decrease intracranial and intraocular pressure (42).

Organomercurial Diuretics—Mercurial diuretics promote the excretion of chloride and sodium by acting in the proximal tubule and the early segment of the distal tubule, presumably by liberating the mercuric ion which reacts with sulfhydryl receptors (40, 43, 44). The loss of chloride may reach such proportions as to produce hypochloremic alkalosis. When this occurs, mercurials lose their effectiveness. Administration of carbonic anhydrase inhibitors or acidifying salts such as ammonium chloride can correct the alkalosis, thereby restoring the mercurials' effect. Potassium loss produced by the mercurials is not as great as that produced by other kaliuretic diuretics (45).

Loop of Henle Diuretics—Ethacrynic acid and furosemide are potent saluretic agents acting on the ascending limb of the loop of Henle and distal tubules (45–48). These agents are effective even in the presence of decreased glomerular filtration, a condition in which other agents such as the thiazides are relatively ineffective. These diuretics produce significant kaliuresis, and their use can lead to hypokalemia. Thus, concurrent administration of supplemental potassium or potassium-sparing agents is often necessary. The chloride loss produced by these diuretics can lead to hypochloremic alkalosis. This condition, however, does not impair their diuretic action since these agents can exert their diuretic effect in the presence of electrolyte and acid–base disturbances. The major difference between ethacrynic acid and furosemide is that the latter has a broader dose–response curve (49).

Distal Tubule Diuretics—*Thiazides*—Although they have a mild initial inhibitory effect on carbonic anhydrase, the main mechanism of action of the thiazide diuretics appears to be direct blocking of sodium reabsorption in the early portion of the distal tubule (cortical-diluting segment) (50). This action results in natriuresis accompanied by marked bicarbonate (only initially), chloride, potassium, and water losses. The intensity of chloruresis produced by the thiazides is greater than that seen with carbonic anhydrase inhibitors. In contrast to the carbonic anhydrase inhibitors and mercurial diuretics, the thiazides remain active even when systemic acidosis or alkalosis is present.

The antihypertensive effect of the thiazides has been attributed to at least two mechanisms: (*a*) sodium depletion and plasma volume reduction, and (*b*) a decrease in peripheral resistance due to arteriolar wall sodium depletion or a direct effect (51). Chlorthalidone, metolazone, and quinethazone have pharmacological activity indistinguishable from that of the thiazides (52).

Aldosterone Antagonists—The mineralocorticoid, aldosterone, acts as a potent antidiuretic agent by increasing the renal tubular reabsorption of chloride, sodium, and water with concurrent potassium loss. The increased retention of salt and water sometimes associated with some pathological states (*e.g.,* congestive heart failure, liver disease, and the nephrotic syndrome) is thought to be due in part to increased aldosterone secretion (53).

Spironolactone blocks the effect of aldosterone by competitive inhibition in the distal portion of the renal tubule (1). This inhibition results in decreased excretion of potassium and decreased reabsorption of sodium and chloride which promotes a mild diuresis. When administered alone, spironolactone exhibits a slow onset of action (3–7 days) and promotes only variable diuresis. Concurrent administration of an agent that acts in the early segment of the distal renal tubule, such as a thiazide diuretic, produces a more predictable diuresis with a faster onset of action than that achieved with spironolactone alone (54). Additionally, spironolactone is useful clinically in decreasing the potassium loss produced by potassium-depleting diuretics. However, the potassium-sparing effect of spironolactone can lead to hyperkalemia, particularly in patients with decreased renal function, which can seriously disrupt therapy and may even be life threatening.

Triamterene—Triamterene acts in the distal portion of the renal tubule, promoting natriuresis and diuresis while conserving potassium. Evidence indicates that this action is not due to aldosterone antagonism, but rather to a blocking of sodium reabsorption and potassium secretion at a site other than where aldosterone exerts its effect (54, 55). As with spironolactone, use of triamterene can lead to hyperkalemia (56).

Carbonic Anhydrase Inhibitors—Carbonic anhydrase catalyzes the hydration of carbon dioxide to carbonic acid in the renal tubule. The enzyme also acts as a catalyst for the dissociation of carbonic acid to carbon dioxide and water. The hydrogen ions produced by the ionization of carbonic acid are available for sodium and potassium exchange or for combination with bicarbonate ions to form carbonic acid and carbon dioxide, thereby perpetuating the cycle (57).

Inhibition of carbonic anhydrase decreases the concentration of hydrogen ion available for exchange. The decreased hydrogen-ion concentration leads to natriuresis and therefore diuresis. The use of a carbonic anhydrase inhibitor does not greatly alter chloride excretion. However, there may be a marked potassium loss with resulting hypokalemia.

The urine, normally acidic, becomes alkaline, and hydrogen ion is retained leading to metabolic acidosis. When acidosis occurs, the patient becomes refractory to the diuretic effect of the carbonic anhydrase inhibitors. The acid–base imbalance must be corrected before these agents are again effective.

Contraindications and Complications

Electrolyte disturbances that can be produced by all commonly employed diuretics include acute sodium depletion, chronic sodium depletion, hypokalemia, hyperkalemia, and chronic dilutional hyponatremia, as well as alterations in calcium, chloride, and magnesium balance (58–60). The effect of the disturbances on the patient is determined by the severity of the imbalance.

Use of diuretics may result in electrolyte imbalance and aggravate hepatic encephalopathy, although there is no evidence that diuretic usage causes the hepatorenal syndrome.

The mercurial diuretics should not be used in acute nephritis as they may intensify the existing renal lesion (61). Caution must be used when administering mannitol or other osmotic diuretics in acute nephritis because they can produce an acute expansion of the extracellular fluid volume with resulting pulmonary edema (55). Mannitol, while useful in the differential diagnosis of acute

oliguria and acute anuria, should not be used in the anuric patient if the first dose is not effective in promoting urine flow. The continued use of mannitol in this case can lead to further renal damage (1).

Drug hypersensitivity to the diuretic agents has been reported frequently (56). Blood dyscrasias are occasionally encountered during diuretic therapy and have been attributed to these agents.

The thiazides are reported to cause pancreatitis in some patients (62). The relationship of this pancreatitis to the decreased glucose tolerance produced mainly in prediabetic patients by ethacrynic acid and the thiazides is not clear (63). The thiazide diuretics also cause hyperglycemia and hyperuricemia.

The mechanism of the ototoxic effect produced by intravenous ethacrynic acid administration may be related to the retention of ototoxic congeners in patients with impaired renal function (7).

Interactions

Aminoglycoside Antibiotics—The aminoglycoside antibiotics including amikacin, gentamicin, kanamycin, neomycin, and streptomycin are all potentially ototoxic. The reported ototoxicity of ethacrynic acid and furosemide constitutes a basis for caution if these drugs are indicated in the treatment of a patient receiving an aminoglycoside antibiotic. Special caution is necessary if one of these drugs is used alone or concurrently in patients with impaired renal function (see *Kanamycin–Ethacrynic Acid*, p. 120).

Anticoagulants—Thiazide diuretics and ethacrynic acid may enhance the effects of the oral anticoagulants (64). However, the clinical importance of the drug interaction is unknown.

Anticonvulsants—Patients receiving anticonvulsant therapy have been found to have a decreased response to furosemide therapy. Although some anticonvulsants may induce microsomal enzymes, this mechanism is not likely to be responsible since furosemide is not metabolized to any great extent. It seems possible that anticonvulsants decrease absorption of furosemide as well as decrease the sensitivity of the renal tubule to the diuretic (65). More clinical studies are necessary to determine the clinical outcome of this drug interaction.

Antihypertensive Agents—The use of an antihypertensive agent such as guanethidine, methyldopa, or a ganglionic blocking agent with diuretics can result in orthostatic hypotension. Reduction of the dose of the antihypertensive drug may be indicated (see *Guanethidine–Hydrochlorothiazide*, p. 88).

Cardiac Glycosides—The concurrent administration of diuretics and a cardiac glycoside is common in the treatment of edema associated with congestive heart failure. The diuretic-induced hypokalemia enhances the cardiotoxicity of the cardiac glycosides.

When taking these drugs concurrently, the patient should be monitored closely for possible hypokalemia. If hypokalemia occurs, possible measures to reduce the incidence of this adverse interaction include: (*a*) administering liquid oral potassium supplements (preferably as the chloride salt), (*b*) placing the patient on a potassium-rich diet, and (*c*) adding a potassium-sparing diuretic to the therapeutic regimen while monitoring the patient closely for signs of hyperkalemia (see *Digitalis–Chlorothiazide*, p. 52).

Hypoglycemics—The hyperglycemic effect of the thiazides, but probably not ethacrynic acid or furosemide, may result in the loss of diabetic control in patients receiving oral hypoglycemics or insulin or controlled with diet alone. In addition, the significant kaliuresis and resulting hypokalemia produced by almost all diuretics may enhance hyperglycemia (66). Appropriate measures to counteract this effect include: (*a*) discontinuing the diuretic, (*b*) increasing the dose of the hypoglycemic agent (including insulin), (*c*) providing potassium supplementation, and/or (*d*) using a potassium-sparing diuretic (see *Chlorpropamide–Hydrochlorothiazide*, p. 40).

Lithium—Limited data indicate that sodium- and potassium-depleting diuretics increase the serum level of lithium. Concurrent use should be avoided whenever possible. Patients receiving these agents concurrently should be monitored closely for symptoms of lithium toxicity (see *Lithium Carbonate–Chlorothiazide*, p. 137).

Nondepolarizing Muscle Relaxants—The hypokalemia produced by the diuretics may result in the loss of deep tendon reflexes and progress to paralysis. It is theoretically possible that the administration of a nondepolarizing muscle relaxant in the presence of marked hypokalemia could produce a more intensive neuromuscular blockade than in a normokalemic patient. Although this interaction potentially exists, there are no reports of its occurrence clinically. Electrolyte determinations should be obtained prior to the use of the nondepolarizing agents and corrective measures taken if appropriate (see *Tubocurarine–Chlorothiazide*, p. 253).

Salicylates—Aspirin reduced the natriuretic effects of spironolactone in normal subjects, but this drug interaction has not been reported in clinical practice. Aspirin did not affect spironolactone's antihypertensive action in a small group of low renin hypertensive patients. Until more clinical data are available for evaluation, patients receiving spironolactone and aspirin concurrently should be monitored closely for symptoms of decreased clinical response to spironolactone (see *Spironolactone–Aspirin*, p. 223).

Uricosurics—Thiazide diuretics frequently produce an elevation of the plasma level of uric acid by a mechanism not yet fully understood, but it may be due to contraction of plasma volume. Although clinical gout occurs rarely in previously nongouty patients, the possibility of thiazides disrupting the control of gouty patients receiving uricosuric therapy must be considered (see *Probenecid–Chlorothiazide*, p. 208).

References

(1) C. L. Gantt, "Diuretic Therapy," *Rational Drug Ther.*, *6*, 1 (August 1972).
(2) W. G. Walker, "Indications and Contraindications for Diuretic Therapy," *Ann. N.Y. Acad. Sci.*, *139*, 481 (1966).
(3) E. C. Perez-Stable and B. J. Materson, "Diuretic Drug Therapy of Edema," *Med. Clin. N. Amer.*, *55*, 359 (1971).
(4) J. L. Anderton and P. Kincaid-Smith, "Diuretics. II. Clinical Considerations," *Drugs*, *1*, 141 (1971).
(5) P. J. Cannon *et al.*, "Ethacrynic Acid Effectiveness and Mode of Diuretic Action in Man," *Circulation*, *31*, 5 (1965).
(6) R. H. Lloyd-Mostyn and I. J. Lord, "Ototoxicity of Intravenous Frusemide," *Lancet*, *ii*, 1156 (1971).
(7) V. K. G. Pillay *et al.*, "Transient and Permanent Deafness following Treatment with Ethacrynic Acid in Renal Failure," *Lancet*, *i*, 77 (1969).
(8) A. C. Newell, "Ethacrynic Acid in the Treatment of Ambulatory Patients," *Med. J. Aust.*, *1*, 320 (1970).
(9) D. J. Ginsberg *et al.*, "Metabolic Studies with the Diuretic Triamterene in Patients with Cirrhosis and Ascites," *N. Engl. J. Med.*, *271*, 1229 (1964).
(10) D. E. Hutcheon, "Effects of Antikaluretic Diuretics on Biochemical Complications of Thiazide Therapy," *Pharmacologist*, *9*, 196 (1967).
(11) A. B. Cohen, "Hyperkalemic Effects of Triamterene," *Ann. Intern. Med.*, *65*, 521 (1966).
(12) S. L. Fine and R. I. Levy, "Ethacrynic Acid in Acute Pulmonary Edema," *N. Engl. J. Med.*, *273*, 583 (1965).
(13) K. K. Gupta *et al.*, "Frusemide in Acute Pulmonary Oedema," *Lancet*, *i*, 1386 (1967).
(14) M. Lesch *et al.*, "Controlled Study Comparing Ethacrynic Acid to Mercaptomerin in the Treatment of Acute Pulmonary Edema," *N. Engl. J. Med.*, *279*, 115 (1968).

(15) "Textbook of Medicine," P. B. Beeson and W. McDermott, Eds., Saunders, Philadelphia, PA 19105, 1975, pp. 1346–1350.

(16) S. Sherlock et al., "Complications of Diuretic Therapy in Hepatic Cirrhosis," Lancet, i, 1049 (1966).

(17) R. M. Myerson, "The Diuretic Effect of Polythiazide in Cirrhosis of the Liver," Curr. Ther. Res., 3, 431 (1961).

(18) P. Vesin et al., "L'Insuffisance Venale Fonctionnelle du Cirrhotique Ascitique. Etude Critique du Role Diuretiques," Bull. Mem. Soc. Med. Hop. Paris, 113, 778 (1962).

(19) "Current Therapy," H. F. Conn, Ed., Saunders, Philadelphia, PA 19105, 1975, pp. 477–480.

(20) H. P. McDonald, Jr., and R. K. Waterhouse, "Chronic Renal Failure from Urological Diseases: Treatment by Sodium Balancing and Low-Protein Diet of High Biological Value," J. Urol., 103, 262 (1970).

(21) J. F. Maher and G. E. Schreiner, "Studies on Ethacrynic Acid in Patients with Refractory Edema," Ann. Intern. Med., 62, 15 (1965).

(22) R. Muth, "Diuretic Properties of Furosemide in Renal Disease," Ann. Intern. Med., 69, 249 (1968).

(23) "Metolazone," Med. Lett., 16, 77 (1974).

(24) K. G. Barry et al., "Mannitolization I. The Prevention and Therapy of Oliguria Associated with Cross-Clamping of the Abdominal Aorta," Surgery, 50, 335 (1961).

(25) J. L. Dawson, "Jaundice and Anoxic Renal Damage: Protective Effect of Mannitol," Brit. Med. J., 1, 810 (1964).

(26) A. Boda et al., "The Influence of Mannitol on Electrolyte and Water Excretion following Trauma," Surgery, 52, 188 (1968).

(27) J. B. Mann and H. R. Giamore, "Reversal of Mannitol-Fast Oliguria by Intravenous Ethacrynic Acid," Proc. Amer. Soc. Nephathol., 1, 44 (1967).

(28) R. M. Kennedy and L. E. Earley, "Profound Hyponatremia Resulting from a Thiazide-Induced Decrease in Urinary Diluting Capacity in a Patient with Primary Polydipsia," N. Engl. J. Med., 282, 1185 (1970).

(29) C. T. Dollery et al., "Actions of Chlorothiazide in Hypertension," Proc. Roy. Soc. Med., 53, 592 (1960).

(30) W. A. Freyburger et al., "Antidiuretic Properties of Hypotensive Agents, with Special Reference to N,N-Diallylmelamine-N-oxide (U-20388)," Pharmacologist, 8, 182 (1966).

(31) R. F. Spark and J. C. Melby, "Aldosterone in Hypertension. The Spironolactone Response Test," Ann. Intern. Med., 69, 685 (1968).

(32) J. J. Brown et al., "Spironolactone in Hyperaldosteronism," Brit. Med. J., 4, 688 (1969).

(33) R. F. Spark and J. C. Melby, "Hypertension and Low Plasma Renin Activity: Presumptive Evidence for Mineralocorticoid Excess," Ann. Intern. Med., 75, 831 (1971).

(34) R. E. Spiekerman et al., "Potassium-Sparing Effects of Triamterene in the Treatment of Hypertension," Circulation, 34, 524 (1966).

(35) H. S. Assali et al., "Diuretic Effect of Chlorothiazide in Toxemia of Pregnancy," J. Lab. Clin. Med., 52, 423 (1968).

(36) M. D. Lindheimer and A. I. Katz, "Sodium and Diuretics in Pregnancy," N. Engl. J. Med., 288, 891 (1973).

(37) I. MacGillivary, "Bendroflumethiazide and Pregnancy," Amer. J. Obstet. Gynecol., 91, 879 (1965).

(38) A. L. Linton et al., "Forced Diuresis and Haemodialysis in Severe Barbiturate Intoxication," Lancet, i, 1008 (1964).

(39) J. S. Resnick et al., "Acetazolamide Prophylaxis in Hypokalemic Periodic Paralysis," N. Engl. J. Med., 278, 582 (1968).

(40) S. Adler et al., "Intracellular Acid–Base Regulation. I. Response of Muscle Cells to Changes in CO_2 Tension or Extracellular Bicarbonate Concentration," J. Clin. Invest., 44, 8 (1965).

(41) M. Martinez-Maldonado et al., "Diuretics in Nonedematous States. Physiological Basis for the Clinical Use," Arch. Intern. Med., 131, 797 (1973).

(42) "Isosorbide," Med. Lett., 16, 83 (1974).

(43) G. H. Mudge and I. M. Weiner, "The Mechanism of Action of Mercurial and Xanthine Diuretics," Ann. N.Y. Acad. Sci., 71, 344 (1958).

(44) E. J. Cafruny et al., "Effects of the Mercurial Diuretic Mersalyl, on Protein-Bound Sulfhydryl Groups in the Cytoplasm of Rat Kidney Cells," J. Pharmacol., 115, 390 (1955).

(45) E. J. Cafruny et al., "The Pharmacology of Mercurial Diuretics," Ann. N.Y. Acad. Sci., 139, 362 (1966).

(46) D. W. Seldin et al., "Localization of Diuretic Action from the Pattern of Water and Electrolyte Excretion," Ann. N.Y. Acad. Sci., 139, 328 (1966).

(47) W. Suki et al., "The Site of Action of Furosemide and Other Sulfonamide Diuretics in the Dog," J. Clin. Invest., 44, 1458 (1965).

(48) M. Goldberg, "Ethacrynic Acid: Site and Mode of Action," Ann. N.Y. Acad. Sci., 139, 443 (1966).

(49) "The Pharmacological Basis of Therapeutics," 5th ed., L. S. Goodman and A. Gilman, Eds., Macmillan, New York, NY 10022, 1975, p. 835.

(50) S. A. Kleit et al., "Diuretic Therapy—Current Status," Amer. Heart J., 79, 700 (1970).

(51) P. Lund-Johansen, "Hemodynamic Changes in Long-Term Diuretic Therapy of Essential Hypertension, A Comparative Study of Chlorthalidone, Polythiazide and Hydrochlorothiazide," Acta Med. Scand., 187, 509 (1970).

(52) "The Pharmacological Basis of Therapeutics," 5th ed., L. S. Goodman and A. Gilman, Eds., Macmillan, New York, NY 10022, 1975, p. 830.

(53) H. P. Wolff et al., "Role of Aldosterone in Edema Formation," Ann. N.Y. Acad. Sci., 139, 285 (1966).

(54) G. W. Liddle, "Aldosterone Antagonists and Triamterene," Ann. N.Y. Acad. Sci., 139, 466 (1966).

(55) K. D. Gardner, "A Rational Approach to Diuretic Therapy: A Review for Physicians," Hawaii Med. J., 29, 633 (1970).

(56) K. B. Hansen and A. D. Bender, "Changes in Serum Potassium Levels Occurring in Patients Treated with Triamterene and a Triamterene-Hydrochlorothiazide Combination," Clin. Pharmacol. Ther., 8, 392 (1967).

(57) K. C. Leibman et al., "Nature of the Inhibition of Carbonic Anhydrase by Acetazolamide and Benzthiazide," J. Pharmacol. Exp. Ther., 131, 271 (1964).

(58) W. G. Walker, "Indications and Contraindications for Diuretic Therapy," Ann. N.Y. Acad. Sci., 139, 481 (1966).

(59) W. N. Suki et al., "Mechanism of the Effect of Thiazide Diuretics on Calcium and Uric Acid," Clin. Res., 15, 78 (1967).

(60) F. E. Demartini et al., "Effect of Ethacrynic Acid on Calcium and Magnesium Excretion," Proc. Soc. Exp. Biol. Med., 124, 320 (1967).

(61) L. E. Earley, "Diuretics," N. Engl. J. Med., 276, 966 (1967).

(62) A. L. Cornish et al., "Effects of Chlorothiazide on the Pancreas," N. Engl. J. Med., 265,
673 (1961).

(63) A. P. Shapiro et al., "Effect of Thiazides on
Carbohydrate Metabolism in Patients with
Hypertension," N. Engl. J. Med., 265, 1028
(1961).

(64) J. Koch-Weser and E. M. Sellers, "Drug
Interactions with Coumarin Anticoagulants,"
N. Engl. J. Med., 285, 547 (1971).

(65) S. Ahmad, "Renal Insensitivity to Frusemide
Caused by Chronic Anticonvulsant Therapy,"
Brit. Med. J., 3, 657 (1974).

(66) F. W. Wolff et al., "A New Form of Experimental Diabetes," Diabetes, 12, 335 (1963).

Hypoglycemic Therapy

Diabetes mellitus may be classified into two general types. The ketoacidosis-prone (juvenile and growth-onset) type usually develops early in life and is generally characterized by a greatly reduced capacity to produce insulin. The ketoacidosis-resistant (maturity-onset) type is most likely to occur in adult life, is most frequently seen in persons over 40 years of age, and is characterized by a gradual onset of symptoms. Although patients with maturity-onset diabetes often have fasting insulin levels which are normal or near normal, these patients are unable to metabolize glucose adequately. This situation results in prolonged, elevated serum glucose levels after glucose ingestion which are characteristic of the disease. Many ketoacidosis-prone and some ketoacidosis-resistant diabetic patients are referred to as "labile" or "brittle" diabetics because their condition is unstable and difficult to manage.

Obesity is generally a contributing factor to maturity-onset diabetes mellitus. Weight reduction resulting from proper diet often produces a marked improvement in symptoms in many diabetic patients. Heredity also appears to be an important factor in the development of diabetes mellitus. A family history of diabetes is noted with many diabetic patients. Periodic screening for diabetes is recommended for individuals having a family history of the disease. Statistics also indicate that there are more diabetics among mothers giving birth to large babies [i.e., 4.54 kg (10 lb)] than among mothers giving birth to smaller babies. Additionally, there seems to be a positive correlation between a large birth weight and the eventual development of diabetes mellitus.

Characteristics of Diabetes

Diabetes mellitus is caused by an insufficient supply of insulin or interference with the action of insulin in the body although other factors may also be involved. Since insulin plays an important role in the utilization and storage of glucose, a decrease in its activity can lead to excessive amounts of glucose in the blood (hyperglycemia) and the excretion of glucose in the urine (glycosuria).

Symptoms of the diabetic state include polyuria, polydipsia, polyphagia, weight loss, visual disturbances, pruritus, pain in the hands and feet, weakness, fatigue, drowsiness, and slow healing of cuts and scratches. Not all of these symptoms will be experienced by every diabetic patient. Some will only have several while others (hidden diabetics) may not have any apparent symptoms.

Failure to control the diabetic state may lead to serious complications such as metabolic acidosis and coma. Acidosis can result from the accumulation of ketone bodies (ketosis) such as acetoacetic acid, acetone, and β-hydroxybutyric acid. These substances are produced in larger quantities when the body, unable to utilize glucose, breaks down fat and protein to supply energy.

Even when diabetes is "successfully" controlled, many long-term complications may arise. Diabetic retinopathy is one of the leading causes of blindness in the United States. Arteriosclerosis is commonly seen in diabetic patients. The impaired circulation that results from this condition often leads to ulceration of the extremities, poor wound healing, and gangrene. Additionally, angina pectoris and myocardial infarction resulting from compromised coronary blood flow are very common in older diabetic patients. Renal failure and peripheral nerve dysfunction may also result.

Laboratory Tests

Normally, the concentration of glucose in the blood or serum is 60–110 mg/100 ml (mg%). When blood levels exceed this range, chemical hyperglycemia exists. Several methods have been utilized in the screening for and diagnosis of diabetes. The 2-hr postglucose blood sugar determination is often used for screening purposes. Blood is drawn 2 hr after a 100-g glucose load or after a meal containing 100 g of carbohydrate has been ingested. An alternative, but perhaps less satisfactory, approach is the 2-hr postprandial blood sugar determination.

There are variations in the standard glucose values that have been used as the basis for screening and diagnosis. These variations result from the fact that different methods of analysis are used and different values are being measured (e.g., serum glucose values are generally 15 mg/100 ml higher than whole blood values). Furthermore, uniform opinion does not exist as to what glucose levels, determined by a particular method, suggest the possibility of diabetes.

The glucose tolerance test may be used to clarify results obtained in the screening procedures. The patient should have eaten a full diet with sufficient carbohydrate content for 3 days. Prior to the test, the patient fasts after midnight, and then a fasting blood sample and urine specimen are obtained. A solution containing 100 g of glucose (or 1.75 g/kg) is ingested, and blood and urine glucose levels are determined at appropriate intervals (*e.g.*, 30, 60, 90, 120, and 180 min after ingestion of the solution). If excessive glucose remains in the blood for a prolonged period, diabetes may be suspected.

The United States Public Health Service has developed a "point system" for the detection of diabetes based on whole blood glucose concentrations. The points are designated as follows: fasting $>$ 100 mg% $=$ 1 point; 1 hr $>$ 170 mg% $=$ 0.5 point; 2 hr $>$ 120 mg% $=$ 0.5 point; and 3 hr $>$ 110 mg% $=$ 1 point. A total of 2 points is necessary for the diagnosis of diabetes (1). These criteria may need to be adjusted to account for the influence of age on blood glucose.

If the oral glucose tolerance test is not definitive, other tests such as the intravenous glucose tolerance test [which eliminates the possibility of irregular gastrointestinal (GI) absorption], oral and intravenous tolbutamide tolerance tests, and a cortisone glucose tolerance test may be performed.

It is important to recognize that many factors can alter serum glucose levels and may lead to a mistaken interpretation of laboratory results. Many drugs, particularly corticosteroids and thiazide diuretics, produce this effect; preferably, they should be discontinued prior to the test to avoid interference.

Treatment

The goals of diabetic management include correction of the metabolic disturbances with diet and drugs, attainment and maintenance of ideal body weight, and prevention of complications associated with the disease or its therapy. Successful control can be achieved in most patients with relatively little disturbance of their normal activities.

Diet—Some form of dietary regulation is necessary in all diabetic patients. Many mild cases, particularly in elderly patients, respond to dietary control alone. If the patient can be maintained symptom free, this treatment is preferred. Since obesity is often a contributing factor to the development of diabetes, weight reduction which can be accomplished by use of a controlled diet is an important objective. Increased activity and physical training have marked effects on utilization of body fuels which are independent of insulin concentration. Both to correct the physiological changes of obesity

and to achieve negative caloric balance, increasing the daily level of physical activity in those with limited activity is of benefit (2).

Even when body weight is normal, certain dietary guidelines should be observed. Dietary requirements vary depending on factors such as the severity of the disease and physical activity, as well as weight. Adherence to a diet need not be an ordeal for the diabetic patient. A number of guides (3, 4) have been developed for these patients; they provide tables of food values as well as menu guides that include a wide selection of foods. For the most successful control, the patient should eat meals at regular times and should not skip meals or eat between them.

Insulin—The use of a pancreatic extract (containing insulin) in a diabetic patient by Banting and Best in 1922 represented a dramatic breakthrough in the treatment of diabetes mellitus. Subsequent studies showed that insulin has a molecular weight of about 6000 and is made up of two chains of amino acids joined together by disulfide linkages. Later work (5) led to a complete synthesis of human insulin. Although much information has been gathered concerning its nature and activity, many questions pertaining to its biosynthesis and secretion remain unresolved.

Insulin therapy usually is required for ketoacidosis-prone and labile diabetics and in those ketoacidosis-resistant diabetics whose condition is not controlled by diet alone. In addition, insulin may be needed during periods of stress (*e.g.*, surgery, infection, or injury) by mild diabetic patients being treated with diet alone or with oral agents. Therefore, it is important that all diabetic patients be familiar with insulin and its administration. It is also generally recommended that insulin be used in place of an oral hypoglycemic during pregnancy. (Table I describes various preparations of insulin.)

Sulfonylurea Derivatives—Because of the need to give insulin preparations parenterally, the introduction of the oral hypoglycemic agents was greeted enthusiastically. Most experience has been with the sulfonylurea derivatives of which four are available (acetohexamide, chlorpropamide, tolazamide, and tolbutamide). Although chemically related to the anti-infective sulfonamide derivatives, these agents are devoid of antibacterial activity.

The principal mechanism by which the sulfonylureas reduce serum glucose levels involves stimulation of the release of endogenous insulin from functional β-cells of the pancreas. Therefore, they are usually of value in the treatment of ketoacidosis-resistant (maturity-onset) diabetic patients who still possess some β-cell function. Other mechanisms, however, are probably also involved.

Although the therapeutic management of each patient must be individualized, the most likely candidates for successful therapy with a sulfonylurea derivative are those diabetics whose condition has developed after age 40 and who require less than 40 units of insulin daily. The sulfonylureas are of little value in treating ketoacidosis-prone diabetic subjects because of the significantly reduced capacity of these patients to secrete insulin.

Many diabetic patients are currently being adequately controlled with the use of a sulfonylurea derivative. However, a study (6) involving tolbutamide has raised questions as to the safety of this therapy. This investigation, known as The University Group Diabetes Program, has suggested that there is a greater risk of death from cardiovascular disease with tolbutamide therapy than with dietary control alone or diet and insulin therapy combined. As a result of these findings, the Food and Drug Administration has recommended (7) that the use of tolbutamide and other sulfonylurea derivatives should be limited to those patients with symptomatic maturity-onset nonketotic diabetes that cannot be adequately controlled by diet or weight loss alone and in whom the use of insulin is impractical or unacceptable. Although the evidence pre-

Table I—PROPERTIES OF VARIOUS PREPARATIONS OF INSULIN[a]

Preparation	Appearance	Protein Modifier	Approximate Time of Onset[b], hr	Approximate Duration of Action[b], hr	Compatible Mixed With
Fast acting					
Insulin injection USP (regular insulin)	Clear solution	None	1	6	All preparations
Insulin injection USP "Insulin made from zinc-insulin crystals" (regular insulin)	Clear solution	None	1	8	All preparations
Prompt insulin zinc suspension USP [c]	Cloudy suspension	None	1	14	Insulin zinc suspension
Intermediate acting					
Isophane insulin suspension USP (NPH insulin, isophane insulin)	Cloudy suspension	Protamine	2	24	Insulin injection
Insulin zinc suspension USP [d]	Cloudy suspension	None	2	24	Insulin injection, prompt insulin zinc suspension
Globin zinc insulin injection USP	Clear solution	Globin	2	18	— —
Long acting					
Protamine zinc insulin suspension USP	Cloudy suspension	Protamine	7	36	Insulin injection
Extended insulin zinc suspension USP [e]	Cloudy suspension	None	7	36	Insulin injection, prompt insulin zinc suspension

[a] Adapted with permission from "The Pharmacological Basis of Therapeutics," 5th ed., L. S. Goodman and A. Gilman, Eds., Macmillan, New York, NY 10022, 1975, p. 1517. [b] These figures are representative. The values may be expected to vary over a relatively wide range, depending on the dose and the individual patient. [c] Semilente. [d] Lente. [e] Ultralente.

sented has been challenged (8), it points out the need for careful evaluation of therapy and the need for continuing studies to answer the questions that have been raised. The FDA has proposed new labeling requirements for the hypoglycemic agents that include special warnings on cardiovascular mortality (9).

Of the sulfonylurea derivatives, tolbutamide is the most widely used. It is the shortest acting of the group and twice-daily administration is probably preferable, although satisfactory results have been reported with the administration of one daily dose in the morning. This drug is bound to plasma proteins and is subsequently oxidized to carboxytolbutamide, an inactive metabolite which is the major excretory product.

Acetohexamide is metabolized, in part, to hydroxyhexamide which, in contrast to carboxytolbutamide, possesses hypoglycemic activity greater than its parent compound (10). It is suggested that once-daily dosage is adequate in patients receiving 1 g or less/day, whereas patients who need 1.5 g/day usually benefit from twice-daily dosage (before the morning and evening meals).

Tolazamide, a newer sulfonylurea, is said to provide adequate control in some diabetics who are not responsive to other oral agents. Its duration of action may be slightly longer than that of acetohexamide. It is converted in the body to several metabolites that possess hypoglycemic activity (10), although less than that of the parent compound. When the daily dose exceeds 500 mg, the dose should be divided and given twice daily.

Chlorpropamide is the longest acting of the sulfonylureas, having a half-life of about 36 hr (10). It is more highly bound to plasma proteins than the other sulfonylureas and, although it had generally been assumed that chlorpropamide is not metabolized to a significant degree, more current evidence (11) suggests otherwise. It is usually administered in a single daily dose, although divided doses have been utilized to minimize GI intolerance.

Hypoglycemia is the most frequent adverse reaction seen with the sulfonylureas, occurring most often with chlorpropamide (12). Improper patient selection or overdosage is usually responsible.

Other reactions are usually infrequent and mild and include GI disturbances (anorexia, nausea, vomiting, and abdominal pain), dermatological reactions (erythema, urticaria, and photosensitivity), hematopoietic disorders (leukopenia and, rarely, agranulocy-

tosis), and hepatic reactions (cholestatic jaundice). Intolerance to alcohol (disulfiram-like reaction) also has been noted. The incidence of adverse effects is higher with chlorpropamide than with the other sulfonylureas (13).

The sulfonylureas must be used cautiously, if at all, in patients with hepatic or renal impairment since these organs have an important role in the metabolism and excretion of such agents. Their use during pregnancy is not recommended because of a lack of knowledge regarding their teratogenic potential.

Some patients, whose diabetic states have been adequately controlled by a sulfonylurea for even long periods, experience secondary failure. A number of reasons may be responsible for this occurrence including progressive worsening of the disease, an adaptive response of the body resulting in increased metabolism and excretion of the drug, improper selection of patients, poor adherence to diet, and inadequate dosage or failure to take medication. Use of a different sulfonylurea or phenformin may restore adequate control in these situations.

Biguanide Derivatives—Phenformin is chemically and pharmacologically different from the sulfonylureas. There has been considerable controversy as to the mechanism by which it exhibits its hypoglycemic effect and no conclusions have been reached; however, it apparently does not stimulate the release of insulin from the pancreas. Unlike the sulfonylureas, phenformin does not exhibit a hypoglycemic effect in patients without diabetes.

Phenformin is used in the treatment of ketoacidosis-resistant diabetes in a manner similar to the sulfonylureas. The results of The University Group Diabetes Program investigation (14) with phenformin suggest that its use also should be limited to those situations described for the sulfonylureas. It may be useful in some patients who do not respond to sulfonylurea therapy (primary or secondary failures) because of its different mechanism of action. The use of phenformin with a sulfonylurea is sometimes effective in ketoacidosis-resistant diabetics unresponsive to either agent alone.

The half-life of phenformin is 3 hr. The hypoglycemic effect may be prolonged to between 6 and 14 hr with the use of timed-release formulations.

GI disturbances are commonly associated with phenformin therapy. These effects can be minimized by reducing the dose or by using timed-release capsules. An unpleasant metallic taste is often a warning signal of impending GI reactions. GI symptoms may be particularly evident after the ingestion of excessive quantities of alcohol. Weakness, malaise, and weight loss may result from continued therapy.

Ketonuria has developed with phenformin therapy even when serum glucose values are relatively normal. When these values are normal, a decrease in phenformin dosage or an increased dietary intake of carbohydrates may be indicated. The condition should not be interpreted as a need for insulin until serum and urine glucose determinations have been made.

Severe and occasionally fatal lactic acidosis has occurred in patients receiving phenformin. However, because most of these patients had some degree of renal or cardiovascular impairment which could result in increased lactic acid levels, the contribution of phenformin to the development of this condition is questionable. Since the clinical picture of lactic acidosis is similar to that of diabetic ketoacidosis, it is important to distinguish which condition is actually present. Additional studies of lactate kinetics in diabetic patients with mild lactic acidosis showed a correlation between lactate turnover and oxidation. Phenformin disturbs this relationship by interfering with cellular aerobic metabolism, resulting in overproduction and underutilization of lactic acid. These findings suggest that the site of metabolic derangement leading to lactic acidosis is outside the liver (15).

Interactions

Difficulties in controlling a diabetic patient with one of the hypoglycemic agents can frequently arise when therapy with a second drug is initiated. Certain drugs cause an increase while others decrease serum glucose levels. If this effect is significant, the dose of the hypoglycemic agent (whether insulin, phenformin, or a sulfonylurea) may have to be adjusted to compensate for the altered response.

Although there is considerable variation in the nature and severity of these interactions, most interactions can be prevented by knowledge of the potential problems of such concurrent therapy or corrected rather readily once they do occur by recognition of the symptoms of the altered response and use of appropriate measures to correct the situations that result (*e.g.*, changing the dose of the hypoglycemic agent).

Although diabetes is a chronic disorder and complications usually occur, most patients can be controlled adequately by diet or with available medication with minimal difficulty.

Concurrent use of hypoglycemic agents and other drugs may alter the normal hypoglycemic response by several mechanisms. Aspirin and sulfonamides may displace sulfonylureas from plasma protein binding sites resulting in an enhanced hypoglycemic response. Clinical data on these interactions are not conclusive but indicate that patients receiving these agents concurrently should be monitored closely (see *Chlorpropamide–Aspirin*, p. 36, and *Tolbutamide–Sulfaphenazole*, p. 250).

Phenylbutazone may inhibit the excretion of the sulfonylureas and a downward adjustment of the sulfonylurea dosage may be indicated (see *Tolbutamide–Phenylbutazone*, p. 247).

Allopurinol, chloramphenicol, and dicumarol inhibit the metabolism of the oral hypoglycemics, resulting in an increased half-life and hypoglycemic action (see *Chlorpropamide–Allopurinol*, p. 35; *Tolbutamide–Chloramphenicol*, p. 243; and *Tolbutamide–Sulfaphenazole*, p. 250).

Monoamine oxidase inhibitors exert a hypoglycemic action by impairing insulin release and inhibiting hepatic gluconeogenesis. Patients maintained on hypoglycemic agents should be monitored closely for symptoms of hypoglycemia when monoamine oxidase inhibitors are added to the drug regimen since a decrease in hypoglycemic dosage may be necessary (see *Insulin–Phenelzine*, p. 110).

Glucocorticoids, phenytoin (diphenylhydantoin), and the thiazide diuretics may cause an increase in the serum glucose level. This effect may not be significant in all patients but may, in some cases, contribute to a loss of diabetic control (see *Chlorpropamide–Hydrochlorothiazide*, p. 40; *Insulin–Phenytoin*, p. 112; and *Chlorpropamide–Cortisone*, p. 38).

Alcohol (in doses as small as 70 ml of 100-proof whiskey) lowers serum glucose levels by suppressing gluconeogenesis and modifying β-cell function which results in significant hypoglycemia (see *Tolbutamide–Alcohol*, p. 240). Concurrent use of alcohol and phenformin has been associated with the development of lactic acidosis (see *Phenformin–Alcohol*, p. 177).

Propranolol interferes with carbohydrate metabolism and poses definite risks of hypoglycemia and possibly hyperglycemia. The risk is further complicated by propranolol's blockade of the warning symptoms of hypoglycemia and the compensatory reaction to this metabolic imbalance (see *Insulin–Propranolol,* p. 114).

References

(1) Q. R. Remein and H. L. Wilkerson, "The Efficiency of Screening Tests for Diabetes," *J. Chron. Dis., 16,* 6 (1961).

(2) "Diabetes Mellitus: Diagnosis and Treatment," vol. III, S. S. Fajans and K. E. Sussman, Eds., American Diabetes Association, Inc., New York, NY 10017, 1971, p. 78.

(3) "Guide for the Diabetic," Eli Lilly and Co., Indianapolis, Ind.

(4) "If You Have Diabetes," Pfizer Laboratories Division, New York, N.Y.

(5) P. G. Katsoyannis, "The Chemical Synthesis of Human and Sheep Insulin," *Amer. J. Med., 40,* 652 (1966).

(6) The University Group Diabetes Program, "A Study of the Effects of Hypoglycemic Agents on Vascular Complications in Patients with Adult-Onset Diabetes, Part 1: Design Methods, and Baseline Characteristics, Part 2: Mortality Results," *Diabetes, 19,* suppl. 2, 747, 785 (1970).

(7) "Oral Hypoglycemic Drug Labeling," *FDA Drug Bull.,* May 1972.

(8) *Clin-Alert,* No. 179, Science Editors, Inc., Louisville, KY 40209, 1972.

(9) *Fed. Reg.,* 40 (130), 28587, July 7, 1975.

(10) "The Pharmacological Basis of Therapeutics," 5th ed., L. S. Goodman and A. Gilman, Eds., Macmillan, New York, NY 10022, 1975, p. 1521.

(11) P. M. Brotherton *et al.,* "A Study of the Metabolic Fate of Chlorpropamide in Man," *Clin. Pharmacol. Ther., 10,* 505 (1969).

(12) "Manual of Medical Therapeutics," 20th ed., M. G. Rosenfeld, Ed., Little, Brown, Boston, Mass., 1971, p. 372.

(13) *Ibid.,* p. 373.

(14) G. L. Knatterud *et al.,* "Effects of Hypoglycemic Agents on Vascular Complications in Patients with Adult-Onset Diabetes. IV. A Preliminary Report on Phenformin Results," *J. Amer. Med. Ass., 217,* 777 (1971).

(15) G. L. Searle and M. D. Siperstein, "Lactic Acidosis Associated with Phenformin Therapy," *Diabetes, 24,* 741 (1975).

Hypolipidemic Therapy

The rationale for pharmacological management of hyperlipoproteinemia has yet to be established. For pharmacological management of secondary hyperlipoproteinemias, elevations in plasma lipoprotein levels are generally resolved with treatment of the underlying disease. Drug therapy of primary hyperlipoproteinemias is primarily concerned with atherosclerotic or ischemic cardiovascular disease. The incidence of coronary heart disease was greater in patients with elevated levels of plasma cholesterol (1, 2), triglycerides (3), low density lipoprotein, and very low density lipoprotein (4–6) than in persons with normal levels.

Although conclusive evidence has yet to be presented that lowering plasma lipoprotein levels decreases the incidence and progression of coronary heart disease, the fact that hyperlipoproteinemia is related to the pathogenesis of this condition justifies efforts toward pharmacological management of elevated plasma lipoprotein levels.

Drugs that exert either an inhibiting effect on lipoprotein synthesis or a stimulating effect on lipoprotein degradation or clearance are useful for treating primary hyperlipoproteinemias, particularly those associated with the initiation and progression of ischemic vascular or atherosclerotic heart disease.

The more commonly used agents may be divided into those that reduce serum very low density lipoprotein levels (clofibrate and niacin) and those that reduce serum low density lipoprotein levels (cholestyramine, clofibrate, colestipol, dextrothyroxine, neomycin, niacin, and β-sitosterol). The use of drug therapy and dietary control is often essential for effective management of hyperlipoproteinemia. Restriction of caloric intake may often aid the reduction of plasma very low density lipoprotein levels while substitution of unsaturated fats for saturated fats may aid reduction of plasma low density lipoprotein levels.

Therapeutic Indications

Primary hyperlipoproteinemias were classified based on plasma lipoprotein patterns and physiological findings (7). This classification of hyperlipoproteinemias might be an oversimplification of hyperlipidemic disorders, but it is useful in discussing the hypolipidemic agents.

For Type I (fat-induced or exogenous) hyperlipoproteinemia, none of the drugs currently available is effective. Type I hyperlipoproteinemia is characterized by elevated fasting levels of chylomicrons. The chylomicronemia is further increased by ingestion of fat. High triglyceride and normal cholesterol levels are present in the plasma. Upon high-speed centrifugation, the plasma contains a creamy upper layer and a clear lower layer.

Type II (familial) hyperlipoproteinemia may be subdivided into Type II-A and Type II-B. Type II-A is characterized by high levels of β-lipoproteins which correspond to low density lipoproteins. After centrifugation of plasma, the plasma is generally clear. Elevated cholesterol with normal levels of triglycerides is present. Type II-B is a combination of Type II-A and Type IV hyperlipoproteinemias. For the treatment of Type II-A, cholestyramine, colestipol, dextrothyroxine, β-sitosterol, and, questionably, clofibrate and niacin are effective. For the treatment of Type II-B, cholestyramine and clofibrate may be effective.

Type III hyperlipoproteinemia is characterized by the presence of an abnormal β-lipoprotein which corresponds to very low density lipoprotein. Elevations of plasma triglycerides and cholesterol levels are present. The plasma appears turbid after centrifugation. Induction of hyperlipoproteinemia can occur with carbohydrate ingestion.

Type IV hyperlipoproteinemia is characterized by increased pre-β-lipoprotein very low density lipoproteins. Upon high-speed centrifugation, the plasma is turbid. Cholesterol and triglyceride levels are elevated and carbohydrate reduction occurs.

Type V hyperlipoproteinemia is characterized by increased chylomicrons and pre-β-lipoproteins (Types I and IV). The plasma is turbid with a creamy upper layer upon high-speed centrifugation. Both cholesterol and triglyceride levels are elevated. For Types III, IV, and V hyperlipoproteinemias, clofibrate and niacin may be effective.

In Types I and V, the abnormality theoretically involves those mechanisms responsible for chylomicron clearance while Types II, III, and IV presumably involve endogenous influence on lipoprotein synthesis and/or clearance.

Heparin is effective in decreasing plasma triglyceride and chylomicron levels by release of lipoprotein lipase. Estrogens also were shown to be effective in the lowering of very low density lipoprotein levels in patients with elevated very low density lipoprotein levels. However, estrogen and heparin are of little value for the treatment of hyperlipoproteinemia alone.

Pharmacological Mechanisms

The major lipids found in serum consist of triglycerides, free cholesterol, cholesterol esters, phospholipids, and free fatty acids. Each of these, except free fatty acids, is a lipid–protein complex which may be separated into four categories (Table I) based on density gradients (8).

Plasma lipoproteins are produced primarily in the liver and are then released to the plasma. The lipid component can be synthesized locally in the liver or can enter the liver from the plasma. Plasma lipids are derived from either intestinal uptake and release of lipids of dietary origin as circulating chylomicrons or from circulating free fatty acids released from adipose tissue. Hyperlipoproteinemia can, therefore, be expected to be caused by increased lipoprotein synthesis or reduced removal of circulating lipoproteins.

Secondary hyperlipoproteinemia is associated with demonstrable underlying disease processes such as hypothyroidism, diabetes mellitus, pancreatitis, glycogen storage disease, nephrotic disease, myxedema, and alcoholism. Primary hyperlipoproteinemias, on the other hand, include either those of idiopathic origin or those that are due to malfunctions in lipoprotein turnover mechanisms.

Antibiotics—Administration of neomycin (1.5–2.0 g) reduced the mean serum cholesterol level by 22% (9). Lowering of serum cholesterol levels is probably mediated through antibacterial mechanisms affecting the intestinal flora. Binding of neomycin to bile acids is thought to be another mechanism.

The antihyperlipoproteinemic effects of amphotericin, candicidin, filipin, and nystatin were studied after oral administration to dogs (10). The range of percent decrease in serum cholesterol levels was from 3 to 50. As for neomycin, the suggestion is put forward that these changes are dependent on antibiotic effects on intestinal bacterial flora.

Cholestyramine—Cholestyramine, the chloride salt of an anion-exchange resin, decreases circulating cholesterol levels markedly. Triglyceride levels are affected negligibly.

The mechanism of action of cholestyramine has been described in detail (11). The resin binds bile acids both *in vivo* and *in vitro*. Bile is sequestered in the gastrointestinal (GI) tract, preventing reabsorption and promoting fecal excretion, thus interfering with the enterohepatic cycle of bile acids. An eightfold increase in bile acid excretion was reported after cholestyramine administration (13.3 g/day) and an 11-fold increase was found when the dose was increased to 20 g/day (12). This interference of bile reabsorption would be expected to promote oxidation of hepatic and circulatory cholesterol to bile acids, thus lowering serum cholesterol levels.

The initial blockade of the enterohepatic circulation of sterols can, however, cause an initial increase in cholesterol production that may be sufficient to elevate serum levels. This elevation is due to release of feedback inhibition mechanisms which inhibit cholesterol synthesis. A decrease in serum cholesterol levels occurs when synthesis fails to balance loss, and it continues until a new steady-state equilibrium is established. Cholestyramine (24–36 g/day) administration reduced serum cholesterol levels while phospholipid levels fell slightly and triglyceride levels were not reduced at all (13). The amount of feces, fecal fat, and fecal nitrogen increased in all subjects studied. The effect of cholestyramine on the excretion of cholesterol-4-^{14}C was reported (14). With a dose of 200 mg/day, a 16% reduction in total serum cholesterol occurred in 1 week and an 80% reduction occurred in 2 months. The prompt increase in fecal bile acid excretion at the onset of therapy was followed by a compensatory increase in cholesterol synthesis and a possi-

Table I—CATEGORIES OF MAJOR LIPIDS IN PLASMA

Lipoprotein	Density	Major Lipid Component
Chylomicrons	0.95	Triglyceride
Very low density (VLD)	0.95–1.006	Triglyceride
Low density (LD)	1.006–1.063	Cholesterol ester
High density (HD)	1.063–1.21	Phospholipid

ble shift of cholesterol from extravascular pools into the circulating and hepatic pools. A 24% decline in serum cholesterol levels was reported in patients with Type II hyperlipoproteinemia (15). Patients with other types had no response to cholestyramine.

The recommended oral dose of cholestyramine is 4 g three times daily. Large doses (30 g/day) can induce moderate degrees of malabsorption (12).

Clofibrate—The primary effect of clofibrate is exerted upon very low density lipoproteins. A reduction in cholesterol and total lipid levels was demonstrated in the plasma of rats (16). More recent studies indicate that circulating triglyceride levels are reduced more effectively than are cholesterol levels.

The effect of clofibrate on Type III hyperlipoproteinemia was reported to be twice that exerted on Type II hyperlipoproteinemia (17). In Type II hyperlipoproteinemia, circulating cholesterol levels were decreased 28% and circulating triglyceride levels were decreased 44%. When clofibrate was combined with dietary management, additional improvement in plasma cholesterol and triglyceride levels occurred.

In one study (18), 75% of the patients had at least a 25% reduction of triglyceride levels with long-term clofibrate therapy. A 15% reduction of serum cholesterol levels was obtained in 50% of the patients. Maximum effect was reported for cholesterol and triglycerides which correspond to pre-β-lipoproteins (19). The effect of clofibrate on the hyperlipidemia of puromycin aminonucleoside-induced nephrosis was reported to include reduction of serum cholesterol, β-lipoproteins, and triglycerides (20).

Clofibrate is well absorbed from the GI tract, is present in plasma as chlorophenoxyisobutyric acid, and is strongly bound to albumin. The average plasma half-life is 12 hr. Clofibrate is excreted predominantly as a conjugated glucuronide into the urine. The mechanism of action of clofibrate has yet to be clearly defined.

Reduced free fatty acid levels were shown in plasma following clofibrate administration (21). The hypolipidemic effect was attributed to reduced free fatty acid transport, possibly due to displacement of free fatty acid from a common binding site on the albumin molecule, as well as to decreased availability of hepatic carbohydrate due to interference with the production of glucose from protein. This mechanism is consistent with the increase in liver protein and reduction in liver glycogen observed

in dogs and rats during clofibrate treatment (22).

The possible significance of the competitive interaction of clofibrate with dextrothyroxine, 17-ketosteroids, pyridoxine, and tryptophan for anionic binding sites on serum albumin was discussed (20). Displaced thyroxine and tryptophan could accumulate in the liver, causing increased synthesis of mitochondrial α-glycerophosphate dehydrogenase as well as the coenzyme nicotinamide adenine dinucleotide. These increases would theoretically increase L-α-glycerophosphate degradation to dihydroxyacetone phosphate, thereby shunting intermediates of triglyceride and phospholipid synthetic pathways into glycolytic pathways. Conversion of acetate-^{14}C into cholesterol in rat liver slices was reported to be reduced by 30–50% (16). It was suggested that metabolic or other actions of endogenous steroids were induced, thus implying augmentation of endogenous control mechanisms.

Clofibrate decreased the conversion of acetate-^{14}C to cholesterol by 75% (23). This finding was attributed to an inhibition of hepatic synthesis of cholesterol which presumably occurred between acetate and mevalonate. Inhibition of the transfer of triglycerides from the liver to plasma was theorized (24). An increase in liver weight was reported to be due to increased protein and phospholipid. This increase was associated with decreased cholesterol and glycerol concentrations. The failure to transfer was related to inhibition of lipid synthesis, reduced production of protein which was required for transport, and a direct inhibition of the transport process.

The mode of action of clofibrate may be mediated *via* increased oxidation or removal of triglyceride rather than by affecting its rate of synthesis (25). This mechanism was based on the observation that the half-life of isotopically labeled triglyceride was markedly shortened after drug administration (25).

Other studies (26) demonstrated an effect on fractional turnover rate of ^{14}C-labeled cholesterol. In addition, free fatty acid turnover and labeled incorporation rates of plasma triglyceride were measured during ^{14}C-labeled palmitate infusion. The suggestion was made that the triglyceride-reducing properties of clofibrate were due to enhanced peripheral clearance.

The recommended dose of clofibrate is 2 g/day administered in four divided doses or 1 g twice a day. Side effects (19, 27) include nausea, vomiting, diarrhea, drowsiness, giddiness, dermatological manifestations, weakness, myalgia, malaise, and acute muscle cramps with elevation of serum creatinine phosphokinase and glutamic oxaloacetic transaminase.

Dextrothyroxine—Thyroid hormones have been advocated for use in the therapy of hyperlipoproteinemia. The most effective analog for clinical use is the dextro isomer of the thyroid hormone. In contrast, the natural hormone (levothyroxine) causes an increase in basal metabolic rate (28) and myocardial metabolism to such an extent, in doses required for lowering of plasma lipoproteins, that its clinical use is precluded. The main action of dextrothyroxine is to lower low density lipoprotein and cholesterol levels. Plasma cholesterol levels are reported to be lowered by approximately 20% in clinically effective doses (6, 28, 29).

The mechanism of action involves both an increase in cholesterol synthesis which occurs in combination with an increased excretion or degradation rate (28, 30, 31). Turnover studies using isotopically labeled low density lipoprotein demonstrated decreased low density lipoprotein levels due to an increased rate of fractional catabolism and a reduced biological half-life which exceeded the increased rate of cholesterol synthesis (32). By using labeled cholesterol, a fall in the plasma cholesterol level related to increased clearance was demonstrated (31). Increased sterol excretion in feces was reported (28, 31).

During the initial stages of therapy, serum cholesterol levels may increase and decrease until a new steady state is established. This result depends on the integrated effect of dextrothyroxine on cholesterol synthesis, absorption, excretion, and degradation.

Reported clinical doses of dextrothyroxine range from 1 to 11 mg/day (6, 28, 29). Initial dosage should begin with 1–2 mg/day with a slow stepwise increase until plasma cholesterol levels decrease.

Reported side effects include development of a hypermetabolic state, hyperthyroidism, angina, and myocardial infarction (28, 29, 33). Signs of increased basal metabolic rate, anginal pain, and tachypnea indicate the need for lowered doses. Hypothyroid patients required only one-third of the euthyroid dose to achieve hypocholesterolemic effects (29).

Thyroid drugs should not be used in the presence of myocardial disease.

Estrogens—Estrogens have been shown to effect lowering of very low density lipoprotein levels in patients with elevated serum very low density lipoprotein levels (34) and cholesterol concentrations decreased by 50% (35).

The side effects of estrogens, which include clotting, impotence, and gynecomastia, make their usefulness minimal. An exception is the use of estrogens for the treatment of hyperlipoproteinemias with another primary condition, such as in female patients.

Heparin—Intravenous administration of heparin causes release of lipoprotein lipase from tissues. There is an associated decrease of serum triglycerides (very low density lipoprotein) and chylomicrons (36).

The application of heparin is severely limited and not practical due to the fact that its effect is short lived, and heparin must be given intravenously.

Niacin—Lowered serum cholesterol levels were reported following niacin administration (37). A 20% decrease in plasma triglyceride levels was found after treatment for 1 day with 1 g of niacin (38). Reduction of serum cholesterol levels required 4 days at this dose level. It may thus be assumed that both cholesterol and triglyceride levels are reduced, with temporal variation being present.

The mechanism of action of niacin may involve depression of plasma free fatty acid levels due to reduced mobilization of free fatty acids from adipose tissues. The epinephrine-induced rise in plasma free fatty acid levels was diminished by niacin (39). The mechanism of the effect on free fatty acids is related to inhibition of lipolysis in adipose tissue and diminished hepatic production of very low density lipoproteins (38). Diminished formation and release of hepatic triglycerides can be associated with the inhibitory effect of niacin on cyclic adenosine-3,5-monophosphate (40), which is an integral component of lipolytic pathways.

Reduction of cholesterol is suggested to be due to reduced conversion of very low density lipoproteins to low density lipoproteins (38). This mechanism is based on the assumption that the low density lipoprotein is the skeleton of the very low density lipoprotein which remains after transport of triglycerides to the periphery is complete.

Increased fecal excretion of endogenous neutral steroids (41), perhaps associated with inhibition of absorption of dietary cholesterol, has been demonstrated. Isotope studies also indicate that increased mobilization and reduced synthesis of cholesterol are enhanced.

Dose requirements are generally 1.5–6 g/day po in three divided doses. A direct dose–response relationship was demonstrated (42). The maximum response occurred at doses of 6 g/day.

Large doses of niacin are needed to achieve the metabolic effects described. The large doses administered over long periods frequently induce toxic symptoms (42, 43), which include cutaneous flushing, pruritus, nausea, vomiting, diarrhea, and signs of hepatic involvement such as jaundice, decreased sulfobromophthalein retention, abnormal cephalin flocculation, thymol turbidity, and increased serum transaminase values. Prolonged use may cause histopathological liver changes, including fibrosis and cholangiolitis. Glucose tolerance may be decreased, demanding caution in diabetics and preclinical diabetics.

Miscellaneous—Colestipol is a synthetic insoluble polymer of tetraethylenepentamine and epichlorohydrin which is not absorbed in the intestinal tract when administered orally (44). The main effect of colestipol is to decrease plasma low density lipoprotein and cholesterol levels. The cholesterol-lowering activity of colestipol is associated with its bile acid-binding properties. Increased fecal excretion induced an initial increase in cholesterol synthesis. Decreased plasma levels are observed when a new steady-state relationship between hepatic and plasma cholesterol pools develops.

The oral dose in clinical trials was 4–5 g/day. Side effects are minimal; however, the possibility of malabsorption, diarrhea, or constipation should be considered.

The cholesterol-lowering activity of β-sitosterol has been studied (45–47). β-Sitosterol is a naturally occurring plant sterol which closely resembles cholesterol in chemical structure, but which differs markedly in its absorption from the intestinal tract. Plasma low density lipoprotein and cholesterol levels are reduced after oral administration of β-sitosterol, but triglyceride levels are unaffected.

Orally administered β-sitosterol acts by decreasing cholesterol absorption in the intestinal tract. Theoretically, the mechanism may involve interference of the enzymatic process required for cholesterol esterification and hindrance of cholesterol transport out of mucosal cells, blockade of absorption by competing for fatty acids and bile salts, or displacement of cholesterol from bile salts and formation of insoluble mixed crystals with β-sitosterol. As with other agents which affect cholesterol and bile acid, absorption and an initial increase in cholesterol synthesis may result in elevated plasma cholesterol levels before a new steady state with lower plasma levels is established. Oral doses range from 12 to 25 g/day. Toxic effects are minimal, but observation for signs of malabsorption, diarrhea, and constipation is indicated.

Contraindications

Cholestyramine—This drug is contraindicated in patients with complete obstruction of the bile ducts.

Clofibrate—Clofibrate is contraindicated in patients with impaired hepatorenal function. Also, it should not be used in female patients where the possibility of pregnancy exists.

Dextrothyroxine—Dextrothyroxine is contraindicated in euthyroid patients with organic heart diseases including angina pectoris, cardiac arrhythmias, congestive heart failure, myocardial infarction, and hypertensive cardiovascular disease or advanced hepatorenal disease. It also is contraindicated in nursing mothers or pregnant females. Dextrothyroxine should not be given to patients with a history of iodism.

Estrogens—These drugs are contraindicated in patients with known or suspected carcinoma of the breast or genital organs, unless specifically indicated as a therapeutic agent. It is also contraindicated in thrombophlebitis, pulmonary embolism, and liver disorders.

Heparin—This drug is contraindicated in the presence of hemorrhagic blood dyscrasias, increased capillary fragility, subacute bacterial endocarditis, recent surgical procedures involving the cranium or intracranial hemorrhage, ulcerative or granulomatous lesions and extensive denudation of skin, and GI hemorrhage.

Niacin—Niacin is contraindicated in patients with a history of peptic ulcer, diabetes mellitus, or impaired liver function.

Interactions

Cholestyramine—Cholestyramine binds organic acids, including drugs such as aspirin, chlorothiazide, phenobarbital, tetracycline, and some digitalis glycosides. Also, it interferes with the absorption of digoxin, phenylbutazone, thyroid, and warfarin (see *Digoxin–Cholestyramine*, p. 62; *Phenylbutazone–Cholestyramine*, p. 185; *Thyroid–Cholestyramine*, p. 239; and *Warfarin–Cholestyramine*, p. 278).

Cholestyramine may interfere with the absorption of vitamin D and other fat-soluble vitamins (48). Abnormalities involving vitamin K absorption or liver function have not been reported.

Clofibrate—Sensitivity to coumarin anticoagulants is increased, indicating the need for sequential prothrombin time determinations when clofibrate and coumarin derivatives are administered concurrently (see *Warfarin–Clofibrate*, p. 280).

Dextrothyroxine—Dextrothyroxine may interact with clofibrate to cause enhancement of each drug's hypolipidemic effects, but the clinical outcome of the drug interaction is unknown.

The anticoagulant response of warfarin or other oral anticoagulants may be enhanced by thyroid-type compounds (see *Warfarin–Thyroid*, p. 301). Also, thyroxine and other related substances may increase the response to imipramine and shorten the time necessary for the response of imipramine to occur (see *Imipramine–Thyroid*, p. 101).

References

(1) M. M. Gertler et al., "The Interrelationships of Serum Cholesterol, Cholesterol Esters and Phospholipids in Health and in Coronary Disease," *Circulation, 2*, 205 (1950).

(2) W. B. Kannel et al., "The Coronary Profile: 12-Year Follow-Up in the Framingham Study," *J. Occup. Med., 9*, 611 (1967).

(3) M. J. Albrink and E. B. Mann, "Serum Triglycerides in Coronary Artery Disease," *Arch. Intern. Med., 103*, 4 (1959).

(4) J. W. Gofman et al., "Blood Lipids and Human Atherosclerosis," *Circulation, 2*, 161 (1950).

(5) D. P. Barr et al., "Protein-Lipid Relationships in Human Plasma II. In Atherosclerosis and Related Conditions," *Amer. J. Med., 11*, 480 (1951).

(6) E. H. Strisower et al., "Treatment of Hyperlipidemias," *Amer. J. Med., 45*, 488 (1968).

(7) D. S. Fredrickson et al., "Fat Transport in Lipoproteins—An Integrated Approach to Mechanisms and Disorders," *N. Engl. J. Med., 276*, 34, 94, 148, 215, 273 (1967).

(8) H. A. Eder, "The Lipoproteins of Human Serum," *Amer. J. Med., 23*, 269 (1957).

(9) P. Samuel et al., "Long-Term Reduction of Serum Cholesterol Levels of Patients with Atherosclerosis by Small Doses of Neomycin," *Circulation, 35*, 938 (1967).

(10) C. P. Schaffner and H. W. Gordon, "The Hypocholesterolemic Activity of Orally Administered Polyene Macrolides," *Proc. Nat. Acad. Sci. USA, 61*, 36 (1968).

(11) D. M. Tennent et al., "Plasma Cholesterol Lowering Action of Bile Acid Binding Polymers in Experimental Animals," *J. Lipid Res., 1*, 469 (1960).

(12) S. A. Hashim et al., "Cholestyramine Resin Therapy for Hypercholesteremia: Clinical and Metabolic Studies," *J. Amer. Med. Ass., 192*, 289 (1965).

(13) R. P. Howard et al., "Effect of Cholestyramine Administration on Serum Lipids and on Nitrogen Balance in Familial Hypercholesterolemia," *J. Lab. Clin. Med., 68*, 12 (1966).

(14) R. B. Morre et al., "The Effect of Cholestyramine on Fecal Excretion of Intravenously Administered Cholesterol-4-C^{14} and Its Degradation Products in Hypercholesterolemic Patients," *J. Clin. Invest., 47*, 1664 (1968).

(15) H. J. Fallon and J. W. Woods, "Response of of Hyperlipoproteinemia to Cholestyramine Resin," *J. Amer. Med. Ass., 204*, 1161 (1968).

(16) J. M. Thorp and W. S. Waring, "Modification of Metabolism and Distribution of Lipids by Ethyl Chlorophenoxyisobutyrate," *Nature, 194*, 948 (1962).

(17) R. I. Levy et al., "Drug and Dietary Management of Types II and III Hyperlipoproteinemia. Two Forms of 'Familial Hypercholesterolemia'," *Circulation, 36*, 171 (1967).

(18) D. B. Hunninghake et al., "Long-Term Effects of Clofibrate (Atromid-S) on Serum Lipids in Man," *Circulation, 39*, 675 (1969).

(19) M. F. Oliver, "Atromid-S and Atromid," *Practitioner, 192*, 424 (1964).

(20) K. D. Edwards et al., "Studies on the Pharmacological Control of Hyperlipemia in Experimental Nephrotic Syndrome," *Biochem. Pharmacol., 19*, 2719 (1970).

(21) A. M. Barrett and J. M. Thorp, "Studies on the Mode of Action of Clofibrate: Effects on Hormone-Induced Changes in Plasma Free Fatty Acids, Cholesterol, Phospholipids and Total Esterified Fatty Acids in Rats and Dogs," *Brit. J. Pharmacol. Chemother., 32*, 381 (1968).

(22) D. S. Platt and J. M. Thorp, "Changes in the Weight and Composition of the Liver in the Rat, Dog and Monkey Treated with Ethyl Chlorophenoxyisobutyrate," *Biochem. Pharmacol., 15*, 915 (1966).

(23) D. R. Avoy et al., "Effects of α-p-Chlorophenoxyisobutyryl Ethyl Ester (CPIB) with and without Androsterone on Cholesterol Biosynthesis in Rat Liver," *J. Lipid Res., 6*, 369 (1965).

(24) D. L. Azarnoff et al., "Studies with Ethyl Chlorophenoxyisobutyrate (Clofibrate)," *Metabolism, 14*, 959 (1965).

(25) N. Spirtz, "Effects of Ethyl-α-p-chlorophenoxyisobutyrate (CPIB) on Endogenous Hyperglyceridemia," *Circulation, 32*, suppl. 2, 201 (1965).

(26) P. J. Nestel et al., "The Effect of Chlorophenoxyisobutyric Acid and Ethinyl Estradiol on Cholesterol Turnover," *J. Clin. Invest., 44*, 891 (1965).

(27) T. Langer and R. I. Levy, "Acute Muscular Syndrome Associated with Administration of Clofibrate," *N. Engl. J. Med., 279*, 856 (1968).

(28) N. G. Schneeberg et al., "Reduction of Serum Cholesterol by Sodium Dextrothyroxine in Euthyroid Subjects," *Ann. Intern. Med., 56*, 265 (1962).

(29) G. S. Boyd and M. F. Oliver, "The Effect of Certain Thyroxine Analogues on Serum Lipids in Human Subjects," *J. Endocrinol., 21*, 33 (1960).

(30) D. Kritchevsky, "Influence of Thyroid Hormones and Related Compounds on Cholesterol Biosynthesis and Degradation: A Review," *Metabolism, 9*, 984 (1960).

(31) T. A. Miettinen, "Mechanism of Serum Cholesterol Reduction by Thyroid Hormones in Hypothyroidism," *J. Lab. Clin. Med., 71*, 537 (1968).

(32) K. W. Walton et al., "The Significance of Alterations in Serum Lipids in Thyroid Dysfunction. II. Alterations of the Metabolism and Turnover of ^{131}I-Low Density Lipoproteins in Hypothyroidism and Thyrotoxicosis," *Clin. Sci., 29*, 217 (1965).

(33) E. M. Jepson, "Long-Term Trial of D-Thyroxine in Hypercholesterolaemia," *Brit. Med. J.*, *1*, 1446 (1963).

(34) C. J. Glueck *et al.*, "Amelioration of Hypertriglyceridaemia, by Progestational Drugs in Familial Type-V Hyperlipoproteinaemias," *Lancet*, *i*, 1290 (1969).

(35) E. M. Russ *et al.*, "Influence of Gonadal Hormones on Protein Lipid Relationships in Human Plasma," *Amer. J. Med.*, *19*, 4 (1955).

(36) D. S. Fredrickson *et al.*, "Lipolytic Activity of Post-Heparin Plasma in Hyperglyceridemia," *J. Lipid Res.*, *4*, 24 (1963).

(37) R. Atlschul *et al.*, "Influence of Nicotinic Acid on Serum Cholesterol in Man," *Arch. Biochem. Biophys.*, *54*, 558 (1955).

(38) L. A. Carlson *et al.*, "Effect of Nicotinic Acid on Plasma Lipids in Patients with Hyperlipoproteinemia during the First Week of Treatment," *J. Atheroscler. Res.*, *8*, 667 (1968).

(39) L. A. Carlson and L. Oro, "The Effect of Nicotinic Acid on the Plasma Free Fatty Acids; Demonstration of a Metabolic Type of Sympathicolysis," *Acta Med. Scand.*, *172*, 641 (1962).

(40) R. W. Butcher *et al.*, "Effects of Lipolytic and Antipolytic Substances on Adenosine 3',5'-Monophosphate Levels in Isolated Fat Cells," *J. Biol. Chem.*, *243*, 1705 (1968).

(41) T. A. Miettinen, "Effect of Nicotinic Acid on Catabolism and Synthesis of Cholesterol in Man," *Clin. Chem. Acta*, *20*, 43 (1968).

(42) K. G. Berge *et al.*, "Hypercholesteremia and Nicotinic Acid. A Long Term Study," *Amer. J. Med.*, *31*, 24 (1961).

(43) W. B. Parsons, Jr., "Treatment of Hypercholesteremia by Nicotinic Acid. Progress Report with Review of Studies Regarding Mechanism of Action," *Arch. Intern. Med.*, *107*, 639 (1961).

(44) T. M. Parkinson *et al.*, "Effects of Colestipol (U-26,597A), a New Bile Acid Sequestrant, on Serum Lipids in Experimental Animals and Man," *Atherosclerosis*, *11*, 531 (1970).

(45) J. V. Farquhar *et al.*, "The Effect of β-Sitosterol on Serum Lipids of Young Men with Arteriosclerotic Heart Disease," *Circulation*, *14*, 77 (1956).

(46) M. M. Best and C. H. Duncan, "Modification of Abnormal Serum Lipid Patterns in Atherosclerosis by Administration of Sitosterol," *Ann. Intern. Med.*, *45*, 614 (1956).

(47) S. M. Grundy *et al.*, "The Interaction of Cholesterol Absorption and Cholesterol Synthesis in Man," *J. Lipid Res.*, *10*, 304 (1969).

(48) W. G. Thompson and G. R. Thompson, "Effect of Cholestyramine on the Absorption of Vitamin D_3 and Calcium," *Gut*, *10*, 717 (1969).

Muscle Relaxant Therapy *

Drugs that produce a flaccid paralysis of skeletal muscle through a selective inhibition of the neuromuscular junction are termed muscle relaxants. This type of drug action was first described in 1856 to account for the toxic action of South American arrow poison or curare (1), but it remained an academic curiosity until the 1930's (2). Curare was first used clinically as a relaxant in spasticity and in the treatment of tetanus (3). This use was followed by the application of curare as an adjunct to pentylenetetrazol shock therapy in 1940 (4) and as a muscle relaxant supplement to general anesthesia in 1942 (5). This latter application proved to be quite successful and subsequently has become the major clinical use of the alkaloids of curare and several synthetic agents.

Therapeutic Indications

The primary therapeutic application of the myoneural blocking drugs is to produce a flaccid skeletal muscle relaxation as a supplement to general anesthesia (6, 7). The depth of anesthesia can be lightened significantly when these drugs are used without sacrifice of adequate muscle relaxation, and surgical procedures can be performed more rapidly and efficiently with less depressant effect on the patient.

Relaxation of Skeletal Muscle Spasticity Associated with Trauma—This application has ranged from a temporary relief of the spasticity and pain associated with whip-lash injury to an effective relaxation allowing orthopedic manipulation such as correction of dislocation and fracture alignment. These drugs also have been used as aids in the differential diagnosis of the pain associated with either nerve root compression or muscle splinting. Differentiation of joint immobilization due to either muscle spasm or organic change is facilitated by these agents.

Diagnosis of Myasthenia Gravis—A patient with myasthenia gravis is extremely sensitive to the competitive neuromuscular blocking agents, and small doses of these drugs may be used to diagnose the borderline case. This use has been largely replaced by acetylcholinesterase inhibitors or the short-acting neuromuscular stimulant edrophonium which improve the patient's strength rather than intensifying the weakness (8).

*This discussion concerns the skeletal muscle relaxant drugs such as succinylcholine and tubocurarine.

Relaxation of Respiratory Muscle Guard— Effective use has been made of the myoneural blockers to facilitate trachael intubation and endoscopy in unanesthetized patients. These muscle relaxants are also used in respiratory intensive care units to facilitate controlled respiration.

Prevention of Trauma Associated with Convulsions—A less frequent use of these drugs has been to "soften" the excessive muscle contractions of convulsive disorders, tetanus, and shock therapy to prevent dislocation and fracture.

Their use in reducing hyperkinesia associated with cerebral palsy, paraplegia, chorea, and athetosis has been disappointing and should no longer be considered. The control of these symptoms can be achieved more efficiently with the centrally acting muscle relaxants without loss of voluntary movement.

Pharmacological Mechanisms

These muscle relaxants owe their primary pharmacological action to their ability to interfere with the normal transmission processes which occur at the junction of the motor nerve termination on skeletal muscle fibers. This junction is a contiguous nerve to muscle connection, with small projections of the motor nerve terminal fitted into invaginations of the postjunctional muscle membrane. The motor nerve innervating this junctional site is cholinergic (9) and is thus considered to transmit nerve action potential excitation to the muscle membrane through acetylcholine release.

The current concept of neurochemical transmission can be applied to this junction. Acetylcholine is synthesized within the motor axon and is stored, in bound form, within small intra-axonal vesicles. Motor nerve action potentials cause these vesicles to move toward the inner surface of the nerve terminal membrane. The acetylcholine storage vesicles rupture on contact with the terminal membrane, releasing the bound acetylcholine complex actively across the membrane. Free acetylcholine is thus liberated into the junctional space. This functional release of acetylcholine requires not only nerve action potentials, but the presence of a proper balance of ionic calcium (Ca^{+2}) as well (10). The facilitory action of calcium is effectively antagonized by magnesium ions, by some local anesthetics, and possibly by some polypeptide antibiotics.

The postjunctional muscle membrane contains receptor sites which react rather specifically with free acetylcholine. According to Waser (11), these receptors are anionic groups which combine with the cationic quaternary ammonium portion of acetylcholine under the influence of strong coulombic forces. The receptor membrane also contains estrophilic groups which bind the carbonyl portion of the acetylcholine molecule through nucleophilic attraction (12). The combination of acetylcholine with these receptor sites results in a prompt depolarization of the postjunctional muscle membrane. The intensity of the depolarization and the ability of the motor nerve to produce contractile activity are dependent on the number of receptors occupied by acetylcholine molecules (11).

Depolarization is a reversal of the resting state electrical negativity which exists on the inner surface of the membrane compared to the outer membrane surface. This negative polarity (potential) is produced by a selective ionic permeability mechanism within the membrane which actively excludes ionic sodium and retains potassium ions within the cell. Depolarization is produced by a breakdown in this normal membrane resistance to ionic permeability and is associated with a rapid influx of sodium ions and a slower efflux of potassium ions. The resting state negative polarity of from 60 to 90 mv is rapidly neutralized by the inflow of sodium ions.

The reversal of membrane polarity induced by the released acetylcholine is, at first, localized at the postjunctional receptor membrane. This localized depolarization is called the end-plate potential. If the end-plate potential achieves a certain level of intensity (excitability threshold), the breakdown of membrane resistance to ionic movement spreads to the adjacent muscle membrane; the initial depolarization of the postjunctional membrane then becomes propagated as an action potential which spreads spontaneously over the muscle membrane (13). Membrane depolarization is soon followed by an activation of the contractile elements.

While the phenomenon of depolarization is occurring, the membrane is refractory. That is, it cannot be reexcited (redepolarized) by additional acetylcholine. Recovery to a reexcitable state requires that normal membrane polarity be reestablished by the return of membrane resistance to sodium-ion entrance into the cell. Recovery (re-

polarization) of the neuromuscular junction begins almost simultaneously with the release of acetylcholine by the attraction of the mediator to acetylcholinesterase, an enzyme located on or near the postjunctional membrane. The combination of acetylcholine with acetylcholinesterase results in a rapid hydrolytic destruction of the mediator and a restoration of postjunctional membrane excitability. Thus, as the muscle is contracting, the receptor membrane is repolarizing to an excitable condition with the restoration of normal ionic gradients.

From this brief review of the now generally accepted processes of neuromuscular transmission, it can be deduced that muscle contractions and tonus will fail should a defect occur in the ability of the motor nerve to either synthesize, store, or release acetylcholine. A failure in one or all of these presynaptic processes is felt to be responsible for the symptoms of myasthenia gravis. Transmission failure occurs if the combination of the released acetylcholine with the end-plate receptors is prevented or if the repolarization processes of the postjunctional membrane are inhibited or slowed. The muscle relaxant drugs alter the neuromuscular transmission mechanisms which occur after the normal release of acetylcholine, although there is evidence that some of these drugs also depress the quantitative release of acetylcholine (14).

The drugs that produce muscle relaxation by blocking neuromuscular transmission do so by one of two primary mechanisms: by competition with acetylcholine for postjunctional membrane receptors and by persistent postjunctional membrane depolarization.

The competitive neuromuscular blockers are the alkaloids of curare, metocurine (dimethyl tubocurarine) and tubocurarine, and the synthetic agents, benzoquinonium, gallamine triethiodide, and pancuronium. The competitive drugs have a strong affinity for the receptor sites on the postjunctional membrane and effectively compete with the released acetylcholine for these functional sites. They do not produce an effect *per se* after receptor occupation, but they do prevent the membrane from being depolarized by acetylcholine. As the transmission block proceeds with these drugs, there is a gradual diminution in both the amplitude and duration of the end-plate potential. When the latter is depressed to about 70% of the normal value, the end-plate potential remains completely localized and muscle activity fails (6, 7, 9).

The transmission failure produced by the competitive blockers can be reversed by a proper excess of acetylcholine at the postjunctional membrane. A competitive excess of mediator is best achieved by using drugs which inhibit acetylcholinesterase (anticholinesterase), such as neostigmine and physostigmine. Competitive neuromuscular block also can be reversed by drugs that produce a selective cholinergic stimulation of the postjunctional membrane. Such drugs include ambenonium, edrophonium, neostigmine, and pyridostigmine which stimulate neuromuscular transmission as well as inhibit acetylcholinesterase (9).

The persistent membrane-depolarizing class of myoneural blocking drugs is exemplified by decamethonium and succinylcholine. These drugs also have an affinity for the end-plate receptors; but unlike the competitive blockers, their combination with these receptors results in an immediate and persistent membrane depolarization. This first effect is termed the phase I or membrane unstabilization phase of a depolarizing transmission blockade. This phase is not unlike the action produced by an excess of acetylcholine at this site, which can occur under the influence of excessive doses of anticholinesterase drugs and organophosphate insecticides.

The phase I depolarization produced by the depolarizing blocking drugs results in a brief period of muscle stimulation—observed as fasciculations and tremor—prior to paralysis. The end-plate potential produced is similar to that caused by released acetylcholine, but it is significantly more prolonged. Repolarization does occur, but slowly, and only to about 50% of the initial resting level while the drug is combined with the membrane receptors. This slow shift to a partially repolarized state is termed phase II block, nondepolarizing block, or desensitization block. In this phase, neuromuscular transmission is still prevented, but the neuromuscular stimulant drugs, which effectively antagonize the competitive blockers and significantly exacerbate the depolarizing paralysis while in phase I, will now reverse the transmission failure. This shift from the phase I to a phase II receptor membrane observed with the depolarizing drugs is not completely understood, but it is important in terms of antagonizing the neuromuscular block produced.

Both types of neuromuscular blockers have a selectivity for the end-plate receptors of skeletal muscle, but they do produce other pharmacological actions (6, 7). This activity, which may contribute to side effects and toxic manifestations, includes ganglionic transmission blockade (the curarines especially), histamine and heparin release from tissue mast cells and circulating basophils (curarines and succinylcholine), and both postganglionic cholinergic (muscarinic) receptor antagonism (gallamine triethiodide) and stimulation (benzoquinonium, decamethonium, and succinylcholine).

Response Variants

Several factors (6, 7, 15) can result in an exaggerated response to an average dose of these muscle relaxant drugs, apart from the normal 3–4% patient variation. The most significant factors are those that enhance the neuromuscular depression with a resultant prolonged paresis and apnea. Some factors can be considered as definite contraindications to the use of muscle relaxants and others only as therapeutic cautions.

Repeated Dosage—The response of the postjunctional membrane to repeated doses of the two types of neuromuscular blocking drugs is distinctly different. The competitive blockers show a cumulative effect and the depolarizing drugs show a partial tachyphylaxis. Supplemental dosage of the competitive muscle relaxants should thus be reduced by 30–50%. Even though a complete paralysis persists only about 10 min following effective doses of tubocurarine, it should be noted that a partial neuromuscular blockade and end-plate sensitivity to this drug continue for an additional 30–40 min.

A second dose of succinylcholine, on the other hand, is observed to produce a less intense paralysis and there is a gradual reduction in the degree of muscle relaxation when the drug is given by continuous infusion. This progressive decrease in muscle relaxation observed with the depolarizing blockers is due to the shift to a phase II block, with the end-plate membrane becoming insensitive to additional depolarization. Even though the degree of muscle relaxation with successive doses of succinylcholine is reduced, the duration of transmission block appears to become progressively longer.

Biotransformation—With the exception of succinylcholine which is a substrate for plasma and liver pseudocholinesterase, the neuromuscular depressants are highly charged molecules with little exposure to biotransformation enzymes. The curarines are metabolized to a small extent, but decamethonium and gallamine triethiodide are excreted in urine almost entirely unchanged.

The curarines, however, bind rather extensively to plasma and tissue protein. In fact, serum levels of free tubocurarine initially decline rather rapidly because of plasma protein binding. This brief and rapid decrease is then followed by a much slower rate of decline as the drug is excreted in both urine and bile. Only a small amount of that excreted is in the form of metabolites.

Renal function is thus an important factor in the duration and intensity of muscle relaxation produced by decamethonium and gallamine triethiodide. Even though the kidney is the primary excretory organ for tubocurarine, sufficient amounts can be excreted in the bile to allow use of the drug in anuric patients.

Hepatic integrity is a significant factor in the duration and degree of muscle relaxation produced by succinylcholine. This drug is hydrolyzed extensively (90%) by liver pseudocholinesterase in two steps: first, to the monocholine derivative and then to succinic acid and choline. The latter degradation step is about six times slower than the first metabolic reaction. The duration of muscle relaxation produced by this drug is thus prolonged in patients with sufficient hepatic parenchymal damage to prevent synthesis of this enzyme (hypoproteinemia) or in the rare patient with congenital enzyme deficiency. In addition, the monocholine metabolite, in contrast to the parent succinyldicholine, is a weak competitive blocker of neuromuscular transmission. The slower rate of metabolism of succinylmonocholine could lead to an accumulation of this derivative and an intensification of muscle paralysis if succinyldicholine is given in large or repetitive doses.

Myasthenia Gravis—A patient with this condition is considered a doubtful recipient of either type of neuromuscular blocking drug. The sensitivity of the myasthenic patient to the competitive blocking drugs sharply restricts the selection of an effective dose without respiratory muscle failure. The neuromuscular block produced by the competitive agents is also more difficult to antagonize. The myasthenic patient does not appear to be more sensitive to the depolarizing muscle relaxants, but the block produced by these drugs reaches phase II much faster and the risk of a prolonged apnea is increased. In either case, any drug which would add to muscle weakness or to the depression of an already insufficient myoneural transmission should either be avoided or used with care.

Myotonia—Individuals with this syndrome should not be given depolarizing drugs. These patients are very sensitive to the muscle stimulation effect of these drugs and to an increase in plasma potassium levels. Decamethonium and succinylcholine increase the myotonia not only by end-plate depolarization but also by release of intracellular potassium. The exaggerated muscle tonus produced can prevent both spontaneous and controlled ventilation.

Ionic Balance Factors—Changes in ionic balance may alter the muscle relaxation produced by both classes of muscle relaxant drugs. The most often reported problem is associated with changes in either calcium or potassium levels.

Calcium-ion balance is required for a normal function of both the motor nerve ending and the postjunctional muscle membrane. A deficiency or an excess of calcium results in a depressed neuromuscular transmission. A lowered membrane calcium level is accompanied by a decrease in the quantity of acetylcholine released by the motor nerve, but it facilitates the entrance of sodium into an unstable postjunctional membrane. Thus, there is a tendency to tetany, even with a partial motor nerve failure and muscle weakness.

An elevated calcium level, on the other hand, while increasing the quantity of acetylcholine released per nerve action potential, decreases the end-plate membrane excitability. The neuromuscular blocking drugs, especially the competitive type, may add to the myasthenia produced by calcium-ion alteration. This effect has been reported as a prolonged neuromuscular block in dehydrated patients with hypocalcemia and in patients with carcinoma (especially of the lung) who are reported to be hypercalcemic.

Hypokalemia sufficient to produce neuromuscular membrane hyperpolarization (depressed excitability) definitely enhances the competitive blocking drugs, but the block produced by the depolarizing blocking drugs is not materially affected with the exception that phase II block may be faster in onset (7). The depolarizing muscle relaxants liberate potassium from skeletal muscle in sufficient amounts to produce hyperkalemia. Decamethonium (4 mg) and succinylcholine (100 mg) were reported to elevate plasma potassium levels about 0.5 mEq/liter in normal individuals (16). Incidences of cardiac arrest and cardiovascular collapse have followed the use of succinylcholine in patients with severe burns, massive trauma, hemiplegia, and paraplegia. These individuals respond to the depolarizing blocking drugs with an exaggerated potassium loss and much more severe hyperkalemia (16, 17).

Side Effects—The extrajunctional pharmacology of these muscle relaxants is sufficient to warrant therapeutic caution in some patients. The cholinergic stimulation produced by benzoquinonium and succinylcholine would make the use of these drugs difficult in patients with a detached retina or with glaucoma. Both drugs elevate intraocular pressure by producing a sustained contraction of the extraocular muscle. The cholinergic stimulation produced by these two drugs would also make their use potentially dangerous in persons with existing heart block.

The curarines, because of their propensity to release histamine, should be used carefully in patients with bronchial asthma. This problem may not be significant, however, since epinephrine levels are also elevated. Histamine release is not a problem with gallamine triethiodide, but this drug produces a significant incidence of tachycardia and hypertension.

Interactions

The use of neuromuscular blocking drugs has led to complications (6, 7, 15) as a result of interactions with therapeutic or industrial chemicals. Since these muscle relaxants are used only in a clinic or hospital setting, any interaction becomes a therapeutic complication rather than a life and death situation away from expert medical attention.

The most prevalent therapeutic complication encountered with these muscle relaxant drugs is an exaggerated neuromuscular transmission depression when used with other drugs or chemicals which add to this depression. This complication may be observed with drugs which have a similar neuromuscular depressant activity as a side effect or, by some which may indirectly increase the blocking effect of the muscle relaxants *per se*. The problems reported are observed as a more difficult to reverse or as a prolonged neuromuscular depression with a greater respiratory muscle involvement (prolonged apnea following surgery). Occasionally, the problem of "recurarization" is reported when drugs are administered in the recovery room to patients who have not fully recovered from the actions of the relaxant drugs used in surgery.

A more rare incidence of therapeutic complications involves the extrajunctional pharmacology of the muscle relaxants. Again, this is observed almost entirely as a problem in surgical patients receiving drugs which enhance these pharmacological actions.

Anticholinesterase Drugs and Chemicals— These interactions could be a potential complication but apparently do not occur frequently. There is an occasional incidence of prolonged apnea in the postsurgical patient overzealously treated with anticholinesterase drugs as an antagonist of competitive neuromuscular depression. This treatment converts the competitive blockade to a depolarizing depression of neuromuscular transmission due to acetylcholine accumulation.

A more frequent interaction problem is concerned with the use of succinylcholine in patients who have received the more persistent anticholinesterase drugs prior to surgery. Such drugs include echothiophate and isoflurophate as topically applied miotics. In this complication, the muscle relaxation produced by succinylcholine is both intensified and prolonged. A similar problem would exist if the patient had been exposed to toxic concentrations of the organophosphate insecticides (*e.g.,* malathion and parathion).

Drugs Having a Competitive Neuromuscular Blocking Action—Some general anesthetics and antibiotics have a competitive neuromuscular blocking action that enhances the muscle relaxation produced by the curarines and gallamine triethiodide. An additive effect with the depolarizing blocking drugs is also possible if the neuromuscular depression produced by these muscle relaxant drugs has progressed to a phase II block, but this complication has not been clearly shown.

Anesthetics—The most frequent interaction reported is associated with the use of tubocurarine as an adjunct to ether anesthesia. This anesthetic agent has sufficient competitive neuromuscular blocking activity to prolong the muscle paralysis produced by curarines and gallamine triethiodide. Other general anesthetics reported to enhance the competitive blocking drugs are cyclopropane, enflurane, fluroxene, halothane, and methoxyflurane.

This interaction cannot be considered a major clinical problem since the intensified neuromuscular block can still be reversed by neostigmine or avoided by reducing the dose of muscle relaxant.

Antibiotics—The aminoglycoside and polypeptide antibiotics have been reported frequently to enhance the neuromuscular blocking action of the competitive and, occasionally, the depolarizing blocking drugs (see *Tubocurarine–Neomycin*, p. 254). The antibiotic implicated most is neomycin, but incidences with colistin, gentamicin, kanamycin, polymyxin B, streptomycin, and viomycin have also been reported.

Drugs which Alter Ionic Balance or Muscle Excitability—A few incidences of muscle relaxant enhancement have occurred when the competitive neuromuscular blocking drugs have been given to patients treated with large doses of diuretics. This problem occurs as a result of the hypokalemia induced by those diuretics that produce a comparatively greater potassium loss. The diuretics most often implicated are chlorthalidone, ethacrynic acid, furosemide, and the thiazides (see *Tubocurarine–Chlorothiazide*, p. 253). Competitive neuromuscular block enhancement requires hypokalemia of sufficient magnitude to produce a hyperpolarized postjunctional muscle membrane. Although this drug interaction is not supported by clinical evidence, the patient's electrolyte balance should be monitored closely prior to the use of the muscle relaxant.

A hyperpolarized postjunctional muscle membrane is also produced when local anesthetics are given intravenously or when repetitive doses of quinine or quinidine and the β-adrenergic blocking drugs (such as propranolol) are used (see *Tubocurarine–Quinidine*, p. 259, and *Tubocurarine–Propranolol*, p. 257). These drugs enhance the neuromuscular block produced by the competitive muscle relaxants.

Extrajunctional Interactions—The histamine-releasing actions of the curarines tend to produce bronchoconstriction in some patients. However, neither this complication nor an additive effect with other known agents that cause bronchoconstriction has been reported frequently. A more often observed problem with the curarines is a precipitation of a hypotensive crisis in patients treated with other ganglionic or adrenergic antagonists.

The autonomic receptor pharmacology of the other muscle relaxants also could be a potential problem, but again it has not been reported frequently. The selective vagolytic tachycardia produced (*e.g.*, by gallamine triethiodide) could be significantly enhanced by anticholinergic therapy. Such drugs include glutethimide, meperidine, and some phenothiazines and tricyclic antidepressant drugs as well as those with a primary atropine-like pharmacology. Conversely, benzoquinonium and succinylcholine produce a muscarinic receptor stimulation with bradycardia. This secondary pharmacological action of these muscle relaxants is of sufficient magnitude to be avoided in patients with a depressed myocardium (pathological or drug induced). It may be important to note that succinylcholine-induced bradycardia is enhanced by cyclopropane and halothane, but it is prevented by thiopental sodium.

Diazepam has been reported to increase the intensity and to prolong the duration of neuromuscular blockade produced by gallamine triethiodide (see *Gallamine Triethiodide–Diazepam*, p. 75), but the clinical significance of this drug interaction has not been established.

References

(1) C. Bernard, "Analyse Physiologique des Proprietes des Systemes Musculaire et Nerveux au Moyer du Curare," *C. R. Acad. Sci.*, **43**, 825 (1856).

(2) R. C. Gill, "Curare: Misconceptions Regarding the Discovery and Development of the Present Form of Curarizing Drugs," *J. Physiol.*, **141**, 425 (1958).

(3) R. West, "Curare in Man," *Proc. Roy. Soc. Med.*, **25**, 1107 (1932).

(4) A. E. Bennett, "Preventing Traumatic Complications in Convulsive Shock Therapy by Curare," *J. Amer. Med. Ass.*, **114**, 322 (1940).

(5) H. R. Griffith and G. E. Johnson, "The Use of Curare in General Anesthesia," *Anesthesiology*, **3**, 418 (1942).

(6) "The Pharmacological Basis of Therapeutics," 5th ed., L. S. Goodman and A. Gilman, Eds., Macmillan, New York, NY 10022, 1975, p. 575.

(7) "Drill's Pharmacology in Medicine," 4th ed., J. R. DiPalma, Ed., McGraw-Hill, New York, N.Y., 1971, p. 735.

(8) "The Pharmacological Basis of Therapeutics," 5th ed., L. S. Goodman and A. Gilman, Eds., Macmillan, New York, NY 10022, 1975, pp. 462–463.

(9) F. G. Standaert and W. F. Riker, Jr., "The Consequences of Cholinergic Drug Actions on Motor Nerve Terminals," *Ann. N.Y. Acad. Sci.*, **144**, 517 (1967).

(10) R. P. Rubin, "The Role of Calcium in the Release of Neurotransmitter Substances and Hormones," *Pharmacol. Rev.*, **22**, 389 (1970).

(11) P. G. Waser, "Receptor Localization by Autoradiographic Technics," *Ann. N.Y. Acad. Sci.*, **144**, 737 (1967).

(12) R. B. Barlow, "Steric Aspects of Drug Action," *Biochem. Soc. Symp.*, **19**, 46 (1960).

(13) "Drill's Pharmacology in Medicine," 4th ed., J. R. DiPalma, Ed., McGraw-Hill, New York, N.Y., 1971, pp. 742–748.

(14) W. F. Riker, Jr., and M. Okamoto, "Pharmacology of Motor Nerve Terminals," *Ann. Rev. Pharmacol.*, **9**, 173 (1969).

(15) "Muscle Relaxants," F. F. Foldes, Ed., F. A. Davis Co., Philadelphia, Pa., 1966.

(16) R. P. Belin and C. I. Karleen, "Cardiac Arrest in the Burned Patient following Succinyldicholine Administration," *Anesthesiology, 27*, 516 (1966).

(17) R. I. Mazze *et al.*, "Hyperkalemia and Cardiovascular Collapse following Administration of Succinylcholine to the Traumatized Patient," *Anesthesiology, 31*, 540 (1969).

Sedative–Hypnotic Therapy

Sedatives and hypnotics comprise one of the largest and most popular categories of drugs. This discussion covers alcohol, barbiturates, chloral hydrate, and other drugs traditionally classified as sedatives.

The purpose of sedative therapy is to reduce anxiety or tension without interfering with the normal activities of the patient. The sedation produced can alleviate anxiety associated with neuroses or the anxiety that often accompanies somatic disease. Sedatives are generally more useful in emotionally upset or neurotic individuals than in psychotic patients.

Therapeutic Indications

It is nearly axiomatic that small doses of hypnotic drugs produce sedation, and large doses produce more profound central nervous system (CNS) depression.

There are excellent benefits to be derived from the use of sedatives and/or hypnotics in acute or chronic distress. Even in the presence of pain, their antianxiety activity can bring a measure of relief, despite their lack of analgesic activity in normal therapeutic doses. However, in uncontrolled pain, they may bring about confusion and agitation. Problems arise from their use when they become the vehicle in which the patient escapes his or her problems.

Their true clinical usefulness depends to a large degree on the patient's general attitude toward drugs (1). Some patients are so afraid of drugs that they prefer some degree of insomnia to any hypnotic or will respond to subtherapeutic doses. Other patients may even respond to a placebo that satisfies their psychic need for medication. However, in a study of hypnotic doses of chloral betaine, diphenhydramine, and pentobarbital *versus* a placebo in humans, the hypnotics demonstrated better hypnosis as well as producing more side effects (2). Other studies (3–5) also established the general clinical superiority of hypnotic sedatives over placebos. In an epidemiological study of the clinical effects of chloral hydrate, diphenhydramine, pentobarbital, and secobarbital, satisfactory responses were found in 60–80% of the 4177 patients studied with a low incidence (1.8–5.6%) of adverse reactions (6). All patients recovered promptly when the drugs were discontinued.

It is important to recognize the effects that psychic factors have on the efficacy of sedative–hypnotics. It also was suggested that hypnotics should be given on an interrupted basis to lessen the probability of tolerance and habituation and to allow the prescribing of sublethal amounts of drugs (7). Frequently, doses must be individualized and reevaluated.

No single hypnotic is superior in all aspects. Chloral hydrate and paraldehyde are among the oldest hypnotics and continue to be clinically useful. Because of the unpleasant taste of paraldehyde and the pungent odor it imparts to exhaled breath, it is not as popular as chloral hydrate. Drugs such as the barbiturates, ethchlorvynol, flurazepam, glutethimide, methaqualone, and methyprylon are effective hypnotics with about the same indications as chloral hydrate and paraldehyde.

In choosing a sedative, the practitioner is faced with about the same situation as in choosing a hypnotic. There are numerous effective drugs with essentially small therapeutic differences. Newer compounds such as the benzodiazepines are safer for the potentially suicidal patient than the barbiturates because of their wider margin of safety. Chlordiazepoxide has an impressive margin of safety when taken in suicidal attempts (8). Although a satisfactory therapeutic response may be obtained with many currently used sedative drugs, the practitioner's choice can be important relative to potential drug interactions, dependence potential, margin of safety, and whether or not the patient will take the medication continuously or intermittently. The latter factor can influence the previous factors.

Pharmacological Mechanisms

Although drugs of this class act at all levels in the CNS, the reticular-activating system is especially sensitive to the depressant effects of the sedative–hypnotics. The effects on the reticular-activating system appear to be responsible for the sedative–hypnotics' sleep-inducing properties (9).

The clinical effects of sedative–hypnotics are typified by the barbiturates. They are rapidly absorbed after oral administration and distributed throughout the body. Normal hypnotic doses can reduce motor performance (10), judgment (11, 12), and the performance of simple intellectual tasks (13). It is unclear whether their action is at the cellular or synaptic level (9), and many theories exist as to how they produce their effects. The barbiturates have anticonvulsant activity, a property which may be shared, to varying degrees, by other sedative–hypnotic drugs.

Many hypnotic drugs stimulate the production of hepatic microsomal enzymes, forming the basis of many drug interactions of this class. The CNS depression that they produce also accounts for a substantial number of potentially serious interactions with other drugs producing CNS depression. Alcohol is a primary culprit in this regard. Although the classic "Mickey Finn" of chloral hydrate and alcohol has not been substantiated clinically, the interaction of alcohol with CNS depressant drugs can be serious.

The microsomal enzyme-inducing properties of barbiturates and other sedative–hypnotics are well known (14). Microsomal enzyme induction can begin to appear after the inducing drug has been given for 2 days (15), but more commonly it takes about 7 days (16, 17). After discontinuation of the microsomal enzyme-inducing drug, the time for enzyme activity to return to normal varies around a 1-month period (18). It has been shown that phenobarbital increases the rate of synthesis and decreases the breakdown of mouse microsomal protein (19). Phenobarbital had a similar effect on rat microsomal phospholipid (20). Phenobarbital also was shown to produce a 20–40% increase in liver microsomal protein (21–23). The physiological significance of enhanced liver growth and function produced by microsomal enzyme-inducing drugs is not known (14). However, many drug interactions occur due to the unintentional rapid metabolism of drugs given concurrently with microsomal enzyme-inducing drugs.

Contraindications

Barbiturates are contraindicated in conditions of idiosyncrasy or hypersensitivity, acute intermittent porphyria, and renal impairment for those drugs largely excreted *via* the kidneys (*e.g.,* aprobarbital, barbital, and phenobarbital). They are also contraindicated in potentially suicidal patients and in patients with demonstrated addiction potential.

Caution should be used for patients with severe respiratory depression or hypofunctional thyroid or adrenal glands. Hepatic malfunction is not an absolute contraindication unless the malfunction is severe, in which case these drugs might accumulate to toxic levels.

The nonbarbiturate chloral hydrate is contraindicated in severe renal, hepatic, or cardiac disease and gastritis or gastric or duodenal ulceration. Paraldehyde is contraindicated in gastritis or gastric or duodenal ulceration (when given by mouth), in hepatic insufficiency, and in colitis (when administered rectally). Idiosyncrasy or hypersensitivity is a contraindication for all of these agents.

Alcohol Interactions

Anticoagulants—The incidental use of small to moderate amounts of alcohol in patients receiving oral anticoagulants is not contraindicated. However, in chronic heavy alcohol users with liver dysfunction, anticoagulant activity may be altered. In these patients, frequent determinations of prothrombin time are necessary, and sudden changes in alcohol consumption should be avoided (see *Warfarin–Alcohol*, p. 265).

Aspirin—Concurrent ingestion of aspirin and alcohol may enhance occult blood loss and gastric damage induced by aspirin. These agents should be avoided in patients with a history of gastrointestinal (GI) bleeding. There is no evidence that concurrent use of these drugs is more harmful than either drug alone, but the potential toxicity of either agent requires that concurrent use be avoided whenever possible (see *Aspirin–Alcohol*, p. 16).

Barbiturates—Concurrent ingestion of barbiturates and alcohol leads to an intensification of their CNS depressant effects. Patients should be informed that even moderate amounts of alcohol (90–120 ml of 100-proof whiskey) will impair their ability to drive or operate hazardous machinery and that this danger is increased when barbiturates are given concurrently (see *Phenobarbital–Alcohol*, p. 180).

Benzodiazepines—Benzodiazepines and alcohol, when taken concurrently, cause an intensification of the CNS effects of each drug. Patients receiving a benzodiazepine should be warned to avoid alcohol and to use caution when driving or operating hazardous machinery (see *Diazepam–Alcohol*, p. 47).

Chloral Hydrate—Concurrent ingestion of chloral hydrate and alcohol results in a greater CNS depression than when either agent is taken alone. Occasionally, subjects receiving chloral hydrate may develop a vasodilation reaction after they ingest alcohol. All patients ingesting these agents concurrently should be warned of these possible effects (see *Chloral Hydrate–Alcohol*, p. 20).

Guanethidine—Alcohol may enhance the antihypertensive effects of guanethidine. Patients treated with guanethidine should be cautioned that they may experience symptoms of postural hypotension and syncope and that alcohol may intensify these effects (see *Guanethidine–Alcohol*, p. 79).

Hypoglycemics—Diabetic patients treated with phenformin should avoid ingestion of alcoholic beverages because concurrent use may cause hypoglycemic reactions or lead to life-threatening lactic acidosis with shock. Some patients receiving phenformin also experience a pronounced anorexia and intolerance to alcohol. Patients should be cautioned about the severe effects resulting from concurrent ingestion of these agents (see *Phenformin–Alcohol*, p. 177).

Insulin-dependent diabetic patients should be discouraged from excessive alcohol intake because of the possibility of precipitating a life-threatening hypoglycemic crisis. The concurrent use of insulin and alcohol by alcoholic patients has led to two deaths and three instances of permanent mental impairment. In each case, patients stabilized on insulin were found comatose or semiconscious from hypoglycemia caused by consumption of excessive amounts of alcohol (see *Tolbutamide–Alcohol*, p. 240).

Sulfonylureas and alcohol interact by multiple mechanisms and cause unpredictable fluctuations in serum glucose levels. Alcohol ingestion may also precipitate a disulfiram-like reaction (*e.g.*, flushing, headache, palpitations, and a feeling of breathlessness) in patients stabilized on a sulfonylurea (particularly chlorpropamide). Diabetic patients receiving sulfonylureas should abstain from drinking alcohol, and they should be warned about the severe effects resulting from concurrent ingestion of these agents (see *Tolbutamide–Alcohol*, p. 240).

Meprobamate—Meprobamate and alcohol can enhance the CNS depressant effect of each drug. This effect is usually mild if alcohol intake is moderate (90–120 ml of 100-proof whiskey) and meprobamate is taken in a single dose of 200–400 mg. However, these effects become more pronounced if meprobamate is taken chronically. Patients taking meprobamate should avoid alcohol and use caution when driving or operating hazardous machinery (see *Meprobamate–Alcohol*, p. 145).

Phenytoin—Alcohol has been demonstrated to induce microsomal enzymes that metabolize phenytoin (diphenylhydantoin) (24), but this study was done on chronic alcoholics. Moderate alcohol intake should

pose few problems, but epileptic patients who chronically consume alcohol to excess should be observed closely if receiving phenytoin.

Propoxyphene—Propoxyphene and alcohol ingested together in large quantities may result in dangerous respiratory and CNS depression attributable to their additive depressant effects. However, it is unlikely that such effects will occur after administration of therapeutic doses of propoxyphene and moderate amounts of alcohol (90–120 ml of 100-proof whiskey). Patients ingesting both agents should be warned about the harmful effects and cautioned about driving or operating hazardous machinery (see *Propoxyphene–Alcohol*, p. 210).

Barbiturate Interactions

Alkalinizers—Alkalinization of the urine could shorten the biological half-life of the weakly acidic barbiturates by rendering a greater proportion of the barbiturate ionized and therefore less readily absorbed from renal tubular fluid. This interaction is of questionable significance except for slowly metabolized barbiturates such as phenobarbital. The pKa of phenobarbital is sufficiently lower than the other common barbiturates and falls so close to the physiological pH of body fluids that sodium bicarbonate may be used to alkalinize the urine to produce greater renal clearance of phenobarbital in overdosage. The pKa's of other barbiturates are sufficiently high relative to extracellular fluid and urine that alkalinization has little effect on the amount excreted.

Antacids—The effects of barbiturates may be diminished by administration of antacids. If gastric pH were increased significantly by an antacid, the possibility exists that absorption of weakly acidic barbiturates could be slowed by decreasing the amount of absorbable unionized barbiturate in the stomach. However, this potential interaction has not been documented clinically.

Anticoagulants—Barbiturates significantly reduce the effectiveness of the oral anticoagulants probably because of enzyme induction (see *Warfarin–Phenobarbital*, p. 291).

Chlorpromazine—The hydroxylation of drugs such as chlorpromazine is increased after chronic treatment with barbiturates. In doses of 300–1200 mg/day, the primary mode of metabolism for chlorpromazine is hydroxylation. Concurrent administration of phenobarbital with chlorpromazine in large doses to humans increased the rate of chlorpromazine elimination over that of chlorpromazine alone. The effects of smaller doses of this drug on metabolism of chlorpromazine have not been established (see *Phenobarbital–Chlorpromazine*, p. 183).

CNS Depressants—Phenobarbital enhances the CNS depressant effects of alcohol and antihistamines (see *Phenobarbital–Alcohol*, p. 180, and *Chlorcyclizine–Phenobarbital*, p. 23).

Hypoglycemics—Sulfonylurea hypoglycemics (chlorpropamide) may theoretically enhance the CNS action of barbiturates, but evidence of clinical significance is lacking. However, these drugs should be used together cautiously until such an interaction is proven not to occur.

Reserpine—Although animal data showed that reserpine tends to decrease the anticonvulsant effects of barbiturates, other research showed that reserpine can enhance their sedative effects. However, the clinical reports about this drug interaction are inconclusive (see *Thiopental–Reserpine*, p. 236).

Steroids—Barbiturates may induce the metabolism of endogenous and exogenous hydrocortisone (cortisol) to the polar 6β-hydroxycortisol and nonpolar compounds such as 17-hydroxycorticosteroids. Barbiturates also induce the metabolism of dexamethasone and may decrease its therapeutic effectiveness. This drug interaction may be clinically significant in steroid-dependent patients (see *Dexamethasone–Phenobarbital*, p. 42).

Miscellaneous—The interaction implicating phenobarbital as inducing hepatic microsomal enzymes to enhance phenytoin (diphenylhydantoin) or tricyclic antidepressant metabolism is of unproven clinical significance in normal dosage regimens. In both situations, normal observation by the practitioner would be satisfactory, although chronic and/or large-dose therapy would require closer monitoring than usual (see *Phenytoin–Phenobarbital*, p. 205, and *Nortriptyline–Phenobarbital*, p. 161).

Enzyme induction is implicated in reported cases of reduced griseofulvin efficacy, although phenobarbital also may reduce the absorption of griseofulvin (see *Griseofulvin–Phenobarbital*, p. 77).

Other Sedative–Hypnotic Interactions

Analgesics—The CNS depressant effects of narcotic analgesics, in particular, theoretically may be enhanced by concurrent administration with other CNS depressant drugs. Such an interaction would be desirable in allaying anxiety associated with pain and explains why sedative drugs are given often with opiate analgesics. Although

clinical documentation is lacking, the dose of the narcotic analgesic may need to be reduced when administered concurrently with other CNS depressants.

Anesthetics—The typical reaction would theoretically be enhanced CNS depression resulting in longer recovery times after anesthesia. In fact, the CNS depressant properties of certain phenothiazines and narcotics are used for preoperative sedation, so such interactions may be clinically useful.

Anticoagulants—In general, CNS depressants lead to decreased serum levels of oral anticoagulants by stimulating microsomal enzyme production. However, this is not true in all cases. Glutethimide is particularly implicated in enzyme induction, and the dosage of oral anticoagulants must be adjusted upward accordingly. Conversely, if glutethimide is given chronically with oral anticoagulants to a patient stabilized on the anticoagulant, withdrawal of the enzyme-inducing drug would probably result in increased levels of oral anticoagulant if the dose were not readjusted (see *Warfarin–Glutethimide*, p. 284).

Other sedative–hypnotics such as ethchlorvynol have been implicated as inducing hepatic microsomal enzymes that metabolize oral anticoagulants more rapidly, but sufficient clinical documentation is not available. The short-term use of chloral hydrate with warfarin is an exception to the general rule of enzyme induction. Chloral hydrate may, in fact, cause a transient, but clinically insignificant, enhancement of the hypoprothrombinemic effect of the oral anticoagulants (see *Warfarin–Chloral Hydrate*, p. 273). It is wise to monitor prothrombin time regardless of what other drugs the patient is taking and attempt to stabilize drug intake and therapeutic response.

Antidepressants—Ethchlorvynol may cause transient delirium when used concurrently with amitriptyline; however, the clinical significance of this interaction remains to be determined.

Monoamine oxidase inhibitors marketed in the United States are used as antidepressants, with the exception of pargyline which is used for its antihypertensive properties. Drugs such as furazolidone (an anti-infective) also produce monoamine oxidase inhibition. The action of chloral hydrate may possibly be prolonged by hepatic microsomal enzyme inhibition by the monoamine oxidase inhibitors (see *Chloral Hydrate–Furazolidone*, p. 22). It is well known that the monoamine oxidase inhibitors affect many more enzymes than monoamine oxidase, so any

CNS depressant should be suspected of interacting with them.

Antihypertensives—CNS depressants tend to improve the effects of antihypertensive drugs by controlling the anxiety or tension component of high blood pressure. Caution would be warranted in giving high doses of either class of drug, but normal therapeutic doses should pose few problems for the practitioner aware of the possible consequences.

Psychotropic Agents—Psychotropic agents such as the benzodiazepines, phenothiazines, and tricyclic antidepressants almost invariably tend to produce drowsiness. Therefore, the same precautions that would be used in prescribing CNS depressants with other drowsiness-producing drugs should be observed. Awareness and recognition of overlapping CNS effects of these agents should help to avert potential problems.

References

(1) "Drugs of Choice, 1974–1975," W. Modell, Ed., Mosby, St. Louis, Mo., 1974, p. 237.

(2) H. Jick et al., "Clinical Effects of Hypnotics. I. A Controlled Trial," J. Amer. Med. Ass., 209, 2013 (1969).

(3) L. Lasagna, "A Study of Hypnotic Drugs in Patients with Chronic Disease," J. Chron. Dis., 3, 122 (1956).

(4) J. M. Hinton, "A Comparison of the Effects of Six Barbiturates and a Placebo on Insomnia and Motility in Psychiatric Patients," Brit. J. Pharmacol., 20, 319 (1963).

(5) S. S. Bloomfield et al., "A Method for the Evaluation of Hypnotic Agents in Man. The Comparative Hypnotic Effects of Secobarbital, Methaqualone and Placebo in Normal Subjects and in Psychiatric Patients," J. Pharmacol. Exp. Ther., 156, 375 (1967).

(6) S. Shapiro et al., "Clinical Effects of Hypnotics. II. An Epidemiological Study," J. Amer. Med. Ass., 209, 2016 (1969).

(7) L. E. Hollister, in "Clinical Pharmacology," 1st ed., K. L. Melmon and H. F. Morrelli, Eds., Macmillan, New York, NY 10022, 1972.

(8) G. Zbinden et al., "Experimental and Clinical Toxicology of Chlordiazepoxide (Librium)," Toxicol. Appl. Pharmacol., 3, 619 (1961).

(9) "The Pharmacological Basis of Therapeutics," 5th ed., L. S. Goodman and A. Gilman, Eds., Macmillan, New York, NY 10022, 1975, pp. 105–108.

(10) C. O. Kornetsky et al., "Comparison of Psychological Effects of Certain Centrally Acting Drugs in Man," AMA Arch. Neurol. Psychiat., 77, 318 (1957).

(11) S. Goldstone et al., "Effect of Quinalbarbitone, Dextroamphetamine and Placebo on Apparent Time," Brit. J. Psychol., 49, 324 (1958).

(12) G. M. Smith and H. K. Beecher, "Amphetamine, Secobarbital and Athletic Performance III: Quantitative Effects on Judgment," J. Amer. Med. Ass., 172, 623 (1960).

(13) A. B. Goldstein et al., "Effects of Secobarbital and of d-Amphetamine on Psychomotor Performance of Normal Subjects," J. Pharmacol. Exp. Ther., 130, 55 (1960).

(14) A. H. Conney, "Pharmacological Implications of Microsomal Enzyme Induction," Pharmacol. Rev., 19, 317 (1967).

(15) M. Corn, "Effect of Phenobarbital and Glutethimide on the Biological Half-Life of Warfarin," Thromb. Diath. Haemorrh., 16, 606 (1966).

(16) S. A. Cucinell et al., "The Effect of Chloral Hydrate on Bishydroxycoumarin Metabolism," J. Amer. Med. Ass., 197, 366 (1968).

(17) D. S. Robinson and M. G. MacDonald, "The Effect of Phenobarbital Administration on the Control of Coagulation Achieved during Warfarin Therapy in Man," J. Pharmacol. Exp. Ther., 153, 250 (1966).

(18) M. G. MacDonald et al., "The Effects of Phenobarbital, Chloral Betaine, and Glutethimide Administration on Warfarin Plasma Levels and Hypoprothrombinemic Response in Man," Clin. Pharmacol. Ther., 10, 80 (1969).

(19) L. Shuster and H. Jick, "The Turnover of Microsomal Protein in the Livers of Phenobarbital-Treated Mice," J. Biol. Chem., 241, 5361 (1966).

(20) J. L. Holtzman and J. R. Gillette, "The Effect of Phenobarbital on the Synthesis of Microsomal Phospholipid in Female and Male Rats," Biochem. Biophys. Res. Commun., 24, 639 (1966).

(21) A. H. Conney et al., "Adaptive Increases in Drug-Metabolizing Enzymes Induced by Phenobarbital and Other Drugs," J. Pharmacol. Exp. Ther., 130, 1 (1960).

(22) A. H. Conney and A. G. Gilman, "Puromycin Inhibition of Enzyme Induction by 3-Methylcholanthrene and Phenobarbital," J. Biol. Chem., 238, 3682 (1963).

(23) H. Remmer and H. J. Merker, "Drug-Induced Changes in the Liver Endoplasmic Reticulum: Association with Drug Metabolizing Enzymes," Science (N.Y.), 142, 1657 (1963).

(24) R. M. H. Kater et al., "Increased Rate of Clearance of Drugs from the Circulation of Alcoholics," Amer. J. Med. Sci., 258, 35 (1969).

Uricosuric Therapy

Uricosuric agents are, by definition, compounds that increase the excretion of uric acid in the urine. Normally, individuals excrete between 0.2 and 0.7 g of uric acid/day and maintain serum levels of approximately 5 mg%. Uric acid is reabsorbed and secreted by the kidney through an active process. Drugs that block the reabsorption of uric acid from the urine to the serum increase the excretion of uric acid and thus are termed uricosuric agents.

Therapeutic Indications

Uricosuric agents are indicated when hyperuricacidemic conditions exist. The uric acid precipitates as sodium urate crystals if the concentration of uric acid exceeds its solubility product. Crystal formation may be seen in the subcutaneous tissues, joints, renal parenchyma, and renal pelvis (1). Inflammation and severe pain may accompany these conditions, and death may result from damage to the kidneys (2). Uricosuric agents decrease the concentration of uric acid in the serum and prevent the formation of more urate crystals. The uricosurics also produce an equilibrium which favors dissolution of the urate crystals already present (3).

Pharmacological Mechanisms

The reabsorption and secretion of organic acids as anions require an active energy-utilizing process. Compounds such as dinitrophenol that block adenosine triphosphate formation can reduce the capacity of the transport system. The anion probably binds to the carrier enzyme and is then transported to the other side of the cell. It is then released into the lumen of either the kidney tubule or the blood vessel, depending on the direction of the transport (3). The capacity of this system to transport these substances is limited, and there are separate transport systems for anionic and cationic forms (4).

Uric acid and the uricosuric agents may compete for a common transport mechanism. The uricosuric agent may have a greater affinity for the carrier system, or it may simply dilute the uric acid and competitively prevent its reabsorption (3). Evidence indicates that some uricosuric agents are transported into the lumen of the tubule by the transport mechanism but are reabsorbed back into the plasma farther down the nephron unit (3).

Low doses of uricosuric agents produce retention of uric acid. Low doses of certain uricosuric agents (e.g., aspirin at 1–2 g/day) inhibit only the secretion of uric acid from the serum to the urine, resulting in the retention of the metabolite and a possible exacerbation of the gouty condition. Higher doses of the same agent (aspirin at 5–6 g/day) inhibit the reabsorption of uric acid from the urine to the plasma and produce the uricosuric effect (3).

Contraindications

Uricosuric drugs cause gastric irritation including nausea and vomiting. Cautious use is recommended in patients with a history of peptic ulcers or impaired renal function.

Uricosuric agents cause a sudden flooding of the renal tubule with poorly soluble uric acid which may result in urate stone formation. The overall risk of urate stone formation during uricosuric therapy can be assessed by measurement of the 24-hr uric acid excretion. If this excretion exceeds 900 mg before treatment, it is probably best to avoid uricosuric agents. In these situations, the use of a xanthine oxidase inhibitor along with alkalinization of the urine might be indicated. To minimize the chance of stone formation, uricosuric therapy is initiated with small doses and gradually the dose is increased over 2 weeks to maintenance levels. If full-dose therapy is to be used initially, it is suggested that the urine be alkalinized with sodium bicarbonate (10–15 g/day) and that the fluid intake exceed 3 liters/day (5).

The use of uricosuric agents is usually contraindicated during an acute attack of gout. Uricosuric agents tend to mobilize additional urate microcrystals into the synovial fluids and arthritic pain is exacerbated (5).

Hypersensitivities including rash and fever are occasionally noted, but blood dyscrasias are rare. Overdoses may result in central nervous system stimulation and convulsions. Death is due to respiratory paralysis (6).

Interactions

Aminophylline—Aminophylline theoretically can reduce the net effect of allopurinol inhibition of xanthine oxidase. However, there are no data to support this possibility and a clinically significant drug interaction probably does not occur (see *Allopurinol–Aminophylline,* p. 3).

Anti-Infectives—Probenecid, particularly in high doses, decreases the renal clearance of nitrofurantoin and increases the serum level of the anti-infective drug. The drug interaction may lead to nitrofurantoin-induced toxicity or decreased nitrofurantoin efficacy as a urinary tract anti-infective agent (see *Nitrofurantoin–Probenecid,* p. 159).

Probenecid also may increase the serum level of penicillin and the drug interaction has been used successfully to treat venereal disease (see *Penicillin–Probenecid,* p. 175).

Probenecid may inhibit the renal excretion of aminosalicylic acid and result in toxic reactions to the anti-infective drug (7, 8). The drug interaction may be clinically significant and a reduction in the dose of aminosalicylic acid may be necessary.

The renal clearance of the cephalosporins is also reduced by probenecid (9, 10). However, the clinical significance of this drug interaction has not been established.

Probenecid may also increase the serum levels of dapsone (11), although the clinical significance of this drug interaction is unknown.

Aspirin—Aspirin antagonizes the ability of probenecid and sulfinpyrazone to increase the renal excretion of uric acid and to reduce serum urate levels. These interactions appear to be clinically significant (see *Sulfinpyrazone–Aspirin,* p. 226).

Diuretics—Long-term use of chlorothiazide and other thiazide diuretics frequently causes mild uric acid retention and diminishes the uricosuric effects of probenecid. However, the clinical significance of the drug interaction has not been established (see *Probenecid–Chlorothiazide,* p. 208).

Indomethacin—Concurrent administration of probenecid causes an approximately twofold increase in serum indomethacin levels. The mechanism of this interaction is competition between indomethacin and probenecid at the renal tubular excretion site. The increase may result in enhanced clinical effectiveness of indomethacin but also may result in increased toxic reactions to the drug (see *Indomethacin–Probenecid,* p. 108).

Iron—Allopurinol has inhibited iron metabolism in animal studies, but this effect was not observed in humans or in other animal studies (see *Allopurinol–Iron,* p. 5).

Mercaptopurine—The administration of allopurinol inhibits the enzymatic oxidation of mercaptopurine within 24 hr when concurrently administered in therapeutic doses. The drug interaction is clinically significant and requires an immediate reduction in the mercaptopurine dose (see *Mercaptopurine–Allopurinol,* p. 148).

Sulfonylureas—Allopurinol may increase the serum half-life of oral sulfonylureas. Although the evidence is limited, this drug interaction appears to be clinically significant (see *Chlorpropamide–Allopurinol,* p. 35).

Uricosurics—Concurrent administration of allopurinol and probenecid may decrease the clinical effectiveness of allopurinol, but the clinical significance of this drug interaction has not been established (see *Allopurinol–Probenecid,* p. 6).

References

(1) E. Calkins, "Rational Drug Therapy," vol. 5, no. 2, Saunders, Philadelphia, Pa., 1971, p. 5.
(2) W. Boyd, "An Introduction to the Study of Disease," 6th ed., Lea and Febiger, Philadelphia, Pa., 1971, p. 539.
(3) "The Pharmacological Basis of Therapeutics," 5th ed., L. S. Goodman and A. Gilman, Eds., Macmillan, New York, NY 10022, 1975, pp. 860–866.
(4) A. Goldstein *et al.,* "Principles of Drug Action," 1st ed., Hoeber, New York, NY 10016, 1969, pp. 198–199.
(5) S. E. Goldfinger, "Treatment of Gout," *N. Engl. J. Med., 285,* 1303 (1971).
(6) S. McKinney *et al.,* "Benemid *p*-(Di-*n*-propylsulfamyl) benzoic Acid: Toxicologic Properties," *J. Pharmacol. Exp. Ther., 102,* 208 (1951).
(7) W. P. Bogee and F. W. Pitts, "Influence of *p*-(Di-*N*-Propylsulfamyl)-benzoic acid (Benemid) on Para-Aminosalicylic (PAS) Plasma Concentrations," *Amer. Rev. Tuberc., 61,* 862 (1970).
(8) D. T. Carr *et al.,* "Concentrations of PAS and Tuberculostatic Potency of Serum after Administration of PAS with or without Benemid," *Proc. Staff Meet. Mayo Clin., 27,* 209 (1952).
(9) S. B. Tuano *et al.,* "Cephaloridine versus Cephalothin: Relation of the Kidney to Blood Level Differences after Parenteral Administration," *Antimicrob. Ag. Chemother., 6,* 101 (1966).
(10) B. R. Meyers *et al.,* "Cephalexin: Microbiological Effects and Pharmacologic Parameters in Man," *Clin. Pharmacol. Ther., 10,* 810 (1969).
(11) C. S. Goodwin and G. Sparell, "Inhibition of Dapsone Excretion by Probenecid," *Lancet, ii,* 884 (1969).

Vitamin Therapy

Vitamins are organic catalysts of exogenous origin that are intimately related to the enzyme systems. They frequently function as coenzymes in many biochemical reactions and customarily are divided into two groups: the fat-soluble and the water-soluble vitamins. The fat-soluble vitamins are A, D, E, and K; the water-soluble vitamins include the B group and vitamin C.

In general, the substantiated use for vitamins is in the treatment of vitamin deficiencies or avitaminosis. Avitaminosis may be due to one of two conditions (1): (a) The supply of vitamins provided by an individual's diet is inadequate; this condition is known as primary deficiency and is prevalent in underdeveloped countries. (b) The supply of vitamins is adequate, but the vitamin cannot be properly utilized by the body. This state is termed secondary conditioned deficiency due to one or more of the following: malabsorption, excessive demand, and/or reduced storage facilities including protein binding and transfer to the active sites.

Aside from clear cases of avitaminosis, controversy surrounds the use of vitamins. In general, nutritionists as well as some medical practitioners believe that many individuals have a mild vitamin deficiency in which the avitaminosis symptoms are absent yet the individual functions at a reduced level biochemically. This belief is apparently widespread as evidenced by the large consumption of vitamin supplements.

The claimed benefits of supplementing the diet in cases where a vitamin deficiency is not evident range from ensuring that the diet contains adequate amounts of vitamins and general "toning" of the body to claims of virility and longevity in the case of vitamin E (2). In spite of the apparent general acceptance of this form of vitamin usage, a sound scientific or medical basis does not exist to substantiate this form of therapy except as a prophylactic measure to prevent avitaminosis.

Vitamin A

Therapeutic Indications—Lack of vitamin A in the diet leads to degeneration of the epithelial tissue lining the mucous membranes in the respiratory and digestive tracts as well as in the lacrimal and salivary glands. The vitamin appears to be necessary for the stability of the lipoprotein membrane of the cell and of the subcellular particles (3–5).

Xerophthalmia may occur due to lack of lacrimal gland secretion. This condition may lead to keratomalacia with ulceration and subsequent blindness. Night blindness is a common symptom of vitamin A deficiency. The vitamin participates in synthesis of mucopolysaccharides and release of a protease affecting dissolution of the cartilaginous matrix.

Causes of vitamin A deficiency are inadequate dietary intake, impaired absorption or storage, failure to convert carotene into vitamin A, or rapid depletion of the body's reserves (6). Impairment of absorption or storage is seen in dysentery, celiac disease, cystic fibrosis of the pancreas, ulcerative colitis, pancreatectomy, obstruction of the biliary ducts, and cirrhosis of the liver. Conversion of carotenes to the vitamin may be impaired in diabetes mellitus and hyperthyroidism.

Deficiency symptoms should be treated by giving doses of up to 25,000 IU/day (1 IU = 0.344 μg trans-vitamin A acetate). In xerophthalmia, 5000 IU/kg/day for 5 days should be the initial dose (7, 8). In severe cases, parenteral doses of 75,000 IU should be given, followed by 75,000 IU orally in conjunction with antibiotic therapy. Several reports (9, 10) suggested massive oral doses (200,000 IU of vitamin A and 50–200 IU of vitamin E) in an oil solution administered every 6 months as an emergency measure to prevent blindness due to vitamin A deficiency in persons from developing countries.

The vitamin has been used topically as an aid in wound healing (11).

Pharmacological Mechanisms—The vitamin A aldehydes, retinal and dehydroretinal, together with the protein opsin form the light-sensitive pigments in the rods and cones of the retina. In terrestrial animals, rhodopsin (visual purple) and iodopsin are the main pigments (12, 13). The action of vitamin A is to promote resynthesis of visual purple. The vitamin also acts to maintain the integrity of epithelial tissue by preventing metaplasia of the stratified squamous type. This effect is believed to occur by stabilizing sulfhydryl groups in proteins.

Contraindications and Toxicity—No well-documented contraindications have been reported, although toxic effects due to overdosage, which include lethargy, malaise, abdominal pain, headaches, excessive sweating, dryness of skin, hyperkeratosis, alopecia, and brittle nails, are not uncommon (14, 15).

Carotenoid deposits may color the soles of the feet, palms of the hands, and the nasolabial folds yellow. Retarded growth and early epiphyseal closure may occur in children whose mothers received excessive doses of vitamin A. Topical application has resulted in local irritation and hypopigmentation (16).

Vitamin A is stored in the liver and kidney and to some extent in the lungs. The storage capacity of young growing individuals is greater than that of the adult. This greater capacity probably explains the higher incidence of vitamin toxicity in children. To prevent vitamin A toxicity in apparently normal individuals, it is recommended that a daily adult dose of 5000 IU not be exceeded. In pregnancy, this amount can be raised to 6000 IU and during lactation to 8000 IU. For infants and children, the dose should be reduced to 1500 and 2500 IU, respectively.

Interactions—Reversal of corticosteroid-induced impairment of wound healing has been reported after topical application of the vitamin (17). The mechanism for this interaction has not been established. Vitamin A does not appear to enhance wound healing in patients not receiving corticosteroids. Adverse effects of this form of therapy have not been reported, and the effect of systemic administration of vitamin A on wound healing has not been established. High doses of the vitamin elevate sedimentation rate and prothrombin time measurements and decrease leukocyte and erythrocyte counts. Decreased absorption of vitamin A may occur with concomitant administration of mineral oil (18–20). It was reported that women receiving oral contraceptives have increased levels of vitamin A (21, 22). However, the clinical significance of these effects has not been established.

Vitamin B Complex: Cyanocobalamin (B$_{12}$)

Therapeutic Indications—Cyanocobalamin deficiency results in pernicious anemia but is usually not due to straightforward dietary deficiency of the vitamin. A defect that impairs secretion of intrinsic factor by the stomach is probably the major cause of the deficiency. Inadequate dietary intake, inadequate ileal absorption (malabsorption syndrome, ileitis, tuberculosis, or ileal resection), and interference with absorption by bacteria or fish tapeworm can also cause the deficiency.

The minimum daily requirement is 1.0–2.5 μg, but the normal body content of 4 mg

or more must be restored in the treatment of pernicious anemia (23). When cyanocobalamin is injected, 75–80% of a single 200–1000-μg dose may be excreted in the urine. This loss is reduced to 50% with hydroxocobalamin (24). Initial therapy consists of 100 μg im every other day for 2 weeks and then monthly for the lifetime of the patient. Since the vitamin is nontoxic, many practitioners will administer 1000 μg/injection (23). Oral cyanocobalamin–intrinsic factor preparations are not recommended since most patients become refractory (23). Persons with pernicious anemia due to a dietary lack of the vitamin respond to as little as 0.1 mg of cyanocobalamin by injection (25). Doses of 2–4 mg are needed to replace body stores, and then 1.5 μg/day will maintain the patient. Recommended daily dietary allowances are 5 μg for adults, 6 μg for the elderly, and 8 μg during pregnancy (26). An increased need for cyanocobalamin may exist in women using oral contraceptives (27).

Pharmacological Mechanisms—Cyanocobalamin acts as a coenzyme in various biological reactions, is located in the mitochondria of the cell, and is believed to be involved in protein and carbohydrate metabolism. Cyanocobalamin stimulates the reticulocytes, thus playing an important role in hematopoiesis in that, together with folic acid, it is involved in the formation of deoxyribonucleotides from ribonucleotides. Cyanocobalamin is absorbed from the ileum with the aid of intrinsic factor, a mucoprotein of the gastric juice (28). Malabsorption of the vitamin has been observed in chronic pancreatic insufficiency (29). The half-life of intravenously administered cyanocobalamin in the serum is about 6 days (30). Small doses of a few micrograms are retained in the body but large doses (milligrams) are rapidly excreted in the urine.

Contraindications and Toxicity—No contraindications have been reported.

Interactions—Aminosalicylic acid causes a decrease in vitamin absorption (31). The mechanism for this has not been established. Chloramphenicol-treated patients may respond poorly to cyanocobalamin therapy since chloramphenicol interferes with erythrocyte maturation (32–35). Neomycin reduces cyanocobalamin absorption, and colchicine apparently increases this phenomenon by an unknown mechanism (36, 37).

Vitamin B Complex: Folic Acid

Therapeutic Indications—Macrocytic anemia is the main manifestation of folic acid deficiency in humans. Megaloblastic anemia occurs in pregnancy because of the mother's increased need for the vitamin. In sprue and other malabsorption syndromes, there is a folate deficiency because of impaired absorption and often megaloblastic anemia is present.

In general, folic acid deficiency is caused by: (a) inadequate dietary intake (infants, alcoholics, and cirrhotic patients), (b) disturbances of intestinal absorption (malabsorption syndrome or resection of the jejunum), (c) increased requirement [pregnancy, chronic hemolytic anemia, malignant disease, or use of oral contraceptives (27)], and (d) disturbances of folic acid metabolism.

A dietary folic acid intake of 5 μg/day or less results in a deficiency (38). The recommended daily dietary allowances are 400 μg of folic acid for adults with an additional 100 μg during lactation and 400 μg during pregnancy. The daily minimum requirement of adults is probably about 50 μg (39).

In megaloblastic anemia due to dietary deficiency of folic acid, 250–5000 μg of folic acid/day is sufficient for normalization (23, 40). During pregnancy, prophylactic doses of folic acid (100–500 μg) are recommended. If anemia develops during pregnancy, 5 mg of folic acid/day should be administered (23).

Pharmacological Mechanisms—Tetrahydrofolic acid (derived from folic acid metabolically) is an important carrier of one-carbon units derived from histidine and serine which are required for the synthesis of purines and methionine (41). In folic acid deficiency, the primary effect is a disturbance of the doubling of DNA in the nucleus during cell division.

Contraindications and Toxicity—High doses (>100 μg/day) as a supplement may mask the appearance of anemia in patients with cyanocobalamin deficiency but are inadequate for protection from subacute degenerative neurological changes (26).

Folic acid is not considered to be toxic even in large doses.

In treatment employing folic acid antagonists, folic acid should be given in a reduced form such as leucovorin (folinic acid) (see *Methotrexate–Leucovorin*, p. 154) (42).

Interactions—A case of a patient with folic acid deficiency was reported in which chloramphenicol antagonized the response to folic acid therapy, presumably by interfering with erythrocyte maturation (32). Folic acid administration interfered with the action of pyrimethamine in the treatment of toxoplasmosis (43). Concurrent folate administration with hydantoins may cause an increase in metabolism of hydantoins. Long-term high-dose anticonvulsant therapy may contribute to marginal folate deficiency (see *Phenytoin–Folic Acid*, p. 197).

Vitamin B Complex: Niacin

Therapeutic Indications—A deficiency of this vitamin leads to pellagra. This disease is associated with a corn (maize) diet but occasionally occurs in chronic alcoholism, cirrhosis of the liver, chronic diarrhea, diabetes mellitus, and neoplasms. Niacin acts as a vasodilator and has been used in angina, migraine, and Meniere's disease, in doses of 25 mg or more four times a day. Niacin, in doses of 1.0–1.5 g three times a day with meals, is employed to lower serum cholesterol triglyceride and, to a lesser extent, phospholipid levels. These doses cause undesirable side effects and long-term benefits of this therapy have yet to be confirmed. In severe niacin deficiency, 300–500 mg of niacinamide should be given in daily oral doses of 50–100 mg (44). To prevent pellagra, a daily intake of 6.6 mg/1000 kcal consumed should be maintained. During pregnancy, this dose should be increased by 2 mg/day and during lactation by 7 mg/day.

Pharmacological Mechanisms — Niacin functions as a component of coenzymes of numerous dehydrogenases important in glycolysis and tissue respiration. Niacin is detoxified to nicotinuric acid and requires coenzyme A. Cholesterol synthesis also requires coenzyme A; therefore, niacin may reduce the amount of coenzyme A available for cholesterol synthesis (45).

Niacin is synthesized from tryptophan by intestinal bacteria. In the body, about 1 mg of niacin is formed from every 60 mg of ingested tryptophan (44, 46).

Contraindications and Toxicity—High doses (>3 g/day) can cause impairment of hepatic function with jaundice (47–50) and should be administered only with extreme caution. Niacin is regarded, however, as nontoxic in the usual therapeutic range.

Interactions—Interactions with other drugs have not been reported; however, large doses elevate cephalin flocculation test measurements.

Vitamin B Complex: Pantothenic Acid

Therapeutic Indications—Pantothenic acid is part of coenzyme A and is involved in the release of energy from carbohydrates. The human pantothenic acid requirement is unknown but human needs are probably met with an intake of 5–10 mg/day, an amount normally present in the diet. Pantothenic acid is so widely distributed in foods that deficiency is practically unknown in humans. The "burning feet" syndrome accompanied by severe paresthesia and great tenderness of the feet experienced by World War II prisoners on poor diets was believed to be due in part to pantothenic acid deficiency. Pantothenic acid was reported to be effective against the neurotoxicity of streptomycin (51). Pantothenic acid in the form of pantothenyl alcohol (250–500 mg) has been used prophylactically after major abdominal surgery to minimize the possibility of paralytic ileus. However, the value of this treatment has been questioned (52).

Interactions—Dexpanthenol, a form of pantothenic acid, may prolong the neuromuscular blocking effects of succinylcholine. However, this effect was not substantiated by controlled studies (see *Succinylcholine–Dexpanthenol*, p. 225).

Vitamin B Complex: Pyridoxine (B$_6$)

Therapeutic Indications—Pyridoxine is necessary for the metabolism of amino acids and is an essential part of the enzyme glycogen phosphorylase. The symptoms of pyridoxine deficiency vary with age and include seborrheic and desquamative dermatitis of the mouth and eyes, intertrigo of the breasts and inguinal region of women, stomatitis and glossitis, irritability, depression, somnolence, nausea, and impairment of sensitivity to vibration and positional change (53, 54).

Spontaneous deficiency in humans is rare. A deficiency of pyridoxine in infants results in hyperirritability, convulsions, and anemia. This deficiency is believed to be due to an inborn error of metabolism, leading to a dependency on a high intake of the vitamin. It is seen during the first 7 days of life and leads to convulsions; unless treated, the child may be mentally retarded (55, 56). A genetic defect is probably the cause of pyridoxine-deficiency anemia. The recommended allowance for adults is 2 mg/day with a daily protein intake of 100 g. The requirement of the vitamin increases with protein intake (20 μg/g of protein) (26). An additional 500 μg/day is recommended during pregnancy. An increased need for pyridoxine appears to exist in women using oral contraceptives (27, 57).

When pyridoxine deficiency is due entirely to reduced intake, the recommended daily dose will reverse the deficiency. Pyridoxine-dependent convulsions in infants should be treated with 2–15 mg/day of pyridoxine (58). In pyridoxine-deficiency anemia, the dose should be 10 mg/day; in pyridoxine-sensitive anemia, it should be 500 mg/day (59, 60).

Pharmacological Mechanisms—The term vitamin B$_6$ refers to three pyridine derivatives (pyridoxal, pyridoxamine, and pyridoxine); all are interconverted metabolically in humans. Vitamin B$_6$ is a coenzyme (61). Pyridoxamine phosphate and pyridoxal phosphate act as coenzymes in transamination reactions important for the breakdown of γ-aminobutyric acid in the brain and for oxalate metabolism. Pyridoxal phosphate is the coenzyme in the decarboxylation of amino acids and also is involved in various reactions of tryptophan metabolism. This reaction forms the basis of the tryptophan-loading test for diagnosis of vitamin B$_6$ deficiency.

Interactions—It has been observed that pyridoxine reverses the levodopa-induced improvement in parkinsonism. In the presence of a peripheral dopa decarboxylase inhibitor, pyridoxine appears to enhance the clinical response to levodopa. The mechanism for these interactions is not known. Pyridoxine and vitamin preparations containing pyridoxine should be avoided in patients receiving levodopa (see *Levodopa–Pyridoxine*, p. 131).

A deficiency develops with high doses of isoniazid (62) and hydralazine (63). These drugs apparently lead to increased requirements for pyridoxine; however, the mechanism of this interaction is not well understood. Patients on a poor diet taking these drugs develop a pyridoxine-deficiency neuropathy. In such cases, 100 mg/day of pyridoxine should be given as concurrent therapy.

Although there is some evidence indicating that pyridoxine may interfere with the activity of isoniazid, concurrent administration of the two drugs does not appear to alter the clinical effectiveness of isoniazid in eradicating tubercle bacilli in humans (see *Isoniazid–Pyridoxine*, p. 118).

Vitamin B Complex: Riboflavin (B$_2$)

Therapeutic Indications—Ariboflavinosis leads to lesions of the lips, mouth, eyes, skin, and genitalia (64). The most common lesions are angular stomatitis and cheilosis of the lips. The deficiency symptoms usually disappear after several days of oral administration at a dosage level of 5 mg two or three times daily (44). Recommended daily requirements (26) are 1.7 mg for men and 1.5 mg for women. An additional 300 μg is recommended for women in the second and third trimesters of pregnancy and an additional 500 μg during lactation. The minimum requirement to prevent clinical signs of deficiency is 300 μg/1000 kcal consumed in adults.

Pharmacological Mechanisms—In the form of flavin mononucleotide and flavin adenine dinucleotide, riboflavin functions as a coenzyme or prosthetic group of the flavoproteins. These substances have an important function in biological oxidations and respiration. Riboflavin, in combination with protein, is necessary to prevent recurrent skin lesions (46). Riboflavin is synthesized by the intestinal flora, especially when poorly digestible carbohydrates are present in large amounts. Free riboflavin is converted in the intestinal mucosa into flavin mononucleotide which is transformed into flavin adenine dinucleotide in the liver.

Riboflavin was shown to be absorbed by a specialized transport rather than by passive diffusion (65). Large doses of riboflavin may not be absorbed quantitatively due to rapid movement past the absorption sites.

Contraindications and Toxicity—No contraindications are known. Since riboflavin is not appreciably stored in the body, excessive intake results in increased urinary excretion rather than toxicity.

Interactions—No interactions with other drugs have been reported.

Vitamin B Complex: Thiamine (B$_1$)

Therapeutic Indications—A deficiency of thiamine causes beriberi. This disease is common in Asia with rice-eating people. In the United States, thiamine deficiency is seen in alcoholics and may lead to Wernicke's disease and Korsakoff's psychosis.

Beriberi may be classified as wet, dry, or infantile. Treatment is with 10–20 mg of thiamine/day by injection until clinical improvement is seen and then with 10 mg/day po. Infantile beriberi is treated with 5 mg/day im for 4 days. Thiamine, 10 mg po twice a day, may be given to the mother if the child is being breast fed. The recommended daily allowance for thiamine is 400 μg/1000 kcal consumed for all ages, with an added allowance of 200 μg/day during the second and third trimesters of pregnancy and 400 μg/day during lactation (26).

Pharmacological Mechanisms—Thiamine pyrophosphate functions in carbohydrate metabolism as a coenzyme in the decarboxylation of α-keto acids and in transketolase reactions (66). Thiamine pyrophosphate plays an important part in the production

of stimuli in the peripheral nerves and in the recovery process after stimulation (67).

Thiamine is absorbed by an active process (68) but not stored. The tissue of individuals on high thiamine intake soon becomes saturated, and the vitamin is excreted in increased quantities in the urine. High oral doses of thiamine may not be absorbed quantitatively due to saturation of the active transport process or rapid removal from the site of absorption.

Contraindications and Toxicity—No known toxicity exists.

Interactions—No substantiated drug interactions have been reported.

Vitamin C: Ascorbic Acid

Therapeutic Indications—A deficiency of ascorbic acid leads to scurvy. Claims have been made for the efficacy of large doses of ascorbic acid in preventing the common cold, but this claim has not been substantiated by well-controlled clinical trials. In infants, ascorbic acid doses of 20 mg/day will prevent scurvy. In infants with scurvy, 25 mg should be given four times a day; in adults, 100–200 mg five or six times a day is adequate (69). The daily adult dietary allowances recommended by the Food and Nutrition Board (26) are 60 mg for males and 55 mg for females, with an additional 5 mg/day during lactation and pregnancy. An increased need for ascorbic acid may exist in women using oral contraceptives (27). Continual oral administration of aspirin results in a decrease in plasma and leukocyte levels of ascorbic acid to levels just in excess of those associated with the production of scurvy (see *Ascorbic Acid–Aspirin*, p. 12). Since the clinical results of this effect have not been documented, supplemental ascorbic acid as routine therapy is not warranted.

Pharmacological Mechanisms—Ascorbic acid has many functions in the body and its role in metabolism has been summarized by the Food and Nutrition Board (26): (*a*) oxidation of phenylalanine and tyrosine *via para*-hydroxyphenylpyruvate, (*b*) hydroxylation of aromatic compounds, (*c*) conversion of folic acid to folinic acid, (*d*) regulation of the respiratory cycle in mitochondria and microsomes, (*e*) hydrolysis of alkyl monothioglycosides, (*f*) development of odontoblasts and other specialized cells including collagen and cartilage. and (*g*) maintenance of the mechanical strength of blood vessels, particularly the venules.

Contraindications and Toxicity—None has been reported; ascorbic acid toxicity is relatively low. High doses may be taken without the development of toxic effects. After saturation is reached, the vitamin is excreted in the urine in proportion to dose.

However, high doses of ascorbic acid tend to acidify the urine, thus affecting the elimination of weak acids and bases. Acid urine may cause precipitation of urate and cystine stones in the urinary tract. Very large doses of ascorbic acid, therefore, should be avoided in patients with a tendency to gout, to formation of urate stones, or to cystinuria (70).

Interactions—Ascorbic acid-induced acidic urine increases the possibility of aminosalicylic acid and sulfonamide crystalluria (32) and decreases the tubular reabsorption of tricyclic antidepressants (71) and amphetamines (72). Large doses of ascorbic acid cause false-positive results when Benedict's solution is used as a test for glycosuria (73, 74) and a false-negative urinary glucose oxidase dip-stick test for glycosuria (75). In addition, large doses of ascorbic acid were reported to destroy substantial amounts of dietary cyanocobalamin (76) and increase the absorption of elemental iron (see *Ferrous Sulfate–Ascorbic Acid*, p. 72).

There have been isolated reports that large doses of ascorbic acid may counteract the hypoprothrombinemic effect of warfarin, but no studies have supported this observation adequately (see *Warfarin–Ascorbic Acid*, p. 268).

Vitamin D

Therapeutic Indications—Vitamin D is necessary for the proper calcification of bone. A deficiency during childhood leads to rickets or, later in life, to osteomalacia.

Vitamin D deficiency can occur due to lack of intake through poor diet, impaired absorption (idiopathic steatorrhea or celiac disease), and lack of exposure to sunlight in conjunction with reduced intake.

To prevent rickets or osteomalacia, 400 IU/day for children and pregnant or lactating women is required. No allowance is set for normal adults but intake should not exceed 400 IU (1 IU = 25 μg of crystalline ergocalciferol). In the treatment of rickets or osteomalacia due to a simple deficiency of vitamin D, 3000 IU/day po is usually adequate. In cases of impaired absorption in infants and children, the dose should be given intramuscularly. High vitamin D doses (50,000 IU/day) (77) are required in primary vitamin D-resistant rickets. Maintenance doses may range from 1000 to 50,000 IU/day depending upon the individual.

Pharmacological Mechanisms—The activity of vitamin D is closely related to that of the parathyroid hormone and of calcitonin. All three factors are necessary for maintenance of calcium balance and a normal serum calcium level (78, 79). Vitamin D is also believed to be responsible for formation of the calcium transport system in bone cells (78). In rats, vitamin D increased calcium absorption in the intestine (80), and a vitamin D-dependent calcium-binding protein was isolated from the intestinal mucosa of chicks (81).

Vitamin D_3 (cholecalciferol) is formed photochemically from 7-dehydrocholesterol, which in turn is formed from cholesterol (82). In humans, ingested vitamin D or that formed in the skin is rapidly absorbed and transported almost quantitatively to its active sites (83, 84). Bile is necessary for oral absorption. Vitamin D is rapidly metabolized and widely distributed throughout the body.

Vitamin D_3 becomes much more active after hydroxylation by liver enzymes to 25-hydroxycholecalciferol. This compound is further transformed by a kidney enzyme into 1,25-dihydroxycholecalciferol which is still more active. Pseudo-vitamin D-deficient rickets (Prader's syndrome or autosomal recessive vitamin D-dependent rickets) is caused by a deficiency of the enzyme responsible for the latter transformation. These metabolites are not commercially available for clinical use.

Contraindications and Toxicity—Overdosage causes mobilization of bound calcium in the skeleton and increases the serum calcium level. This calcium is taken up by soft tissue, especially the kidney, resulting in nephrocalcinosis and metastatic calcification of other soft tissue such as blood vessels, myocardium, lungs, and skin. The symptoms of hypervitaminosis D include loss of appetite, gastrointestinal (GI) disturbances, head and joint pains, and muscular weakness. These symptoms are reversible, but if untreated, death may occur due to kidney failure. Toxic effects of the vitamin are seen in the adult when doses exceed 1000–3000 IU/kg/day after several months. In infants, hypercalcemia may occur with total daily doses of 3000–4000 IU (85). Because supplementary vitamin D is added to many foods, an intake well above the recommended dose is common.

Interactions—The vitamin may interfere with serum cholesterol measurements (86) and has been found to elevate serum and urine calcium, protein, and inorganic phosphate determinations and to lower alkaline phosphatase measurements.

Phenytoin (diphenylhydantoin) has been reported to increase the metabolic inactivation of vitamin D and decrease the half-life of vitamin D in the body, possibly resulting in hypocalcemia and, less commonly, clinical osteomalacia or rickets (see *Vitamin D–Phenytoin,* p. 261). Long-term high-dose barbiturate anticonvulsant therapy has been reported to decrease the effects of vitamin D, *i.e.,* hypocalcemia (87–89) and the possible development of osteomalacia (90–93). This effect was reversed by treatment with vitamin D (94).

Vitamin E

Therapeutic Indications—Since vitamin E is found widely in foods eaten by humans, it is difficult to identify a specific deficiency disease caused by lack of this vitamin. Humans whose dietary habits are such that vitamin E intake is greatly reduced usually suffer from malnutrition and diseases such as kwashiorkor which mask the effects of vitamin E deficiency. Newborn animals, including human infants, may be deficient in vitamin E because placental transfer is negligible. This deficiency may be the cause of macrocytic and hemolytic anemia in infants (95–98). Human milk, however, is rich in tocopherol (2–5 mg of α-tocopherol/liter) and within 4–6 weeks, breast-fed infants have normal serum vitamin E levels.

Tocopherols are poorly absorbed from the small intestine and require bile for absorption. Probably only 35% of the tocopherol in food is absorbed, the remainder being excreted in the feces (98). Conditions interfering with fat absorption (biliary disease, pancreatic insufficiency, or mineral oil ingestion) will further reduce the amount of tocopherol absorbed. Vitamin E therapy is usually not instituted based upon an established deficiency but rather because the individual is believed to have less than optimum vitamin E intake. The belief that vitamin E will reduce sterility or that it is useful in the prevention and treatment of heart disease in humans has not been substantiated by carefully controlled experiments.

In the absence of definite information about human needs for vitamin E, it is difficult to make a recommendation in terms of dietary intake. It is estimated (26) that healthy adults require 10–30 mg of α-tocopherol/day (1 IU = 1 mg of *dl*-α-tocopherol acetate). The minimal requirement of an infant is probably 500 μg/kg, an amount normally absorbed from the breast milk (99).

Pharmacological Mechanisms—The tocopherols are believed to act as antioxidants *in vivo,* thus protecting the body from random free-radical reactions and therefore playing a role in membrane permeability and stability. Lack of vitamin E causes symptoms which vary with species. These symptoms include muscular paralysis, encephalomalacia, and interference with gestation (2). No common denominator has been established for the physiological function of tocopherol or the reasons for species specificity and tissue susceptibility.

Contraindications and Toxicity—No known contraindications exist. Little is known about the effects of excessive intake of tocopherol in humans, but there is no clearly documented evidence of toxicity.

One case report suggested that vitamin E may enhance oral anticoagulant activity and cause hemorrhage in vitamin K-deficient patients (100).

Vitamin H: Biotin

Therapeutic Indications—Biotin is essential for warm-blooded animals. It acts as a coenzyme in carbon dioxide fixation and transcarboxylation reactions. Biotin deficiency does not occur in humans except under very abnormal circumstances. It is formed by intestinal flora in large quantities. The biotin requirements in humans are unknown. Biotin has been used to treat seborrheic dermatitis in young children (101), which is probably due to a deficiency of biotin in breast milk plus loss due to constant diarrhea. Biotin is nontoxic to animals and humans. In experimental biotin deficiency, doses of 150–300 μg/day reverse the deficiency (102). No contraindications have been reported.

Interactions—Interactions with other drugs are unknown.

Vitamin K

Therapeutic Indications—Vitamin K deficiency causes hypoprothrombinemia, marked by excessive prothrombin time and a tendency for bleeding. The K vitamins [phytonadione (K_1), menaquinone (K_2), and menadione (K_3)] are necessary for the maintenance of prothrombin. Phytonadione is the drug of choice for oral anticoagulant overdosage, in bleeding esophageal varices, and in bleeding due to interference with the activity of vitamin K-dependent clotting factors (II, VII, IX, and X).

The Food and Nutrition Board (26) has not established a daily allowance for vitamin K; the amounts obtained from the intestinal flora and from a normal diet are sufficient to maintain normal prothrombin levels. However, an exception is a newborn infant whose mother's body levels were lacking in vitamin K. It is generally believed that vitamin K administration to newborn infants decreases the incidence of neonatal hemorrhage, especially in premature infants with anorexia (26). For such infants, a single dose of 500–1000 μg sc or im is recommended (103). If the mother has been treated with anticoagulants, the dose should be doubled.

In mild bleeding associated with excessive prolongation of prothrombin time, the oral administration of 5–10 mg of phytonadione is recommended (23). For moderate bleeding, 10–20 mg is given intramuscularly; if hemorrhage is severe, 10–25 mg may be given slowly intravenously. In the cirrhotic patient with massive upper GI bleeding, 25–50 mg of phytonadione given intramuscularly or intravenously is a valuable adjunct to therapy (23).

Pharmacological Mechanisms—Vitamin K is involved in the blood coagulation mechanism. It affects the formation of prothrombin factors VII and IX and possibly factor V (104). The vitamin is believed to act by promoting the formation of the quaternary protein structure (105).

Bile is necessary for optimal absorption of the vitamin. Menadione and synthetic water-soluble preparations are absorbed without bile. Any defect in intestinal absorption of fats (steatorrhea, biliary fistula, bile duct obstruction, sprue, celiac disease, or pancreatic fibrosis) may lead to vitamin K deficiency.

Contraindications and Toxicity—Excessive doses of synthetic vitamin K have led to hemolytic anemia and kernicterus in the infant (106). This effect is believed due to competitive inhibition of bilirubin glucuronidation or protein binding displacement. Doses above 5 mg of vitamin K should not be given to the newborn.

Interactions—Oral anticoagulants are vitamin K antagonists, and, therefore, concurrent therapy is irrational except in the treatment of anticoagulant overdosage (see *Warfarin–Vitamin K,* p. 303). Large doses of vitamin K decrease bilirubin test measurements. Concurrent oral administration with mineral oil may decrease the vitamin's absorption (107). The administration of actinomycin to vitamin K-deficient chicks impaired the prothrombin response after treatment with vitamin K_3 (108).

References

(1) W. Boyd, "An Introduction to the Study of Disease," 6th ed., Lea and Febiger, Philadelphia, Pa., 1971, p. 58.

(2) "Vitamin E," *Med. Lett., 13,* 97 (1971).

(3) J. A. Lucy and J. T. Dingle, "Fat-Soluble Vitamins and Biological Membranes," *Nature, 204,* 156 (1964).

(4) G. Wolf, "Some Thoughts on the Metabolic Role of Vitamin A," *Nutr. Rev., 20,* 161 (1962).

(5) G. Wolf, "Hypervitaminosis A, Experimental Induction in the Human Subject," *Biochem. J., 90,* 35P (1964).

(6) B. M. Kagan and R. S. Goodhart, in "Modern Nutrition in Health and Disease," 3rd ed., M. G. Wohl and R. S. Goodhart, Eds., Lea and Febiger, Philadelphia, Pa., 1964, p. 341.

(7) T. Moore, "The Pathology of Vitamin A Deficiency," *Vitam. Horm., 18,* 499 (1960).

(8) D. S. McLaren, "Xerophthalmia: A Neglected Problem," *Nutr. Rev., 22,* 289 (1964).

(9) J. C. Bauernfeind *et al.,* "Vitamins A and E Nutrition via Intramuscular or Oral Route," *Amer. J. Clin. Nutr., 27,* 234 (1974).

(10) J. A. Olson, "The Prevention of Childhood Blindness by the Administration of Massive Doses of Vitamin A," *Isr. J. Med. Sci., 8,* 1199 (1972).

(11) L. Prutkin, "Wound Healing and Vitamin A Acid," *Acta Dermato–Venereol., 52,* 489 (1972).

(12) G. Wald, "The Visual Function of the Vitamin A," *Vitam. Horm., 18,* 417 (1960).

(13) H. J. Dartnall and K. Tansley, "Physiology of Vision: Retinal Structure and Visual Pigments," *Ann. Rev. Physiol., 25,* 433 (1963).

(14) R. W. Hillman, "Hypervitaminosis A: Experimental Induction in the Human Subject," *Amer. J. Clin. Nutr., 4,* 603 (1956).

(15) J. Soler-Bechara and J. L. Soscia, "Chronic Hypervitaminosis A. Report of a Case in an Adult," *Arch. Intern. Med., 112,* 462 (1963).

(16) A. M. Kligman *et al.,* "Postscript to Vitamin A Acid Therapy for Acne Vulgaris," *Arch. Dermatol., 107,* 296 (1973).

(17) H. P. Ehrlich *et al.,* "The Effects of Cortisone and Anabolic Steroids on the Tensile Strength of Healing Wounds," *Ann. Surg., 170,* 203 (1969).

(18) A. E. Mahle and H. M. Patton, "Carotene and Vitamin A Metabolism in Man. Their Excretion and Plasma Level as Influenced by Orally Administered Mineral Oil and a Hydrophilic Mucilloid," *Gastroenterology, 9,* 44 (1947).

(19) A. C. Curtis and R. S. Balmer, "The Prevention of Carotene Absorption by Liquid Petrolatum," *J. Amer. Med. Ass., 113,* 1785 (1939).

(20) A. C. Curtis and E. M. Kline, "Influence of Liquid Petrolatum on Blood Content of Carotene in Human Beings," *Arch. Intern. Med., 63,* 54 (1939).

(21) J. Wild *et al.,* "Vitamin A, Pregnancy and Oral Contraceptives," *Brit. Med. J., 1,* 57 (1974).

(22) M. H. Briggs, "Vitamin A and the Teratogenic Risks of Oral Contraceptives," *Brit. Med. J., 3,* 170 (1974).

(23) "Manual of Medical Therapeutics," 19th ed., J. W. Smith, Ed., Little, Brown, Boston, Mass., 1969.

(24) V. Herbert and L. W. Sullivan, "Activity of Coenzyme B_{12} in Man," *Ann. N.Y. Acad. Sci., 112,* 855 (1964).

(25) H. C. Heinrich and E. E. Gabbe, "Metabolism of the Vitamin B_{12} Coenzyme in Rats and Man," *Ann. N.Y. Acad. Sci., 112,* 871 (1964).

(26) Food and Nutrition Board, Recommended Dietary Allowances, 7th ed., National Academy of Sciences–National Research Council, Publication No. 1694, Washington, D.C., 1969.

(27) R. C. Theuer, "Effect of Oral Contraceptive Agents on Vitamin and Mineral Needs: A Review," *J. Reprod. Med., 8,* 13 (1972).

(28) G. B. J. Glass, "Gastric Intrinsic Factor and Its Function in the Metabolism of Vitamin B_{12}," *Physiol. Rev., 43,* 529 (1963).

(29) C. Matuchansky, "Vitamin B_{12} Malabsorption in Chronic Pancreatitis," *Gastroenterology, 67,* 406 (1974).

(30) J. F. Adams, "Biological Half-Life of Vitamin B_{12} in Plasma," *Nature, 198,* 200 (1963).

(31) O. Heinwaara and I. P. Palva, "Malabsorption of Vitamin B_{12} during Treatment with *para*-Aminosalicylic Acid. A Preliminary Report," *Acta Med. Scand., 175,* 469 (1964).

(32) F. H. Meyers et al., "Review of Medical Pharmacology," 2nd ed., Lange Medical Publications, Los Altos, Calif., 1970, p. 475.

(33) J. L. Scott et al., "A Controlled Double Blind Study of the Hematologic Toxicity of Chloramphenicol," *N. Engl. J. Med., 272,* 1137 (1965).

(34) R. M. Jiji et al., "Chloramphenicol and Its Sulfamoyl Analogue. Report of Reversible Erythropoietic Toxicity in Healthy Volunteers," *Arch. Intern. Med., 111,* 70 (1963).

(35) P. Saidi et al., "Effect of Chloramphenicol on Erythropoiesis," *J. Lab. Clin. Med., 57,* 247 (1961).

(36) W. W. Faloon and R. B. Chodos, "Vitamin B_{12} Absorption Studies Using Colchicine, Neomycin and Continuous Vitamin B_{12} Administration," *Gastroenterology, 56,* 1251 (1969).

(37) E. D. Jacobson et al., "An Experimental Malabsorption Syndrome Induced by Neomycin," *Amer. J. Med., 28,* 524 (1960).

(38) V. Herbert, "A Palatable Diet for Producing Experimental Folate Deficiency in Man," *Amer. J. Clin. Nutr., 12,* 17 (1963).

(39) V. Herbert, "Minimal Daily Adult Folate Requirement," *Arch. Intern. Med., 110,* 649 (1962).

(40) C. S. Davidson and J. H. Jandl, "On the Daily Allowance for Folic Acid," *Amer. J. Clin. Nutr., 7,* 711 (1959).

(41) M. Friedkin, "Enzymatic Aspects of Folic Acid," *Ann. Rev. Biochem., 32,* 185 (1963).

(42) L. Delmonte and T. H. Jukes, "Folic Acid Antagonists in Cancer Chemotherapy," *Pharmacol. Rev., 14,* 91 (1962).

(43) "Pyrimethamine," Section 8:40, "American Hospital Formulary Service," American Society of Hospital Pharmacists, Washington, D.C., April 1960.

(44) G. A. Goldsmith, in "Nutrition," vol. 2, G. H. Beaton and E. W. McHenry, Eds., Academic, New York, N.Y., 1964, p. 109.

(45) H. Schon, "Effect of Nicotinic Acid on the Cholesterol Contents of Rat Livers," *Nature, 182,* 534 (1958).

(46) M. K. Horwitt, in "Modern Nutrition in Health and Disease," 3rd ed., M. G. Wohl and R. S. Goodhart, Eds., Lea and Febiger, Philadelphia, Pa., 1964, p. 380.

(47) R. M. Kohn and M. Montes, "Hepatic Fibrosis following Long Acting Nicotinic Acid Therapy: A Case Report," *Amer. J. Med. Sci., 258,* 94 (1969).

(48) A. U. Rivin, "Jaundice Occurring during Nicotinic Acid Therapy for Hypercholesteremia," *J. Amer. Med. Ass., 170,* 2088 (1959).

(49) W. O. Pardue, "Severe Liver Dysfunction during Nicotinic Acid Therapy," *J. Amer. Med. Ass., 175,* 137 (1961).

(50) A. H. Baggenstos et al., "Fine Structural Changes in the Liver in Hypercholesteremic Patients Receiving Long-Term Nicotinic Acid Therapy," *Mayo Clin. Proc., 42,* 385 (1967).

(51) I. Murray, "Pantothenic Acid and Biotin," *Practitioner, 182,* 50 (1959).

(52) R. H. Girdwood, "Patient Care in the Age of Science," *Brit. Med. J., 2,* 631 (1963).

(53) R. W. Vilter et al., "The Effect of Vitamin B_6 Deficiency Induced by Desoxypyridoxine in Human Beings," *J. Lab. Clin. Med., 42,* 335 (1953).

(54) R. W. Vilter, "Vitamin B_6 in Medical Practice," *J. Amer. Med. Ass., 159,* 1210 (1955).

(55) D. B. Coursin, "Vitamin B_6 Metabolism in Infants and Children," *Vitam. Horm., 22,* 755 (1964).

(56) C. R. Scriver, "Vitamin B_6-Dependency and Infantile Convulsions," *Pediatrics, 26,* 62 (1960).

(57) A. R. Doberenz et al., "Vitamin B_6 Depletion in Woman Using Oral Contraceptives as Determined by Erythrocyte Glutamic-Pyruvic Transaminase Activities," *Proc. Soc. Exp. Biol. Med., 137,* 1100 (1971).

(58) H. Cramer, "Pyridoxin-Dependent Convulsions in Infants. Metabolic–Genetic Epilepsy," *Deut. Med. Wochenschr., 87,* 1577 (1962).

(59) D. L. Horrigan and J. W. Harris, "Pyridoxine-Responsive Anemia: Analysis of 62 Cases," *Advan. Intern. Med., 12,* 103 (1964).

(60) J. W. Harris and D. L. Horrigan, "Pyridoxine-Responsive Anemia—Prototype and Variations on the Theme," *Vitam. Horm., 22,* 721 (1964).

(61) M. Dixon and E. C. Webb, "Enzymes," 2nd ed., Longmans, London, England, 1964, p. 410.

(62) J. P. Biehl and R. W. Vitler, "Effects of Isoniazid on Pyridoxine Metabolism," *J. Amer. Med. Ass., 156,* 1549 (1954).

(63) N. H. Raskin and R. A. Fishman, "Pyridoxine-Deficiency Neuropathy Due to Hydralazine," *N. Engl. J. Med., 273,* 1182 (1965).

(64) A. Keys et al., "The Performance of Normal Young Men on Controlled Thiamine Intakes," *J. Nutr., 26,* 399 (1943).

(65) G. Levy and W. J. Jusko, "Factors Affecting the Absorption of Riboflavin in Man," *J. Pharm. Sci., 55,* 285 (1966).

(66) P. Handlar, "Hypovitaminosis K," *Fed. Proc., 17,* suppl. 2, 31 (1958).

(67) A. Van Muralt, "The Role of Thiamine in Neurophysiology," *Ann. N.Y. Acad. Sci., 98,* 499 (1962).

(68) A. B. Morrison and J. A. Campbell, "Factors Influencing the Excretion of Oral Test Doses of Thiamine and Riboflavin by Human Subjects," *J. Nutr., 72,* 435 (1960).

(69) G. A. Goldsmith, "Human Requirements for Vitamin C and Its Use in Clinical Medicine," *Ann. N.Y. Acad. Sci., 92,* 230 (1961).

(70) "Vitamin C and the Common Cold," *Med. Lett., 12,* 105 (1970).

(71) F. Sjoqvist, "The pH-Dependent Excretion of Monomethylated Tricyclic Antidepressants," *Clin. Pharmacol. Ther., 10,* 826 (1969).

(72) M. Rowland, "Amphetamine Blood and Urine Levels in Man," *J. Pharm. Sci., 58,* 508 (1969).

(73) "Vitamin C—Were the Trials Well Controlled and Are Large Doses Safe?" *Med. Lett., 13,* 46 (1971).

(74) M. P. Elking and H. F. Karat, "Drug Induced Modifications of Laboratory Test Values," *Amer. J. Hosp. Pharm., 25,* 484 (1968).

(75) K. A. B. Kristensen, "I.V. Tetracycline and 'Dip-Stick' Urine Test," *N. Engl. J. Med., 283,* 660 (1970).

(76) V. H. Herbert and E. Jacob, "Few Conditions Require Massive Doses of Vitamins," *J. Amer. Med. Ass., 229,* 1850 (1974).

(77) E. Kodieck, in "Proceedings of a Conference on the Transfer of Calcium and Strontium across Biological Membranes," R. H. Wasserman, Ed., Academic, New York, N.Y., 1963, p. 185.

(78) H. F. DeLuca, "Mechanism of Action and Metabolic Fate of Vitamin D," *Vitam. Horm., 25,* 315 (1967).

(79) M. T. Harrison, "Interrelationships of Vitamin D and Parathyroid Hormone in Calcium Homeostasis," *Postgrad. Med. J., 40,* 497 (1964).

(80) D. Schachter *et al.,* "Active Transport of Calcium by Intestine: Action and Bio-assay of Vitamin D," *Amer. J. Physiol., 200,* 1263 (1961).

(81) R. H. Wasserman *et al.,* "Vitamin D-Dependent Calcium Binding Protein. Purification and Some Properties," *J. Biol. Chem., 243,* 3978 (1968).

(82) M. Glover *et al.,* "Provitamin D_3 in Tissues and the Conversion of Cholesterol to 7-Dehydrocholesterol In Vivo," *Biochem. J., 51,* 1 (1952).

(83) E. M. Cruickshank *et al.,* "The Vitamin D Content of Tissues of Rats Irradiated with Ultraviolet Light," *Proc. Nutr. Soc., 14,* VIII (1955).

(84) H. Bekemeier, "Vitamin D der Haut," Huber, Berne, Germany, 1966.

(85) Committee on Nutrition, American Academy of Pediatrics, *Pediatrics, 31,* 512 (1963).

(86) R. J. Henry, "Clinical Chemistry: Principles and Techniques," Hoeber Medical Division, Harper and Row, New York, N.Y., 1964, p. 861.

(87) A. Richens and D. J. F. Rowe, "Disturbance of Calcium Metabolism by Anticonvulsant Drugs," *Brit. Med. J., 4,* 73 (1970).

(88) R. Kruse, "Osteopathien bei Antiepileptischer Langzeittherapie (Vorläufige Mitteilung)," *Mschr. Kinderheilk, 116,* 378 (1968).

(89) C. E. Dent *et al.,* "Osteomalacia with Long-Term Anticonvulsant Therapy in Epilepsy," *Brit. Med. J., 4,* 69 (1970).

(90) C. Christiansen *et al.,* "Incidence of Anticonvulsant Osteomalacia and Effect of Vitamin D: Controlled Therapeutic Trial," *Brit. Med. J., 4,* 695 (1973).

(91) T. J. Hahn, "Anticonvulsant Therapy and Vitamin D," *Ann. Intern. Med., 78,* 308 (1973).

(92) J. Linde and J. Molholm Hansen, "Vitamin D in Patients on Anticonvulsants," *Brit. Med. J., 2,* 547 (1974).

(93) J. T. F. Rowe and T. C. B. Stamp, "Anticonvulsant Osteomalacia and Vitamin D," *Brit. Med. J., 2,* 392 (1974).

(94) C. Christiansen *et al.,* "Effect of Vitamin D on Bone Mineral Mass in Normal Subjects and in Epileptic Patients on Anticonvulsants: A Controlled Therapeutic Trial," *Brit. Med. J., 2,* 208 (1973).

(95) A. S. Majaj, "Vitamin E-Responsive Macrocytic Anemia in Protein–Calorie Malnutrition. Measurements of Vitamin E, Folic Acid, Vitamin C, Vitamin B_{12} and Iron," *Amer. J. Clin. Nutr., 18,* 362 (1966).

(96) F. A. Oski and L. A. Barness, "Vitamin E Deficiency: A Previously Unrecognized Cause of Hemolytic Anemia in the Premature Infant," *J. Pediat., 70,* 211 (1967).

(97) J. H. Ritchie *et al.,* "Edema and Hemolytic Anemia in Premature Infants. A Vitamin E Deficiency Syndrome," *N. Engl. J. Med., 279,* 1185 (1968).

(98) G. Klatskin and D. W. Molander, "The Chemical Determination of Tocopherol in Feces, and the Fecal Excretion of Tocopherol in Man," *J. Lab. Clin. Med., 39,* 802 (1952).

(99) H. M. Nitowsky *et al.,* "Vitamin E Requirements of Human Infants," *Vitam. Horm., 20,* 559 (1962).

(100) J. L. Corrigan and F. I. Marcus, "Coagulopathy Associated with Vitamin E Ingestion," *J. Amer. Med. Ass., 230,* 1300 (1974).

(101) A. Nisenson, "Seborrheic Dermatitis of Infants and Leiner's Disease: A Biotin Deficiency," *J. Pediat., 51,* 537 (1957).

(102) V. P. Sydenstricker *et al.,* "Observations on 'Egg White Injury' in Man and Its Cure with Biotin Concentrate," *J. Amer. Med. Ass., 118,* 1199 (1942).

(103) Committee on Nutrition, American Academy of Pediatrics, Report of Commission on Nutrition, "Vitamin K Compounds and Their Water Soluble Analogs: Use in Therapy and Prophylaxis in Pediatrics," *Pediatrics, 28,* 501 (1961).

(104) A. J. Aballi *et al.,* "Coagulation Studies Disease of the Newborn Period. III. Hemorrhagic Disease of the Newborn," *Amer. J. Dis. Child., 97,* 524 (1959).

(105) B. C. Johnson, "Dietary Factors and Vitamin K," *Nutr. Rev., 22,* 225 (1964).

(106) R. M. Wynn, "The Obstetric Significance of Factors Affecting the Metabolism of Bilirubin, with Particular Reference to the Role of Vitamin K," *Obstet. Gynecol. Surv., 18,* 333 (1963).

(107) C. T. Javert and C. Macri, "Prothrombin Concentration and Mineral Oil," *Amer. J. Obstet. Gynecol., 42,* 409 (1941).

(108) R. E. Olson, "Vitamin K Induced Prothrombin Formation: Antagonism by Actinomycin D," *Science, 145,* 926 (1964).

Laboratory Tests and Clinical Values:
Tables

Table I—WHOLE BLOOD, SERUM, AND PLASMA (CHEMISTRY) *

Test	Material	Normal Value
Acetoacetic acid, qualitative	Serum	Negative
quantitative	Serum	0.2–1.0 mg/100 ml
Acetone, qualitative	Serum	Negative
quantitative	Serum	0.3–2.0 mg/100 ml
Albumin, quantitative	Serum	3.2–4.5 g/100 ml (salt fractionation)
		3.2–5.6 g/100 ml by electrophoresis
		3.8–5.0 g/100 ml by dye binding
Alcohol	Serum or whole blood	Negative
Aldolase	Serum	Adults: 3–8 Sibley–Lehninger units/100 ml at 37°
		Children: Approximately two times adult levels
		Newborn: Approximately four times adult levels
Alpha-amino acid nitrogen	Serum	3–6 mg/100 ml
δ-Aminolevulinic acid	Serum	0.01–0.03 mg/100 ml
Ammonia	Plasma	20–150 µg/100 ml (diffusion)
		40–80 µg/100 ml (enzymatic method)
		12–48 µg/100 ml (resin method)
Amylase	Serum	60–160 Somogyi units/100 ml
Argininosuccinic lyase	Serum	0–4 units/100 ml
Arsenic	Whole blood	< 3 µg/100 ml
Ascorbic acid (vitamin C)	Plasma	0.6–1.6 mg/100 ml
	Whole blood	0.7–2.0 mg/100 ml
Barbiturates	Serum, plasma, or whole blood	Negative
Base excess	Whole blood	Males: −3.3 to +1.2
		Females: −2.4 to +2.3
Base, total	Serum	145–160 mEq/liter
Bicarbonate	Plasma	21–28 mmole/liter
Bile acids	Serum	0.3–3.0 mg/100 ml
Bilirubin	Serum	Up to 0.3 mg/100 ml (direct or conjugated)
		0.1–1.0 mg/100 ml (indirect or unconjugated)
		Total: 0.1–1.2 mg/100 ml
		Newborns total: 1–12 mg/100 ml
Blood gases		
pH		7.38–7.44 arterial
		7.36–7.41 venous
pCO₂		35–40 mm Hg arterial
		40–45 mm Hg venous
pO₂		95–100 mm Hg arterial

Continued on next page

* These tables of normal values were adapted with permission from "Todd-Sanford Clinical Diagnosis by Laboratory Methods," I. Davidsohn and J. B. Henry, Eds., Saunders, Philadelphia, PA 19105

Table I—continued

Test	Material	Normal Value
Bromide	Serum	0–5 mg/100 ml
Calcium	Serum	Ionized: 4.2–5.2 mg/100 ml 2.1–2.6 mEq/liter or 50–58% of total Total: 9.0–10.6 mg/100 ml 4.5–5.3 mEq/liter Infants: 11–13 mg/100 ml
Carbon dioxide (CO_2 content)	Whole blood, arterial	19–24 mmole/liter
	Plasma or serum, arterial	21–28 mmole/liter
	Whole blood, venous	22–26 mmole/liter
	Plasma or serum, venous	24–30 mmole/liter
CO_2 combining power	Plasma or serum, venous	24–30 mmole/liter
CO_2 partial pressure (pCO_2)	Whole blood, arterial	35–40 mm Hg
	Whole blood, venous	40–45 mm Hg
Carbonic acid	Whole blood, arterial	1.05–1.45 mmole/liter
	Whole blood, venous	1.15–1.50 mmole/liter
	Plasma, venous	1.02–1.38 mmole/liter
Carboxyhemoglobin (carbon monoxide hemoglobin)	Whole blood	Suburban nonsmokers: < 1.5% saturation of hemoglobin Smokers: 1.5–5.0% saturation Heavy smokers: 5.0–9.0% saturation
Carotene, beta	Serum	40–200 μg/100 ml
Cephalin cholesterol flocculation	Serum	Negative to 1+ after 24 hr 2+ or less after 48 hr
Ceruloplasmin	Serum	23–50 mg/100 ml
Chloride	Serum	95–103 mEq/liter
Cholesterol, total	Serum	150–250 mg/100 ml (varies with diet and age)
Cholesterol, esters	Serum	65–75% of total cholesterol
Cholinesterase Pseudocholinesterase	Erythrocytes Plasma	0.65–1.00 pH unit 0.5–1.3 pH units 8–18 IU/liter at 37°
Citric acid	Serum or plasma	1.7–3.0 mg/100 ml
Congo red test	Serum or plasma	> 60% after 1 hr
Copper	Serum or plasma	Males: 70–140 μg/100 ml Females: 85–155 μg/100 ml
Cortisol	Plasma	8 a.m.–10 a.m.: 5–25 μg/100 ml 4 p.m.–6 p.m.: 2–18 μg/100 ml

Table I—continued

Test	Material	Normal Value
Creatine	Serum or plasma	Males: 0.2–0.6 mg/100 ml Females: 0.6–1.0 mg/100 ml
Creatine phosphokinase (CPK)	Serum	Males: 55–170 units/liter at 37° Females: 30–135 units/liter at 37°
Creatinine	Serum or plasma	0.6–1.2 mg/100 ml
Creatinine clearance (endogenous)	Serum or plasma and urine	Males: 123 ± 16 ml/min Females: 97 ± 10 ml/min
Cryoglobulins	Serum	Negative
Cyanocobalamin (vitamin B_{12})	Serum	Males: 200–800 pg/ml Females: 100–650 pg/ml
Electrophoresis, protein	Serum	

		percent	*g/100 ml*
	Albumin	52–65	3.2–5.6
	Alpha-1	2.5–5.0	0.1–0.4
	Alpha-2	7.0–13.0	0.4–1.2
	Beta	8.0–14.0	0.5–1.1
	Gamma	12.0–22.0	0.5–1.6

Test	Material	Normal Value
Fats, neutral	Serum or plasma	0–200 mg/100 ml
Fatty acids, total free	Serum Plasma	9–15 mmole/liter 300–480 μEq/liter
Fibrinogen	Plasma	200–400 mg/100 ml
Fluoride	Whole blood	< 0.05 mg/100 ml
Folate	Serum Erythrocytes	5–25 ng/ml (bioassay) 166–640 ng/ml (bioassay)
Galactose	Whole blood	Adults: none Children: < 20 mg/100 ml
Gamma globulin	Serum	0.5–1.6 g/100 ml
Globulins, total	Serum	2.3–3.5 g/100 ml
Glucose, fasting	Serum or plasma Whole blood	70–110 mg/100 ml 60–100 mg/100 ml
Glucose tolerance, oral	Serum or plasma	Fasting: 70–110 mg/100 ml 30 min: 30–60 mg/100 ml above fasting 60 min: 20–50 mg/100 ml above fasting 120 min: 5–15 mg/100 ml above fasting 180 min: fasting level or below
Glucose tolerance, intravenous	Serum or plasma	Fasting: 70–110 mg/100 ml 5 min: maximum of 250 mg/100 ml 60 min: significant decrease 120 min: below 120 mg/100 ml 180 min: fasting level
Glucose-6-phosphate dehy- drogenase (G-6-PD)	Erythrocytes	250–500 units/10^9 cells 1200–2000 mIU/ml of packed erythrocytes
γ-Glutamyl transpeptidase	Serum	2–39 units/liter
Glutathione	Whole blood	24–37 mg/100 ml
Growth hormone	Serum	< 10 ng/ml
Guanase	Serum	< 3 nmole/ml/min

Continued on next page

Table I—continued

Test	Material	Normal Value
Haptoglobin	Serum	100–200 mg/100 ml as hemoglobin-binding capacity
Hemoglobin	Serum or plasma	Qualitative: negative Quantitative: 0.5–5.0 mg/100 ml
Hemoglobin	Whole blood	Males: 13.5–18.0 g/100 ml Females: 12.0–16.0 g/100 ml
Hemoglobin A_2	Whole blood	1.5–3.5% of total hemoglobin
α-Hydroxybutyric dehydrogenase	Serum	140–350 units/ml
17-Hydroxycorticosteroids	Plasma	Males: 7–19 μg/100 ml Females: 9–21 μg/100 ml After 25 USP units im of adrenocorticotropic hormone: 35–55 μg/100 ml
Immunoglobulins	Serum	
IgG		800–1600 mg/100 ml
IgA		50–250 mg/100 ml
IgM		40–120 mg/100 ml
IgD		0.5–3.0 mg/100 ml
IgE		0.01–0.04 mg/100 ml
Insulin	Plasma	11–240 μIU/ml (bioassay) 4–24 μunit/ml (radioimmunoassay)
Insulin tolerance	Serum	Fasting: glucose of 70–110 mg/100 ml 30 min: fall to 50% of fasting level 90 min: fasting level
Iodine, butanol extraction (BEI)	Serum	3.5–6.5 μg/100 ml
protein bound (PBI)	Serum	4.0–8.0 μg/100 ml
Iron, total	Serum	50–150 μg/100 ml
Iron-binding capacity	Serum	250–450 μg/100 ml
Iron saturation	Serum	20–55%
Isocitric dehydrogenase	Serum	50–250 units/ml
Ketone bodies	Serum	Negative
17-Ketosteroids	Plasma	25–125 μg/100 ml
Lactic acid	Whole blood (venous)	5–20 mg/100 ml
	Whole blood (arterial)	3–7 mg/100 ml
Lactate dehydrogenase (LDH)	Serum	80–120 Wacker units 150–450 Wroblewski units 71–207 IU/liter
Lactate dehydrogenase isoenzymes	Serum	Anode: LDH_1 17–27% LDH_2 27–37% LDH_3 18–25% LDH_4 3–8% Cathode: LDH_5 0–5%
Lactate dehydrogenase (heat stable)	Serum	30–60% of total

Table I—continued

Test	Material	Normal Value
Lactose tolerance	Serum	Serum glucose changes are similar to those seen in a glucose tolerance test
Lead	Whole blood	0–50 μg/100 ml
Leucine aminopeptidase (LAP)	Serum	Males: 80–200 Goldbarg-Rutenburg units/ml Females: 75–185 Goldbarg-Rutenburg units/ml
Lipase	Serum	0–1.5 Cherry–Crandall units/ml 14–280 mlU/ml
Lipids, total	Serum	400–800 mg/100 ml
cholesterol		150–250 mg/100 ml
triglycerides		10–190 mg/100 ml
phospholipids		150–380 mg/100 ml
fatty acids		9.0–15.0 mmole/liter
neutral fat		0–200 mg/100 ml
phospholipid phosphorus		8.0–11.0 mg/100 ml
Lithium	Serum	Negative Therapeutic level: 0.5–1.5 mEq/liter
Long-acting thyroid-stimulating hormone (LATS)	Serum	None
Luteinizing hormone (LH)	Plasma	Males: < 11 mlU/ml Females: midcycle peak > three times baseline value Premenopausal: < 25 mlU/ml Postmenopausal: > 25 mlU/ml
Macroglobulins, total	Serum	70–430 mg/100 ml
Magnesium	Serum	1.5–2.5 mEq/liter 1.8–3.0 mg/100 ml
Methemoglobin	Whole blood	0–0.24 g/100 ml 0.4–1.5% of total hemoglobin
Mucoprotein	Serum	80–200 mg/100 ml
Nonprotein nitrogen (NPN)	Serum or plasma Whole blood	20–35 mg/100 ml 25–50 mg/100 ml
5′-Nucleotidase	Serum	0–1.6 units
Ornithine carbamyl transferase (OCT)	Serum	8–20 mlU/ml
Osmolality	Serum	280–295 mOsm/liter
Oxygen		
pressure (pO_2)	Whole blood, arterial	95–100 mm Hg
content	Whole blood, arterial	15–23 volumes %
saturation	Whole blood, arterial	94–100%
pH	Whole blood, arterial	7.38–7.44
	Whole blood, venous	7.36–7.41
	Serum or plasma, venous	7.35–7.45

Continued on next page

Table I—continued

Test	Material	Normal Value
Phenylalanine	Serum	Adults: < 3.0 mg/100 ml Newborns (term): 1.2–3.5 mg/100 ml
Phosphatase, acid, total	Serum	0–1.1 units/ml (Bodansky) 1–4 units/ml (King–Armstrong) 0.13–0.63 unit/ml (Bessey–Lowry) 1.4–5.5 units/ml (Gutman–Gutman) 0–0.56 unit/ml (Roy) 0–6.0 units/ml (Shinowara–Jones–Reinhart)
Phosphatase, alkaline, total	Serum	Adults: 1.5–4.5 units/100 ml (Bodansky) 4–13 units/100 ml (King–Armstrong) 0.8–2.3 units/ml (Bessey–Lowry) 15–35 units/ml (Shinowara–Jones–Reinhart) Children: 5.0–14.0 units/100 ml (Bodansky) 3.4–9.0 units/ml (Bessey–Lowry) 15–30 units/100 ml (King–Armstrong)
Phospholipid phosphorus	Serum	8–11 mg/100 ml
Phospholipids	Serum	150–380 mg/100 ml
Phosphorus, inorganic	Serum	Adults: 1.8–2.6 mEq/liter 3.0–4.5 mg/100 ml Children: 2.3–4.1 mEq/liter 4.0–7.0 mg/100 ml
Potassium	Plasma	3.8–5.0 mEq/liter
Proteins, total	Serum	6.0–7.8 g/100 ml
albumin		3.2–4.5 g/100 ml
globulin		2.3–3.5 g/100 ml
Protoporphyrin	Erythrocytes	15–50 μg/100 ml
Pyruvate	Whole blood	0.3–0.9 mg/100 ml
Salicylates	Serum	Negative Therapeutic level: 20–25 mg/100 ml
Sodium	Plasma	136–142 mEq/liter
Sulfate, inorganic	Serum	0.2–1.3 mEq/liter 0.9–6.0 mg/100 ml as SO_4
Sulfhemoglobin	Whole blood	Negative
Sulfobromophthalein (bromsulfonphthalein, BSP) (5 mg/kg)	Serum	< 6% retention after 45 min
Sulfonamides	Serum or whole blood	Negative
Testosterone	Serum or plasma	Males: 400–1200 ng/100 ml Females: 30–120 ng/100 ml
Thiocyanate	Serum	Negative
Thymol flocculation	Serum	0–5 units

Table I—continued

Test	Material	Normal Value	
Thyroid hormone tests	Serum	Expressed as Thyroxine	Expressed as Iodine
T_4 (by column)		5.0–11.0 μg/100 ml	3.2–7.2 μg/100 ml
T_4 (by competitive binding–Murphy–Pattee)		6.0–11.8 μg/100 ml	3.9–7.7 μg/100 ml
free T_4		0.9–2.3 ng/100 ml	0.6–1.5 ng/100 ml
T_3 (resin uptake)		25–38 relative % uptake	
thyroxine-binding globulin (TBG)		10–26 μg/100 ml (expressed as T_4 uptake)	
Transaminases: GOT	Serum	8–33 units/ml	
GPT	Serum	1–36 units/ml	
Triglycerides	Serum	10–190 mg/100 ml	
Urea nitrogen	Serum	8–18 mg/100 ml	
Urea clearance	Serum and urine	Maximum clearance: 64–99 ml/min Standard clearance: 41–65 ml/min or more than 75% of normal clearance	
Uric acid	Serum	Males: 2.1–7.8 mg/100 ml Females: 2.0–6.4 mg/100 ml	
Vitamin A	Serum	15–60 μg/100 ml	
Vitamin A tolerance	Serum	Fasting: 15–60 μg/100 ml 3 or 6 hr after 5000 units vitamin A/kg: 200–600 μg/100 ml 24 hr: fasting values or slightly above	
Unsaturated cyanocobalamin-binding capacity	Serum	1000–2000 pg/ml	
Xylose absorption	Serum	25–40 mg/100 ml between 1 and 2 hr; in malabsorption, maximum approximately 10 mg/100 ml Dose: Adult: 25 g D-xylose Children: 0.5 g/kg D-xylose	
Zinc	Serum	50–150 μg/100 ml	
Zinc sulfate turbidity	Serum	< 12 units	

Table II—URINE

Test	Type of Specimen	Normal Value
Acetoacetic acid	Random	Negative
Acetone	Random	Negative
Addis count	12-hr collection	White blood cells and epithelial cells: 1,800,000/12 hr Red blood cells: 500,000/12 hr Hyaline casts: 0–5000/12 hr
Albumin, qualitative	Random	Negative
quantitative	24 hr	10–100 mg/24 hr

Continued on next page

Table II—continued

Test	Type of Specimen	Normal Value
Aldosterone	24 hr	2–26 μg/24 hr
Alkapton bodies	Random	Negative
Alpha-amino acid nitrogen	24 hr	100–290 mg/24 hr
δ-Aminolevulinic acid	Random	Adults: 0.1–0.6 mg/100 ml
		Children: < 0.5 mg/100 ml
	24 hr	1.5–7.5 mg/24 hr
Ammonia nitrogen	24 hr	20–70 mEq/24 hr
		500–1200 mg/24 hr
Amylase	2 hr	35–260 Somogyi units/hr
Arsenic	24 hr	< 50 μg/liter
Ascorbic acid (vitamin C)	Random	1–7 mg/100 ml
	24 hr	> 50 mg/24 hr
Bence Jones protein	Random	Negative
Beryllium	24 hr	< 0.05 μg/24 hr
Bilirubin, qualitative	Random	Negative
Blood, occult	Random	Negative
Borate	24 hr	< 2 mg/liter
Calcium, qualitative (Sulkowitch)	Random	1+ turbidity
quantitative	24 hr	Average diet: 100–250 mg/24 hr
		Low calcium diet: < 150 mg/24 hr
		High calcium diet: 250–300 mg/24 hr
Catecholamines	Random	0–14 μg/100 ml
	24 hr	< 100 μg/24 hr (varies with activity)
Chloride	24 hr	110–250 mEq/24 hr
Concentration test (Fishberg)	Random after fluid restriction	Specific gravity: > 1.025
		Osmolality: > 850 mOsm/liter
Copper	24 hr	0–30 μg/24 hr
Coproporphyrin	Random	Adults: 3–20 μg/100 ml
	24 hr	50–160 μg/24 hr
		Children: 0–80 μg/24 hr
Creatine	24 hr	Males: 0–40 mg/24 hr
		Females: 0–100 mg/24 hr
		Higher in children and during pregnancy
Creatinine	24 hr	Males: 20–26 mg/kg/24 hr
		1.0–2.0 g/24 hr
		Females: 14–22 mg/kg/24 hr
		0.8–1.8 g/24 hr
Cystine, qualitative	Random	Negative
Cystine and cysteine	24 hr	10–100 mg/24 hr
Diacetic acid	Random	Negative
Epinephrine	24 hr	0–20 μg/24 hr
Estrogens, total	24 hr	Males: 5–18 μg/24 hr
		Females: Ovulation: 28–100 μg/24 hr
		Luteal peak: 22–105 μg/24 hr
		At menses: 4–25 μg/24 hr
		Pregnancy: Up to 45,000 μg/24 hr
		Postmenopausal: 14–20 μg/24 hr

Table II—continued

Test	Type of Specimen	Normal Value
Estrogens, fractionated	24 hr	Nonpregnant, midcycle
Estrone (E1)		2–25 μg/24 hr
Estradiol (E2)		0–10 μg/24 hr
Estriol (E3)		2–30 μg/24 hr
Fat, qualitative	Random	Negative
FIGLU (N-formiminoglutamic acid)	24 hr	< 3 mg/24 hr After 15 g of L-histidine: 4 mg/8 hr
Fluoride	24 hr	< 1 mg/24 hr
Follicle-stimulating hormone (FSH)	24 hr	Adults: 6–50 mouse uterine units (MUU)/24 hr Prepubertal: < 10 MUU/24 hr Postmenopausal: > 50 MUU/24 hr
Fructose	24 hr	30–65 mg/24 hr
Glucose, qualitative	Random	Negative
quantitative:	24 hr	
copper-reducing substances		0.5–1.5 g/24 hr
total sugars		Average: 250 mg/24 hr
glucose		Average: 130 mg/24 hr
Gonadotropins, pituitary (FSH and LH)	24 hr	10–50 MUU/24 hr
Hemoglobin	Random	Negative
Homogentisic acid	Random	Negative
Homovanillic acid (HVA)	24 hr	< 15 mg/24 hr
17-Hydroxycorticosteroids	24 hr	Males: 5.5–14.5 mg/24 hr Females: 4.9–12.9 mg/24 hr Lower in children After 25 USP units im of adreno-corticotropic hormone: a two- to fourfold increase
5-Hydroxyindoleacetic acid (5-HIAA), qualitative	Random	Negative
quantitative	24 hr	< 9 mg/24 hr
Indican	24 hr	10–20 mg/24 hr
Ketone bodies	Random	Negative
17-Ketosteroids	24 hr	Males: 8–15 mg/24 hr Females: 6–11.5 mg/24 hr Children: 12–15 years, 5–12 mg/24 hr < 12 years, < 5 mg/24 hr After 25 USP units im of adreno-corticotropic hormone: 50–100% increase
Androsterone		Males: 2.0–5.0 mg/24 hr Females: 0.8–3.0 mg/24 hr
Etiocholanolone		Males: 1.4–5.0 mg/24 hr Females: 0.8–4.0 mg/24 hr
Dehydroepiandrosterone		Males: 0.2–2.0 mg/24 hr Females: 0.2–1.8 mg/24 hr
11-Ketoandrosterone		Males: 0.2–1.0 mg/24 hr Females: 0.2–0.8 mg/24 hr

Continued on next page

Table II—continued

Test	Type of Specimen	Normal Value
11-Ketoetiocholanolone		Males: 0.2–1.0 mg/24 hr Females: 0.2–0.8 mg/24 hr
11-Hydroxyandrosterone		Males: 0.1–0.8 mg/24 hr Females: 0.0–0.5 mg/24 hr
11-Hydroxyetiocholanolone		Males: 0.2–0.6 mg/24 hr Females: 0.1–1.1 mg/24 hr
Lactose	24 hr	12–40 mg/24 hr
Lead	24 hr	$< 100 \ \mu g/24$ hr
Magnesium	24 hr	6.0–8.5 mEq/24 hr
Melanin, qualitative	Random	Negative
3-Methoxy-4-hydroxymandelic acid (VMA)	24 hr	Adults: 1.5–7.5 mg/24 hr Infants: 83 μg/kg/24 hr
Mucin	24 hr	100–150 mg/24 hr
Myoglobin, qualitative	Random	Negative
quantitative	24 hr	< 1.5 mg/liter
Osmolality	Random	500–800 mOsm/liter
Pentoses	24 hr	2–5 mg/kg/24 hr
pH	Random	4.6–8.0
Phenolsulfonphthalein (PSP)	Urine, timed after 6 mg iv of phenolsulfon-phthalein: 15 min 30 min 60 min 120 min	 20–50% dye excreted 16–24% dye excreted 9–17% dye excreted 3–10% dye excreted
Phenylpyruvic acid, qualitative	Random	Negative
Phosphorus	Random	0.9–1.3 g/24 hr
Porphobilinogen, qualitative	Random	Negative
quantitative	24 hr	0–2.0 mg/24 hr
Potassium	24 hr	40–80 mEq/24 hr
Pregnancy tests	Concentrated morning speci-men	Positive in normal pregnancies or with tumors producing chorionic gonadotropin
Pregnanediol	24 hr	Males: 0–1 mg/24 hr Females: 1–8 mg/24 hr Peak: 1 week after ovulation Pregnancy: 60–100 mg/24 hr Children: negative
Pregnanetriol	24 hr	Males: 1.0–2.0 mg/24 hr Females: 0.5–2.0 mg/24 hr Children: < 0.5 mg/24 hr
Protein, qualitative	Random	Negative
quantitative	24 hr	10–100 mg/24 hr
Reducing substances, total	24 hr	0.5–1.5 mg/24 hr
Sodium	24 hr	80–180 mEq/24 hr
Solids, total	24 hr	55–70 g/24 hr Decreases with age to 30 g/24 hr

Table II—continued

Test	Type of Specimen	Normal Value
Specific gravity	Random	1.016–1.022 (normal fluid intake)
		1.001–1.035 (range)
Sugars (excluding glucose)	Random	Negative
Titratable acidity	24 hr	20–50 mEq/24 hr
Urea nitrogen	24 hr	6–17 g/24 hr
Uric acid	24 hr	250–750 mg/24 hr
Urobilinogen	2 hr	0.3–1.0 Ehrlich unit
	24 hr	0.05–2.5 mg/24 hr or
		0.5–4.0 Ehrlich units/24 hr
Uropepsin	Random	15–45 units/hr
	24 hr	1500–5000 units/24 hr
Uroporphyrins, qualitative	Random	Negative
quantitative	24 hr	10–30 μg/24 hr
Vanillylmandelic acid (VMA)	24 hr	1.5–7.5 mg/24 hr
Volume, total	24 hr	600–1600 ml/24 hr
Zinc	24 hr	0.15–1.2 mg/24 hr

Table III—HEMATOLOGY

Test	Normal Value
Blood volume	Males: 69 ml/kg
	Females: 65 ml/kg
Coagulation tests	
Bleeding time (Ivy)	1–6 min
Bleeding time (Duke)	1–3 min
Clot retraction	½ the original mass in 2 hr
Dilute blood clot lysis time	Clot lyses between 6 and 10 hr at 37°
Euglobin clot lysis time	Clot lyses between 2 and 6 hr at 37°
Partial thromboplastin time (PTT)	60–70 sec
Kaolin activated	35–50 sec
Prothrombin time	12–14 sec
Venous clotting time	
Three tubes	5–15 min
Two tubes	5–8 min
Complete blood count (CBC)	
Hematocrit	Males: 40–54%
	Females: 38–47%
Hemoglobin	Males: 13.5–18.0 g/100 ml
	Females: 12.0–16.0 g/100 ml
Red cell count	Males: 4.6–6.2 $\times$ 10^6/μl
	Females: 4.2–5.4 $\times$ 10^6/μl
White cell count	4500–11,000/μl
Erythrocyte indexes	
Mean corpuscular volume (MCV)	82–98 μm^3
Mean corpuscular hemoglobin (MCH)	27–31 pg
Mean corpuscular hemoglobin concentration (MCHC)	32–36%

Continued on next page

Table III—continued

Test	Normal Value
Hemoglobin A$_2$	1.5–3.5%
Hemoglobin F	< 2%

Osmotic fragility

% NaCl	% Lysis (fresh)	% Lysis (after 24-hr incubation at 37°)
0.20		95–100
0.30	97–100	85–100
0.35	90–99	75–100
0.40	50–95	65–100
0.45	5–45	55–95
0.50	0–6	40–85
0.55	0	15–70
0.60		0–40
0.65		0–10
0.70		0–5
0.75		0

Test	Normal Value
Plasma volume	Males: 39 ml/kg Females: 40 ml/kg
Platelet count	150,000–400,000/μl
Reticulocyte count	0.5–1.5% 25,000–75,000 cells/μl
Sedimentation rate (ESR) (Westergren)	Males under 50 years: < 15 mm/hr Males over 50 years: < 20 mm/hr Females under 50 years: < 20 mm/hr Females over 50 years: < 30 mm/hr
Viscosity	1.4–1.8 times water
White blood cell differential (adult)	*Mean Percent*
Segmented neutrophils	56%
Bands	3%
Eosinophils	2.7%
Basophils	0.3%
Lymphocytes	34%
Monocytes	4%
Whole blood clot lysis time	None in 24 hr

Table IV—SEROLOGY

Test	Normal Value
Antibovine milk antibodies	Negative
Antidesoxyribonuclease (ADNAase)	< 1:20
Antinuclear antibodies (ANA)	< 1:10
Antistreptococcal hyaluronidase (ASH)	< 1:256
Antistreptolysin O (ASLO)	< 160 Todd units
Australia antigen	*see* Hepatitis-associated antigen
Brucella agglutinins	< 1:80
Coccidioidomycosis antibodies	Negative

Table IV—continued

Test	Normal Value
Cold agglutinins	< 1:32
Complement, C'3	100–170 mg/100 ml
C-Reactive protein (CRP)	0
Fluorescent treponemal antibodies (FTA)	Nonreactive
Hepatitis-associated antigen (HAA or HBAg)	Negative
Heterophile antibodies	< 1:56
Histoplasma agglutinins	< 1:8
Latex fixation	Negative
Leptospira agglutinins	Negative
Ox cell hemolysin	< 1:480
Rheumatoid factor	
sensitized sheep cell	< 1:160
latex fixation	< 1:80
bentonite particles	< 1:32
Streptococcal MG agglutinins	< 1:20
Thyroid antibodies	
antithyroglobulin	< 1:32
antithyroid microsomal	< 1:56
Toxoplasma antibodies	< 1:4
Trichina agglutinins	0
Tularemia agglutinins	< 1:80
Typhoid agglutinins	
O	< 1:80
H	< 1:80
VDRL	Nonreactive
Weil–Felix (Proteus OX-2, OX-K, and OX-19 agglutinins)	Fourfold rise in titer between acute convalescent sera

Table V—CEREBROSPINAL FLUID

Test or Constituent	Normal Value
Albumin	10–30 mg/100 ml
Albumin : globulin ratio	1.6–2.2
Calcium	2.1–2.9 mEq/liter
Cell count	0–8 cells/μl
Chloride	Adults: 118–132 mEq/liter Children: 120–128 mEq/liter
Colloidal gold curve	0001111000
Globulins, qualitative (Pandy)	Negative
quantitative	6–16 mg/100 ml
Glucose	45–75 mg/100 ml
Lactate dehydrogenase (LDH)	Approximately $\frac{1}{10}$ of serum level
Protein, total cerebrospinal fluid	15–45 mg/100 ml
ventricular fluid	8–15 mg/100 ml

Continued on next page

Table V—continued

Test or Constituent	Normal Value
Protein electrophoresis	
Prealbumin	4.1 ± 1.2%
Albumin	62.4 ± 5.6%
Alpha-1 globulin	5.3 ± 1.2%
Alpha-2 globulin	8.2 ± 2.0%
Beta globulin	12.8 ± 2.0%
Gamma globulin	7.2 ± 1.1%
Xanthochromia	Negative

Table VI—AMNIOTIC FLUID

	Normal Value	
Test	**Early Gestation (Before 28 Weeks)**	**Term**
Appearance	Clear	Clear or slightly opalescent
Absorbance difference at 450 nm	< 0.05	< 0.02
Albumin	0.04	0.05
Bilirubin	< 0.075 mg/100 ml	< 0.025 mg/100 ml
Chloride	Approximately equal to serum chloride	Generally 1–3 mEq/liter lower than serum chloride
Creatinine	0.8–1.1 mg/100 ml	1.8–4.0 mg/100 ml (generally greater than 2.0 mg/100 ml)
Estriol	Below 10 μg/100 ml	> 60 μg/100 ml
Osmolality	Approximately equal to serum osmolality	< 250 mOsm/liter
pCO_2	33–55 mm Hg	42–55 mm Hg (increases toward term)
pH	7.12–7.38	6.91–7.43 (decreases toward term)
Protein, total	0.60 ± 0.24 g/100 ml	0.26 ± 0.19 g/100 ml
Sodium	Approximately equal to serum sodium	Generally 7–10 mEq/liter lower than serum sodium
Staining, cytologic		
oil red O	< 10%	> 50%
nile blue sulfate	0	> 20%
Urea	18.0 ± 5.9 mg/100 ml	30.3 ± 11.4 mg/100 ml
Uric acid	3.72 ± 0.96 mg/100 ml	9.9 ± 2.23 mg/100 ml
Volume	450–1200 ml	500–1400 ml (increases toward term)

Table VII—GASTRIC FLUID

Test	Normal Value
Fasting residual volume	20–100 ml
pH	< 2.0
Basal acid output (BAO)	0–6 mEq/hr
Maximal acid output (MAO) after histamine stimulation	5–40 mEq/hr
BAO:MAO ratio	< 0.4

Table VIII—SEMINAL FLUID

Test	Normal Value
Liquefaction	Within 20 min
Morphology	$> 70\%$ normal, mature spermatozoa
Motility	$> 60\%$
pH	> 7.0 (average 7.7)
Sperm count	60–150 million/ml
Volume	1.5–5.0 ml

Table IX—SYNOVIAL FLUID

Test	Normal Value
Blood-synovial fluid glucose difference	< 10 mg/100 ml
Differential cell count	Granulocytes $< 25\%$ of nucleated cells
Fibrin clot	Absent
Mucin clot	Abundant
Nucleated cell count	< 200 cells/μl
Viscosity	High
Volume	< 3.5 ml

Table X—MISCELLANEOUS

Test	Specimen	Normal Value
Bile, qualitative	Random stool	Negative in adults; positive in children
Chloride	Sweat	4–60 mEq/liter
Clearances	Serum and timed urine	
creatinine, endogenous		115 ± 20 ml/min
diodrast		600–720 ml/min
inulin		100–150 ml/min
PAH		600–750 ml/min
Diagnex blue (tubeless gastric analysis)	Urine	Free acid present
Fat	Stool, 72 hr	Total fat: < 5 g/24 hr and 10–25% of dry matter Neutral fat: 1–5% of dry matter Free fatty acids: 5–13% of dry matter Combined fatty acids: 5–15% of dry matter
Nitrogen, total	Stool, 24 hr	10% of intake or 1–2 g/24 hr
Sodium	Sweat	10–80 mEq/liter
Trypsin activity	Random, fresh stool	Positive (2+ to 4+)
Thyroid ^{131}I uptake		7.5–25% in 6 hr
Urobilinogen, qualitative	Random stool	Positive
quantitative	Stool, 24 hr	40–200 mg/24 hr 30–280 Ehrlich units/24 hr

Evaluations
of
Drug
Interactions:
Index

Information on a suspected drug interaction can be located most quickly using the *nonproprietary drug name.* All suspected drug interactions discussed in EDI are listed by their nonproprietary name as follows:

Amitriptyline
−Alcohol, 1
−Bethanidine, 83

This listing is reversed to allow access to desired drug interaction information by using the nonproprietary name of either interacting drug:

Alcohol
−Amitriptyline, 1

When a major *drug trade name* is used to find the suspected drug interaction, the entry for this term refers to the nonproprietary drug name:

Elavil Hydrochloride—see Amitriptyline

When a *"class like"* term (*e.g.,* Tricyclic antidepressants) is used to find the suspected interaction, the entry for this term refers to the nonproprietary names of the drugs in that class:

Tricyclic antidepressants—*see*
Amitriptyline, Desipramine, Doxepin,
Imipramine, Nortriptyline,
Protriptyline

Index entries followed by (R) direct the reader to the Recommendations section of the Monograph first. Drugs discussed in the Recommendations section primarily involve agents that are not chemically and pharmacologically related to the title drugs but that may be expected to interact in a similar manner. Since these drugs might be considered as alternative therapy, their interactions with the title drugs, if they occur, are included for completeness. Entries followed by (SI) direct the reader to the Supplemental Information for a brief discussion of the interaction. For example:

Alcohol
−Ethchlorvynol, 47 (R)
−Phenytoin, 444 (SI)

A

Acenocoumarol
–Acetaminophen, 263
–Acetohexamide, 245
–Alcohol, 265
–Allopurinol, 366 (SI)
–Aluminum ions, 266
–Aminosalicylic acid, 363 (SI)
–Amitriptyline, 364 (SI), 375 (SI)
–Antihistamines, 282
–Antipyrine, 295 (R)
–Ascorbic acid, 268
–Aspirin, 270
–Barbiturates, 291
–Benzodiazepines, 276
–Carbamazepine, 366 (SI)
–Carisoprodol, 288
–Chloral betaine, 273
–Chloral hydrate, 273
–Chloramphenicol, 364 (SI),
   390 (SI)
–Chlormezanone, 288
–Chlorphenesin, 288
–Chlorpropamide, 245
–Cholestyramine, 278
–Cinchophen, 297
–Clofibrate, 280
–Desipramine, 364 (SI), 375 (SI)
–Dextrothyroxine, 301
–Diazoxide, 366 (SI)
–Disulfiram, 366 (SI)
–Doxepin, 364 (SI), 375 (SI)
–Estrogens, 365 (SI)
–Ethacrynic acid, 364 (SI),
   418 (SI)
–Ethchlorvynol, 365 (SI)
–Ethotoin, 193
–Fluoxymesterone, 289
–Glucagon, 366 (SI)
–Glutethimide, 284
–Griseofulvin, 285
–Haloperidol, 401 (SI)
–Heparin, 362 (SI)
–Ibuprofen, 343 (SI)
–Imipramine, 364 (SI), 375 (SI)
–Indomethacin, 286
–Insulin, 245 (R)
–Kanamycin, 390 (SI)
–Levothyroxine, 301
–Liothyronine, 301
–Liotrix, 301
–Magnesium ions, 266
–Mefenamic acid, 344 (SI),
   363 (SI)
–Menadione, 303
–Mephenytoin, 193
–Meprobamate, 288
–Mercaptopurine, 366 (SI)
–Methandrostenolone, 289
–Methocarbamol, 288
–Methylphenidate, 366 (SI)
–Methyltestosterone, 289
–Methyprylon, 284
–Nalidixic acid, 364 (SI),
   390 (SI)
–Neomycin, 364 (SI), 390 (SI)
–Norethandrolone, 289
–Nortriptyline, 364 (SI), 375 (SI)
–Oxandrolone, 289
–Oxymetholone, 289
–Oxyphenbutazone, 295
–Phenformin, 365 (SI)
–Phenylbutazone, 295

–Phenytoin, 193
–Phthalylsulfathiazole, 364 (SI),
   390 (SI)
–Phytonadione, 303
–Primidone, 193
–Propylthiouracil, 366 (SI)
–Protriptyline, 364 (SI), 375 (SI)
–Quinidine, 297
–Quinine, 297
–Rifampin, 364 (SI), 390 (SI)
–Salicylates, 270
–Stanozolol, 289
–Streptomycin, 390 (SI)
–Sulfachlorpyridazine, 364 (SI),
   390 (SI)
–Sulfadiazine, 364 (SI), 390 (SI)
–Sulfamerazine, 364 (SI),
   390 (SI)
–Sulfameter, 364 (SI), 390 (SI)
–Sulfamethazine, 364 (SI),
   390 (SI)
–Sulfamethizole, 364 (SI),
   390 (SI)
–Sulfamethoxazole, 364 (SI),
   390 (SI)
–Sulfamethoxypyridazine, 364
   (SI), 390 (SI)
–Sulfaphenazole, 364 (SI),
   390 (SI)
–Sulfapyridine, 364 (SI),
   390 (SI)
–Sulfasalazine, 364 (SI),
   390 (SI)
–Sulfinpyrazone, 295 (R)
–Sulfisoxazole, 364 (SI),
   390 (SI)
–Tetracyclines, 299
–Thiazides, 364 (SI), 418 (SI)
–Thyroglobulin, 301
–Thyroid, 301
–Thyroxine fraction, 301
–Tolazamide, 245
–Tolbutamide, 245
–Triclofos, 273
–Tybamate, 288
–Vitamin C, 268
–Vitamin E, 367 (SI)
–Vitamin K, 303
Acetaminophen
–Acenocoumarol, 263
–Alcohol, 16 (R)
–Anisindione, 263
–Dicumarol, 263
–Diphenadione, 263
–Methotrexate, 150 (R)
–Phenindione, 263
–Phenprocoumon, 263
–Warfarin, 263
Acetazolamide
–Methenamine, 391 (SI)
Acetohexamide
–Acenocoumarol, 245
–Alcohol, 240
–Allopurinol, 35
–Anisindione, 245
–Aspirin, 36
–Barbiturates, 445 (SI)
–Betamethasone, 38
–Chloramphenicol, 243
–Chlorthalidone, 40
–Cortisone, 38
–Dexamethasone, 38
–Dicumarol, 245
–Diphenadione, 245
–Ethacrynic acid, 40 (R)

–Ethotoin, 112 (R)
–Fludrocortisone, 38
–Fluprednisolone, 38
–Furosemide, 40 (R)
–Hydrocortisone, 38
–Isocarboxazid, 110 (R)
–Mebanazine, 110 (R)
–Mephenytoin, 112 (R)
–Meprednisone, 38
–Methylprednisolone, 38
–Metolazone, 40
–Oxyphenbutazone, 247
–Paramethasone, 38
–Pargyline, 110 (R)
–Phenelzine, 110 (R)
–Phenindione, 245
–Phenprocoumon, 245
–Phenylbutazone, 247
–Phenytoin, 112 (R)
–Prednisolone, 38
–Prednisone, 38
–Propranolol, 114 (R)
–Quinethazone, 40
–Salicylates, 36
–Spironolactone, 40 (R)
–Sulfinpyrazone, 247
–Sulfonamides, 250
–Thiazides, 40
–Tranylcypromine, 110 (R)
–Triamcinolone, 38
–Triamterene, 40 (R)
–Warfarin, 245
Acetophenazine
–Alcohol, 402 (SI)
–Aluminum ions, 25
–Amitriptyline, 375 (SI),
   402 (SI)
–Amphetamine, 27
–Barbiturates, 183
–Benztropine, 30
–Bethanidine, 81
–Biperiden, 30
–Cycrimine, 30
–Debrisoquin, 81
–Desipramine, 375 (SI), 402 (SI)
–Dextroamphetamine, 27
–Doxepin, 375 (SI), 402 (SI)
–Guanethidine, 81
–Imipramine, 375 (SI), 402 (SI)
–Levodopa, 122
–Magnesium ions, 25
–Methamphetamine, 27
–Methyldopa, 81 (R)
–Methylphenidate, 27
–Nortriptyline, 375 (SI), 402 (SI)
–Pentylenetetrazol, 402 (SI)
–Phenmetrazine, 27
–Picrotoxin, 402 (SI)
–Piperazine, 34
–Procyclidine, 30
–Propranolol, 355 (SI)
–Protriptyline, 375 (SI), 402 (SI)
–Trihexyphenidyl, 30
Acetyldigitoxin
–Amiloride, 61
–Amphotericin B, 409 (SI)
–Anisotropine, 65
–Barbiturates, 409 (SI)
–Belladonna alkaloids, 65
–Calcium ions, 50
–Chlorthalidone, 52
–Cholestyramine, 62
–Colestipol, 62
–Dicyclomine, 65   *continued*

Acetyldigitoxin *(cont.)*
  –Ethacrynic acid, 52 (R)
  –Ethotoin, 57
  –Furosemide, 52 (R)
  –Glycopyrrolate, 65
  –Heparin, 409 (SI)
  –Hexocyclium, 65
  –Isopropamide, 65
  –Mephenytoin, 57
  –Mercaptomerin, 52
  –Methantheline, 65
  –Methscopolamine, 65
  –Metolazone, 52
  –Oxyphencyclimine, 65
  –Oxyphenonium, 65
  –Phenytoin, 57
  –Pipenzolate, 65
  –Piperidolate, 65
  –Polyamine-methylene resin, 62
  –Propantheline, 65
  –Quinethazone, 52
  –Rauwolfia alkaloids, 58
  –Spironolactone, 61
  –Thiazides, 52
  –Triamterene, 61
  –Tridihexethyl, 65
Acetylsalicylic acid—*see* Aspirin
Achromycin—*see* Tetracycline
Acid–Base Balance Therapy, 327
Actasal—*see* Choline salicylate
Actomol—*see* Mebanazine
Acylanid—*see* Acetyldigitoxin
Adapin—*see* Doxepin
Adrenaline Chloride—*see*
  Epinephrine
Adrenergics—*see* Amphetamine,
  Cyclopentamine,
  Dextroamphetamine,
  Dopamine, Ephedrine,
  Epinephrine, Isoproterenol,
  Levarterenol, Metaraminol,
  Methamphetamine,
  Methoxamine,
  Methylphenidate,
  Phenylephrine,
  Phenylpropanolamine,
  Pseudoephedrine, Tyramine
Adrenergic Therapy, 332
Adrenocorticosteroids—*see*
  Betamethasone, Cortisone,
  Dexamethasone,
  Fludrocortisone,
  Fluprednisolone,
  Hydrocortisone,
  Meprednisone,
  Methylprednisolone,
  Paramethasone, Prednisolone,
  Prednisone, Triamcinolone
Adroyd—*see* Oxymetholone
Akineton—*see* Biperiden
Alcohol
  –Acenocoumarol, 265
  –Acetaminophen, 16 (R)
  –Acetohexamide, 240
  –Amitriptyline, 1
  –Anisindione, 265
  –Aspirin, 16
  –Barbiturates, 180
  –Benzodiazepines, 47
  –Bethanidine, 79
  –Carisoprodol, 145
  –Chloral betaine, 20
  –Chloral hydrate, 20
  –Chlormezanone, 145
  –Chlorphenesin, 145

  –Chlorpropamide, 240
  –Debrisoquin, 79
  –Desipramine, 1
  –Dicumarol, 265
  –Diphenadione, 265
  –Doxepin, 1
  –Ethchlorvynol, 47 (R), 145 (R),
    180 (R)
  –Furazolidone, 389 (SI)
  –Glutethimide, 47 (R), 145 (R),
    180 (R)
  –Guanethidine, 79
  –Haloperidol, 402 (SI)
  –Imipramine, 1
  –Insulin, 240 (R)
  –Meprobamate, 145
  –Methaqualone, 47 (R), 145 (R),
    180 (R)
  –Methocarbamol, 145
  –Metronidazole, 158
  –Nortriptyline, 1
  –Phenformin, 177
  –Phenindione, 265
  –Phenothiazines, 402 (SI)
  –Phenprocoumon, 265
  –Phenytoin, 371 (SI), 444 (SI)
  –Propoxyphene, 210
  –Protriptyline, 1
  –Salicylates, 16
  –Tolazamide, 240
  –Tolbutamide, 240
  –Triclofos, 20
  –Tybamate, 145
  –Warfarin, 265
Aldactone—*see* Spironolactone
Aldomet—*see* Methyldopa
Allobarbital
  –Acenocoumarol, 291
  –Acetohexamide, 445 (SI)
  –Acetyldigitoxin, 409 (SI)
  –Alcohol, 180
  –Amitriptyline, 161
  –Anisindione, 291
  –Antihistamines, 23
  –Betamethasone, 42
  –Chlorpropamide, 445 (SI)
  –Cortisone, 42
  –Desipramine, 161
  –Deslanoside, 409 (SI)
  –Dexamethasone, 42
  –Dicumarol, 291
  –Digitalis, 409 (SI)
  –Digitoxin, 409 (SI)
  –Digoxin, 409 (SI)
  –Diphenadione, 291
  –Doxepin, 161
  –Ethotoin, 205
  –Fludrocortisone, 42
  –Fluprednisolone, 42
  –Gitalin, 409 (SI)
  –Griseofulvin, 77
  –Haloperidol, 183 (R)
  –Hydrocortisone, 42
  –Imipramine, 161
  –Lanatoside C, 409 (SI)
  –Mephenytoin, 205
  –Meprednisone, 42
  –Methylprednisolone, 42
  –Nortriptyline, 161
  –Ouabain, 409 (SI)
  –Paramethasone, 42
  –Phenindione, 291
  –Phenothiazines, 183
  –Phenprocoumon, 291
  –Phenytoin, 205

  –Prednisolone, 42
  –Prednisone, 42
  –Primidone, 205
  –Propranolol, 95
  –Protriptyline, 161
  –Rauwolfia alkaloids, 236
  –Thiothixene, 183 (R)
  –Tolazamide, 445 (SI)
  –Tolbutamide, 445 (SI)
  –Triamcinolone, 42
  –Vitamin D, 455 (SI)
  –Warfarin, 291
Allopurinol
  –Acenocoumarol, 366 (SI)
  –Acetohexamide, 35
  –Aminophylline, 3
  –Anisindione, 366 (SI)
  –Azathioprine, 148
  –Chlorpropamide, 35
  –Dicumarol, 366 (SI)
  –Diphenadione, 366 (SI)
  –Dyphylline, 3
  –Iron, 5
  –Mercaptopurine, 148
  –Oxtriphylline, 3
  –Phenindione, 366 (SI)
  –Phenprocoumon, 366 (SI)
  –Probenecid, 6
  –Sulfinpyrazone, 6 (R)
  –Theobromine, 3
  –Theophylline, 3
  –Thioguanine, 148
  –Tolazamide, 35
  –Tolbutamide, 35
  –Warfarin, 366 (SI)
Alpen—*see* Ampicillin
Alphadrol—*see* Fluprednisolone
Alphaprodine
  –Isocarboxazid, 142
  –Pargyline, 142
  –Phenelzine, 142
  –Tranylcypromine, 142
Alseroxylon
  –Acetyldigitoxin, 58
  –Amitriptyline, 99
  –Amphetamines, 67
  –Barbiturates, 236
  –Chloroform, 220
  –Cinchophen, 219
  –Cyclopropane, 220
  –Desipramine, 99
  –Deslanoside, 58
  –Digitalis, 58
  –Digitoxin, 58
  –Digoxin, 58
  –Doxepin, 99
  –Enflurane, 220
  –Ephedrine, 67
  –Ether, 220
  –Ethyl chloride, 220
  –Fluroxene, 220
  –Gitalin, 58
  –Halopropane, 220
  –Halothane, 220
  –Imipramine, 99
  –Lanatoside C, 58
  –Levarterenol, 67 (R)
  –Metaraminol, 67 (R)
  –Methoxamine, 67 (R)
  –Methoxyflurane, 220
  –Methylphenidate, 67
  –Nitrous oxide, 220
  –Nortriptyline, 99
  –Ouabain, 58
  –Phenylephrine, 67 (R)

continued

Cardioquin—*see* Quinidine
Carisoprodol
–Acenocoumarol, 288
–Alcohol, 145
–Amitriptyline, 147
–Anisindione, 288
–Desipramine, 147
–Dicumarol, 288
–Diphenadione, 288
–Doxepin, 147
–Imipramine, 147
–Nortriptyline, 147
–Phenindione, 288
–Phenprocoumon, 288
–Protriptyline, 147
–Warfarin, 288
Carphenazine
–Alcohol, 402 (SI)
–Aluminum ions, 25
–Amitriptyline, 375 (SI),
  402 (SI)
–Amphetamine, 27
–Barbiturates, 183
–Benztropine, 30
–Bethanidine, 81
–Biperiden, 30
–Cycrimine, 30
–Debrisoquin, 81
–Desipramine, 375 (SI),
  402 (SI)
–Dextroamphetamine, 27
–Doxepin, 375 (SI), 402 (SI)
–Guanethidine, 81
–Imipramine, 375 (SI), 402 (SI)
–Levodopa, 122
–Magnesium ions, 25
–Methamphetamine, 27
–Methyldopa, 81 (R)
–Methylphenidate, 27
–Nortriptyline, 375 (SI), 402 (SI)
–Pentylenetetrazol, 402 (SI)
–Phenmetrazine, 27
–Picrotoxin, 402 (SI)
–Piperazine, 34
–Procyclidine, 30
–Propranolol, 355 (SI)
–Protriptyline, 375 (SI), 402 (SI)
–Trihexyphenidyl, 30
Catecholamines—*see* Dopamine,
  Epinephrine, Isoproterenol,
  Levarterenol, Metaraminol,
  Methoxamine, Nylidrin,
  Phenylephrine, Tyramine
Cedilanid—*see* Lanatoside C
Cedilanid-D—*see* Deslanoside
Cefadyl—*see* Cephapirin
Cefazolin
–Furosemide, 391 (SI)
–Probenecid, 392 (SI), 448 (SI)
–Sulfinpyrazone, 392 (SI)
Celestone—*see* Betamethasone
Cephalexin
–Furosemide, 391 (SI)
–Probenecid, 392 (SI), 448 (SI)
–Sulfinpyrazone, 392 (SI)
Cephaloglycin
–Furosemide, 391 (SI)
–Probenecid, 392 (SI), 448 (SI)
–Sulfinpyrazone, 392 (SI)
Cephaloridine
–Furosemide, 391 (SI)
–Probenecid, 392 (SI), 448 (SI)
–Sulfinpyrazone, 392 (SI)
Cephalosporins—*see* Cefazolin,
  Cephalexin, Cephaloglycin,

Cephaloridine, Cephalothin,
  Cephapirin, Cephradine
Cephalothin
–Furosemide, 391 (SI)
–Probenecid, 392 (SI), 448 (SI)
–Sulfinpyrazone, 392 (SI)
Cephapirin
–Furosemide, 391 (SI)
–Probenecid, 392 (SI), 448 (SI)
–Sulfinpyrazone, 392 (SI)
Cephradine
–Furosemide, 391 (SI)
–Probenecid, 392 (SI), 448 (SI)
–Sulfinpyrazone, 392 (SI)
Chel-Iron—*see* Iron
Chemestrogen—*see* Benzestrol
Chemotherapeutic drugs—*see*
  Cytarabine, Mercaptopurine,
  Methotrexate
Chloral betaine
–Acenocoumarol, 273
–Alcohol, 20
–Anisindione, 273
–Dicumarol, 273
–Diphenadione, 273
–Phenindione, 273
–Phenprocoumon, 273
–Warfarin, 273
Chloral hydrate
–Acenocoumarol, 273
–Alcohol, 20
–Amitriptyline, 161 (R)
–Anisindione, 273
–Desipramine, 161 (R)
–Dicumarol, 273
–Diphenadione, 273
–Doxepin, 161 (R)
–Furazolidone, 22
–Nortriptyline, 161 (R)
–Phenindione, 273
–Phenprocoumon, 273
–Protriptyline, 161 (R)
–Warfarin, 273
Chloramphenicol
–Acenocoumarol, 364 (SI),
  390 (SI)
–Acetohexamide, 243
–Anisindione, 364 (SI), 390 (SI)
–Chlorpropamide, 243
–Clindamycin, 133
–Cyanocobalamin, 450 (SI)
–Decamethonium, 254 (R)
–Dicumarol, 364 (SI), 390 (SI)
–Diphenadione, 364 (SI),
  390 (SI)
–Folic acid, 450 (SI)
–Gallamine triethiodide, 254 (R)
–Lincomycin, 133
–Methotrexate, 395 (SI)
–Metocurine, 254 (R)
–Pancuronium, 254 (R)
–Penicillins, 168
–Phenindione, 364 (SI),
  390 (SI)
–Phenprocoumon, 364 (SI),
  390 (SI)
–Phenytoin, 371 (SI), 390 (SI)
–Succinylcholine, 254 (R)
–Tolazamide, 243
–Tolbutamide, 243
–Tubocurarine, 254 (R)
–Vitamin B, 450 (SI)
–Warfarin, 364 (SI), 390 (SI)
Chlorcyclizine
–Acenocoumarol, 282
–Anisindione, 282

–Barbiturates, 23
–Dicumarol, 282
–Diphenadione, 282
–Phenindione, 282
–Phenprocoumon, 282
–Propranolol, 213
–Warfarin, 282
Chlordiazepoxide
–Acenocoumarol, 276
–Alcohol, 47
–Amitriptyline, 8
–Anisindione, 276
–Decamethonium, 75
–Desipramine, 8
–Dicumarol, 276
–Diphenadione, 276
–Doxepin, 8
–Gallamine triethiodide, 75
–Imipramine, 8
–Levodopa, 124
–Nortriptyline, 8
–Pancuronium, 75
–Phenindione, 276
–Phenprocoumon, 276
–Protriptyline, 8
–Succinylcholine, 75
–Tubocurarine, 75
–Warfarin, 276
Chlormezanone
–Acenocoumarol, 288
–Alcohol, 145
–Amitriptyline, 147
–Anisindione, 288
–Desipramine, 147
–Dicumarol, 288
–Diphenadione, 288
–Doxepin, 147
–Imipramine, 147
–Nortriptyline, 147
–Phenindione, 288
–Phenprocoumon, 288
–Protriptyline, 147
–Warfarin, 288
Chloroform
–Amphetamine, 90
–Bacitracin, 70 (R)
–Clindamycin, 70 (R)
–Colistin, 70
–Decamethonium, 347 (SI),
  439 (SI)
–Dihydrostreptomycin, 70
–Ephedrine, 90
–Epinephrine, 90
–Ethotoin, 200
–Gallamine triethiodide,
  347 (SI), 439 (SI)
–Gentamicin, 70
–Isoproterenol, 90
–Kanamycin, 70
–Levarterenol, 90
–Mephentermine, 90
–Mephenytoin, 200
–Metaraminol, 90
–Methoxamine, 90
–Metocurine, 347 (SI), 439 (SI)
–Neomycin, 70
–Pancuronium, 347 (SI),
  439 (SI)
–Phenylephrine, 90
–Phenytoin, 200
–Polymyxin, 70 (R)
–Primidone, 200
–Rauwolfia alkaloids, 220
–Streptomycin, 70
–Succinylcholine, 347 (SI),
  439 (SI)

continued

continued

continued

Digitoxin *(cont.)*
–Dicyclomine, 65
–Ethacrynic acid, 52 (R)
–Ethotoin, 57
–Furosemide, 52 (R)
–Glycopyrrolate, 65
–Heparin, 409 (SI)
–Hexocyclium, 65
–Isopropamide, 65
–Mephenytoin, 57
–Mercaptomerin, 52
–Methantheline, 65
–Methscopolamine, 65
–Metolazone, 52
–Oxyphencyclimine, 65
–Oxyphenonium, 65
–Phenytoin, 57
–Pipenzolate, 65
–Piperidolate, 65
–Polyamine-methylene resin, 62
–Propantheline, 65
–Quinethazone, 52
–Rauwolfia alkaloids, 58
–Spironolactone, 61
–Thiazides, 52
–Triamterene, 61
–Tridihexethyl, 65
Digoxin
–Amiloride, 61
–Amphotericin B, 409 (SI)
–Anisotropine, 65
–Barbiturates, 409 (SI)
–Belladonna alkaloids, 65
–Calcium ions, 50
–Chlorthalidone, 52
–Cholestyramine, 62
–Colestipol, 62
–Dicyclomine, 65
–Ethacrynic acid, 52 (R)
–Ethotoin, 57
–Furosemide, 52 (R)
–Glycopyrrolate, 65
–Heparin, 409 (SI)
–Hexocyclium, 65
–Isopropamide, 65
–Mephenytoin, 57
–Mercaptomerin, 52
–Methantheline, 65
–Methscopolamine, 65
–Metolazone, 52
–Oxyphencyclimine, 65
–Oxyphenonium, 65
–Phenytoin, 57
–Pipenzolate, 65
–Piperidolate, 65
–Polyamine-methylene resin, 62
–Propantheline, 65
–Quinethazone, 52
–Rauwolfia alkaloids, 58
–Spironolactone, 61
–Thiazides, 52
–Triamterene, 61
–Tridihexethyl, 65
Dihydrostreptomycin
–Chloroform, 70
–Cyclopropane, 70
–Decamethonium, 254
–Enflurane, 70
–Ether, 70
–Ethyl chloride, 70
–Gallamine triethiodide, 254
–Halopropane, 70
–Halothane, 70
–Methoxyflurane, 70
–Metocurine, 254
–Nitrous oxide, 70

–Pancuronium, 254
–Succinylcholine, 254
–Trichloroethylene, 70
–Trichloromonofluoromethane, 70
–Tubocurarine, 254
Dilantin—*see* Phenytoin
Dilor—*see* Dyphylline
Dimenhydrinate
–Acenocoumarol, 282
–Anisindione, 282
–Barbiturates, 23
–Dicumarol, 282
–Diphenadione, 282
–Phenindione, 282
–Phenprocoumon, 282
–Propranolol, 213
–Warfarin, 282
Dimetane—*see* Brompheniramine
Dimethyl tubocurarine—*see* Metocurine
Dipaxin—*see* Diphenadione
Diphenadione
–Acetaminophen, 263
–Acetohexamide, 245
–Alcohol, 265
–Allopurinol, 366 (SI)
–Aluminum ions, 266
–Aminosalicylic acid, 363 (SI)
–Amitriptyline, 364 (SI), 375 (SI)
–Antihistamines, 282
–Antipyrine, 295 (R)
–Ascorbic acid, 268
–Aspirin, 270
–Barbiturates, 291
–Benzodiazepines, 276
–Carbamazepine, 366 (SI)
–Carisoprodol, 288
–Chloral betaine, 273
–Chloral hydrate, 273
–Chloramphenicol, 364 (SI), 390 (SI)
–Chlormezanone, 288
–Chlorphenesin, 288
–Chlorpropamide, 245
–Cholestyramine, 278
–Cinchophen, 297
–Clofibrate, 280
–Desipramine, 364 (SI), 375 (SI)
–Dextrothyroxine, 301
–Diazoxide, 366 (SI)
–Disulfiram, 366 (SI)
–Doxepin, 364 (SI), 375 (SI)
–Estrogens, 365 (SI)
–Ethacrynic acid, 364 (SI), 418 (SI)
–Ethchlorvynol, 365 (SI)
–Ethotoin, 193
–Fluoxymesterone, 289
–Glucagon, 366 (SI)
–Glutethimide, 284
–Griseofulvin, 285
–Haloperidol, 401 (SI)
–Heparin, 362 (SI)
–Ibuprofen, 343 (SI)
–Imipramine, 364 (SI), 375 (SI)
–Indomethacin, 286
–Insulin, 245 (R)
–Kanamycin, 390 (SI)
–Levothyroxine, 301
–Liothyronine, 301
–Liotrix, 301
–Magnesium ions, 266
–Mefenamic acid, 344 (SI), 363 (SI)
–Menadione, 303

–Mephenytoin, 193
–Meprobamate, 288
–Mercaptopurine, 366 (SI)
–Methandrostenolone, 289
–Methocarbamol, 288
–Methylphenidate, 366 (SI)
–Methyprylon, 284
–Nalidixic acid, 364 (SI), 390 (SI)
–Neomycin, 364 (SI), 390 (SI)
–Norethandrolone, 289
–Nortriptyline, 364 (SI), 375 (SI)
–Oxandrolone, 289
–Oxymetholone, 289
–Oxyphenbutazone, 295
–Phenformin, 365 (SI)
–Phenylbutazone, 295
–Phenytoin, 193
–Phthalylsulfathiazole, 364 (SI), 390 (SI)
–Phytonadione, 303
–Primidone, 193
–Propylthiouracil, 366 (SI)
–Protriptyline, 364 (SI), 375 (SI)
–Quinidine, 297
–Quinine, 297
–Rifampin, 364 (SI), 390 (SI)
–Salicylates, 270
–Stanozolol, 289
–Streptomycin, 390 (SI)
–Sulfachlorpyridazine, 364 (SI), 390 (SI)
–Sulfadiazine, 364 (SI), 390 (SI)
–Sulfamerazine, 364 (SI), 390 (SI)
–Sulfameter, 364 (SI), 390 (SI)
–Sulfamethazine, 364 (SI), 390 (SI)
–Sulfamethoxazole, 364 (SI), 390 (SI)
–Sulfamethoxypyridazine, 364 (SI), 390 (SI)
–Sulfaphenazole, 364 (SI), 390 (SI)
–Sulfapyridine, 364 (SI), 390 (SI)
–Sulfasalazine, 364 (SI), 390 (SI)
–Sulfinpyrazone, 295 (R)
–Sulfisoxazole, 364 (SI), 390 (SI)
–Tetracyclines, 299
–Thiazides, 364 (SI), 418 (SI)
–Thyroglobulin, 301
–Thyroid, 301
–Thyroxine fraction, 301
–Tolazamide, 245
–Tolbutamide, 245
–Triclofos, 273
–Tybamate, 288
–Vitamin C, 268
–Vitamin E, 367 (SI)
–Vitamin K, 303
Diphenhydramine
–Acenocoumarol, 282
–Anisindione, 282
–Barbiturates, 23
–Dicumarol, 282
–Diphenadione, 282
–Phenindione, 282
–Phenprocoumon, 282
–Propranolol, 213
–Warfarin, 282
Diphenicillin
–Aspirin, 166
–Chloramphenicol, 168
–Decamethonium, 254 (R)
–Erythromycin, 173
–Gallamine triethiodide, 254 (R)

continued

continued

continued

continued

Methamphetamine *(cont.)*
–Phenothiazines, 27
–Phenytoin, 204
–Primidone, 204
–Propoxyphene, 212
–Protriptyline, 375 (SI)
–Rauwolfia alkaloids, 67
–Tranylcypromine, 188
Methandrostenolone
–Acenocoumarol, 289
–Aminopyrine, 165
–Anisindione, 289
–Antipyrine, 165
–Dicumarol, 289
–Diphenadione, 289
–Oxyphenbutazone, 165
–Phenindione, 289
–Phenprocoumon, 289
–Phenylbutazone, 165
–Sulfinpyrazone, 165
–Warfarin, 289
Methantheline
–Acetyldigitoxin, 65
–Deslanoside, 65
–Digitalis, 65
–Digitoxin, 65
–Digoxin, 65
–Gitalin, 65
–Lanatoside C, 65
–Ouabain, 65
Methapyrilene
–Acenocoumarol, 282
–Anisindione, 282
–Barbiturates, 23
–Dicumarol, 282
–Diphenadione, 282
–Phenindione, 282
–Phenprocoumon, 282
–Propranolol, 213
–Warfarin, 282
Methaqualone
–Alcohol, 47 (R), 145 (R), 180 (R)
Metharbital
–Acenocoumarol, 291
–Acetohexamide, 445 (SI)
–Acetyldigitoxin, 409 (SI)
–Alcohol, 180
–Amitriptyline, 161
–Anisindione, 291
–Antihistamines, 23
–Betamethasone, 42
–Chlorpropamide, 445 (SI)
–Cortisone, 42
–Desipramine, 161
–Deslanoside, 409 (SI)
–Dexamethasone, 42
–Dicumarol, 291
–Digitalis, 409 (SI)
–Digitoxin, 409 (SI)
–Digoxin, 409 (SI)
–Diphenadione, 291
–Doxepin, 161
–Ethotoin, 205
–Fludrocortisone, 42
–Fluprednisolone, 42
–Gitalin, 409 (SI)
–Griseofulvin, 77
–Haloperidol, 183 (R)
–Hydrocortisone, 42
–Imipramine, 161
–Lanatoside C, 409 (SI)
–Mephenytoin, 205
–Meprednisone, 42
–Methylprednisolone, 42
–Nortriptyline, 161
–Ouabain, 409 (SI)

–Paramethasone, 42
–Phenindione, 291
–Phenothiazines, 183
–Phenprocoumon, 291
–Phenytoin, 205
–Prednisolone, 42
–Prednisone, 42
–Primidone, 205
–Propranolol, 95
–Protriptyline, 161
–Rauwolfia alkaloids, 236
–Thiothixene, 183 (R)
–Tolazamide, 445 (SI)
–Tolbutamide, 445 (SI)
–Triamcinolone, 42
–Vitamin D, 455 (SI)
–Warfarin, 291
Methenamine
–Acetazolamide, 391 (SI)
–Thiazides, 391 (SI)
Methicillin
–Aspirin, 166
–Chloramphenicol, 168
–Decamethonium, 254 (R)
–Erythromycin, 173
–Gallamine triethiodide, 254 (R)
–Metocurine, 254 (R)
–Pancuronium, 254 (R)
–Probenecid, 175
–Salicylates, 166
–Succinylcholine, 254 (R)
–Tetracyclines, 170
–Tubocurarine, 254 (R)
Methocarbamol
–Acenocoumarol, 288
–Alcohol, 145
–Amitriptyline, 147
–Anisindione, 288
–Desipramine, 147
–Dicumarol, 288
–Diphenadione, 288
–Doxepin, 147
–Imipramine, 147
–Nortriptyline, 147
–Phenindione, 288
–Phenprocoumon, 288
–Protriptyline, 147
–Warfarin, 288
Methohexital
–Acenocoumarol, 291
–Acetohexamide, 445 (SI)
–Acetyldigitoxin, 409 (SI)
–Alcohol, 180
–Amitriptyline, 161
–Anisindione, 291
–Antihistamines, 23
–Betamethasone, 42
–Chlorpropamide, 445 (SI)
–Cortisone, 42
–Desipramine, 161
–Deslanoside, 409 (SI)
–Dexamethasone, 42
–Dicumarol, 291
–Digitalis, 409 (SI)
–Digitoxin, 409 (SI)
–Digoxin, 409 (SI)
–Diphenadione, 291
–Doxepin, 161
–Ethotoin, 205
–Fludrocortisone, 42
–Fluprednisolone, 42
–Gitalin, 409 (SI)
–Griseofulvin, 77
–Haloperidol, 183 (R)
–Hydrocortisone, 42
–Imipramine, 161

–Lanatoside C, 409 (SI)
–Mephenytoin, 205
–Meprednisone, 42
–Methylprednisolone, 42
–Nortriptyline, 161
–Ouabain, 409 (SI)
–Paramethasone, 42
–Phenindione, 291
–Phenothiazines, 183
–Phenprocoumon, 291
–Phenytoin, 205
–Prednisolone, 42
–Prednisone, 42
–Primidone, 205
–Propranolol, 95
–Protriptyline, 161
–Rauwolfia alkaloids, 236
–Thiothixene, 183 (R)
–Tolazamide, 445 (SI)
–Tolbutamide, 445 (SI)
–Triamcinolone, 42
–Vitamin D, 455 (SI)
–Warfarin, 291
Methotrexate
–Acetaminophen, 150 (R)
–Aminobenzoic acid, 395 (SI)
–Aspirin, 150
–Chloramphenicol, 395 (SI)
–Cytarabine, 151
–Indomethacin, 150 (R)
–Leucovorin, 154
–Phenytoin, 395 (SI)
–Salicylates, 150
–Sulfonamides, 156
–Tetracyclines, 395 (SI)
Methoxamine
–Bethanidine, 186
–Chloroform, 90
–Cyclopropane, 90
–Debrisoquin, 186
–Enflurane, 90
–Ether, 90
–Ethyl chloride, 90
–Fluroxene, 90
–Furazolidone, 10
–Guanethidine, 186
–Halopropane, 90
–Halothane, 90
–Isocarboxazid, 188
–Methoxyflurane, 90
–Nitrous oxide, 90
–Pargyline, 188
–Phenelzine, 188
–Rauwolfia alkaloids, 67 (R)
–Tranylcypromine, 188
–Trichloroethylene, 90
–Trichloromonofluoromethane,
  90
Methoxyflurane
–Amphetamine, 90
–Bacitracin, 70 (R)
–Clindamycin, 70 (R)
–Colistin, 70
–Decamethonium, 347 (SI),
  439 (SI)
–Dihydrostreptomycin, 70
–Ephedrine, 90
–Epinephrine, 90
–Ethotoin, 200
–Gallamine triethiodide, 347
  (SI), 439 (SI)
–Gentamicin, 70
–Isoproterenol, 90
–Kanamycin, 70
–Levarterenol, 90
–Mephentermine, 90

Minocycline *(cont.)*
–Chloroform, 234
–Decamethonium, 254 (R)
–Dicumarol, 299
–Diphenadione, 299
–Enflurane, 234
–Ethyl chloride, 234
–Fluroxene, 234
–Gallamine triethiodide, 254 (R)
–Halopropane, 234
–Halothane, 234
–Iron, 231
–Magnesium ions, 227
–Methotrexate, 395 (SI)
–Methoxyflurane, 234
–Metocurine, 254 (R)
–Pancuronium, 254 (R)
–Penicillins, 170
–Phenindione, 299
–Phenprocoumon, 299
–Sodium bicarbonate, 392 (SI)
–Succinylcholine, 254 (R)
–Trichloroethylene, 234
–Trichloromonofluoromethane, 234
–Tubocurarine, 254 (R)
–Warfarin, 299
Miradon—see Anisindione
Moban—see Molindone
Moderil—see Rescinnamine
Mogadon—see Nitrazepam
Molindone
–Bethanidine, 81 (R)
–Debrisoquin, 81 (R)
–Guanethidine, 81 (R)
–Methyldopa, 81 (R)
Monoamine oxidase inhibitors—
see Isocarboxazid, Pargyline, Phenelzine, Tranylcypromine
Monotheamin—see Theophylline
Morestin—see Estrone
Morphine
–Isocarboxazid, 142
–Pargyline, 142
–Phenelzine, 142
–Tranylcypromine, 142
Motrin—see Ibuprofen
Multifuge Citrate—see Piperazine
Muscle relaxants—*see*
Decamethonium, Gallamine triethiodide, Metocurine, Pancuronium, Succinylcholine, Tubocurarine
Muscle Relaxant Therapy, 435
Mychel—see Chloramphenicol
Mycifradin Sulfate—see Neomycin
Myciguent—see Neomycin
Mylanta—see Aluminum ions
Myodigin—see Digitoxin
Mysoline—see Primidone

N

Nafcillin
–Aspirin, 166
–Chloramphenicol, 168
–Decamethonium, 254 (R)
–Erythromycin, 173
–Gallamine triethiodide, 254 (R)
–Metocurine, 254 (R)
–Pancuronium, 254 (R)
–Probenecid, 175
–Salicylates, 166

–Succinylcholine, 254 (R)
–Tetracyclines, 170
–Tubocurarine, 254 (R)
Nalidixic acid
–Acenocoumarol, 364 (SI), 390 (SI)
–Anisindione, 364 (SI), 390 (SI)
–Dicumarol, 364 (SI), 390 (SI)
–Diphenadione, 364 (SI), 390 (SI)
–Phenindione, 364 (SI), 390 (SI)
–Phenprocoumon, 364 (SI), 390 (SI)
–Warfarin, 364 (SI), 390 (SI)
Nalline Hydrochloride—see Nalorphine
Nalorphine
–Isocarboxazid, 142
–Pargyline, 142
–Phenelzine, 142
–Tranylcypromine, 142
Nandrolone
–Aminopyrine, 165
–Antipyrine, 165
–Oxyphenbutazone, 165
–Phenylbutazone, 165
–Sulfinpyrazone, 165
Naqua—see Trichlormethiazide
Narcotics—*see* Alphaprodine, Anileridine, Codeine, Dextromethorphan, Hydrocodone, Hydromorphone, Levorphanol, Meperidine, Methadone, Morphine, Nalorphine, Oxycodone, Oxymorphone
Nardil—see Phenelzine
Naturetin—see Bendroflumethiazide
Nebcin—see Tobramycin
Nebs—see Acetaminophen
Nembutal—see Pentobarbital
Neobiotic—see Neomycin
Neomycin
–Acenocoumarol, 364 (SI), 390 (SI)
–Ampicillin, 76
–Anisindione, 364 (SI), 390 (SI)
–Carbenicillin, 76
–Chloroform, 70
–Cyanocobalamin, 450 (SI)
–Cyclopropane, 70
–Decamethonium, 254
–Dicumarol, 364 (SI), 390 (SI)
–Diphenadione, 364 (SI), 390 (SI)
–Enflurane, 70
–Ethacrynic acid, 120
–Ether, 70
–Ethyl chloride, 70
–Fluroxene, 70
–Furosemide, 120
–Gallamine triethiodide, 254
–Halopropane, 70
–Halothane, 70
–Methoxyflurane, 70
–Metocurine, 254
–Nitrous oxide, 70
–Pancuronium, 254
–Penicillin, 76
–Phenindione, 364 (SI), 390 (SI)
–Phenprocoumon, 364 (SI), 390 (SI)
–Succinylcholine, 254
–Trichloroethylene, 70

–Trichloromonofluoromethane, 70
–Tubocurarine, 254
–Vitamin B, 450 (SI)
–Warfarin, 364 (SI), 390 (SI)
Neo-Synephrine Hydrochloride—
see Phenylephrine
Neothylline—see Dyphylline
Neuromuscular relaxants—*see*
Decamethonium, Gallamine triethiodide, Metocurine, Pancuronium, Succinylcholine, Tubocurarine
Neurondia—see Barbital
Nitrazepam
–Acenocoumarol, 276
–Alcohol, 47
–Amitriptyline, 8
–Anisindione, 276
–Decamethonium, 75
–Desipramine, 8
–Dicumarol, 276
–Diphenadione, 276
–Doxepin, 8
–Gallamine triethiodide, 75
–Imipramine, 8
–Levodopa, 124
–Nortriptyline, 8
–Pancuronium, 75
–Phenindione, 276
–Phenprocoumon, 276
–Protriptyline, 8
–Succinylcholine, 75
–Tubocurarine, 75
–Warfarin, 276
Nitrofurantoin
–Probenecid, 159
–Sulfinpyrazone, 159
Nitrous oxide
–Amphetamine, 90
–Bacitracin, 70 (R)
–Clindamycin, 70 (R)
–Colistin, 70
–Decamethonium, 347 (SI), 439 (SI)
–Dihydrostreptomycin, 70
–Ephedrine, 90
–Epinephrine, 90
–Gallamine triethiodide, 347 (SI), 439 (SI)
–Gentamicin, 70
–Isoproterenol, 90
–Kanamycin, 70
–Levarterenol, 90
–Mephentermine, 90
–Metaraminol, 90
–Methoxamine, 90
–Metocurine, 347 (SI), 439 (SI)
–Neomycin, 70
–Pancuronium, 347 (SI), 439 (SI)
–Phenylephrine, 90
–Polymyxin, 70 (R)
–Rauwolfia alkaloids, 220
–Streptomycin, 70
–Succinylcholine, 347 (SI), 439 (SI)
–Tetracyclines, 70 (R)
–Tubocurarine, 347 (SI), 439 (SI)
–Viomycin, 70
Noctec—see Chloral hydrate
Noludar—see Methyprylon
Norepinephrine—see Levarterenol
Norethandrolone
–Acenocoumarol, 289
–Aminopyrine, 165

continued

continued

Phenindione *(cont.)*
  –Phenytoin, 193
  –Phthalylsulfathiazole, 364 (SI)
    390 (SI)
  –Phytonadione, 303
  –Primidone, 193
  –Propylthiouracil, 366 (SI)
  –Protriptyline, 364 (SI), 375 (SI)
  –Quinidine, 297
  –Quinine, 297
  –Rifampin, 364 (SI), 390 (SI)
  –Salicylates, 270
  –Stanozolol, 289
  –Streptomycin, 390 (SI)
  –Sulfachlorpyridazine, 364 (SI),
    390 (SI)
  –Sulfadiazine, 364 (SI), 390 (SI)
  –Sulfamerazine, 364 (SI),
    390 (SI)
  –Sulfameter, 364 (SI), 390 (SI)
  –Sulfamethazine, 364 (SI),
    390 (SI)
  –Sulfamethizole, 364 (SI),
    390 (SI)
  –Sulfamethoxazole, 364 (SI),
    390 (SI)
  –Sulfamethoxypyridazine,
    364 (SI), 390 (SI)
  –Sulfaphenazole, 364 (SI),
    390 (SI)
  –Sulfapyridine, 364 (SI), 390 (SI)
  –Sulfasalazine, 364 (SI), 390 (SI)
  –Sulfinpyrazone, 295 (R)
  –Sulfisoxazole, 364 (SI), 390 (SI)
  –Tetracyclines, 299
  –Thiazides, 364 (SI), 418 (SI)
  –Thyroglobulin, 301
  –Thyroid, 301
  –Thyroxine fraction, 301
  –Tolazamide, 245
  –Tolbutamide, 245
  –Triclofos, 273
  –Tybamate, 288
  –Vitamin C, 268
  –Vitamin E, 367 (SI)
  –Vitamin K, 303
Phenmetrazine
  –Haloperidol, 27 (R)
  –Phenothiazines, 27
Phenobarbital
  –Acenocoumarol, 291
  –Acetohexamide, 445 (SI)
  –Acetyldigitoxin, 409 (SI)
  –Alcohol, 180
  –Amitriptyline, 161
  –Anisindione, 291
  –Antihistamines, 23
  –Betamethasone, 42
  –Chlorpropamide, 445 (SI)
  –Cortisone, 42
  –Desipramine, 161
  –Deslanoside, 409 (SI)
  –Dexamethasone, 42
  –Dicumarol, 291
  –Digitalis, 409 (SI)
  –Digitoxin, 409 (SI)
  –Digoxin, 409 (SI)
  –Diphenadione, 291
  –Doxepin, 161
  –Ethotoin, 205
  –Fludrocortisone, 42
  –Fluprednisolone, 42
  –Folic acid, 197 (R)
  –Gitalin, 409 (SI)
  –Griseofulvin, 77
  –Haloperidol, 183 (R)

  –Hydrocortisone, 42
  –Imipramine, 161
  –Lanatoside C, 409 (SI)
  –Mephenytoin, 205
  –Meprednisone, 42
  –Methylprednisolone, 42
  –Nortriptyline, 161
  –Ouabain, 409 (SI)
  –Paramethasone, 42
  –Phenindione, 291
  –Phenothiazines, 183
  –Phenprocoumon, 291
  –Phenytoin, 205
  –Prednisolone, 42
  –Prednisone, 42
  –Primidone, 205
  –Propranolol, 95
  –Protriptyline, 161
  –Rauwolfia alkaloids, 236
  –Thiothixene, 183 (R)
  –Tolazamide, 445 (SI)
  –Tolbutamide, 445 (SI)
  –Triamcinolone, 42
  –Vitamin D, 455 (SI)
  –Warfarin, 291—
Phenothiazines—*see*
    Acetophenazine,
    Butaperazine, Carphenazine,
    Chlorpromazine,
    Fluphenazine,
    Mesoridazine, Perphenazine,
    Piperacetazine,
    Prochlorperazine, Promazine,
    Thiopropazate, Thioridazine,
    Trifluoperazine,
    Triflupromazine
Phenprocoumon
  –Acetaminophen, 263
  –Acetohexamide, 245
  –Alcohol, 265
  –Allopurinol, 366 (SI)
  –Aluminum ions, 266
  –Aminosalicylic acid, 363 (SI)
  –Amitriptyline, 364 (SI), 375 (SI)
  –Antihistamines, 282
  –Antipyrine, 295 (R)
  –Ascorbic acid, 268
  –Aspirin, 270
  –Barbiturates, 291
  –Benzodiazepines, 276
  –Carbamazepine, 366 (SI)
  –Carisoprodol, 288
  –Chloral betaine, 273
  –Chloral hydrate, 273
  –Chloramphenicol, 364 (SI),
    390 (SI)
  –Chlormezanone, 288
  –Chlorphenesin, 288
  –Chlorpropamide, 245
  –Cholestyramine, 278
  –Cinchophen, 297
  –Clofibrate, 280
  –Desipramine, 364 (SI), 375 (SI)
  –Dextrothyroxine, 301
  –Diazoxide, 366 (SI)
  –Disulfiram, 366 (SI)
  –Doxepin, 364 (SI), 375 (SI)
  –Estrogens, 365 (SI)
  –Ethacrynic acid, 364 (SI),
    418 (SI)
  –Ethchlorvynol, 365 (SI)
  –Ethotoin, 193
  –Fluoxymesterone, 289
  –Glucagon, 366 (SI)
  –Glutethimide, 284
  –Griseofulvin, 285

  –Haloperidol, 401 (SI)
  –Heparin, 362 (SI)
  –Ibuprofen, 343 (SI)
  –Imipramine, 364 (SI), 375 (SI)
  –Indomethacin, 286
  –Insulin, 245 (R)
  –Kanamycin, 390 (SI)
  –Levothyroxine, 301
  –Liothyronine, 301
  –Liotrix, 301
  –Magnesium ions, 266
  –Mefenamic acid, 344 (SI),
    363 (SI)
  –Menadione, 303
  –Mephenytoin, 193
  –Meprobamate, 288
  –Mercaptopurine, 366 (SI)
  –Methandrostenolone, 289
  –Methocarbamol, 288
  –Methylphenidate, 366 (SI)
  –Methyltestosterone, 289
  –Methyprylon, 284
  –Nalidixic acid, 364 (SI),
    390 (SI)
  –Neomycin, 364 (SI), 390 (SI)
  –Norethandrolone, 289
  –Nortriptyline, 364 (SI), 375 (SI)
  –Oxandrolone, 289
  –Oxymetholone, 289
  –Oxyphenbutazone, 295
  –Phenformin, 365 (SI)
  –Phenylbutazone, 295
  –Phenytoin, 193
  –Phthalylsulfathiazole,
    364 (SI), 390 (SI)
  –Phytonadione, 303
  –Primidone, 193
  –Propylthiouracil, 366 (SI)
  –Protriptyline, 364 (SI), 375 (SI)
  –Quinidine, 297
  –Quinine, 297
  –Rifampin, 364 (SI), 390 (SI)
  –Salicylates, 270
  –Stanozolol, 289
  –Streptomycin, 390 (SI)
  –Sulfachlorpyridazine, 364 (SI),
    390 (SI)
  –Sulfadiazine, 364 (SI), 390 (SI)
  –Sulfamerazine, 364 (SI),
    390 (SI)
  –Sulfameter, 364 (SI), 390 (SI)
  –Sulfamethazine, 364 (SI),
    390 (SI)
  –Sulfamethizole, 364 (SI),
    390 (SI)
  –Sulfamethoxazole, 364 (SI),
    390 (SI)
  –Sulfamethoxypyridazine,
    364 (SI), 390 (SI)
  –Sulfaphenazole, 364 (SI),
    390 (SI)
  –Sulfapyridine, 364 (SI), 390 (SI)
  –Sulfasalazine, 364 (SI), 390 (SI)
  –Sulfinpyrazone, 295 (R)
  –Sulfisoxazole, 364 (SI), 390 (SI)
  –Tetracyclines, 299
  –Thiazides, 364 (SI), 418 (SI)
  –Thyroglobulin, 301
  –Thyroid, 301
  –Thyroxine fraction, 301
  –Tolazamide, 245
  –Tolbutamide, 245
  –Triclofos, 273
  –Tybamate, 288
  –Vitamin C, 268

Polaramine—see
  Dexchlorpheniramine
Polyamine-methylene resin
  –Acetyldigitoxin, 62
  –Deslanoside, 62
  –Dextrothyroxine, 239
  –Digitalis, 62
  –Digitoxin, 62
  –Digoxin, 62
  –Gitalin, 62
  –Lanatoside C, 62
  –Levothyroxine, 239
  –Liothyronine, 239
  –Liotrix, 239
  –Oxyphenbutazone, 185
  –Phenylbutazone, 185
  –Thyroglobulin, 239
  –Thyroid, 239
  –Thyroxine fraction, 239
Polycillin—see Ampicillin
Polymyxin
  –Chloroform, 70 (R)
  –Cyclopropane, 70 (R)
  –Decamethonium, 254 (R)
  –Enflurane, 70 (R)
  –Ether, 70 (R)
  –Ethyl chloride, 70 (R)
  –Fluroxene, 70 (R)
  –Gallamine triethiodide, 254 (R)
  –Halopropane, 70 (R)
  –Halothane, 70 (R)
  –Methoxyflurane, 70 (R)
  –Metocurine, 254 (R)
  –Nitrous oxide, 70 (R)
  –Pancuronium, 254 (R)
  –Succinylcholine, 254 (R)
  –Trichloroethylene, 70 (R)
  –Trichloromonofluoromethane,
    70 (R)
  –Tubocurarine, 254 (R)
Polythiazide
  –Acenocoumarol, 364 (SI),
    418 (SI)
  –Acetohexamide, 40
  –Acetyldigitoxin, 52
  –Anisindione, 364 (SI), 418 (SI)
  –Bethanidine, 88
  –Chlorpropamide, 40
  –Debrisoquin, 88
  –Decamethonium, 253
  –Dicumarol, 364 (SI), 418 (SI)
  –Digitalis, 52
  –Digitoxin, 52
  –Digoxin, 52
  –Diphenadione, 364 (SI),
    418 (SI)
  –Gallamine triethiodide, 253
  –Gitalin, 52
  –Guanethidine, 88
  –Isocarboxazid, 374 (SI)
  –Lanatoside C, 52
  –Methenamine, 391 (SI)
  –Lithium carbonate, 137
  –Metocurine, 253
  –Ouabain, 52
  –Pancuronium, 253
  –Pargyline, 374 (SI)
  –Phenelzine, 374 (SI)
  –Phenindione, 364 (SI), 418 (SI)
  –Phenprocoumon, 364 (SI),
    418 (SI)
  –Probenecid, 208
  –Procainamide, 355 (SI)
  –Quinidine, 355 (SI)
  –Succinylcholine, 253
  –Tolazamide, 40

  –Tolbutamide, 40
  –Tranylcypromine, 374 (SI)
  –Tubocurarine, 253
  –Warfarin, 364 (SI), 418 (SI)
Potassium iodide—*see* Iodine
Potassium salicylate—*see*
  Salicylates
Prednisolone
  –Acetohexamide, 38
  –Aspirin, 18
  –Barbiturates, 42
  –Chlorpropamide, 38
  –Ethotoin, 45
  –Insulin, 38 (R)
  –Mephenytoin, 45
  –Phenformin, 38 (R)
  –Phenytoin, 45
  –Primidone, 45
  –Salicylates, 18
  –Tolazamide, 38
  –Tolbutamide, 38
  –Vitamin A, 450 (SI)
Prednisone
  –Acetohexamide, 38
  –Aspirin, 18
  –Barbiturates, 42
  –Chlorpropamide, 38
  –Ethotoin, 45
  –Insulin, 38 (R)
  –Mephenytoin, 45
  –Phenformin, 38 (R)
  –Phenytoin, 45
  –Primidone, 45
  –Salicylates, 18
  –Tolazamide, 38
  –Tolbutamide, 38
  –Vitamin A, 450 (SI)
Preludin—see Phenmetrazine
Premarin—see Conjugated
  estrogens
Presamine—see Imipramine
Primidone
  –Acenocoumarol, 193
  –Aminosalicylic acid, 202 (R)
  –Amphetamine, 204
  –Anisindione, 193
  –Barbiturates, 205
  –Betamethasone, 45
  –Chloroform, 200
  –Cortisone, 45
  –Cycloserine, 202 (R)
  –Dexamethasone, 45
  –Dextroamphetamine, 204
  –Dicumarol, 193
  –Diphenadione, 193
  –Disulfiram, 195
  –Enflurane, 200
  –Ethyl chloride, 200
  –Fludrocortisone, 45
  –Fluprednisolone, 45
  –Fluroxene, 200
  –Folic acid, 197
  –Halopropane, 200
  –Halothane, 200
  –Hydrocortisone, 45
  –Isoniazid, 202
  –Meprednisone, 45
  –Methamphetamine, 204
  –Methoxyflurane, 200
  –Methylphenidate, 204
  –Methylprednisolone, 45
  –Paramethasone, 45
  –Phenindione, 193
  –Phenprocoumon, 193
  –Prednisolone, 45
  –Prednisone, 45

  –Triamcinolone, 45
  –Trichloroethylene, 200
  –Trichloromonofluoromethane,
    200
  –Vitamin D, 261
  –Warfarin, 193
Principen—see Ampicillin
Pro-Banthine—see Propantheline
Probenecid
  –Allopurinol, 6
  –Aminosalicylic acid, 392 (SI),
    448 (SI)
  –Aspirin, 226 (R)
  –Cefazolin, 392 (SI), 448 (SI)
  –Cephalexin, 392 (SI), 448 (SI)
  –Cephaloglycin, 392 (SI),
    448 (SI)
  –Cephaloridine, 392 (SI),
    448 (SI)
  –Cephalothin, 392 (SI), 448 (SI)
  –Cephapirin, 392 (SI), 448 (SI)
  –Cephradine, 392 (SI), 448 (SI)
  –Chlorthalidone, 208
  –Dapsone, 392 (SI), 448 (SI)
  –Ethacrynic acid, 208 (R)
  –Furosemide, 208 (R)
  –Heparin, 363 (SI)
  –Indomethacin, 108
  –Metolazone, 208
  –Nitrofurantoin, 159
  –Penicillins, 175
  –Phthalylsulfathiazole, 392 (SI)
  –Quinethazone, 208
  –Rifampin, 392 (SI)
  –Salicylates, 226 (R)
  –Spironolactone, 208 (R)
  –Sulfachlorpyridazine, 392 (SI)
  –Sulfadiazine, 392 (SI)
  –Sulfamerazine, 392 (SI)
  –Sulfameter, 392 (SI)
  –Sulfamethazine, 392 (SI)
  –Sulfamethizole, 392 (SI)
  –Sulfamethoxazole, 392 (SI)
  –Sulfamethoxypyridazine,
    392 (SI)
  –Sulfaphenazole, 392 (SI)
  –Sulfapyridine, 392 (SI)
  –Sulfasalazine, 392 (SI)
  –Sulfisoxazole, 392 (SI)
  –Thiazides, 208
  –Triamterene, 208 (R)
Procainamide
  –Ethacrynic acid, 355 (SI)
  –Furosemide, 355 (SI)
  –Rauwolfia alkaloids, 219 (R)
  –Thiazides, 355 (SI)
Prochlorperazine
  –Alcohol, 402 (SI)
  –Aluminum ions, 25
  –Amitriptyline, 375 (SI), 402 (SI)
  –Amphetamine, 27
  –Barbiturates, 183
  –Benztropine, 30
  –Bethanidine, 81
  –Biperiden, 30
  –Cycrimine, 30
  –Debrisoquin, 81
  –Desipramine, 375 (SI),
    402 (SI)
  –Dextroamphetamine, 27
  –Doxepin, 375 (SI), 402 (SI)
  –Guanethidine, 81
  –Imipramine, 375 (SI), 402 (SI)
  –Levodopa, 122
  –Magnesium ions, 25
  –Methamphetamine, 27

continued

continued

continued

continued

Tranylcypromine *(cont.)*
  −Epinephrine, 188
  −Imipramine, 103
  −Insulin, 110
  −Isoproterenol, 188
  −Levarterenol, 188
  −Levodopa, 128
  −Metaraminol, 188
  −Methamphetamine, 188
  −Methoxamine, 188
  −Methylphenidate, 188
  −Narcotics, 142
  −Nortriptyline, 103
  −Phenylpropanolamine, 188
  −Propranolol, 374 (SI)
  −Protriptyline, 103
  −Pseudoephedrine, 188
  −Thiazides, 374 (SI)
  −Tolazamide, 110 (R)
  −Tolbutamide, 110 (R)
  −Tyramine, 188
Tremin—see Trihexyphenidyl
Triamcinolone
  −Acetohexamide, 38
  −Aspirin, 18
  −Barbiturates, 42
  −Chlorpropamide, 38
  −Ethotoin, 45
  −Insulin, 38 (R)
  −Mephenytoin, 45
  −Phenformin, 38 (R)
  −Phenytoin, 45
  −Primidone, 45
  −Salicylates, 18
  −Tolazamide, 38
  −Tolbutamide, 38
  −Vitamin A, 450 (SI)
Triamterene
  −Acetohexamide, 40 (R)
  −Acetyldigitoxin, 61
  −Bethanidine, 88 (R)
  −Chlorpropamide, 40 (R)
  −Debrisoquin, 88 (R)
  −Deslanoside, 61
  −Digitalis, 61
  −Digitoxin, 61
  −Digoxin, 61
  −Gitalin, 61
  −Guanethidine, 88 (R)
  −Lanatoside C, 61
  −Lithium carbonate, 137 (R)
  −Ouabain, 61
  −Probenecid, 208 (R)
  −Tolazamide, 40 (R)
  −Tolbutamide, 40 (R)
Trichlormethiazide
  −Acenocoumarol, 364 (SI),
    418 (SI)
  −Acetohexamide, 40
  −Acetyldigitoxin, 52
  −Anisindione, 364 (SI), 418 (SI)
  −Bethanidine, 88
  −Chlorpropamide, 40
  −Debrisoquin, 88
  −Decamethonium, 253
  −Dicumarol, 364 (SI), 418 (SI)
  −Digitalis, 52
  −Digitoxin, 52
  −Digoxin, 52
  −Diphenadione, 364 (SI),
    418 (SI)
  −Gallamine triethiodide, 253
  −Gitalin, 52
  −Guanethidine, 88
  −Isocarboxazid, 374 (SI)
  −Lanatoside C, 52

  −Lithium carbonate, 137
  −Methenamine, 391 (SI)
  −Metocurine, 253
  −Ouabain, 52
  −Pancuronium, 253
  −Pargyline, 374 (SI)
  −Phenelzine, 374 (SI)
  −Phenindione, 364 (SI), 418 (SI)
  −Phenprocoumon, 364 (SI),
    418 (SI)
  −Probenecid, 208
  −Procainamide, 355 (SI)
  −Quinidine, 355 (SI)
  −Succinylcholine, 253
  −Tolazamide, 40
  −Tolbutamide, 40
  −Tranylcypromine, 374 (SI)
  −Tubocurarine, 253
  −Warfarin, 364 (SI), 418 (SI)
Trichloroethylene
  −Amphetamine, 90
  −Bacitracin, 70 (R)
  −Clindamycin, 70 (R)
  −Colistin, 70
  −Decamethonium, 347 (SI),
    439 (SI)
  −Dihydrostreptomycin, 70
  −Ephedrine, 90
  −Epinephrine, 90
  −Ethotoin, 200
  −Gallamine triethiodide,
    347 (SI), 439 (SI)
  −Gentamicin, 70
  −Isoproterenol, 90
  −Kanamycin, 70
  −Levarterenol, 90
  −Mephentermine, 90
  −Mephenytoin, 200
  −Metaraminol, 90
  −Methoxamine, 90
  −Metocurine, 347 (SI), 439 (SI)
  −Neomycin, 70
  −Pancuronium, 347 (SI), 439 (SI)
  −Phenylephrine, 90
  −Phenytoin, 200
  −Polymyxin, 70 (R)
  −Primidone, 200
  −Rauwolfia alkaloids, 220
  −Streptomycin, 70
  −Succinylcholine, 347 (SI),
    439 (SI)
  −Tetracyclines, 234
  −Tubocurarine, 347 (SI),
    439 (SI)
  −Viomycin, 70
Trichloromonofluoromethane
  −Amphetamine, 90
  −Bacitracin, 70 (R)
  −Clindamycin, 70 (R)
  −Colistin, 70
  −Decamethonium, 347 (SI),
    439 (SI)
  −Dihydrostreptomycin, 70
  −Ephedrine, 90
  −Epinephrine, 90
  −Ethotoin, 200
  −Gallamine triethiodide,
    347 (SI), 439 (SI)
  −Gentamicin, 70
  −Isoproterenol, 90
  −Kanamycin, 70
  −Levarterenol, 90
  −Mephentermine, 90
  −Mephenytoin, 200
  −Metaraminol, 90
  −Methoxamine, 90

  −Metocurine, 347 (SI), 439 (SI)
  −Neomycin, 70
  −Pancuronium, 347 (SI), 439 (SI)
  −Phenylephrine, 90
  −Phenytoin, 200
  −Polymyxin, 70 (R)
  −Primidone, 200
  −Rauwolfia alkaloids, 220
  −Succinylcholine, 347 (SI),
    439 (SI)
  −Tetracyclines, 234
  −Tubocurarine, 347 (SI), 439 (SI)
  −Viomycin, 70
Triclofos
  −Acenocoumarol, 273
  −Alcohol, 20
  −Anisindione, 273
  −Dicumarol, 273
  −Diphenadione, 273
  −Phenindione, 273
  −Phenprocoumon, 273
  −Warfarin, 273
Triclos—see Triclofos
Tricyclic antidepressants—*see*
    Amitriptyline, Desipramine,
    Doxepin, Imipramine,
    Nortriptyline, Protriptyline
Tridihexethyl
  −Acetyldigitoxin, 65
  −Deslanoside, 65
  −Digitalis, 65
  −Digitoxin, 65
  −Digoxin, 65
  −Gitalin, 65
  −Lanatoside C, 65
  −Ouabain, 65
Trifluoperazine
  −Alcohol, 402 (SI)
  −Aluminum ions, 25
  −Amitriptyline, 375 (SI), 402 (SI)
  −Amphetamine, 27
  −Barbiturates, 183
  −Benztropine, 30
  −Bethanidine, 81
  −Biperiden, 30
  −Cycrimine, 30
  −Debrisoquin, 81
  −Desipramine, 375 (SI), 402 (SI)
  −Dextroamphetamine, 27
  −Doxepin, 375 (SI), 402 (SI)
  −Guanethidine, 81
  −Imipramine, 375 (SI), 402 (SI)
  −Levodopa, 122
  −Magnesium ions, 25
  −Methamphetamine, 27
  −Methyldopa, 81 (R)
  −Methylphenidate, 27
  −Nortriptyline, 375 (SI), 402 (SI)
  −Pentylenetetrazol, 402 (SI)
  −Phenmetrazine, 27
  −Picrotoxin, 402 (SI)
  −Piperazine, 34
  −Procyclidine, 30
  −Propranolol, 355 (SI)
  −Protriptyline, 375 (SI), 402 (SI)
  −Trihexyphenidyl, 30
Triflupromazine
  −Alcohol, 402 (SI)
  −Aluminum ions, 25
  −Amitriptyline, 375 (SI), 402 (SI)
  −Amphetamine, 27
  −Barbiturates, 183
  −Benztropine, 30
  −Bethanidine, 81
  −Biperiden, 30
  −Cycrimine, 30

Evaluations of Drug Interactions SECOND EDITION

ORDER FORM

EVALUATIONS OF DRUG INTERACTIONS
Second Edition

Price:
APhA members $8.75   Non members $12.50

(To receive favored member rate, mailing label from *JAPhA* or *APhA Weekly* must be attached to this order.)

No. of copies @ $ 8.75_____ (APhA members)

@ $12.50_____ (Non members)

☐ Total remittance enclosed $_____ ☐ Bill me
   Orders for less than $20.00 must be prepaid.

For quantity discount schedule (10 or more copies), write to Publications Division.

Order Desk:
American Pharmaceutical Association
2215 Constitution Avenue, N.W., Washington, DC 20037

APhA
MEMBERS:
Attach
mailing label
from
JAPhA
or
APhA Weekly
here.

NAME _____

ADDRESS _____

_____

CITY _____

STATE _____   ZIP _____

(Prices include shipping or mailing at lowest cost surface rate. Allow four weeks for delivery.)